IAC-IARC-WHO Cytopathology Reporting Systems • 1st Edition

WHO Reporting System for Soft Tissue Cytopathology

International Academy of Cytology – International Agency for Research on Cancer – World Health Organization
Joint Editorial Board

THE INTERNATIONAL ACADEMY OF CYTOLOGY 1957

International Agency for Research on Cancer
World Health Organization

Suggested citation
International Academy of Cytology – International Agency for Research on Cancer – World Health Organization Joint Editorial Board. WHO Reporting System for Soft Tissue Cytopathology. Lyon (France): International Agency for Research on Cancer; 2026. (IAC-IARC-WHO cytopathology reporting systems series, 1st ed.; vol. 4). https://publications.iarc.who.int/651.

Sales, rights, and permissions
Print copies are distributed by WHO Press, World Health Organization, 20 Avenue Appia, 1211 Geneva 27, Switzerland
Tel.: +41 22 791 3264; Fax: +41 22 791 4857; email: bookorders@who.int; website: https://whobluebooks.iarc.who.int

To purchase IARC publications in electronic format, see the IARC Publications website (https://publications.iarc.who.int).

First print run (1000 copies)

Updated corrigenda can be found at https://publications.iarc.who.int

IARC Library Cataloguing-in-Publication Data
Names: International Academy of Cytology – International Agency for Research on Cancer – World Health Organization Joint Editorial Board.
Title: WHO reporting system for soft tissue cytopathology / edited by International Academy of Cytology – International Agency for Research on Cancer – World Health Organization Joint Editorial Board.
Description: Lyon: International Agency for Research on Cancer, 2026. | Series: IAC-IARC-WHO cytopathology reporting systems. | Includes bibliographical references and index.
Identifiers: ISBN 9789283245360 (pbk.)
Subjects: MESH: Neoplasms, Connective and Soft Tissue – pathology. | Neoplasms, Connective and Soft Tissue – classification. | Cytodiagnosis – methods.
Classification: NLM QZ 340

The WHO Reporting System for Soft Tissue Cytopathology presented in this book reflects the views of the International Academy of Cytology (IAC) – International Agency for Research on Cancer (IARC) – World Health Organization (WHO) Joint Editorial Board that convened via video conference 22–24 June 2022, as well as subsequent consultation.

The IAC-IARC-WHO Joint Editorial Board

For the complete list of all contributors and their affiliations, see pages 249–250.

WHO Reporting System for Soft Tissue Cytopathology

Edited by	The IAC-IARC-WHO Joint Editorial Board
IAC Pathology Editing	Andrew S. Field
IARC Pathology Review	Dilani Lokuhetty Harshima Wijesinghe Pavitratha Puspanathan
Project Assistant	Asiedua Asante
Assistants	Camille Bou Anne-Sophie Bres Nicole Suty
Copy editing	Jessica Cox Julia Slone-Murphy
Production Editors	Sharon Paul Julia Slone-Murphy
Principal Information Assistant	Alberto Machado
Information Assistants	Catarina Marques Ramon Cierco Jimenez
Layout	Catarina Marques
Printed by	Imprimerie Chirat 42540 Saint-Just-la-Pendue, France
Publisher	International Agency for Research on Cancer (IARC) 25 Av. Tony Garnier, CS 90627 69366 Lyon, CEDEX 07, France

Contents

List of abbreviations

2D, 3D	two-dimensional, three-dimensional
CNB	core needle biopsy
CNS	central nervous system
CT	computed tomography
CXR	chest X-ray
DNA	deoxyribonucleic acid
EBUS	endobronchial ultrasound
EBV	Epstein–Barr virus
EDTA	ethylenediaminetetraacetic acid
EUS	endoscopic ultrasound
FISH	fluorescence in situ hybridization
FNAB	fine-needle aspiration biopsy
H&E	haematoxylin and eosin
HAART	highly active antiretroviral therapy
HIV	human immunodeficiency virus
HPF	high-power field
IAC	International Academy of Cytology
IARC	International Agency for Research on Cancer
ICC	immunocytochemistry
ICD-11	International Classification of Diseases, 11th revision
ICD-O	International Classification of Diseases for Oncology
ISH	in situ hybridization
ITD	internal tandem duplication
KSHV/HHV8	Kaposi sarcoma–associated herpesvirus / human herpesvirus 8
LBC	liquid-based cytopathology
MRI	magnetic resonance imaging
N:C ratio	nuclear-to-cytoplasmic ratio
NGS	next-generation sequencing
Pap	Papanicolaou stain
PCR	polymerase chain reaction
PET	positron emission tomography
PET-CT	positron emission tomography–computed tomography
RNA	ribonucleic acid
ROM	risk of malignancy
ROSE	rapid onsite evaluation
RT-PCR	reverse transcription polymerase chain reaction
SISH	silver in situ hybridization
STNUMP	Soft tissue neoplasm of uncertain malignant potential
TNM	tumour, node, metastasis

Foreword

The classification of tumours can be viewed from many perspectives. To a histopathologist it is all about the histopathological patterns, to a molecular pathologist or geneticist it is all about which genes are affected, and to an epidemiologist it is about the tumours' incidence. The WHO Classification of Tumours series started in the 1960s as a result of the histopathologist's need to make diagnoses by grouping tumours according to their microscopic appearance. The programme now includes contributions from many specialties, including, of course, cytopathology. However, the cytopathologist looks at tumours slightly differently than other specialists do, and although the main classification is helpful, it has become clear that reporting systems using common terminology and established diagnostic categories that assist communication between cytopathologists and clinicians need to be based on entities defined by key diagnostic cytopathological features. These reporting systems have to be truly international, serving the needs of patients worldwide.

The International Academy of Cytology (IAC), a scientific, non-profit organization with members from 49 affiliated cytopathology societies, therefore approached the International Agency for Research on Cancer (IARC) – home to the WHO Classification of Tumours Programme – to see whether it would be possible to produce a complementary series of WHO Reporting Systems for Cytopathology. The two organizations signed a memorandum of understanding in early 2020 and have produced the first three volumes of the series: the WHO Reporting System for Lung Cytopathology; the WHO Reporting System for Pancreaticobiliary Cytopathology; and the WHO Reporting System for Lymph Node, Spleen, and Thymus Cytopathology. This is the WHO Reporting System for Soft Tissue Cytopathology, and four other reporting systems are in progress for breast, kidney and adrenal, liver, and head and neck cytopathology.

Cytopathology is used in the diagnosis of soft tissue lesions, including neoplasms, and it is particularly powerful in low-resource settings. Special histochemical stains and ancillary methods such as immunocytochemistry and in situ hybridization are applicable to smears and cell blocks, which also provide excellent material for NGS. The avoidance of formalin in cytopathological preparations enhances the application of diagnostic molecular techniques, whether simple PCR or NGS.

Just as the WHO Classification of Tumours series (also known as the WHO Blue Books), published in print volumes and as a web resource (https://tumourclassification.iarc.who.int), is an essential tool for standardizing diagnostic practice worldwide and serves as a vehicle for the translation of cancer research into practice, we hope that these first-edition WHO Reporting Systems will fulfil the same role for cytopathology. The key diagnostic cytopathological features listed for each tumour type under the diagnostic categories represent the first international consensus and are described in precise, uniform language. These diagnostic criteria are underpinned by available evidence that has been evaluated and debated by experts in the field. Each entity's section includes discussion of its differential diagnosis based on its cytopathological features so that the Systems can be used worldwide, especially in low-resource settings. This is then followed by discussion of the current best-practice application of ancillary testing on cytopathology material to further the diagnosis. About 40 authors and editors participated in the production of this volume and gave their time freely to this task. We are very grateful for their help; it is a remarkable team effort.

This volume, like those of the WHO Classification of Tumours series, has been led by an editorial board composed of standing and expert members. The standing members include the chair of the WHO Classification of Tumours Editorial Board and others nominated by the IAC. The expert members, selected on the basis of informed bibliometric analysis and advice from the standing members, represent a broad international expertise, as does the authorship group. The diagnostic process is increasingly multidisciplinary, and we are delighted that several radiology and clinical experts have joined us to address specific needs.

In addition to using the International System of Units (SI) for all measurements, we have standardized the genomic nomenclature by using Human Genome Variation Society (HGVS) notation. We have also further standardized our use of units of length, adopting the convention used by the International Collaboration on Cancer Reporting (https://www.iccr-cancer.org) and the UK Royal College of Pathologists (https://www.rcpath.org/), so that the size of tumours is now given exclusively in millimetres (mm) rather than centimetres (cm). This is clearer, in our view, and avoids the use of decimal points – a common source of medical errors.

The goal of this long-term project is to meet the needs of the cytopathology community and enhance the use of FNAB cytopathology to benefit patient care. Like the WHO Classification of Tumours, the WHO Reporting Systems, both the website and the print books, are published on a non-profit basis, with proceeds ploughed directly back into the series to support the costs involved, including production, printing, and distribution. There are substantial discounts available for residents of lower-income countries and trainees. It is of vital importance that cancers continue to be classified and diagnosed according to the same standards internationally so that patients can benefit from multicentre clinical trials and studies, as well as from the results of local research conducted on different continents.

Ian A. Cree, Dilani Lokuhetty, Andrew S. Field, Ravi Mehrotra, Martha Bishop Pitman, Fernando Schmitt

Standing Members of the International Academy of Cytology (IAC) – International Agency for Research on Cancer (IARC) – World Health Organization (WHO) Joint Editorial Board

1

Introduction to the WHO Reporting System for Soft Tissue Cytopathology

Edited by: Field AS, Lazar AJ, Pitman MB

Background

Domanski HA
Field AS
Klijanienko J
Rekhi B

Soft tissue cytopathology is accepted as the first-line approach for following up on previously diagnosed and treated sarcomas, as well as for confirming soft tissue metastases from carcinomas, myeloid tumours, and other sarcomas {1423,1017, 696,1470}. In many institutions, fine-needle aspiration biopsy (FNAB) has been successfully used as an initial diagnostic procedure or as a complement to core needle biopsy (CNB) for the diagnosis of soft tissue masses in the context of a multidisciplinary approach {1509,1017,1470,1458,344,1159,753,1169, 1001,784,705,712,1066,832}. In low-resource settings, FNAB has been used as a readily available, less expensive, and less infrastructure-demanding initial diagnostic test for examination of soft tissue lesions {1041}. Progress in minimally invasive diagnostic procedures, advances in imaging techniques, and the continuously growing array of ancillary tests applied to cytopathological specimens over the past decades have brought widespread acceptance of the use of FNAB in the primary diagnosis of soft tissue lesions globally {1062,342,740}. Important limitations of cytopathology stem from the limited experience of most pathologists in the cytopathological diagnosis of soft tissue tumours {1311,1458,338} and from the lack of a uniform cytopathological nomenclature with a standardized system for reporting soft tissue cytopathology {342,753} similar to those used in other organs systems.

In 2019, an international group of cytopathologists experienced in soft tissue cytopathology was brought together by the International Academy of Cytology (IAC) and began the process of developing such a system. The objectives were to produce a reporting system that would reflect the fifth-edition WHO classification of soft tissue and bone tumours (STB5) {1503}, which is currently undergoing revision to produce the sixth edition (STB6), and to create a basis for a minimally invasive approach to the cytomorphological diagnosis of soft tissue lesions. The development of a standardized reporting system with clearly defined diagnostic categories that can be applied in everyday practice is an essential step to increase and support the use of FNAB in the diagnosis of soft tissue tumours and maximize its synergies with other diagnostic modalities. The WHO Reporting System for Soft Tissue Cytopathology (WHO System) has continued the development of a reporting system, and the members of the expert editorial board acknowledge the work of the members of the IAC group.

In 2020, the IAC signed a memorandum of understanding with the International Agency for Research on Cancer (IARC), which is the WHO agency responsible for developing and promulgating the *WHO Classification of Tumours* series ("the WHO Blue Books"), to develop a series of WHO Reporting Systems for cytopathology {412}. Three other WHO Reporting Systems have been published to date, for cytopathology of the following sites: lung; pancreaticobiliary; and lymph nodes, spleen, and thymus {611,613,612}. The primary aim of this collaboration is to establish universal standardized cytopathology reporting systems for each site, with standardized terminology, as well as to establish by international consensus the key diagnostic cytopathological criteria for entities, to ensure robust cytopathological diagnoses globally, including accommodating and supporting laboratories with limited resources in low- and middle-income countries {412}.

This WHO System is intended to assist cytopathologists in their daily work of interpreting and reporting FNAB samples and to help optimize the appropriate handling and preparation of FNAB material for ancillary studies. The WHO System provides a structured reporting system to facilitate communication between cytopathologists and clinicians, with the fundamental aim of improving patient care {412}. The WHO System is based on a consensus of expert cytopathologists and the published literature of the established key diagnostic cytopathological criteria and the most cost-effective and accurate ancillary tests. Six diagnostic categories are clearly defined and form the reporting structure:

- Insufficient/Inadequate/Non-diagnostic
- Benign
- Atypical
- Soft tissue neoplasm of uncertain malignant potential (STNUMP)
- Suspicious for malignancy
- Malignant

Individual entities are presented with brief clinical, imaging, and histopathological descriptions to assist the cytopathologist, and then the focus is on the cytopathology and its differential diagnosis, followed by a discussion of ancillary tests. The *Definition*, *Clinical features and imaging*, and *Histopathology* subsections correspond closely to STB5 and are following by subsections on *Key diagnostic cytopathological features*, *Discussion and differential diagnosis*, and finally *Ancillary testing*. The differential diagnoses of specific entities focus on their cytopathological criteria so that the WHO System can be used globally. A detailed review of the most recent ancillary testing is presented for each entity.

FNAB is based on high-yield specimens and well-prepared direct smears and cell blocks that rely on the expertise of the FNAB operator. The WHO System includes detailed guides on sampling methods, specimen preparation, and the use of rapid onsite evaluation (ROSE). ROSE increases the cost-effectiveness and efficiency of the triage of FNAB material to optimize the diagnosis based on cytopathology and ancillary tests supporting the multidisciplinary approach.

Specific entities and neoplasms are presented in the "Benign", "STNUMP", and "Malignant" chapters, organized by the pattern and cell-type presentation encountered by the reporting cytopathologist, which is similar to the lineage presentation in STB5. Entities in the WHO System are not the complete equivalent of those presented in the WHO Blue Books, because there is a lack of cytopathological criteria and references for several rare or recently defined soft tissue neoplasms, and because not all soft tissue lesions are amenable to cytopathological examination. Most of these entities are discussed in the introductory sections of the various chapters and in the differential diagnoses of neoplasms with clearly defined cytopathological diagnostic criteria.

The WHO System integrates cytomorphology and the six defined diagnostic categories with lineage-based molecular classifications, in alignment with the soft tissue sections of the forthcoming STB6, which is currently being written and has some changes from the fifth edition. These changes include the renaming of "undifferentiated small round cell sarcomas" as "undifferentiated spindle and small round cell sarcomas", which include Ewing sarcoma as the prototype and other sarcomas defined by specific gene fusions. This forms a bridge between morphology and molecular-based classifications based on specific gene alterations, especially fusions. But the sarcomas other than Ewing sarcoma in this section are not only composed of round cells. Sarcomas with *BCOR* genetic alterations contain an admixture of round and spindle cells, and sarcomas with *EWSR1*::*NFATC2* fusions (now a discrete entity rather than a subtype of what was previously called "round cell sarcoma with *EWSR1*–non-ETS fusions") or with *CIC* rearrangement contain a significant admixture of epithelioid cells {1490,463,199,1174}. *PATZ1*-rearranged sarcomas are now grouped with the tumours of uncertain differentiation, in light of the variable immunohistochemical expression of myogenic and neurogenic markers by the tumours cells {222}.

There are also a number of new entities in STB6, most of which have been described in only a handful (or in some cases no) cytopathological reports {152,1160,1462,1524,1280} and will require the awareness of cytopathologists so as to correlate the diagnosis of these tumours by histopathology and molecular testing with any subsequent cytopathology in the future. The new entities in STB6 include lipoblastoma-like tumour, which enters the differential diagnosis of lipoma and has a *PLAG1* rearrangement {488,510}; calcifying fibrous tumour; *PRRX1*-rearranged fibroblastic tumour; nodular necrotizing fibroblastic sarcoma {1099}; chondroid synoviocytic neoplasm {670}; spindle cell haemangioma with *HMGA2*::NCOR fusion; *SRF*-rearranged myoid neoplasm; *OGT*-rearranged acral mesenchymal neoplasm {800}; acral fibrochondromyxoid tumour {153}; *GLI1*-altered mesenchymal tumour {1280}; superficial FET::ETS neurocristic tumour, which harbours the same fusion event as Ewing sarcoma but with location in skin and superficial soft tissues and an indolent course {440}; kinase-altered spindle cell neoplasms; *NUTM1*-rearranged sarcoma {1565}; and FET::CREB round to epithelioid mesenchymal tumours {313,54, 66,1542,1163,9}.

In the forthcoming STB6, the terminology and status of atypical spindle cell / pleomorphic lipomatous tumour, with its *RB1* gene deletion, and atypical lipomatous tumour / well-differentiated liposarcoma, with its distinctive *MDM2*/*CDK4* amplification, are confirmed, and the cytopathology has been further described {1462}. However, it is recognized that atypical spindle cell / pleomorphic lipomatous tumour can undergo sarcomatous transformation. Undifferentiated pleomorphic sarcoma has been moved to "fibroblastic and myofibroblastic tumours" from "tumours of uncertain differentiation". *YAP1*::*TFE3* haemangioendothelioma has been separated from epithelioid haemangioendothelioma {152}. "NTRK-rearranged spindle cell neoplasm" has been replaced by "kinase-altered spindle cell tumour, including NTRK-rearranged mesenchymal tumour", which includes other tumours showing gene rearrangements such as NTRK rearrangements and *EGFR* internal tandem duplication (ITD), as well as *RET*, *RAF1*, *BRAF*, *ALK*, *ROS1*, and *MET* rearrangements {1524}. "Superficial CD34-positive pleomorphic fibrous tumour" has replaced "superficial CD34-positive fibroblastic tumour", as a better descriptor of this tumour with its *PRDM10* rearrangement {1160}. "*SMAD3*-rearranged fibroblastic tumour" has replaced "*EWSR1*::*SMAD3* tumour" {934}. "Fusion-associated spindle cell rhabdomyosarcoma", including infantile cases characterized by a recurrent *VGLL2*-related fusion {44} and "*MYOD1*-mutant spindle cell sclerosing rhabdomyosarcoma" {1166}, have replaced the single group "spindle cell / sclerosing rhabdomyosarcoma", based on morphology, genetic changes, and importantly clinical outcomes {1180,795}. Another molecular subset of fusion-positive rhabdomyosarcomas, containing epithelioid and spindle cells, with proclivity for bones followed by soft tissues (mostly in the head and neck region), is also included {795}. "Inflammatory leiomyosarcoma" has been renamed "inflammatory rhabdomyoblastic tumour" and grouped with the skeletal muscle tumours {237}. The diagnostic criteria of keratin-positive giant cell–rich tumour with *HMGA2*::*NCOR2* fusion have been refined {12}. A number of entities have been deleted, including deep fibrous histiocytoma and ectomesenchymoma.

These newly defined entities demonstrate the need to further expand the spectrum of soft tissue tumours diagnosable by FNAB cytopathology, assisted in most cases by molecular testing, while at the same time it is crucial to be aware that all molecular test results must be interpreted in a clinical-cytopathological context, particularly when remembering the non-specificity of certain rearrangements (e.g. *EWSR1* rearrangements) and gene fusions (e.g. FET::CREB fusions) {419,1404}.

The role of soft tissue cytopathology

Domanski HA
Klijanienko J

The range of possible origins of a soft tissue swelling is broad, including tumours of mesenchymal origin. The objective of the diagnostic workup of soft tissue lesions is to provide information that will enable optimal treatment planning. As a best practice, all patients presenting with an unexplained deep soft tissue mass or with a superficial soft tissue lesion with a diameter > 50 mm should be referred to a specialized orthopaedic oncology centre in which the management of sarcoma cases is common practice {509}. The diagnostic procedure involves an interdisciplinary joint decision made by an oncologist, a surgeon, a radiologist, a nuclear medicine physician, and a pathologist, who correlate their findings to define an optimal diagnostic strategy {289,158}.

Clinical data and appropriate imaging are essential for the evaluation of soft tissue lesions. In most cases, a biopsy is required for further management, and a biopsy is mandatory for all solid deep-seated tumours, to exclude or establish malignancy and assess the histopathological type and grade of the tumour in cases of sarcoma {1503}.

Over the past decades, CNB and FNAB, or a combination of both, along with an intraprocedural evaluation of FNAB smears or touch preparation of CNB, have largely replaced surgical biopsies in the examination of soft tissue lesions {404,344,788, 1355,1159,683}. CNB through a single tract is currently recommended for obtaining specimens for the diagnosis of most limb and superficial trunk soft tissue tumours {1503}. However, the role of cytopathology in the evaluation of soft tissue lesions has been steadily increasing due to advances in imaging techniques and the growing availability of ancillary tests using small biopsies {1232,1478,281,355,740,335,643,1062,80,198,573, 783,1329}.

The advantages of soft tissue FNAB are good sensitivity and specificity, low morbidity, a reduced time to diagnosis, and a low cost–benefit ratio. FNAB is less invasive and less expensive than either CNB or open biopsy, and it can sample a lesion more extensively.

FNAB is well established and widely used as a first-line approach or as a complementary diagnostic procedure with CNB for the confirmation of metastatic tumours to soft tissue, for the evaluation and documentation of local recurrences and metastases of previously diagnosed sarcomas, and for the initial diagnosis of malignant soft tissue neoplasms {1423, 1017,696,1470,1509,1458,344,1159,753,1169,1001,784,705,712, 1066,832,1311}. FNAB in conjunction with rapid onsite evaluation (ROSE) and specimen triage for cost-effective ancillary testing enables adequacy assessment and guidance for concurrent CNB. FNAB offers a fast, precise, and low-risk diagnostic modality, avoiding invasive and expensive diagnostic procedures and unnecessary excisions {1017,342,753}. The use of ROSE makes confirmation of the malignancy possible in the space of a few minutes in most cases, and consequently can be used to indicate or contraindicate the use of CNB. ROSE is also invaluable for the triaging of samples for ancillary techniques such as molecular and ICC tests, cell block, flow cytometry (in the case of malignant lymphoma), and tissue banking. In the case of distinguishing certain blastemal tumours such as neuroblastoma versus nephroblastoma, ROSE allows confirmation of the need for additional samples of the bone marrow and cerebrospinal fluid, which can then be performed at the same time, particularly in children and adolescents, under the same broad anaesthetic cover.

The majority of palpable soft tissue masses are benign, and the frequency of benign tumours is estimated to be approximately 100 times that of sarcomas {1197}. FNAB of non-neoplastic and clinically non-aggressive soft tissue tumours with benign imaging features has been shown to be a rapid diagnostic procedure, leading to optimal treatment including either local excision or simply watchful waiting {753,1509,338,29,33}. Soft tissue masses presenting as tumours in children, adolescents, and adults frequently require consultation to distinguish between benign and malignant lesions, and they can pose a diagnostic dilemma. In superficial or deep lesions where the clinical and imaging hypothesis that the lesion is benign is confirmed by a simple FNAB, the tumour can be observed or excised {1072,158}.

In many centres, FNAB has been an integral part of the care for patients with soft tissue lesions, and the initial diagnosis (and in some cases the final diagnosis) is based on cytopathology alone integrated with clinical and imaging findings and where necessary ancillary testing {739,352}. This multidisciplinary approach allows the establishment of the diagnosis, the initiation of appropriate treatment and further management, and the avoidance of expensive surgical excision and histopathology – which in low- and middle-income countries may not be available {1041,1397,864,286,1}.

When used as the initial diagnostic test, FNAB has been shown to be highly accurate, with 89–100% sensitivity and 90–100% specificity in distinguishing benign from malignant soft tissue tumours and in documenting recurrences or metastases of previously treated sarcomas {1533,691,1470,1001,320, 420,1311}.

However, there is a limitation to using FNAB for the precise subtyping and grading of soft tissue sarcomas compared to CNB and open biopsy. The overall accuracy of FNAB in making the specific histopathological diagnosis of soft tissue lesions has been shown to be somewhat inferior to that of CNB and open biopsy {712,1066,420}. The diagnosis of rare soft tissue lesions can be difficult, especially with limited material that lacks architectural features, and without ancillary testing. However, ICC and molecular findings can support a specific diagnosis in many cases {1470,1017,1062,342}. When adequate sampling is available, FNAB can accurately define tumour type in 77–97% of cases {1017,176}. In the paediatric age group, FNAB combined with molecular testing and ICC is generally more accurate for subtyping malignant musculoskeletal neoplasms than in adults, because many childhood neoplasms harbour a detectable genetic abnormality {22,21,323,343,463,199}.

The grading of soft tissue sarcomas has been acknowledged as a common limitation in the cytopathological evaluation of soft tissue tumours. The US National Cancer Institute (NCI) and the French Fédération Nationale des Centres de Lutte Contre le Cancer (FNCLCC) systems, based on tumour differentiation, mitotic rate, and necrosis, are the most widely used histopathological grading systems for sarcomas {246}. Assessing these parameters may not always be feasible in FNAB samples {1311, 868,889}. Nevertheless, most sarcomas can be accurately graded in smears when segregated into high and low grades, which is usually sufficient information to plan initial treatment or further management. Weir et al. (1999) {1496} and Ng et al. (2010) {1017} reported 92% and 95% accuracy, respectively, in cytopathological sarcoma grading, and Palmer et al. (2001) {1066} reported 90% correctly graded sarcomas. In a subset of sarcomas, a specific histopathological diagnosis from FNAB smears can determine the corresponding malignancy grade {712,342}.

One important limitation of cytopathology is the limited experience of most practising pathologists in the wide array of soft tissue neoplasms and their morphological heterogeneity, making the cytopathological diagnosis of soft tissue tumours challenging {338,342}. Successful FNAB evaluation requires an experienced cytopathologist and close collaboration between the orthopaedic surgeon, oncologist, and cytopathologist. Complications of a correctly performed FNAB in examination of soft tissue lesions are minor and include small haematomas and localized tenderness. The risk of tumour cell spread in needle tracts is strongly related to the needle size and the number of passes performed; with regular 22–25 gauge needles, the incidence of this complication is exceedingly low {663,125,774}.

Integration of clinical, imaging, and key FNAB cytopathological features with ancillary testing in a diagnostic approach

Domanski HA
Geijer M
Kilpatrick SE
Klijanienko J
Schmitt F

Soft tissue tumours comprise a heterogeneous group of benign, intermediate, and malignant lesions with mesenchymal differentiation. Sarcomas are rare, constituting < 1% of all malignant neoplasms. The frequency of benign soft tissue tumours is estimated to be at least 100 times that of sarcomas. Soft tissue tumours occur in various planes and locations, and 99% of benign soft tissue neoplasms are superficial, whereas two thirds of the extremity and trunk-wall sarcomas are deep-seated. Sarcomas often present complex clinical and morphological features. The optimal diagnostic management of soft tissue lesions is a multimodal evaluation with synthesis of clinical data, imaging, and cytomorphology, supported by ancillary studies when necessary {509}. Patients presenting with a soft tissue lesion or a suspicion of a sarcoma should preferably be referred to specialized orthopaedic oncology centres with access to multidisciplinary expertise {1213,1356,904,882,583,509}. In such centres, oncological, imaging, histopathological and cytopathological, and molecular pathology expertise can be combined in a multidisciplinary team to facilitate the adequate evaluation, therapy, and follow-up of patients with soft tissue neoplasms. This multidisciplinary management favourably influences outcomes for patients with both benign and malignant soft tissue lesions {1305,1035,469,567,680,629}.

Clinical history and clinical examination are important to guide the initial evaluation of soft tissue lesions, including the decision as to whether there is a need for imaging and biopsy, and if so, what type of imaging and biopsy will provide the information necessary to inform further patient care. Relevant clinical characteristics should include the patient's age, sex, clinical history, and family history of cancers and genetic tumour syndromes, as well as the clinical findings, such as tumour site, presentation, duration and type of symptoms, and laboratory test results.

Imaging is an important part of the workup of soft tissue lesions; it helps to determine whether a lesion is benign or malignant, homogeneous or heterogeneous, as well as to identify any notable structures, such as origin from a large nerve trunk {1449, 149,220}. MRI is the main imaging modality in the examination of soft tissue lesions in the extremities, pelvis, and trunk; CT has a role in the evaluation of calcified lesions and pleuropulmonary and retroperitoneal sarcomas {509}. Ultrasound and MRI both provide diagnostic information that assists in distinguishing between benign and malignant soft tissue masses {999}, and combining these two modalities increases diagnostic performance, particularly the specificity {1302}. Nuclear medicine and hybrid imaging such as PET-CT are valuable to detect multiple lesions and evaluate tumour activity.

Most soft tissue tumours require a biopsy for diagnosis, particularly when malignancy cannot be ruled out by clinical or imaging means. A biopsy also provides information regarding the histopathological type of soft tissue tumour and grade of malignancy in cases of sarcoma {509}.

Ideally, an FNAB should be the first biopsy method in the examination of a suspected recurrence or metastasis of a previously treated sarcoma or other malignancies presenting as soft tissue tumours {1423,1017,696}, followed by CNB and excision biopsy when necessary. Depending on local expertise and the site of the lesion, FNAB can be used for the evaluation of primary soft tissue lesions alone in the clinical setting of a multidisciplinary diagnostic team {1470,705,784,1311,1509,1001,1169}, or it can be followed immediately by CNB {1159,344,753,1073}. ICC and molecular analysis performed on cytopathological specimens enhance the role of FNAB {740,281,355,643,1232, 198}, but their use and availability vary between institutions and socioeconomic settings.

The quality of the FNAB procedure and the adequacy of the cytopathological material and its suitability for ancillary tests have a great impact on the efficacy of FNAB of soft tissue neoplasms {1062,335}. ROSE offers significant benefits in terms of controlling the quality and quantity of FNAB samples and for immediately triaging material for ancillary tests {342,22}; it is recommended by the WHO Reporting System for Soft Tissue Cytopathology (WHO System) as best practice for the FNAB and the triaging of cytopathological material.

The nomenclature and classification of soft tissue neoplasms used in daily clinical practice are based on the fifth-edition WHO classification of soft tissue and bone neoplasms {1503}. In cytopathology practice, soft tissue lesions can be classified according to their presumed histogenesis or according to their differentiation towards a predominant cell type based on low-power smear patterns, the cell and tissue fragment architectural features, and the background of the FNAB smears {198,1311,31, 739,413}.

In this WHO System, each entity is placed into a cytopathological pattern and cell type group, such as adipocytic, myxoid, spindle cell, epithelioid, chondro-osseous, pleomorphic, and round cell. Each of these groups presents certain differential diagnoses to the cytopathologist and affects the approach to diagnosis, while the cytopathology of each entity mirrors its histopathology. ICC and molecular genetic tests on FNAB material can then be used to confirm or rule out a specific diagnosis.

Surgery remains the treatment of choice for most high-grade soft tissue sarcomas in adults, with additional radiotherapy or chemotherapy for cases with risk of local recurrence or metastasis. Low-grade sarcomas and many benign soft tissue neoplasms may be treated by surgery alone. In adequate FNAB specimens, it is usually possible to categorize a sarcoma cytomorphologically as low-grade or high-grade {712,1066,1496}. The treatment of some paediatric sarcomas (e.g. small round cell sarcomas) may include neoadjuvant therapy with potentially curative histogenetic-specific chemotherapy protocols; with the use of ancillary tests based on FNAB material, a specific diagnosis can be established in almost all cases {22,463,343,1232}.

However, assessing the parameters for sarcoma grading in histopathological sections and establishing the histopathological diagnosis is not always feasible using FNAB samples {655}. In any case in which FNAB has failed to yield material sufficient for diagnosis or the cytopathological diagnosis does not match the suspected clinical and imaging diagnosis, the imaging findings should be reviewed and correlated, and if suspicion remains high, CNB or simple excision biopsy should be performed before any major surgical or oncological procedure is undertaken.

Diagnostic categories and report structure

Field AS
Domanski HA
Klijanienko J

Diagnostic categories

Each of the categories of the WHO Reporting System for Soft Tissue Cytopathology (WHO System) is associated with a ROM that is directly linked to a recommendation for further diagnostic testing to achieve a specific diagnosis or to refine a differential diagnosis and suggest further management. Specific processes or tumours that have a similar ROM when diagnosed on cytopathology are placed in the same category; for example, inflammatory and benign neoplastic entities are placed in the "Benign" category. The WHO System uses categories to assist communication of the ROM to the clinician, but a specific diagnosis or a differential diagnosis that can be further refined by ancillary testing is the aim of all cytopathology reporting and paramount in the report.

There are six WHO System categories that can be used for direct FNAB smears, LBC, and touch preparations of soft tissue CNB:

- Insufficient/Inadequate/Non-diagnostic
- Benign
- Atypical
- Soft tissue neoplasm of uncertain malignant potential (STNUMP)
- Suspicious for malignancy
- Malignant

Currently there are limited publications defining the ROM for these categories in soft tissue cytopathology, and there is a need for further research using the WHO System to more clearly define the ROM associated with each category.

Individual cytopathologists, as well as departments with more than one cytopathologist, should choose to use either "Insufficient" or "Inadequate" as the term for cases where there is no material for assessment or when there are technical problems that prevent assessment of material on the slides. If there is adequate benign soft tissue material on the smears, then this is described and reported as "Benign". Correlation with the clinical and imaging findings should be carried out wherever possible, and if the material on the slides shows benign material that does not correlate with or explain the imaging or clinical findings, then it is mandatory to include a caveat in the report conclusion, that the material "may not represent the lesion seen on imaging and further diagnostic workup is recommended". This discrepancy may relate to sampling error, particularly with small lesions seen on imaging, or it may reflect the limitations of imaging in accurately distinguishing some soft tissue lesions.

It is recognized that in some cytopathology practices in some parts of the world the term "Non-diagnostic" has been applied to encompass not only cases where there is insufficient or technically obscured material, but also cases where there is benign cytopathological material that does not correlate with or explain the clinical and/or imaging findings. This is the first WHO Reporting System for Soft Tissue Cytopathology , and the expert editorial board accepts that in line with current usage, these cases may in some regions of the world be categorized as "Non-diagnostic" and placed in the "Insufficient/Inadequate" category. However, the term "Non-diagnostic" is not encouraged in soft tissue FNAB. Research into the impact of this approach on the "Insufficient/Inadequate/Non-diagnostic" and "Benign" ROM is required.

If any atypical features are seen in a case showing otherwise insufficient material, the case is regarded as "Atypical" and not "Insufficient".

The "Benign" category includes specific neoplasms and inflammatory processes including suppurative, granulomatous, and specific infectious or inflammatory diseases. If the features are benign but a precise diagnosis cannot be made, the features should be described and a differential diagnosis provided. If the features raise a differential diagnosis that includes a low-grade or high-grade lesion, then the case is placed in the "Atypical" category. As with all categories, correlation with clinical features and wherever possible imaging is mandatory.

The "Atypical" category includes cases where there is scant or poorly prepared cellular material, as well as, importantly, cases with considerable material showing mainly benign cytopathological features but with some features that may raise the possibility of malignancy, for example a spindle cell pattern with low cellularity but moderate nuclear atypia. The ability of individual cytopathologists and their teams to confidently diagnose soft tissue lesions on cytopathology alone varies with local practice and expertise, as well as the expectations and support of their clinical colleagues.

The "Atypical" category is expected to have a relatively low to intermediate ROM and allows for a high negative predictive value for a "Benign" diagnosis, while the "Suspicious for malignancy" category is expected to have a higher ROM and provide for a high positive predictive value, approaching 100% for a "Malignant" categorization. The categories stratify the ROM and allow for the development of recommendations for the further diagnostic workup of the case to achieve as specific a diagnosis as possible, which is the aim of all cytopathology.

The "Soft tissue neoplasm of uncertain malignant potential" ("STNUMP") category encompasses two distinct groups: firstly, cases where the diagnosis of a specific neoplasm can be made and the neoplasm's behaviour (in terms of recurrence, invasiveness, or ability to metastasize) is uncertain, for example solitary fibrous tumour; and secondly, the "STNUMP" category includes tumours with intermediate biological potential and tumours requiring the application of histopathological criteria to determine risk stratification as to their risk of metastasis.

The "Suspicious for malignancy" category includes cases where there is scant, poorly smeared, or poorly prepared and stained material suggestive of malignancy, as well as cases where there is considerable material, some of which appears malignant, but not all features of a particular malignancy are present or there may be discrepant features. The report should specifically describe the features that are suspicious and provide a differential diagnosis of the lesions suspected.

The "Malignant" category is reserved for those cases in which there are unequivocal features of malignancy without any discrepant findings. All cytopathology specimen types are obtained by a sampling technique, and it is not always possible to make a precise diagnosis of a specific soft tissue tumour even with ancillary testing. The precise diagnosis of a primary soft tissue malignancy or metastatic carcinoma or lymphoma involving soft tissue often requires ancillary testing.

The presentation of tumours in this WHO System loosely follows the order found in the sixth-edition WHO classification of soft tissue and bone tumours, but the grouping of tumours is by smear pattern, cell type, and the architectural features of the tissue fragments, reflecting a cytopathologist's diagnostic approach {413}. Tumours that have not been described in the cytopathology literature are not included, and rare tumours with few publications are presented in the differential diagnosis of more common tumours.

Structured reporting

Each cytopathology report on a soft tissue FNAB should have a structured format, with a heading of a specific diagnostic category using the WHO System's standardized terminology and a diagnosis. Structured reporting improves the quality, clarity, and reproducibility of reports within individual pathology departments and between countries, and it will improve patient care and facilitate research and quality assurance measures. Standard guidelines for cell block preparation, ICC, FISH, and flow cytometry in cases of lymphoid lesions, as well as molecular pathology for tests of diagnostic, prognostic, and predictive markers, will improve diagnostic accuracy, reduce cost, and improve patient care. Structured reports are based on key diagnostic cytopathological findings for each lesion, which act as a checklist for the reporting cytopathologist and will also improve reporting.

The essential or core requirements in a cytopathology report are presented here. This is not intended to make any particular format mandatory, but some components are required: the precise location of the lesion; the number of direct smears and amount and type of fluids received; the diagnostic category using the defined terminology of the reporting system; a microscopic description of the key diagnostic features; and a diagnosis, which may be specific or descriptive with a differential diagnosis. The aim of all FNAB cytopathology is to provide as accurate and specific a diagnosis as possible, and if not possible, a differential diagnosis that weights the most likely diagnoses. Supplementary reports of any ancillary tests and their results are also required, wherever possible in an integrated final report and diagnosis. Ancillary tests may change the final category, for example when ICC confirms a malignancy suspected on the cytopathology alone. The diagnostic summary, including site of biopsy, category, and diagnosis, must be clearly delineated and stand out in the report so that it can be easily seen by the patient care team, and it is best placed early on the first page rather than at the end of multiple pages of report.

It is not recommended to use a number in defining a category at any stage. A category number can be included in the body of the report for audit and research purposes but not in the diagnostic summary. Reducing a cytopathology report to a number reduces the information that can be given to the clinician and management team and increases the risk of error.

The diagnostic category states whether there is inadequate material and an "Insufficient/Inadequate/Non-diagnostic" categorization is applicable, or whether there is adequate material and a "Benign", "Atypical", "STNUMP", "Suspicious for malignancy", or "Malignant" category can be applied. But it is recognized that some cytopathologists prefer to include a statement in the report that "there is adequate material for assessment". Other cytopathologists require a statement to be included regarding the degree of cellularity of the material from the target lesion; this assessment of cellularity does not include inflammatory cells except in cases of an inflammatory lesion.

The microscopic description should provide a clear, concise cytopathological description, which usually includes the degree of cellularity and focuses on the presence or absence of key cytopathological diagnostic features. Some cytopathologists prefer to provide a full description of these features; others may prefer, in cases where there is a specific diagnosis, to provide minimal or no description.

The aim of cytopathology is to provide as specific a diagnosis as possible in the vast majority of cases, and this remains the priority. Categories allow the grouping of lesions, including those that are "Atypical", "STNUMP", or "Suspicious for malignancy", and the establishment of a ROM and subsequent management recommendations as part of an algorithm to aid communication with the clinician and further diagnostic management of the patient.

The ancillary tests should always be part of the final cytopathology report, and if ICC, flow cytometry, in situ hybridization, or molecular pathology reports are issued by a different laboratory, then it is recommended that they should be added as a supplementary report to the original cytopathology report, in the interest of having a final all-inclusive integrated report for optimal patient care. The WHO reporting systems for cytopathology are based on the cytomorphology findings for the initial categorization and reporting of the lesion, which can be applied in any well-resourced or low- and middle-income country (LMIC) setting, but they also incorporate the application of appropriate ancillary testing as current best practice. Subsequent ancillary testing may well change the final diagnostic category and provide a specific diagnosis of a particular case.

The standardized cytopathology report

Demographic information

- Patient's name, date of birth, address, patient identifiers / patient episode, date of request, and laboratory accession number
- Referring doctor and contact details

Type of specimen

- FNAB, including FNAB technique; for example, FNAB by palpation alone or ultrasound-guided or endobronchial ultrasound (EBUS)-directed FNAB

Clinical and imaging information

- Precise site, size (mm), imaging (ultrasound, CXR, tomogram, CT, MRI) features

- Previous cytopathology, CNB or excision biopsy results, and other previous biopsy results when available
- History of malignancies that may be presenting as metastases

Diagnostic summary

- Totally in bold, on the first page (if the laboratory information system supports this)
- Each institution should select a term for this main heading, such as "Diagnostic summary" (as used throughout this volume), "Diagnosis", or "Final diagnosis", and use it consistently

Category

- Using the diagnostic category terminology of the WHO System and not a number

Diagnosis

- Inclusion of the exact site of the FNAB in the diagnostic summary is recommended; this information should correlate with the labelling of the specimen jar and the request form; if it does not, the clinician should be contacted
- Specific diagnosis or differential diagnosis

Other information included in the report

Material received

- Number of air-dried slides, number of alcohol-fixed slides
- Type (saline, RPMI medium, formalin, only specimen without diluent, LBC) and volume of fluid received, with description of fluid (colour, presence of blood, viscosity, presence of particulate matter), including any other specimens received and specifically designated for flow cytometry, microbiology and cell block

Details of rapid onsite evaluation (if conducted)

- Number of passes, gauge of needle used, imaging modality used
- The names of those performing the clinical and diagnostic procedures, including the cytopathology biomedical scientist, pathology trainee, or cytopathologist attending the ROSE, are usually not included in the final report, but they should be recorded in digital attachments to the report
- Number of slides processed and stained at ROSE, air-dried and alcohol-fixed, and other specimen types prepared
- The specific verbatim ROSE report provided to the clinician should be documented, as well as the name of the cytopathologist or cytopathology biomedical scientist issuing ROSE; this is usually not included in the final report, but it should be recorded in digital attachments to the report, along with the details of any further procedures following ROSE

Microscopic description

- Optional, but inclusion of a statement of the degree of cellularity (e.g. scant, mildly cellular, moderately cellular, highly cellular) or the specimen quality (e.g. "specimen satisfactory for assessment") is recommended
- Optional to include the key diagnostic cytopathological features where present or absent, but if the final diagnosis is not specific and is based on a differential diagnosis, then a microscopic description is required
- Include a specific diagnosis, or if this is not possible, a discussion of the differential diagnosis, emphasizing the most likely diagnosis; cytopathologists may prefer a subheading or "Comment" at the end of the microscopic description to convey the diagnosis
- If the lesion is "Insufficient/Inadequate/Non-diagnostic", "Atypical", or "Suspicious for malignancy", then the report should include a clear description of what material is present on the slides, and the reason why the material is insufficient, atypical, or suspicious for malignancy should be stated; for the "Atypical" and "Suspicious for malignancy" categories, this may include a discussion of the differential diagnosis

Ancillary testing

- Depending on local practice, the cytopathology report, including its conclusion, can be issued as a final or provisional report, with supplementary information or addenda on ancillary studies to follow and to be added to a final integrated report; or in some cases the cytopathology report can be withheld until ancillary reports are available, in which case best practice includes the cytopathologist immediately contacting the clinician to discuss the case and stating that there is a need for ancillary testing
- Includes all cell block H&E and special stains, ICC, in situ hybridization, and molecular techniques performed on the cell block or direct smear slide scrapings and further stains; the report should state which type of specimen was used for each ancillary test to facilitate continuous quality assurance
- If flow cytometry results are available for cases of lymphoproliferative diseases, and are issued by the same laboratory, then these results should be entered here; or if flow cytometry results are issued by a different laboratory, their results should be added as a supplementary report when available under ancillary testing in the original report
- If a CNB or other surgical biopsy was performed at the same time as the FNAB, the supplementary report should recommend correlation with the surgical report, and its accession number should be stated

Risk of malignancy and diagnostic management recommendations

Domanski HA
Klijanienko J

The goal of establishing a ROM for each category in the WHO Reporting System for Soft Tissue Cytopathology (WHO System) is to supply clinically relevant information by linking each diagnostic category with recommendations for the further diagnostic management and triage of individual cases (see Table 1.01). The ROM for each category is based on the published literature reporting the experience of centres actively involved in the diagnosis and management of a significant number of soft tissue cases. In this first edition of the WHO System, the ROM is extracted from a limited number of studies, because most publications regarding musculoskeletal FNAB are based on a single diagnostic entity or series of both bone and soft tissue tumours with significant heterogeneity regarding primary versus recurrent or metastatic lesions, FNAB technique, use of imaging guidance, and use of ROSE and ancillary testing. The data in these studies are often not sufficient for the calculation of ROM as applied to the WHO System. In addition, there has been no established reporting system for soft tissue FNAB cytopathology, although a seven-category system was proposed in 2021 {753}. The ROM will be the subject of further research and subsequent modification in future editions of the WHO System.

The management of all diagnostic categories requires correlation with clinical and imaging findings, and a multidisciplinary approach is essential for the workup of patients with soft tissue tumours. Intraprocedural evaluation of FNAB smears by ROSE is strongly recommended during the sampling procedure.

The "Insufficient/Inadequate/Non-diagnostic" category includes cases where there is insufficient cytopathological material for assessment due to technical reasons, such as an insufficient number of cells on the smears, poor quality of smears, air-drying artefact in alcohol-fixed Pap-stained or H&E-stained smears, and slow air-drying artefact in air-dried Giemsa-stained smears. Several factors may affect the quality and quantity of FNAB samples: the size, consistency, and location of the mass; its imaging characteristics; and its proximity to the vital structures all have an impact on the quality of the FNAB yield and subsequent biopsy results, as does the inherent nature of the lesion. The expertise and technical skills of the physician who performs the FNAB procedure are a crucial factor, as is the expertise of the cytopathologist, laboratory staff, or other staff who prepare the direct smears for routine examination and triage for ancillary studies {342,29,832}.

In a study of FNAB of soft tissue of 828 patients, the inadequate rate was 3% and the ROM 42%, and this included a CNB with FNAB in all but 2 patients {753}. A retrospective study of FNAB of 301 soft tissue lesions {1001} showed a 7% inadequate rate (with haemangiomas accounting for almost half of the inadequate specimens), with a ROM of 9%. In a study of 1114 soft tissue and bone FNAB specimens, most of which had ROSE, 3% of cases were inadequate, and within that group, 70% were soft tissue lesions {696}. In a retrospective study of 94 bone and 36 soft tissue FNAB specimens, the insufficient rate for soft tissue lesions was 8%, with an estimated ROM of 27.3% {176}. In a recent retrospective study of 2214 cases at one institution, the ROM of an "Insufficient" categorization was 29.87% {460}.

Diagnostic management recommendations for the "Insufficient/Inadequate/Non-diagnostic" category include correlation with the clinical and imaging findings, and in most cases repeat FNAB with ROSE and imaging guidance, especially in deep-seated, cystic, or haemorrhagic or necrotic lesions. In cases where the imaging is uncertain or a suspicious mass remains unresolved by further FNAB, CNB or a surgical biopsy should be recommended.

The majority of palpable soft tissue lesions are benign. The "Benign" category includes cytopathological features of mass-forming inflammatory lesions that can explain the clinical context, as well as benign neoplasms of various types, such as lipomatous, myxoid, spindle cell, epithelioid, and chondro-osseous neoplasms.

Table 1.01 The WHO Reporting System for Soft Tissue Cytopathology: estimated risk of malignancy (ROM) and diagnostic management options by diagnostic category

Diagnostic category	Estimated ROM[a]	Diagnostic management options
Insufficient/Inadequate/Non-diagnostic	30% (9–42%)	CORRELATE. Repeat FNAB, preferably with ROSE.
Benign	2% (0–4%)	CORRELATE. If discrepancy, repeat FNAB and/or CNB. If correlation, review when appropriate.
Atypical	40% (46%)	CORRELATE. Discuss at MDTM. Repeat FNAB and/or CNB and/or surgical biopsy.
STNUMP	51% (20–27%)	CORRELATE. Discuss at MDTM. Repeat FNAB and/or CNB and/or surgical biopsy.
Suspicious for malignancy	68% (71–80%)	CORRELATE. Discuss at MDTM. Consider repeat FNAB to obtain material for ancillary testing, but will usually require CNB and/or surgical biopsy.
Malignant	98% (91–100%)	CORRELATE. Discuss at MDTM. Will usually require CNB and/or surgical biopsy.

CORRELATE, correlate with clinical and imaging findings, and where available with cell block, ICC, FISH, PCR, and NGS findings; MDTM, multidisciplinary team meeting; STNUMP, "Soft tissue neoplasms of uncertain malignant potential".

[a]Estimated ROMs are based on a large retrospective study using the WHO System categories, including the "STNUMP" category, and on a series of other retrospective studies in brackets {753,1001,696,176,1017,705}.

In general, a benign diagnosis is based on evidence-based, established cytopathological criteria and ancillary techniques where required. Wherever possible, the cytopathological categorization of "Benign" should be accompanied by a specific diagnosis, such as lipomatous tumour, nodular fasciitis, ischaemic fasciitis, or myositis ossificans, but precise diagnosis may not always be possible {333,320}.

For superficial or deep soft tissue lesions where the clinical and imaging impression is that a benign lesion or neoplasm is considered most likely, and this is confirmed by FNAB, treatment options depend on the clinical symptoms, size, and anatomical location of the lesion or neoplasm, as well as the precise diagnosis. For asymptomatic benign tumours, such as lipoma or nodular fasciitis, the management options may be to wait and watch, whereas other lesions categorized as "Benign" may require limited or wide excision if causing symptoms {1072,158}. The ROM for the "Benign" category is very low, estimated at 0–3.6% {753,1001,176,1017,705}; it was found to be 2.49% in a large recent study using the WHO System reporting categories {460}. FNAB is highly accurate when used as an initial diagnostic test, with 89–100% sensitivity and 90–100% specificity in distinguishing benign from malignant soft tissue tumours {1533, 691,1470,1001,320,420,1311}; it showed 97.4% sensitivity and 98.2% specificity, depending on various study parameters, in a recent large meta-analysis {188}.

The "Atypical" category includes samples where a specific diagnosis of a benign process or neoplasm cannot be made on the FNAB smears although the cytopathological features appear most likely benign, but some features raise the possibility of an indeterminate or perhaps malignant neoplasm, which cannot be excluded. The cytopathological features that make the smear atypical should always be stated, and (if possible) a differential diagnosis should be provided to enhance correlation with other findings. Most cases represent poorly sampled neoplasms and include smears from myxoid lesions or smears where small numbers of spindle cells show no or low-grade atypia. In a report of 828 patients, the ROM in this category was 46% {753}, and in a recent large retrospective study the ROM was 39.62% {460}.

Diagnostic management recommendations for the "Atypical" category include mandatory correlation with the clinical history and imaging findings. This category requires a cell block and usually ancillary testing, and it most commonly requires repeat FNAB with cell block or CNB whenever this is available and can be used at the site of the neoplasm. Incisional or excisional surgical biopsy may be considered to confirm a benign or malignant lesion. Alternatively, if clinical and imaging findings indicate that the process is highly likely to be a benign reactive or inflammatory lesion, a "watch and wait" approach may be considered.

There is a lack of published data to estimate the ROM for the diagnostic category "Soft tissue neoplasm of uncertain malignant potential" ("STNUMP"). One recent large retrospective study that recategorized reports based on the WHO System categories found a ROM of 51.43% {460}. In the management of cases in this category, every effort should be made to establish a precise diagnosis according to the WHO classification of soft tissue and bone tumours, and this usually requires ancillary tests and correlation between cytopathology and clinical and imaging findings. Further workup can include performing a repeat FNAB (to provide additional smears for cytopathological assessment and particularly to obtain material for cell blocks that can be used for H&E stains, ICC, FISH, and NGS), proceeding to CNB for histopathological material and ancillary testing, or proceeding to incisional biopsy or resection. In some cases, depending on the surgical accessibility of the neoplasm or considerations of patient age and status, observation and clinical follow-up may be used. Ideally, the clinical, imaging, and FNAB findings are assessed and treatment decisions are made by a multidisciplinary team. Risk assessment in some of these tumour types, for example solitary fibrous tumour and gastrointestinal stromal tumour, requires histopathological assessment {310,652}.

The report of an FNAB categorized as "Suspicious for malignancy" should always state what features make the material suspicious and what lesion is suspected, and a differential diagnosis should be provided. In almost all cases where sufficient material is available, ancillary testing is required and may make it possible to render a specific malignant or benign diagnosis. This category supports a high positive predictive value for the "Malignant" category, but it should not be used as the sole basis for initiating therapy. The ROM for the "Suspicious" group was found to be 72% in a study proposing a seven-category system {753} and 80% in another retrospective study of 301 patients {1001}. A recent large retrospective study using the WHO System's six categories found a ROM of 68.42% {460}. The authors of that study made the interesting observation that the ROM varied not only with categorization into the six categories, but also with the FNAB pattern seen, from 3% for lipomatous tumours, which include one of the most common FNAB targets (superficial lipoma), to 62.78% for spindle cell, 78.15% for epithelioid, 84.58% for myxoid, 94.26% for pleomorphic, and 100% for round cell tumours. Further research around this finding will be worthwhile to guide cytopathologists and clinicians.

Close communication with the members of the clinical team and a review of all relevant clinical and imaging findings is mandatory to avoid unnecessary risks. The further workup of the patient to establish as specific a diagnosis as possible in a management plan should be determined within the multidisciplinary team. This may include repeating the FNAB, preferably with ROSE and triaging of material for appropriate ancillary tests; in most cases, CNB, to assess histopathological features, or surgical biopsy, for a definitive histopathological diagnosis, is also required.

The "Malignant" category includes all cases where the material is unequivocally malignant with the key cytopathological features diagnostic of a specific tumour or group of tumours, for example metastatic carcinomas, high-grade lymphomas, or low- or high-grade sarcomas. Ideally, a specific diagnosis should be made, or the case should be categorized as "Malignant" and a differential diagnosis provided. Ancillary testing is usually required to confirm or make a specific diagnosis, for example the use of ICC to diagnose the type and origin of metastatic carcinoma; the use of ICC, FISH, or molecular tests to diagnose the specific type of soft tissue sarcoma (e.g. round cell sarcoma, including Ewing sarcoma; rhabdomyosarcoma; or a spindle cell sarcoma, including a synovial sarcoma); or on uncommon occasions the use of flow cytometry to diagnose a lymphoma involving soft tissues. The estimated ROM for the "Malignant" category is 91–100% based on several retrospective studies {753,1001,176,1017,705}, and it was 97.69% in a recent large retrospective study, which also found that the ROM varied with the cytomorphological pattern as well as with the WHO System categorization {460}. The plan for further management should be determined by the multidisciplinary team and includes workup for distant metastasis. The type of surgical intervention depends on whether the neoplasm is subcutaneous or deep, accessible for excision, small or large, and/or adjacent or even involving vital structures, but wide radical excision is envisaged for the majority of soft tissue sarcomas sited in the extremities, the chest wall, and (in most cases) the intra-abdominal region. The optimal neoadjuvant or adjuvant chemo and/or radiotherapy is tailored to the individual patient and type of malignancy.

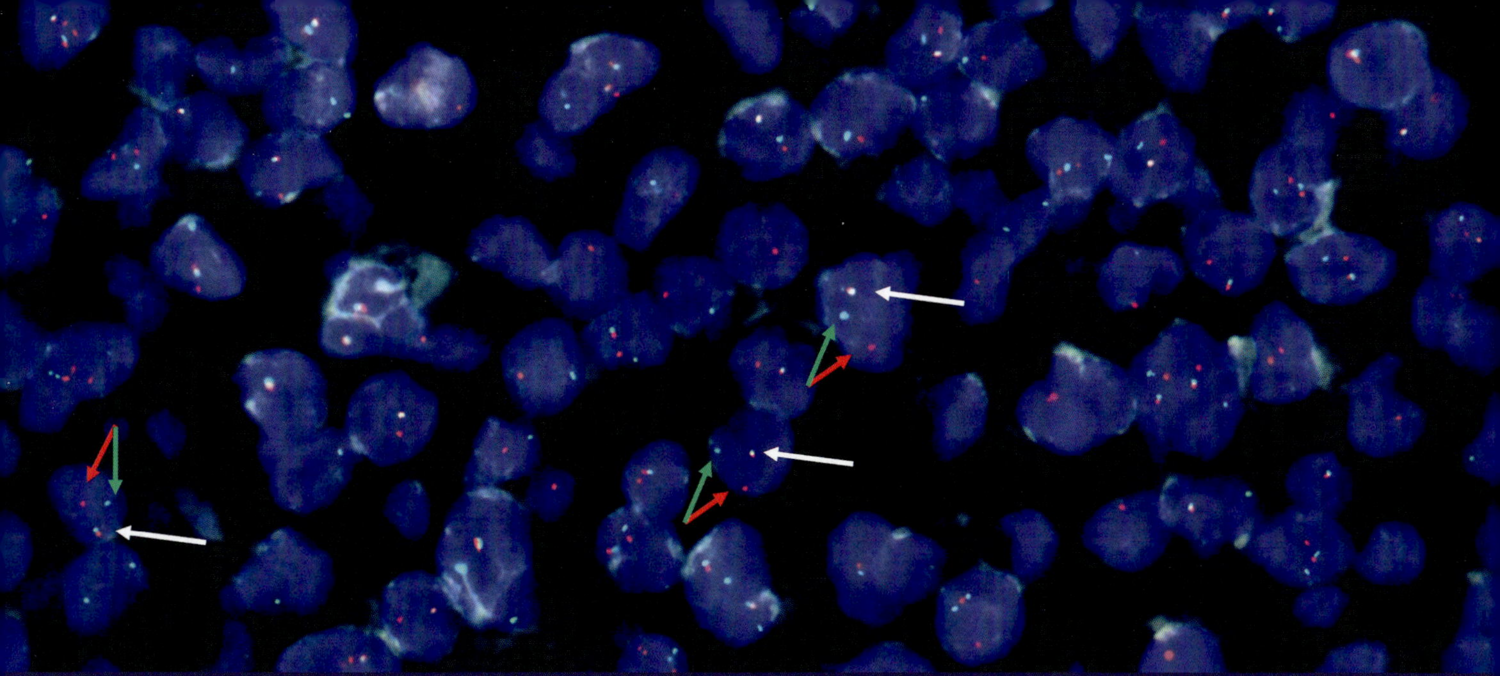

2

Soft tissue cytopathology techniques

Edited by: Lazar AJ, Pitman MB, Qian X, Schmitt F

Introduction

Qian X
Domanski HA

Evaluation of soft tissue masses by FNAB, with or without concurrent CNB, has been increasingly used and has gained greater acceptance in recent years. This has occurred in concert with the rapid development in molecular genetic diagnostics, the massive expansion of sensitive and specific ICC biomarkers, and the maturation of various image-guided needle biopsy techniques, as well as the increasing use of a multidisciplinary approach in patient care. Enhanced by ROSE, which enables immediate triage for flow cytometry, microbiological culture, ICC, and cytogenetic and molecular studies, FNAB is a valuable, cost-effective, and time-sensitive diagnostic modality for soft tissue lesions and neoplasms, especially those with clinical or imaging features suspicious for malignancy. This chapter focuses on the practical approaches of FNAB sampling techniques, ROSE management, effective triage of biopsy material, and various cytopathological preparation methods, as well as the judicious use of ancillary studies {342,1062}.

FNAB techniques and specimen management

Klijanienko J
Domanski HA
Mehrotra R
Qian X

High-quality FNAB material is fundamental to ensuring an accurate diagnosis that can lead to effective management. The quality depends on the technique of sampling, the tumour size, the consistency of the lesion, the location of the lesion, and the proper management of cytopathological material. How and by whom a lesion is biopsied is preferably decided by a multidisciplinary team composed of an oncologist, surgeon, radiologist, and cytopathologist {159}.

Anaesthesia

For sampling superficial lesions in adults, local anaesthesia is optional. Patients usually experience minimal discomfort during the FNAB procedure, but the use of local anaesthesia can reduce patient anxiety as well as any pain. Injection of 1% lidocaine, with or without epinephrine, can be used. For FNAB in children, local anaesthesia with skin cream is recommended, which can be followed with injection of 1% lidocaine if needed. Sedation by inhalation is also an option. Sampling deep lesions may require general anaesthesia.

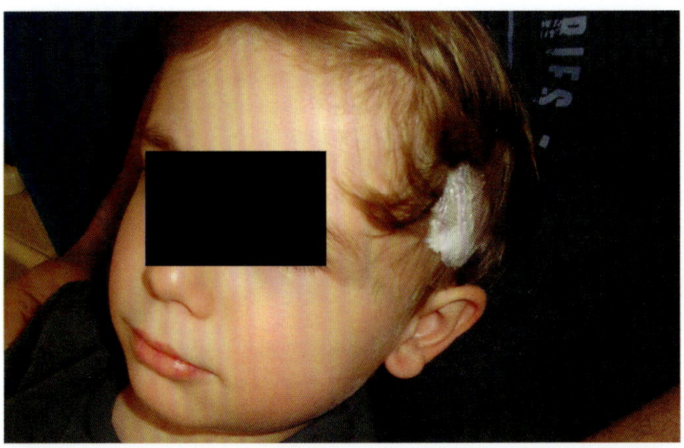

Fig. 2.01 Local skin anesthesia. Histiocytosis X FNAB with local skin anaesthesia.

Needles

Needles of between 22 and 27 gauge are used for FNAB, and as large as 18 gauge for small CNB. The choice of gauge may vary depending on the characteristics of the lesion. Fibrotic lesions are more easily biopsied with a 25–27 gauge needle, while lesions with an abundant myxoid or cellular component are best biopsied with a 22 or 23 gauge needle.

Use of suction

The FNAB technique can be performed with or without suction. In the absence of suction, capillary action is used, and this is generally recognized as comparable to FNAB with suction {1547}. Capillary action is achieved by using the needle by itself and agitating the needle into and back through the target repeatedly, or by attaching the needle to a syringe and withdrawing the syringe plunger to about 2 mL prior to puncture and moving the needle up and down within the target lesion. This technique is most successful with cellular, less fibrotic lesions, as well as vascular lesions that bleed easily. FNAB using suction is useful for cystic lesions and more fibrotic lesions.

FNAB guidance

Superficial and deeper, palpable lesions can be sampled with or without imaging guidance, but ideally there should be initial assessment with ultrasound or other imaging modalities. All deeply located, non-palpable lesions or lesions with complicated anatomical relationships should be sampled using imaging guidance. In this situation, the guidance technique (e.g. ultrasound versus CT) and the point of needle penetration are chosen by the interventional radiologist. Optimally, the needle and its contents should be entrusted to the pathology

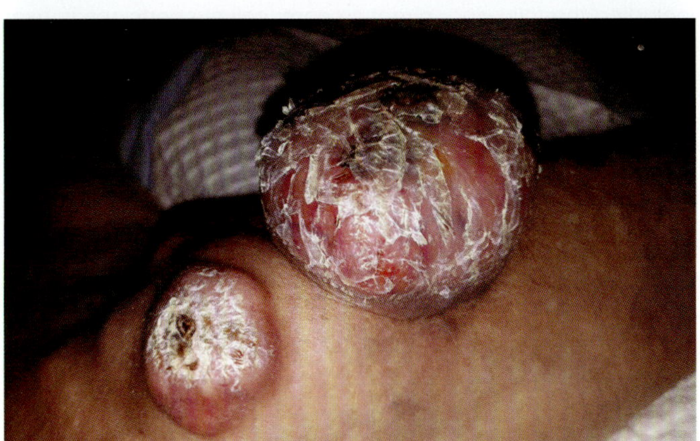

Fig. 2.02 Superficial, clearly malignant lesion. Superficial, easily palpable dermatofibrosarcoma protuberans, which can be punctured without imaging guidance.

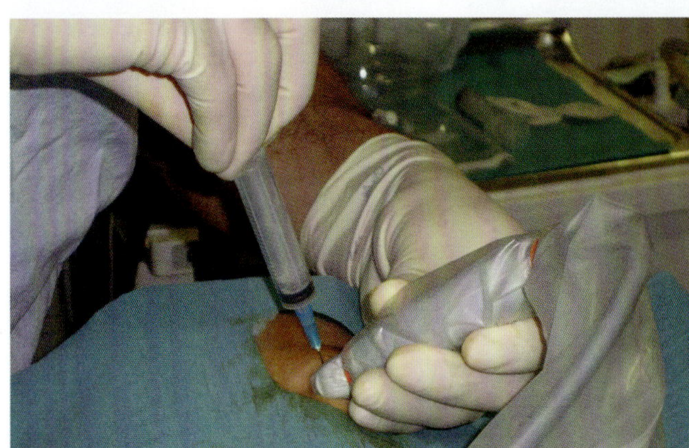

Fig. 2.03 Ultrasound-guided FNAB. Intraorbital rhabdomyosarcoma showing complicated anatomical relationships is biopsied under ultrasound guidance.

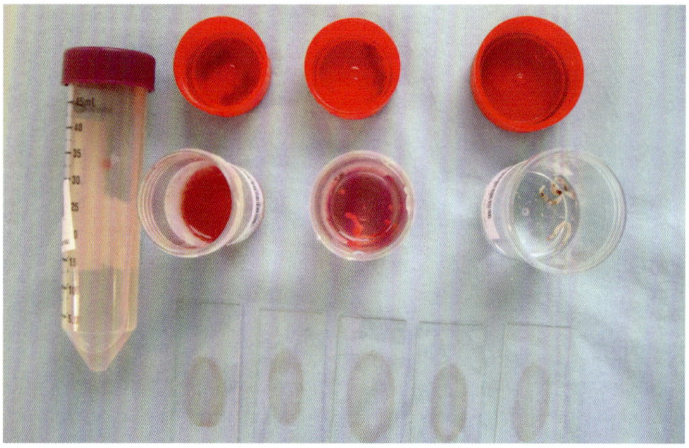

Fig. 2.04 The use of cytopathology material for ancillary techniques. An example of the use of ancillary techniques, including ICC and molecular studies, in Ewing sarcoma. Conventional smears for Giemsa stain, Hanks solution for cell block, ethylenediaminetetraacetic acid (EDTA) cores for cryopreservation, EDTA cell suspension for molecular analyses, and fixed cores for histopathological analysis.

team immediately after each FNAB pass, so that the team can expertly smear the material, stain, perform ROSE, judge the quality of the material, and provide cost-effective and efficient triage {1054}.

Complications

Dissemination of tumour cells in the puncture path has not been reported with the use of a fine needle (22–27 gauge). Dissemination is associated with the use of larger CNB. However, the puncture site and path can be marked with ink, photographed, and excised at the time of surgical resection.

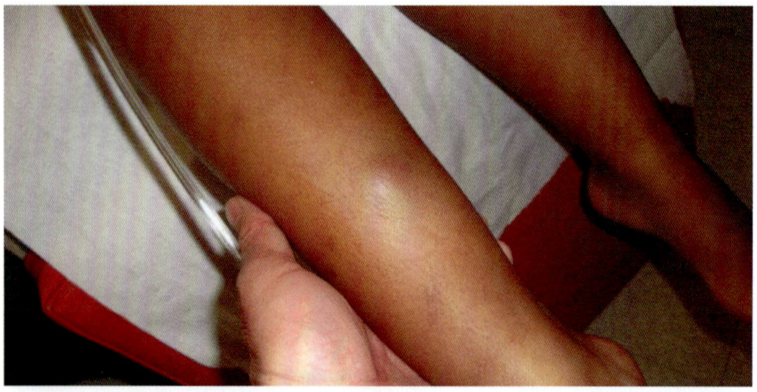

Fig. 2.05 Dermatofibrosarcoma protuberans. A superficial pretibial lesion, which may be easily investigated by FNAB.

Specimen management

The quality of the FNAB material should be evaluated by the pathologist during the procedure and ROSE provided. The cellularity of a given FNAB sample from soft tissue tumours is extremely variable. Tumours that are fibrotic and/or rich in vascularity may yield hypocellular and/or haemodiluted material, respectively. In some instances, low cellularity is characteristic and may be a diagnostic consideration in the differential diagnosis, such as in desmoid tumours or fibromatoses. Inversely, samples from round cell / pleomorphic / blastemal tumours, melanoma, or lymphoma are usually extremely rich in cells {738}.

Fixation and staining

Air-dried, Giemsa-stained smears can be quickly prepared at ROSE. If Pap or H&E staining is planned, smears must be fixed in alcohol immediately after smearing, to avoid air-drying artefact.

Rapid onsite evaluation

ROSE is beneficial for ensuring the adequate quantity and quality of the sample, and it is advised for all soft tissue FNAB. ROSE makes it possible for a cytopathologist to perform the initial provisional cytomorphological diagnosis and determine the quality and quantity of material for both cytopathological assessment and triage for ancillary studies; for example, when a round cell sarcoma is encountered, a portion of the fresh cell suspension may be dedicated for molecular analysis {404}. In addition, ROSE can provide the information that immediate CNB is required. Overall, the use of ROSE increases both the efficiency of small-volume biopsy samples and the accuracy of soft tissue tumour diagnosis on FNAB samples {1259}. If ROSE cannot be performed, cytopathologists should liaise closely with the interventional radiologist to establish a protocol for soft tissue FNAB procedures and the use of material.

Ancillary techniques

The diagnosis of soft tissue tumours frequently requires the use of ancillary techniques. Although ICC can be performed on direct smears or LBC slides, cell block preparations are preferred because most antibodies are validated on formalin-fixed histopathological sections. Molecular studies such as NGS and FISH can be performed on all specimen types with validation, including the following: direct smears; cell suspensions in fixatives; fresh or frozen tissue; and formalin-fixed, paraffin-embedded tissue {461,353,735,645}.

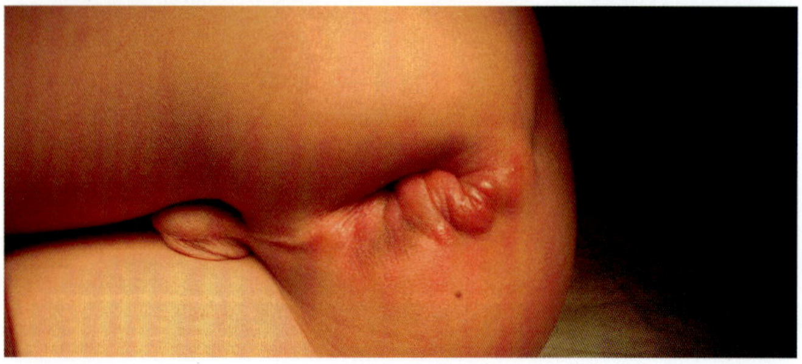

Fig. 2.06 Perianal tumor. Perianal lesions are frequently rhabdomyosarcomas.

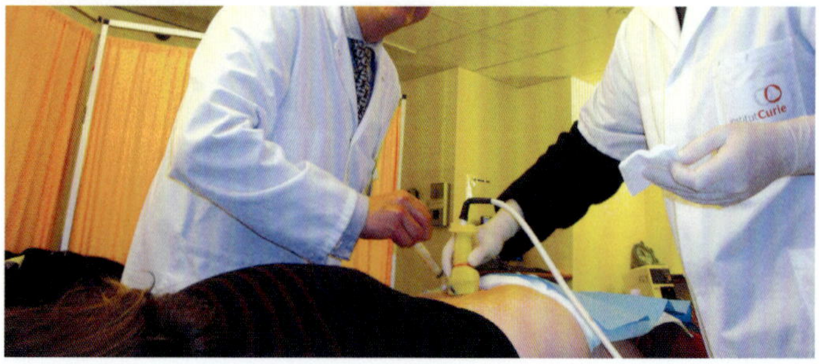

Fig. 2.07 Cooperation between radiologist and pathologist. Optimal sampling of connective tissue tumour is performed by a team composed of radiologist and pathologist.

Imaging guidance of soft tissue FNAB

Domanski HA
Bode-Lesniewska B
Geijer M

Imaging guidance in soft tissue FNAB may be helpful or in some cases mandatory, depending on the skill and preferences of the cytopathologist and interventional radiologist {1418,1470, 1458}. Small localized subcutaneous lesions may be sampled using manual palpation as guidance. Soft tissue lesions that are deep-seated or adjacent to a neurovascular bundle; that are intra-abdominal, pelvic, or intrathoracic; or that for some other reason are difficult to reliably biopsy using manual guidance should be biopsied using imaging guidance.

During the FNAB procedure, the imaging appearance before and after the sampling should be documented, as well as the needle position when the biopsy is actually obtained. If the procedure is performed by a radiologist or clinician, biopsy results are improved if ROSE is used {1455,120,22}.

Ultrasound is a low-cost and readily available modality for biopsy guidance {1208,1338,1535}. Ultrasound of soft tissue lesions can determine their echogenicity, size, vascularity, and relationship with adjacent structures, as well as provide a working differential diagnosis. If guiding fixtures on the transducer are used, lesions at a comparatively large distance from the skin may be biopsied reliably. With ultrasound, it is possible to guide the biopsy needle to parts of a heterogeneous tumour that are not necrotic, and vascularized parts of the tumour may be identified and avoided by using colour or power Doppler. Ultrasound guidance may be used by the cytopathologist or by a radiologist in the radiology department, depending on local expertise and equipment.

CT may be used for all biopsies of soft tissue lesions, but it uses ionizing radiation for imaging {837}. To reduce the radiation dose to the patient and the operator, CT guidance should be reserved for deep-seated lesions and lesions surrounded by complex anatomy. Usually, image guidance with CT is done without intravenous contrast enhancement. However, if the lesion is cystic or heterogeneous or shows other suspicious signs for necrosis, intravenous contrast may be used to delineate the viable parts of the tumour for biopsy.

Biopsies requiring image guidance are usually complex procedures, which may be associated with more risks due to more difficult access routes. With CT, the biopsy tract can be planned beforehand, and the approach can be discussed with the operating surgeon before biopsy if needed. In some cases, lesions detected on MRI may not be visible on CT, which makes CT guidance difficult, with the risk of having a false negative biopsy result. In such cases, hybrid imaging, where previously obtained MRI images are superimposed on the CT image, may be used. In addition, ROSE plays an important role: the immediate feedback helps the operator to decide the best needle path for additional passes or for acquiring a concurrent CNB.

Biopsies in the musculoskeletal system are occasionally done as both an FNAB and a CNB during the same procedure {344, 22}. If repeated FNAB passes are planned, especially in combination with CNB, the patient should receive local anaesthetic at the puncture site and towards the periosteum if a bone biopsy is planned. Some patients may also benefit from a sedative administered some time before the procedure. If a trocar is used for the CNB {794}, a hybrid biopsy may be done, where the trocar is also used to guide the FNAB. This reduces the numbers of both skin passes and biopsy tracts, and it reduces the radiation dose if CT is used for guidance. Such a coaxial biopsy may also be performed using a thicker needle as a guide, through which thin 22 gauge or 25 gauge needles can be inserted, making it easier to perform repeated biopsies of deep-seated lesions.

Rapid onsite evaluation

Ozawa M
Rekhi B

ROSE is a clinical service, offered by cytopathologists, supervised pathology trainees, or well-trained cytotechnologists, that provides immediate feedback regarding an FNAB or touch imprint of a CNB, with the goal of optimizing patient care. ROSE provides numerous benefits, including decreasing the number of passes required for an adequate sample, improving the yield for diagnostic accuracy, optimizing sample triage and allocation of material for ancillary tests, decreasing the likelihood of the need for additional repeat or more invasive diagnostic procedures, and minimizing the delay in diagnosis {166,1259,1290}.

The rarity of soft tissue tumours and the cytomorphological overlap between lesions often creates challenges in their accurate diagnosis, as well as in the grading of sarcomas {1209}. The accuracy of FNAB in distinguishing benign from malignant soft tissue tumours and sarcoma from other malignancies has been shown to be comparable to that of surgical biopsies, with up to 96% sensitivity and 98% specificity {1276,1066,696}. However, tumour heterogeneity, as well as the presence of haemorrhage and/or necrosis in large soft tissue tumours, may result in an insufficient or suboptimal yield. With small or deep-seated lesions, reactive cells surrounding the lesion can mimic neoplasia. The ROM in cases of non-diagnostic FNAB from bone and soft tissue lesions is reported to be as high as 42% in one study {753}.

These issues highlight the importance of ROSE to minimize the likelihood of an inadequate FNAB and to alert the proceduralist to the possible need for additional sampling. The principal rapid stains used for onsite evaluation include Giemsa, toluidine blue, ultrafast Pap, and rapid H&E. Method selection is often influenced by technical considerations, speed, and cost, as well as the operator's preference {17,558}. Triage with ROSE based on the direct smears also allows for allocation of sampled material for routine cytomorphological evaluation, liquid medium preparations, and cell block material for supplemental ancillary studies; for example, a small round cell pattern may warrant triage for molecular testing as well as additional tests including flow cytometry to exclude non-Hodgkin lymphoma {1557,1311}. Touch preparations of CNB carry a risk of damaging fragile cellular material but offer benefits similar to those of ROSE. ICC is the most commonly used technique for the evaluation of tissue type of origin and differentiation, and it is applicable to FNAB material; LBC preparations; cell block or CNB sections; and molecular genetic assays, including cytogenetics, FISH, PCR, and NGS, which are increasingly being employed in soft tissue lesions. However, limited cellularity often requires the prioritization of the samples, and requests for more material at the FNAB procedure can be addressed by ROSE

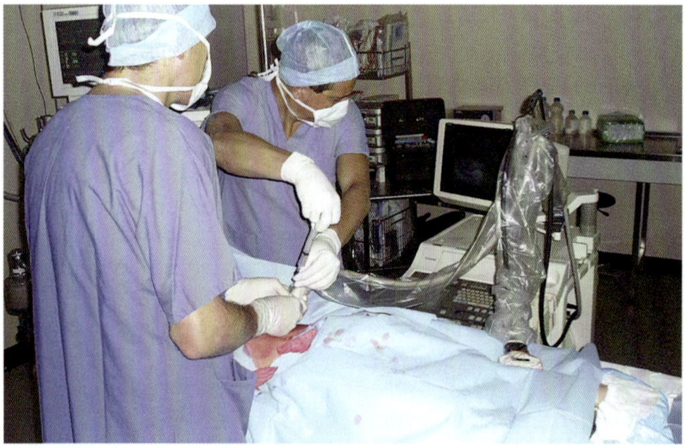

Fig. 2.08 ROSE. FNAB with ultrasound guidance.

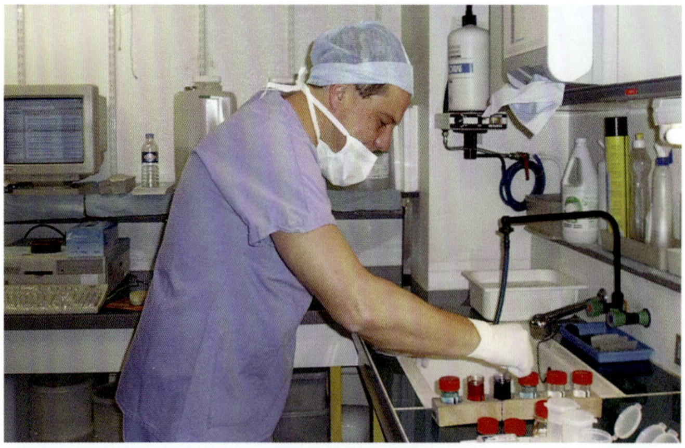

Fig. 2.09 ROSE. Rapid staining using a Giemsa stain of direct smears.

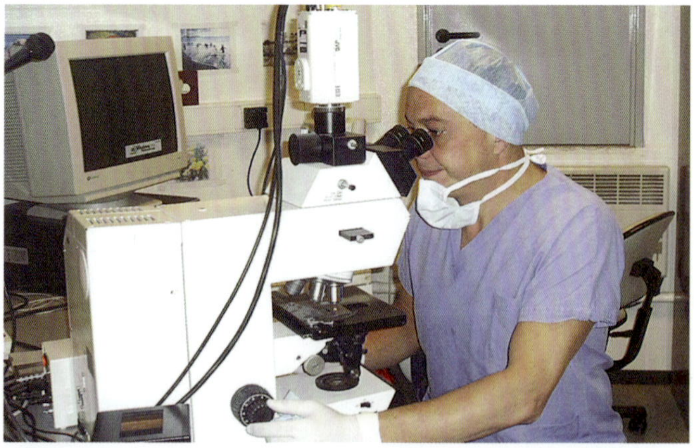

Fig. 2.10 ROSE. Rapid microscopic assessment of the stained direct smears.

Cell preparation methods

Dodd LG
Bode-Lesniewska B
Jain D

FNAB smears are the most common cytopathological specimens procured from soft tissue lesions by palpation of superficial masses or using imaging guidance in deeply sited lesions {420,1470}. Other common preparations are centrifugation smears, cytospin/cytocentrifuge smears, and LBC, any of which can be used, especially for a sample from a cystic or partly cystic lesion or a body cavity effusion fluid that may show involvement by soft tissue sarcomas {202,1283}. In addition, cell blocks and touch smears from CNB can be useful diagnostic specimens and valuable resources for ancillary testing {1470,1240}.

Direct FNAB smears

FNAB material varies in consistency depending on the nature of the lesion sampled. Cystic lesions usually yield fluid that should be processed differently than samples from more solid lesions. If FNAB yields fluid from a large cystic lesion, a repeat FNAB using ultrasound or other imaging guidance to sample solid areas, if any, should be performed. The fluid can be fixed either in ethanol, in the same volume of ethanol as cyst fluid sample, or in a commercially available LBC medium, or the fluid can be processed by cytocentrifuging followed by direct smearing of the deposit for air-dried and alcohol-fixed smears. Post-FNAB needle rinses can also be handled in the same ways.

A variety of smearing techniques are available, which can be used depending on the consistency of the FNAB material. The commonly used technique is to place a drop of material near the frosted end of the slide and use a second slide oriented perpendicular to the first slide as a spreader to gently spread the material down the length of the slide. An alternative technique may be employed if the sample is very thin or bloody, where the diagnostic material is placed in the centre of the slide and another slide is placed longitudinally on the first slide and used to spread the material to produce smears on both slides. Care should be taken to apply gentle and constant pressure while making smears to avoid crushing of cells and to produce evenly spread smears.

The number of FNABs performed on any given lesion depends on many factors, including the operator's expertise, the relative accessibility of the lesion, and the need for image guidance for needle placement. Usually, two to four passes are performed on a given lesion. A small amount of the specimen is placed onto a glass slide and smeared, and the remainder of the specimen can be collected for LBC or cell block preparation. A minimum of two smears can be prepared from the sample on the slide. One of the slides is immediately placed in 96% ethanol for several minutes for fixation and subsequently stained with Pap or H&E, while the other is thoroughly air-dried, stained using the Giemsa stain, and used immediately to assess adequacy and make a provisional diagnostic evaluation using ROSE.

Visual inspection of the material and the suspected diagnosis enables triaging of the sample at ROSE or on arrival in the laboratory. Haemolytic and mucolytic agents are used to pretreat haemorrhagic and mucinous specimens. Sparsely cellular specimens can be processed by cell concentration methods.

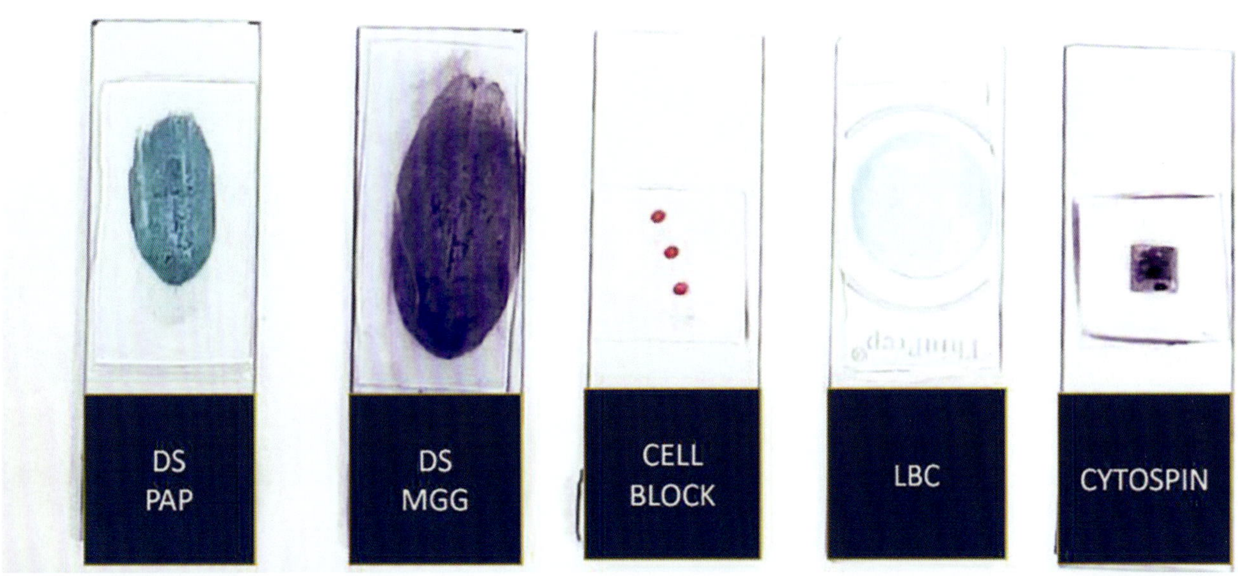

Fig. 2.11 Different types of cytopathology preparations. Direct smear, Pap (DS PAP); direct smear, Giemsa (DS MGG); cell block, H&E; liquid-based cytopathology (LBC); cytospin, Giemsa.

Cytospin preparations

Cytospin preparations are prepared if scant and/or sparsely cellular fluid is produced from the lesion. Body cavity specimens are usually thin and clear and should be spun down at a high-speed cytospin to deposit a monolayer of cells onto the slide. If the fluid is turbid, thick, and opalescent, smears can be prepared from the sediment of simple centrifugation.

Touch imprint preparations

Touch imprints of CNB are easily prepared and can be particularly helpful in hypercellular tumours such as malignant small round cell tumours of soft tissues {1240}. Touch imprint smears are prepared by gently dabbing or rolling the core biopsy of the tissue on the glass slide to cover at least 50–60% of the slide surface. The slide is immediately fixed in 96% ethanol or can be air-dried for Giemsa staining and ROSE. Tumour cells can be procured from touch imprints for downstream molecular analysis or other ancillary techniques {336}. However, vigorous touch preparations may lose tumour cellularity, cause crush artefact of the CNB, and result in reduced DNA content in CNB {1181}.

LBC offers the transportation of the FNAB material in a stable collecting medium {932}. Several commercially available platforms are available, and the specimen is collected into company-specific vials of patented preservative and fixative to generate LBC slides after processing on specific platforms {202}. LBC slide preparations lack the pattern recognition features of direct smears used routinely by cytopathologists and diminish any background.

Cell blocks

Cell blocks can be prepared from FNAB or body cavity fluids, facilitated by ROSE. A dedicated pass can be taken for cell block preparation based on the initial assessment of the lesion. Several methods can be employed, ranging from simple centrifugation, removal of the supernatant, and then use of the sedimentation pellet; to adjuvant-based techniques; to automated cell blocks {625,1005,1329}. Cell blocks are vital resources for performing ancillary techniques such as ICC, in situ hybridization, and molecular testing. It is essential to have a cell block in soft tissue tumour cytopathology, especially in the current era of a growing number of targetable genetic abnormalities in soft tissue tumours.

Introduction: The role of ancillary testing

Bode-Lesniewska B
Kilpatrick SE

Soft tissue tumours are a group of more than 100 mesenchymal entities characterized by a wide range of microscopic patterns, including spindle, myxoid, epithelioid, and pleomorphic, and they often show pronounced intratumoral heterogeneity. The research findings of recent decades have deepened our understanding of the pathogenesis of both benign and malignant soft tissue tumours, and they have revealed a plethora of etiologically important molecular aberrations {1503}. Some of these aberrations are highly specific to particular entities, such as the *STAT6*::*NAB2* translocation in solitary fibrous tumour and rearrangement of the *SS18* gene in synovial sarcoma, whereas others occur in more than one clinically and histopathologically well-defined entity, for example *EWSR1*::*ATF1* in atypical fibrous histiocytoma and clear cell sarcoma, or the *ALK* gene rearrangement in inflammatory myofibroblastic tumour, anaplastic lymphoma, and some lung adenocarcinomas. Reliable surrogate ICC markers have been developed for many of the genetic aberrations, facilitating diagnosis and based on high-quality cytopathological samples {1073,198,643}.

FNAB of soft tissue masses is a minimally invasive diagnostic method, but it has the inherent limitation of small sample size, both as measured in absolute values and in relation to the volume of the studied mass. Sensitive and specific ancillary methods allow the detection of specific diagnostic tumour properties from this limited material {335,1073,198,643,573}. Not only can ICC characterize the line of differentiation, such as by the detection of epithelial, myogenic, neural, or endothelial antigens, but it can also demonstrate, with high accuracy, the changes caused at the protein level by specific genetic aberrations, for example *STAT6* rearrangement, *KIT* mutation, *MDM2* amplification, or *SMARCB1* (*INI1*) inactivation {1250,1073,198,643}. The precise detection of specific mutations either to confirm the ICC findings or to detect mutations that lack an ICC surrogate can be performed with more laborious, time-consuming, and costly molecular methods, i.e. cytogenetic analysis, FISH, PCR, or NGS {704,1464,1195}. ICC and FISH have the advantage of short turnaround times, and NGS provides the advantage of comprehensiveness and, with various platforms, a comparable turnaround time.

All methods applicable to histopathological samples of soft tissue tumours are also applicable to cytopathological material, with the additional advantage of smears for FISH analysis lacking truncation artefact, i.e. whole cells and nuclei are present on the cytopathological slides rather than only the sectioned incomplete cell on the slide of a paraffin-embedded section.

The prerequisite for the application of any ancillary test to FNAB material is that there be sufficient material, quantitatively as well as qualitatively, and that clinical and imaging information be available {740,335}. The triaging of the FNAB for the application of ancillary methods in the context of a soft tissue tumour should be planned before and during the collection of the FNAB, based on the differential diagnosis and ROSE. Direct smears and cell block are sometimes underestimated in their value in the diagnostic workup of soft tissue masses as a source of material {335,1062,1557}.

Flow cytometry

Sewell WA

Flow cytometry is an ancillary technique widely used to assess haematolymphoid disorders in nodal and extranodal tissues {1554,109,1461}, but flow cytometry has a limited role in the assessment of disorders of other cell lineages. Cell-cycle analysis by determination of nuclear DNA has long been used as a prognostic marker in carcinoma {929}. Flow cytometry has also been used to investigate blood for circulating tumour cells {756} and fluids such as pleural effusions for carcinoma cells {1516}. In these cases, the samples contain single abnormal cells in a suspension, which is a requirement of flow cytometry. It is usually straightforward to prepare samples of haematolymphoid disorders into single-cell suspensions, but this is challenging with biopsy material from disorders of soft tissues {806}. Therefore, routine clinical flow cytometry is largely limited to the analysis of haematolymphoid disorders, which can involve soft tissues.

In soft tissue, the commonest haematolymphoid tumour is extranodal lymphoma, and about 30% of lymphomas arise in sites that normally lack lymphocytes {1342}. Plasmacytoma and myeloid sarcoma can also be assessed by flow cytometry {425, 1108}. Haematolymphoid lesions may be suspected because of clinical features or because of the findings of ROSE {640}. If flow cytometry is to be performed on an FNAB, it is optimal to take a dedicated pass. Samples must be placed in a tissue culture medium with or without fetal bovine serum, or if such medium is not available, in saline {1273,292,1272}. If flow cytometry is performed 18–24 hours or more after sample collection, commercial or in-house stabilizing solutions should be used {297,373}. Some protocols recommend storage at 4 °C pending analysis, while others recommend ambient temperature {1273,1272,292}.

Analysis of FNAB samples by flow cytometry involves preparing preferably tens of thousands of cells in suspension, staining them with fluorochrome-labelled antibodies, and running them through a flow cytometer to determine the amount of label on each cell {8}. The antibodies should initially cover key lymphocyte markers. If a suspicious population cannot be identified by these markers, the sample should be assessed for plasma cell and myeloid lineages {1517}. Key markers for the initial detection of haematolymphoid tumours are listed in Table 2.01, and a table of commonly used CD markers and tables of the phenotypes of major B-cell and T-cell lymphomas are presented in the companion volume, the WHO Reporting System for Lymph Node, Spleen, and Thymus Cytopathology {612}. A classification of haematolymphoid tumours is presented in the *Haematolymphoid Tumours* volume of the WHO Classification of Tumours series {1502}.

Table 2.01 Key markers for the initial detection of haematolymphoid tumours

Cell type	Marker(s)
All lineages	CD45
B cell	CD5, CD10, CD19, CD20, kappa, lambda
T cell	CD3, CD4, CD5, CD7, CD8
NK cell	CD16, CD56
Plasma cell	CD38, CD138
Myeloid	CD13, CD33, CD34, KIT (CD117)

Immunocytochemistry

Chebib I
Jo VY

Many soft tissue neoplasms have distinctive immunophenotypes, and the specific diagnosis of most entities requires ancillary testing that commonly includes a panel of ICC markers {198,643, 1073}. Historically, these markers have been combinations of tissue type–specific markers, actin and intermediate filaments, and cluster of differentiation (CD) surface markers to identify a line of differentiation. However, these stains are largely nonspecific and in many cases cannot be used to render definitive interpretations of soft tissue tumours. The recent expansion in specific molecular alterations has allowed for development of antibodies targeting these tumour-defining molecular events. Many of these novel ICC stains identify overexpression or loss of expression of proteins secondary to underlying gene amplification, gene mutation, or gene fusion events. Some tumour-specific markers have been identified by gene expression profiling studies. More recently developed antibodies now target specific mutations or fusion products and serve as reliable surrogate molecular tests.

Preparation

ICC may be performed on FNAB or exfoliative cytopathology samples using several preparation types, including cell block, direct smears, cytospin, and LBC preparations {814,1369,272, 410,442,539,1319,368,1289}. Cell blocks may be prepared using several methods {641,625,758,1005}.

Fixation

Formalin-fixed cell block preparation is the most reliable methodology to perform ICC for soft tissue tumours {814,1369,272,410,442, 539,1319,368,1289}. Markers typically used for soft tissue tumour formalin-fixed histopathology and cell block specimens are unlikely to be validated for alternative cytopathological preparations. Furthermore, most soft tissue tumours require a panel of markers for appropriate classification, and alternative preparations are unlikely to provide sufficient material for complete ancillary workup.

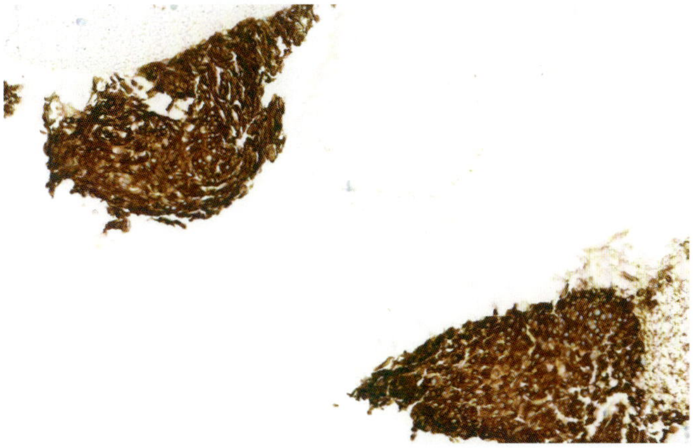

Fig. 2.12 Gastrointestinal stromal tumour. Strong cytoplasmic positivity for KIT (CD117) in gastrointestinal stromal tumour (ICC, KIT [CD117]).

Controls

Regular tissue controls can be used for ICC on cell block preparations. However, laboratories performing ICC on alternative preparations must ensure that the appropriate validations and controls have been developed for that particular cytopathological preparation and are continually monitored. Control slides may be stored at −70 °C without significant loss of antigenicity.

Antigen retrieval

Antigen retrieval can be performed on alternative cytopathology specimens, such as smears and LBC preparations {607,311}. Although some membrane-bound markers may not require retrieval, heat-induced epitope retrieval improves detection, especially for nuclear markers. Protease retrieval may damage epitopes on direct smears.

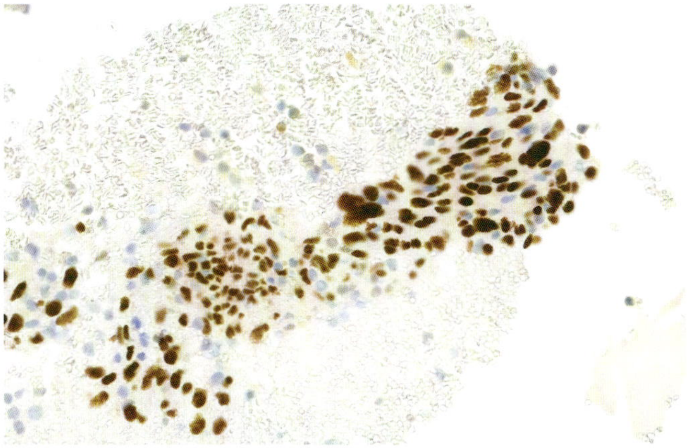

Fig. 2.13 Schwannoma. Nuclear SOX10 positivity in schwannoma (ICC, SOX10).

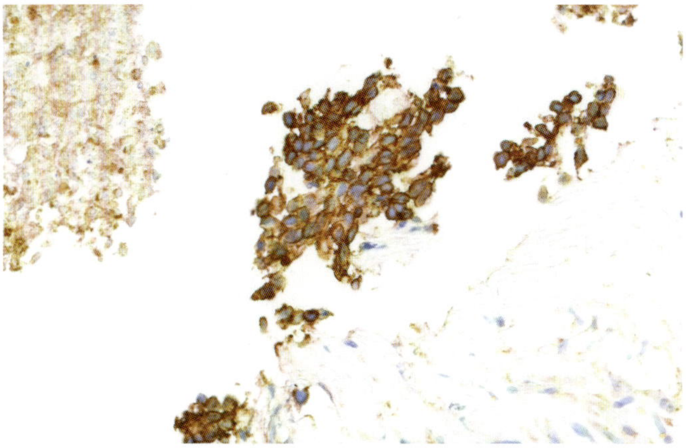

Fig. 2.14 Ewing sarcoma. Strong membranous CD99 positivity in Ewing sarcoma (ICC, CD99).

Performance

Formalin-fixed, paraffin-embedded (FFPE) cell block preparations are the most common FNAB material used for ICC and are largely subject to the same limitations as immunohistochemistry on tissue sections, whereas other cytopathological preparations are constrained by the limited or total lack of validation of cytopathological preparations and lack of appropriate controls {814,1369,272,410,442,539,1319,368,1289}. Direct smear preparations suffer from bloody or proteinaceous backgrounds causing nonspecific staining and from thick or 3D tissue fragments. These specimens may benefit from additional washing steps. Membranous and cytoplasmic markers typically show more nonspecific staining in these settings than do nuclear markers. Stained versus unstained air-dried and alcohol-fixed smears show comparable results {1420,5}.

A subset of antibodies have been reported to be unreliable on non–formalin-fixed preparations, probably due to loss of antigenicity or protein diffusion secondary to alcohol fixation. They include S100, KIT (CD117), calretinin, CD5, inhibin, napsin A, OCT3/4, PAX5, BerEP4, D2-40, and PAX8 {1369,1243}. Although alternative fixation methods have shown comparable ICC expression, formalin fixation provides reproducibility, facilitates standardization, and is available in most laboratories.

Diagnostic applications

Diagnostic applications of the more commonly used markers in soft tissue cytopathology are summarized in Table 2.02, Table 2.03, and Table 2.04 (p. 28), and they are discussed further in the relevant sections. The use of ICC panels requires awareness of the expected immunophenotypes of tumours in a given differential diagnosis that has been established based on the FNAB, as well as of the pitfalls in overlapping or aberrant expression of specific markers. Expression of keratins is seen in many soft tissue neoplasms, including high-grade sarcomas and soft tissue neoplasms with epithelioid morphology. Antibodies for both traditional and lineage-specific transcription

Table 2.02 Immunocytochemical markers for histogenetic tissue differentiation in soft tissue neoplasms

Line of differentiation	Immunocytochemical marker(s)
Epithelial	Keratin, EMA
Smooth muscle	SMA, desmin, caldesmon, calponin
Skeletal muscle	Desmin, MSA, myogenin, MYOD1
Endothelial	CD34, CD31, ERG
Fibroblastic/myofibroblastic	CD34, SMA, desmin
Myoepithelial	Keratin, EMA, S100, GFAP, p63 (40%)
Neural crest	S100, GFAP, SOX10
Perineural	EMA, CD34, claudin-1
Osteoblastic	SATB2
Melanocytic	S100, SOX10, melan-A (MART1), HMB45
Histiocytic	CD68, CD163, PU.1

Table 2.03 Relevant immunocytochemical surrogates for molecular alterations in soft tissue cytopathology (continued on next page)

Alteration type Immunocytochemical marker	Tumour type	Staining pattern
Gene inactivation		
SMARCB1 (INI1)	• Epithelioid sarcoma, extrarenal rhabdoid tumour • Poorly differentiated chordoma • Epithelioid malignant peripheral nerve sheath tumour (~50%) • Epithelioid schwannoma • Myoepithelial tumour (subset)	Loss of nuclear staining
RB1	• Spindle cell / pleomorphic lipoma • Myofibroblastoma • Cellular angiofibroma • Atypical spindle cell / pleomorphic lipomatous tumour	Loss of nuclear staining
SDHB	• Succinate dehydrogenase–deficient gastrointestinal stromal tumour • Paraganglioma	Loss of cytoplasmic staining
PRKAR1A	• Malignant melanotic nerve sheath tumour	Cytoplasmic
Amplification leading to overexpression		
MDM2	• Atypical lipomatous tumour / well-differentiated liposarcoma • Dedifferentiated liposarcoma • Intimal sarcoma	Nuclear
CDK4	• Atypical lipomatous tumour / well-differentiated liposarcoma • Dedifferentiated liposarcoma • Intimal sarcoma	Nuclear
MYC	• Radiation-associated and lymphoedema-associated angiosarcomas	Nuclear
Activating mutations leading to overexpression		
PDGFRA	• Gastrointestinal stromal tumour • Inflammatory fibroid polyp	Membranous, cytoplasmic
β-catenin	• Desmoid fibromatosis	Nuclear

Table 2.03 Relevant immunocytochemical surrogates for molecular alterations in soft tissue cytopathology (continued)

Alteration type		
Immunocytochemical marker	**Tumour type**	**Staining pattern**
Gene fusion leading to overexpression		
Pan-TRK	• Kinase-altered spindle cell tumour, including NTRK-rearranged mesenchymal tumour • Infantile fibrosarcoma • Inflammatory myofibroblastic tumour (subset)	Cytoplasmic, nuclear
ALK	• Inflammatory myofibroblastic tumour (subset) • Epithelioid fibrous histiocytoma	Cytoplasmic
ROS1	• Inflammatory myofibroblastic tumour	Cytoplasmic
STAT6	• Solitary fibrous tumour	Nuclear
DDIT3	• Myxoid liposarcoma	Nuclear
WT1 C-terminus	• Desmoplastic small round cell tumour	Nuclear
FOSB	• Epithelioid haemangioma • Pseudomyogenic haemangioendothelioma	Nuclear
TFE3	• Alveolar soft part sarcoma • *YAP1::TFE3*-associated epithelioid haemangioendothelioma • PEComa (subset)	Nuclear
CAMTA1	• Epithelioid haemangioendothelioma	Nuclear
YAP1 C-terminus	• *YAP1::TFE3*-associated epithelioid haemangioendothelioma	Nuclear
PLAG1	• Lipoblastoma • Myoepithelial neoplasms (mixed tumours) with *PLAG1* rearrangement	Nuclear
HMGA2	• Lipoma (subset) • Atypical lipomatous tumour / well-differentiated liposarcoma • Dedifferentiated liposarcoma • Aggressive angiomyxoma	Nuclear
BCOR	• Sarcomas with *BCOR* genetic alterations • Primitive myxoid mesenchymal tumour of infancy • Clear cell sarcoma of kidney	Nuclear
Cyclin B3 (CCNB3)	• Sarcomas with *BCOR* genetic alterations (subset)	Nuclear
Translocation-specific markers		
SS18::SSX	• Synovial sarcoma	Nuclear
SSX C-terminus	• Synovial sarcoma	Nuclear
PAX3/7::FOXO1	• Alveolar rhabdomyosarcoma	Nuclear
Mutation-specific markers		
BRAF p.V600E	• Glomus tumour (rare subset)	Cytoplasmic
Epigenetic		
H3 p.K28me3 (K27me3)	• Malignant peripheral nerve sheath tumour	Loss of nuclear staining
Overexpression		
NKX2-2	• Ewing sarcoma	Nuclear
NKX3-1	• Mesenchymal chondrosarcoma • *EWSR1/FUS::NFATC2* sarcoma	Nuclear
WT1 and ETV4	• *CIC*-rearranged sarcoma	Nuclear
MUC4	• Low-grade fibromyxoid sarcoma / sclerosing epithelioid fibrosarcoma	Cytoplasmic
DOG1	• Gastrointestinal stromal tumour	Cytoplasmic

factor differentiation-specific markers only identify the line of differentiation and do not distinguish between normal tissue counterparts and benign and malignant neoplasms. However, for some tumour types, the main diagnostic utility of ICC remains determining the line of differentiation, such as for leiomyoma and leiomyosarcoma, which lack recurrent molecular alterations but show expression of the smooth muscle markers SMA, desmin, and caldesmon. Many tumours have distinctive immunophenotypes that can guide appropriate molecular testing once identified. For example, Ewing sarcoma shows diffuse membranous CD99 staining and nuclear staining for NKX2-2 {600}, and the diagnosis can subsequently be confirmed by FISH testing to identify *EWSR1* rearrangement. Other tumour types have so-called "polyphenotypic" profiles, such as desmoplastic small round cell tumour, which is positive for keratins, EMA, desmin, and the C-terminus of WT1 {106,562}. Some highly reliable tumour-specific markers have been identified by gene expression profiling, including DOG1

Table 2.04 Immunocytochemical markers in soft tissue cytopathology (continued on next page)

Category				
	Marker	**Soft tissue tumours**	**Localization**	**Comments**
Tissue differentiation				
	Keratins	• Epithelioid sarcoma, extrarenal rhabdoid tumour • Synovial sarcoma • Malignant peripheral nerve sheath tumour with glandular differentiation • Chordoma • Myoepithelial neoplasm • Desmoplastic small round cell tumour • Pseudomyogenic haemangioendothelioma and vascular tumours with epithelioid morphology • Fibroblastic reticulum cell sarcoma (subset) • Many soft tissue tumours, especially with epithelioid morphology	Cytoplasmic	• Used in ICC panels to differentiate metastatic carcinoma from high-grade sarcoma • May be seen in several high-grade sarcomas and soft tissue neoplasms with epithelioid morphology
	EMA	• Epithelioid sarcoma, extrarenal rhabdoid tumour • Synovial sarcoma • Malignant peripheral nerve sheath tumour with glandular differentiation • Chordoma • Myoepithelial neoplasm • Desmoplastic small round cell tumour • Perineurioma • Many soft tissue tumours, especially with epithelioid morphology	Cytoplasmic	• Used in ICC panels to differentiate metastatic carcinoma from high-grade sarcoma • May be seen in several high-grade sarcomas and soft tissue neoplasms with epithelioid morphology
	SMA, muscle actin, calponin, h-caldesmon	• Tumours with myofibroblastic, myoepithelial, smooth muscle, pericytic, or skeletal muscle differentiation • Glomus tumour • PEComa	Cytoplasmic	• Muscle differentiation may be seen in many soft tissue tumours
	Desmin	• Tumours with smooth muscle, skeletal muscle, or less commonly myofibroblastic or myoepithelial differentiation • Myofibroblastoma • Angiomyofibroblastoma • Cellular angiofibroma (subset) • Atypical spindle cell lipomatous tumour • Lipoblastoma • Angiomatoid fibrous histiocytoma (subset) • Desmoplastic small round cell tumour (dot-like) • Tenosynovial giant cell tumour • Fibroblastic reticulum cell sarcoma	Cytoplasmic	• Muscle differentiation may be seen in several high-grade sarcomas
	S100	• Benign peripheral nerve sheath tumours, including granular cell tumour, and malignant melanotic nerve sheath tumour • Tumours with adipocytic differentiation • Tumours with cartilaginous differentiation • Epithelioid malignant peripheral nerve sheath tumour • Clear cell sarcoma of soft tissue • Myoepithelial neoplasm • Chordoma • Ossifying fibromyxoid tumour • Biphenotypic sinonasal sarcoma • Kinase-altered spindle cell tumour, including NTRK-rearranged mesenchymal tumour • Interdigitating dendritic cell sarcoma • Extraskeletal myxoid chondrosarcoma (subset)	Cytoplasmic, nuclear	• Used in ICC panels to differentiate metastatic melanoma from high-grade undifferentiated sarcoma • Typically weak or negative in conventional malignant peripheral nerve sheath tumour
	SOX10	• Benign peripheral nerve sheath tumours, including granular cell tumour, and malignant melanotic nerve sheath tumour • Epithelioid malignant peripheral nerve sheath tumour • Clear cell sarcoma of soft tissue • Myoepithelial neoplasm	Nuclear	• Used in ICC panels to differentiate metastatic melanoma from high-grade sarcoma • Typically weak or negative in conventional malignant peripheral nerve sheath tumour
	MYOD1, myogenin (MYF4)	• Rhabdomyoma • Rhabdomyosarcoma • Sarcoma with rhabdomyosarcomatous transformation/differentiation • Biphenotypic sinonasal sarcoma	Nuclear	• Positive in any malignancy with rhabdomyosarcomatous transdifferentiation

in gastrointestinal stromal tumour {1501,952} and MUC4 in low-grade fibromyxoid sarcoma {970,359}. As stated above, many ICC markers are now available as testing surrogates for underlying molecular alterations.

Table 2.04 Immunocytochemical markers in soft tissue cytopathology (continued from previous page, continued on next page)

Category				
	Marker	**Soft tissue tumours**	**Localization**	**Comments**
Melanocytic differentiation				
	MITF	• Clear cell sarcoma of soft tissue • PEComa • Granular cell tumour	Nuclear	
	HMB45, melan-A	• Clear cell sarcoma of soft tissue • PEComa • Malignant melanotic nerve sheath tumour	Cytoplasmic	
Cluster differentiation				
	CD1a	• Langerhans cell histiocytosis	Membranous, cytoplasmic	
	CD21	• Follicular dendritic cell sarcoma	Membranous, cytoplasmic	
	CD23	• Follicular dendritic cell sarcoma	Membranous, cytoplasmic	
	CD31	• Tumours with vascular differentiation	Membranous, cytoplasmic	• May be seen in macrophages
	CD34	• Tumours with vascular differentiation • Epithelioid sarcoma • Solitary fibrous tumour • Dermatofibrosarcoma protuberans • Giant cell fibroblastoma • Spindle cell lipoma • Atypical spindle cell lipomatous tumour • Myofibroblastoma • Cellular angiofibroma (subset) • Superficial CD34-positive pleomorphic fibrous tumour • Perineurioma • Neurofibroma • Pleomorphic hyalinizing angiectatic tumour • Kinase-altered spindle cell neoplasms, including NTRK-rearranged mesenchymal tumour	Membranous, cytoplasmic	• May be seen in several soft tissue tumours
	CD35	• Follicular dendritic cell sarcoma	Membranous, cytoplasmic	
	CD99	• Ewing sarcoma • *CIC*-rearranged sarcoma • Sarcomas with *BCOR* genetic alterations • Angiomatoid fibrous histiocytoma • Solitary fibrous tumour • Synovial sarcoma	Membranous, cytoplasmic	
	KIT (CD117)	• Gastrointestinal stromal tumour	Membranous, cytoplasmic	
Vascular differentiation				
	ERG	• Tumours with vascular differentiation • Epithelioid sarcoma • Tumours with cartilaginous differentiation • Ewing sarcoma with *EWSR1::ERG* • *SMAD3*-rearranged fibroblastic tumour • Phosphaturic mesenchymal tumour • *CIC*-rearranged sarcoma (subset)	Nuclear	
	FLI1	• Tumours with vascular differentiation • Ewing sarcoma	Nuclear	• Positive in lymphocytes and lymphoma
	D2-40	• Tumours with lymphatic differentiation	Cytoplasmic	• Expressed in a number of soft tissue tumours, in myoepithelial cells, and in mesothelial cells

Table 2.04 Immunocytochemical markers in soft tissue cytopathology (continued from previous page, continued on next page)

Category				
	Marker	**Soft tissue tumours**	**Localization**	**Comments**
Other				
	WT1	• *CIC*-rearranged sarcoma	Nuclear	• Positive in retroperitoneal smooth muscle neoplasms
	SATB2	• Tumours with osteoblastic differentiation • Sarcomas with *BCOR* genetic alterations • Undifferentiated pleomorphic sarcomas (subset)	Nuclear	
	NKX2-2	• Ewing sarcoma • Mesenchymal chondrosarcoma • Olfactory neuroblastoma	Nuclear	• Positive in rare *CIC*-rearranged sarcoma
	KSHV/HHV8	• Kaposi sarcoma	Nuclear	
	GLUT1	• Perineurioma • Infantile capillary haemangioma	Membranous	
	ETV4	• *CIC*-rearranged sarcoma	Nuclear	
	Claudin-1	• Perineurioma	Membranous	
	MUC4	• Low-grade fibromyxoid sarcoma, sclerosing epithelioid fibrosarcoma • Synovial sarcoma • Malignant peripheral nerve sheath tumour with epithelial differentiation	Membranous, cytoplasmic	• Positive in metastatic carcinoma
	DOG1	• Gastrointestinal stromal tumour	Cytoplasmic	
	TLE1	• Synovial sarcoma • Malignant peripheral nerve sheath tumour • Sarcomas with *BCOR* genetic alterations • Solitary fibrous tumour (subset)	Nuclear	• TLE1 is considered positive when nearly all tumour nuclei are strongly positive
Molecular/mutation-specific markers				
Mutations resulting in cellular localization				
	β-catenin	• Desmoid-type fibromatosis • Sinonasal myopericytoma	Nuclear	
Loss of expression				
	SMARCB1 (INI1)	• Epithelioid sarcoma, extrarenal rhabdoid tumour • Poorly differentiated chordoma • Epithelioid malignant peripheral nerve sheath tumour (subset) • Myoepithelial tumour (subset) • Extraskeletal myxoid chondrosarcoma (poorly differentiated subset, very rare) • Ossifying fibromyxoid tumour (mosaic pattern) • Synovial sarcoma (weak to absent/reduced expression)	Nuclear	• Loss of expression
	RB1	• Spindle cell / pleomorphic lipoma • Myofibroblastoma • Cellular angiofibroma • Atypical spindle cell / pleomorphic lipomatous tumour	Nuclear	• Loss of expression can be difficult to interpret due to weak internal control staining
	H3 p.K28me3 (K27me3)	• Malignant peripheral nerve sheath tumour	Nuclear	• Loss of expression • Positive in Merkel cell carcinoma, ependymoma • May be very weak or negative in synovial sarcoma
	SDH subunits (SDHB)	• Gastrointestinal stromal tumour • Paraganglioma	Cytoplasmic	• Loss of expression
	YAP1 C-terminus	• *YAP1::TFE3*-associated epithelioid haemangioendothelioma	Nuclear	• Loss of expression
	PRKAR1A	• Malignant melanotic nerve sheath tumour	Cytoplasmic	• Loss of expression

Table 2.04 Immunocytochemical markers in soft tissue cytopathology (continued)

Category				
	Marker	**Soft tissue tumours**	**Localization**	**Comments**
Amplification leading to overexpression				
	MDM2	• Atypical lipomatous tumour / well-differentiated liposarcoma • Dedifferentiated liposarcoma • Intimal sarcoma	Nuclear	• Weakly positive in macrophages in fat necrosis • Amplification of the *MDM2* locus may lead to overexpression of CDK4, HMGA2, STAT6, and/or GLI1
	CDK4	• Atypical lipomatous tumour / well-differentiated liposarcoma • Dedifferentiated liposarcoma • Intimal sarcoma	Nuclear	
	MYC	• Radiation-associated or lymphoedema-associated angiosarcomas	Nuclear	
Mutations leading to overexpression				
	PDGFRA	• Gastrointestinal stromal tumour • Inflammatory fibroid polyp	Membranous, cytoplasmic	• Positivity may be seen in fibroblasts, smooth muscle cells, and smooth muscle neoplasm • Increased dilution (1:10 000) improves specificity for gastrointestinal stromal tumours with *PDGFRA* mutations
Translocation leading to overexpression				
	Pan-TRK	• Kinase-altered spindle cell neoplasms, including NTRK-rearranged mesenchymal tumour • Infantile fibrosarcoma • Inflammatory myofibroblastic tumour (subset)	Cytoplasmic, nuclear	
	ALK	• Inflammatory myofibroblastic tumour (subset) • Epithelioid fibrous histiocytoma	Cytoplasmic	• Positive in rhabdomyosarcoma (subset) • Positive in angiomatoid fibrous histiocytoma (subset)
	ROS1	• Inflammatory myofibroblastic tumour	Cytoplasmic	
	STAT6	• Solitary fibrous tumour	Nuclear	• Locus may be amplified in dedifferentiated liposarcoma (subset)
	DDIT3	• Myxoid liposarcoma	Nuclear	
	WT1 C-terminus	• Desmoplastic small round cell tumour	Nuclear	
	FOSB	• Epithelioid haemangioma • Pseudomyogenic haemangioendothelioma	Nuclear	
	TFE3	• Alveolar soft part sarcoma • *YAP1::TFE3*-associated epithelioid haemangioendothelioma • PEComa (subset)	Nuclear	• Positive in granular cell tumour • TFE3 may be weakly expressed in many soft tissue tumours
	CAMTA1	• Epithelioid haemangioendothelioma	Nuclear	
	PLAG1	• Lipoblastoma • Myoepithelial neoplasms with *PLAG1* rearrangement	Nuclear	
	HMGA2	• Lipoma (subset) • Atypical lipomatous tumour / well-differentiated liposarcoma • Dedifferentiated liposarcoma • Aggressive angiomyxoma	Nuclear	• Positive in embryonal rhabdomyosarcoma • Positive in benign fibrous histiocytoma • Positive in nodular fasciitis
	BCOR	• Sarcomas with *BCOR* genetic alterations	Nuclear	• Positive in synovial sarcoma
	Cyclin B3 (CCNB3)	• Sarcomas with *BCOR* genetic alterations (subset)	Nuclear	
Translocation-specific markers				
	SS18::SSX	• Synovial sarcoma	Nuclear	
	SSX C-terminus	• Synovial sarcoma	Nuclear	
Mutation-specific markers				
	BRAF p.V600E	• Glomus tumour (rare subset)	Cytoplasmic	

In situ hybridization

Bode-Lesniewska B
Pantanowitz L

FISH is a well-established in situ hybridization (ISH) method to visualize and diagnose numerical and structural abnormalities in chromosomal DNA. It is widely used in clinical laboratories as a gold standard for identifying deletions, amplifications, and rearrangements of selected genes {1245,892}. The advantage of FISH lies in the low number of tumour cells needed and the fact that alterations can be detected specifically within the neoplastic cells of interest.

Technical requirements

FISH is a robust method that is applicable to almost all types of cytopathological specimens. Targeted evaluation of cells of interest is a prerequisite for reliable FISH results. FISH requires as few as 50–100 tumour cells and permits direct correlation with cytomorphology {1245}. Internal validation of FISH assays is necessary, and external quality assurance is recommended {827,872,689}. All steps of the procedure should be carried out according to the manufacturer's specifications (with some adjustments appropriate to smaller biopsy specimens and preparations), using probes approved by the US Food and Drug Administration (FDA) or other national regulatory body {1111,1205}. Any deviation requires separate validation. The use of adhesive slides with positive electrostatic charge is recommended to prevent cell loss during pretreatment and DNA denaturation {845}. FISH analysis requires a fluorescent microscope with appropriate filters, ideally equipped with an automated stage for precise relocalization of cells of interest. Scoring of FISH signals can be done at the fluorescent microscope or based on high-quality compressed 2D images from z-stacks at the computer screen {1244}. Probes for chromogenic ISH for *MDM2* gene amplification are helpful in the diagnostics of lipomatous neoplasias {875}, whereas this method is less suitable for the detection of gene fusions.

Management of types of cytopathological specimens

A wide range of cytopathological preparations have been used for FISH, including unstained, Pap-stained, Giemsa-stained, and H&E-stained smears, cytospins, and LBC preparations, as well as unstained formalin-fixed, paraffin-embedded (FFPE) cell blocks {1245,1111,1192,129}. Cell blocks are usually preferred for FISH analysis, because they can be handled like surgical pathology specimens. However, the quality of DNA is compromised by formaldehyde fixation due to cross-linking and chemical modifications of nucleotides {1192,845,129}. The wide variety of cell block processing protocols introduces an additional factor of variability {1205,1192}. Besides the lack of formalin fixation, the main advantage of performing FISH on non–cell block cytopathology specimens is that the tumour cells are complete rather than sectioned, and they therefore have intact, non-truncated nuclei containing the true number of signals {1245,845,129,1132}. FISH is also feasible on previously immunostained ethanol-fixed cytopathological slides, for example TTF1-stained slides, as long as autofluorescent diaminobenzidine is avoided as a chromogen {1247}.

Validation is needed in each laboratory to control for potentially interfering factors due to variability in staining and fixation protocols. At least 50 tumour cells should be evaluated, avoiding 3D tissue fragments with overlapping nuclei and areas with necrosis. The best-suited area for FISH analysis should be selected on the stained smears, allowing for efficient use of the probe {1245,845,129,414}. When using the only diagnostic

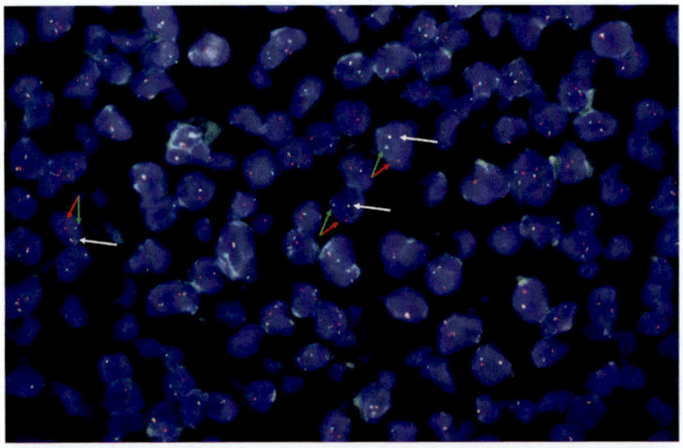

Fig. 2.15 *EWSR1* gene FISH. *EWSR1* gene FISH demonstrating the rearrangement of this gene, which can be seen in numerous soft tissue tumours, including Ewing sarcoma, liposarcoma, and clear cell sarcoma (among others). The break-apart FISH probe demonstrates one fused signal (white arrows) and one split signal (red and green arrows) in the nuclei (blue) of the tumour, indicating the rearrangement of the *EWSR1* gene.

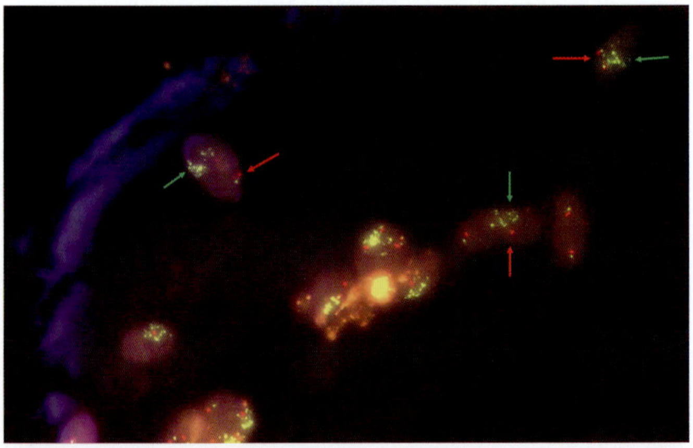

Fig. 2.16 *MDM2* gene amplification on FISH performed on a direct FNAB smear. *MDM2* gene FISH of an FNAB direct smear of a lipomatous mass from the retroperitoneum, demonstrating *MDM2* gene amplification (multiple clustered green *MDM2* gene signals indicated by green arrows, in contrast to isolated 1–2 red centromeric signals per nucleus, indicated by red arrows), rendering the diagnosis of a well-differentiated liposarcoma.

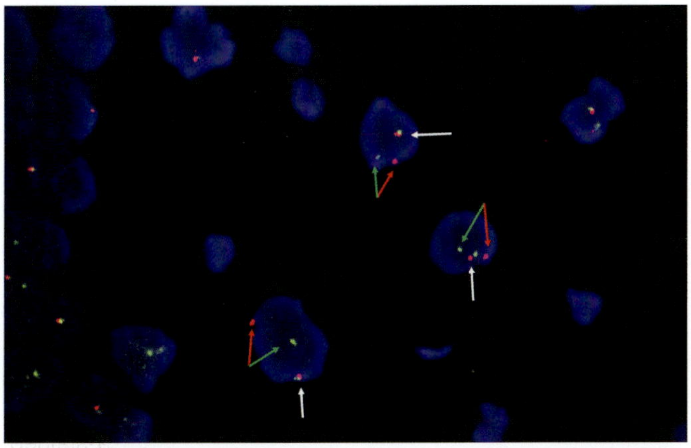

Fig. 2.17 *SS18* gene rearrangement in a primary pleuropulmonary synovial sarcoma. *SS18* gene rearrangement in an FNAB of a pleuropulmonary mass, showing one fused signal (white arrows) and one split signal (red and green arrows) of a break-apart FISH probe.

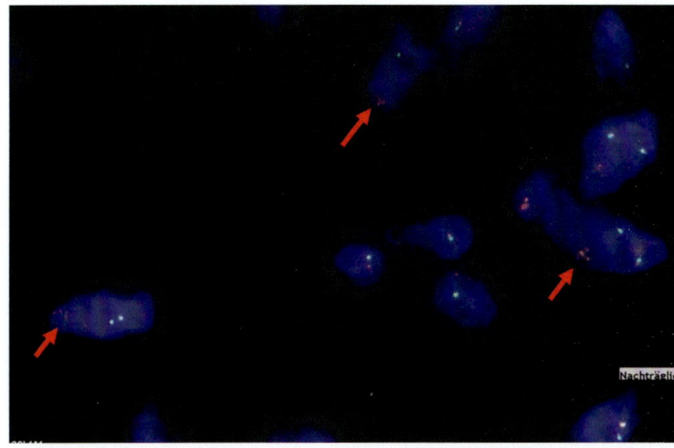

Fig. 2.18 *COL1A1* gene FISH in a dermatofibrosarcoma protuberans. *COL1A1* gene FISH of an FNAB of a direct smear of a superficial mass of the back. The nuclei show one fused signal and one split signal with concomitant amplification of the red signals (red arrows), diagnostic for dermatofibrosarcoma protuberans.

slide in a particular case, capturing images of selected areas or digitally scanning the whole slide prior to the procedure is recommended. When testing for rearrangements, a result is considered positive when > 15% of tumour cells either have isolated 3′ signals in the deletion pattern or have break-apart patterns. However, results within the borderline range (15–20% of cells) should be interpreted with caution because of possible false positive results due to technical factors {1246}.

Fixation

Cytospins and direct smears are particularly well suited for FISH techniques, because the retained 3D nature of the intact nuclei allows the evaluation of the ISH signals, devoid of the truncation artefact typical for cut slides of cell blocks or biopsy samples, and they provide evenly spread samples with isolated, non-overlapping nuclei, which are easily accessible for scoring {1447}. Alcohol-based fixation or air-drying offers better preservation of nucleic acids for hybridization than formalin fixation and paraffin embedding. While formalin fixation is standard for surgical pathology specimens, alcohol fixatives are mostly used for non–cell block cytopathological preparations. The quality of DNA in air-dried or alcohol-fixed cytopathological samples is actually better than that following formaldehyde fixation {1245,1111,845,129,1132}. Fixatives containing acidic components, such as Bouin solution or acidic decalcification solutions, have been shown to yield suboptimal FISH results {1265}.

Controls

Running external or on-slide control specimens is not required for FISH. The presence of signals in all cell nuclei in a specimen serves as the internal control for good hybridization efficiency.

Procedures

The most widely used method of ISH is the application of fluorescent labels for the nucleic acid probes (i.e. FISH), and this is particularly well suited for the detection of gene translocations using break-apart and fusion probes, as well as for enumeration of gene signals, including gene loss, deletion, gain, and amplification. Chromogenic or silver ISH may also be applied to cytopathological specimens in selected situations {447}, including for soft tissue tumours, especially in the context of the detection of gene amplification rather than gene rearrangement {875,1412}.

The steps involved in FISH include slide pretreatment, denaturation of the probe and the slide to obtain single-stranded DNA, hybridization, post-hybridization washes, nuclear DNA counter-staining, and examination and scoring {1245,1185}. There are different protocols for FISH analysis in different types of cytopathological specimens. If smears or cytospins are used, adhesive-coated slides are recommended, to avoid tumour cells floating off during the procedure. In cytopathological specimens, the target cells for FISH evaluation may be sparse and strongly intermixed with benign cells; therefore, in some cases it may be difficult to differentiate benign from malignant cells on the DAPI-counterstained slide after hybridization. This can be resolved by using a relocation software coupled with an automated stage and photo documentation of the cells before uncovering and hybridization of the specimen. This approach improves the sensitivity and specificity of FISH analyses {1245,1111}. There are also fully automated

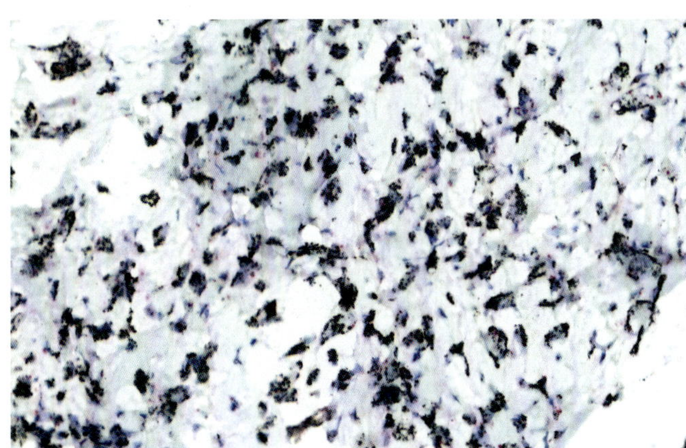

Fig. 2.19 *MDM2* gene amplification in a dedifferentiated liposarcoma of the thigh. Silver in situ hybridization of the *MDM2* gene on the cell block of an FNAB of a deeply located soft tissue mass of the thigh. Amplification of the *MDM2* gene with clusters of *MDM2* gene signals (black) and 1–2 red centromeric CEP12 signals.

FISH systems for scanning and computer-assisted interpretation of FISH images {253,825}.

Diagnostic applications

Depending on the genetic aberration, ISH detects translocations or gene fusions with the application of break-apart or fusion probes, respectively. ISH can also detect gene amplifications, such as *MDM2* amplification in atypical lipomatous tumours and well-differentiated and dedifferentiated liposarcomas, as well as duplications, deletions, insertions, and aneusomies. ISH may also demonstrate the presence of genetic material of a pathogen, for example in EBV-associated smooth muscle tumours.

The appropriate choice of FISH probe is suggested by the differential diagnosis based on the cytopathology of the sample, as well as the ICC and the clinical data {355,1377,1445,958,573, 1503}. The successful application of this approach to FNAB of translocation-associated soft tissue tumours is documented in the literature for several entities, such as Ewing sarcoma {959, 324}, synovial sarcoma {866,697}, alveolar rhabdomyosarcoma {1561}, myxoid liposarcoma {1469}, extraskeletal myxoid chondrosarcoma {1464}, and *CIC*::DUX-rearranged sarcoma {1379}.

Molecular testing

Bode-Lesniewska B
Jo VY
Kilpatrick SE

With the rapidly evolving technology that enables the determination of disease-related genetic aberrations, molecular testing of cytopathological material, which is a minimally invasive tumour sampling technique, is likely to increase to provide cytopathologists and clinicians with accurate diagnostic, prognostic, and treatment predictive information {1144,865, 1112,573,1206,1110,1451}.

Technical requirements

Successful molecular testing of FNAB samples of soft tissue tumours is directly dependent on specimen adequacy. Sequencing-based molecular testing has two basic input requirements: the amount of nucleic acid yield (which is based on the overall cellularity of the specimen) and the ratio of tumour to neoplastic cells or neoplastic nuclear fraction {1207,119}.

Management of types of cytopathological specimens

DNA and RNA can be extracted from different types of routine cytopathological specimens. Different approaches are used for processing the specimens depending on individual laboratory preferences. Any of the resulting cytopathology specimen preparations and stains are suitable for molecular testing {271,626}.

Fixation

Among the preanalytical factors affecting the quality of molecular assays, fixation is key. As a general rule, non–cross-linking fixation using alcoholic reagents (e.g. wet or spray fixatives) or air-drying provides higher-quality nucleic acids than fixation in formalin. In fact, a prolonged fixation time in formalin leads to C>T sequence artefact, a potential pitfall of cell block–based molecular assays {873}. In general, air-dried and ethanol-fixed slides provide high-quality nucleic acids and similar results in terms of DNA quality {119,1207}. Assessment of nucleic acid quantity and quality to assure successful sequencing-based molecular testing requires several techniques to be used in a complementary manner, including spectrophotometer analysis, fluorescence assays, capillary electrophoresis, and quantitative PCR assays {119}.

Controls

The use of control material is an integral component of any type of molecular testing, including NGS. Control samples are a requirement for clinical testing and are used to readily detect sources of error and monitor the overall performance of the assays. For this purpose, positive, negative, and no-template controls are generally used. Each run should also include a sensitivity control to ensure the detection of the target of interest at the lowest limit of detection established for the assay {633}. Clinical laboratories typically derive a set of controls needed to match the specifics of the methods used with respect to the intended clinical use. In this context, the incorporation of controls that reflect the quality of cytological samples, depending on differences in preparation, is also an important consideration. For example, for formalin-fixed, paraffin-embedded (FFPE) cell blocks, controls should be prepared using similar procedures from a well-characterized sample with variants near the limit of detection of the assay.

Procedures

A variety of molecular testing methodologies can be used for assessment of soft tissue tumour cytopathology specimens. These include methods ranging from single-gene–based mutation assays (e.g. Sanger sequencing, pyrosequencing, and real-time PCR), to multiplexed assays, to broad expanded molecular profiling approaches such as NGS. Testing using an expanded NGS panel approach offers the advantage of simultaneously screening multiple genes for a variety of alterations, including single-nucleotide variations, insertion-deletions, copy-number changes, gene fusions, tumour mutation burden, and microsatellite instability, depending on the design of the assay. In the diagnosis of soft tissue tumours, RNA-based gene fusion NGS testing is of particular interest because the procedure combines the simultaneous testing for numerous aberrations, in contrast to single-gene FISH or the single-breakpoint search of Sanger sequencing PCR.

Diagnostic applications

Molecular testing of soft tissue tumour samples is primarily used for diagnostic purposes. Specific gene fusions, point mutations, or amplifications/deletions can be detected either by a dedicated search for a particular aberration with FISH or PCR or as part of a broader panel analysis with NGS {205, 1250}. The development of mutation antibodies, such as KIT (CD117) and β-catenin, and fusion-specific antibodies, as used for identifying synovial sarcoma and myxoid liposarcoma, has improved differential diagnosis and facilitated the choice of the proper molecular study. The detection of any particular mutation must be correlated with the cytopathology and ICC findings, because many mutations are not specific for just one entity, and some, such as *ALK* or *EWSR1* gene fusions, occur in both mesenchymal and non-mesenchymal tumours.

The detection of mutations in one of the involved genes of gastrointestinal stromal tumours, such as *KIT*, *PDGFRA*, or an SDH gene, is not only of diagnostic importance but also of prognostic and predictive value, because these mutations determine the appropriate therapy with tyrosine kinase inhibitors. The complete diagnostic workup of gastrointestinal stromal tumour can be performed on EUS-guided FNAB samples, including the molecular analysis if adequate tumour material is available {498, 493,1558}.

The most common soft tissue entities with gene fusions are presented in Table 2.05, and the most common soft tissue entities associated with gene mutations, deletions, or amplification are presented in Table 2.06.

Table 2.05 The most common soft tissue entities with gene fusions

Soft tissue entity	Gene fusion(s)
Angiomatous fibrous histiocytoma	*EWSR1::CREB1* or *EWSR1::ATF1*
Alveolar rhabdomyosarcoma	*PAX3::FOXO1* or *PAX7::FOXO1*
Alveolar soft part sarcoma	*ASPSCR1::TFE3*
***BCOR*-associated sarcomas**	*BCOR::CCNB3*, *BCOR* internal tandem duplication (ITD)
***CIC*-rearranged sarcoma**	*CIC::DUX4*
Clear cell sarcoma	*EWSR1::ATF1* or *EWSR1::CREB1*
Dermatofibrosarcoma protuberans	*COL1A1::PDGFB*
Desmoplastic small round cell tumour	*EWSR1::WT1*
Epithelioid haemangioma	*FOS* (*c-FOS*) and *FOSB* fusions
Epithelioid haemangioendothelioma	*WWTR1::CAMTA1* or *YAP1::TFE3*
Ewing sarcoma	Fusions of *EWSR1* and a member of the ETS family of transcription factors (most commonly *FLI1*, rarely *ERG*)
Extraskeletal myxoid chondrosarcoma	*NR4A3::EWSR1* or *NR4A3::TAF15*
Infantile fibrosarcoma	*ETV6::NTRK3*
Inflammatory myofibroblastic tumour	*ALK* fusion with various partners (*TPM3*, *TPM4*, *CLTC*, *CARS1*, *ATIC*, *SEC31A* (*SEC31L1*), *PPFIBP1*, *DCTN1*, *EML4*, *PRKAR1A*, *LMNA*, *TFG*, *FN1*, *HNRNPA1*)
Low-grade fibromyxoid sarcoma	*FUS::CREB3L2* or *FUS::CREB3L1*
Mesenchymal chondrosarcoma	*HEY1::NCOA2*
Myxoid liposarcoma	*FUS::DDIT3* or rarely *EWSR1::DDIT3*
Nodular fasciitis	*USP6::MYH9*
PEComa	*TFE3* fusions
Solitary fibrous tumour	*NAB2::STAT6*
Synovial sarcoma	*SS18::SSX1/SSX2/SSX4*
Tenosynovial giant cell tumour	*CSF1* fusions

Table 2.06 The most common soft tissue entities associated with gene mutations, deletions, or amplification

Soft tissue entity	Most common aberration(s)
Angiosarcoma (radiotherapy-associated)	Amplification of *MYC*
Atypical lipomatous tumour / well-differentiated liposarcoma	Amplification of 12q13-p15, including *MDM2* and *CDK4*
Dedifferentiated liposarcoma	Amplification of 12q13-p15, including *MDM2* and *CDK4*
Desmoid fibromatosis	Mutation of *CTNNB1* (encoding β-catenin)
Epithelioid schwannoma	Loss of *SMARCB1* (*INI1*)
Epithelioid sarcoma	Loss of *SMARCB1* (*INI1*)
Gastrointestinal stromal tumour	Mutation of *KIT*, mutation of *PDGFRA*
Intramuscular myxoma	Mutation of *GNAS*
Intimal sarcoma	Amplification of 12q13-p15, including *MDM2* and *CDK4*
Spindle cell / pleomorphic lipoma	Loss of *RB1*
Spindle cell rhabdomyosarcoma	Mutation of *MYOD1*

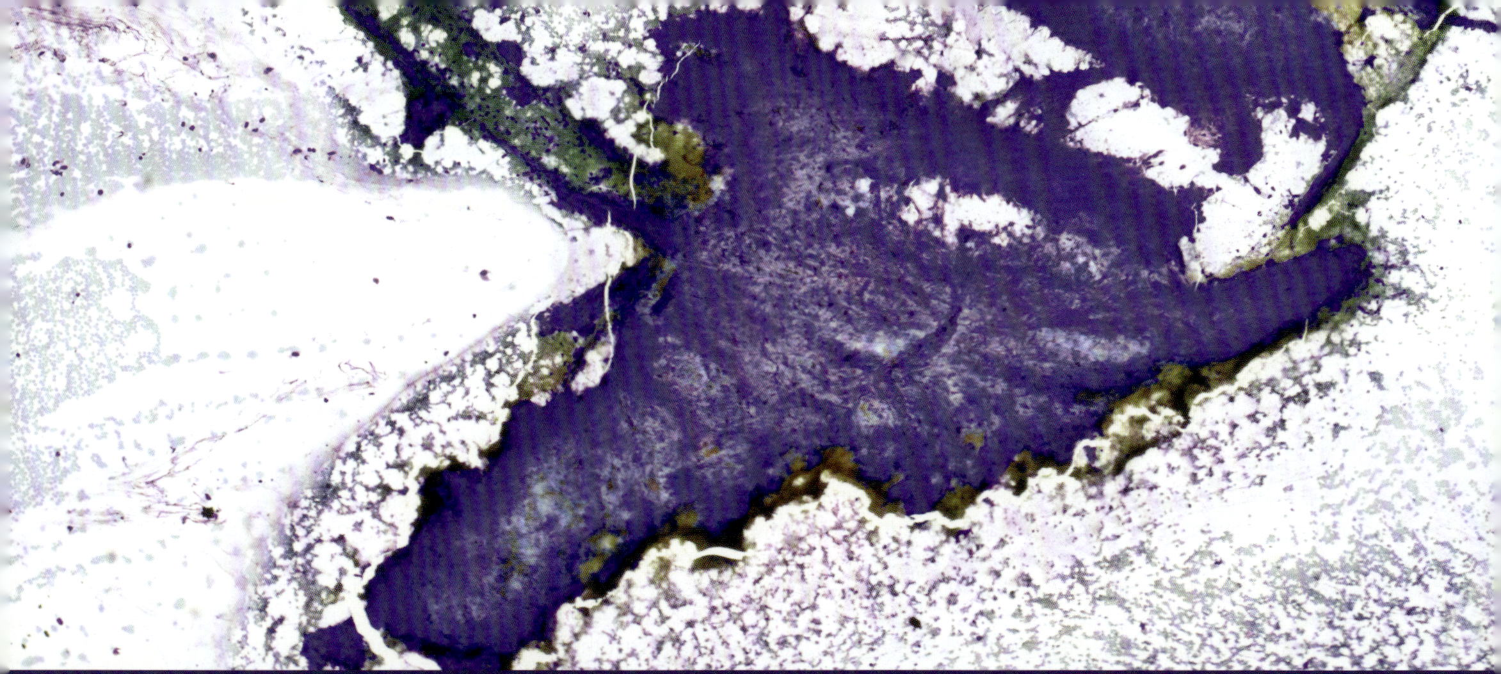

3

Diagnostic category: Insufficient/Inadequate/Non-diagnostic

Edited by: Domanski HA, Pitman MB, Schmitt F

Introduction

Bode-Lesniewska B
Field AS
Monaco SE
Raymond WA
Rekhi B
Teot LA

A categorization of "Insufficient/Inadequate/Non-diagnostic" is used to convey to the patient care team that the specimen provided no useful information concerning the targeted lesion and that additional sampling is necessary. The precise terminology for this category has been controversial, and the terms provided have been used interchangeably and inconsistently among institutions, which has resulted in all three terms being offered as options for this category. An institution should choose one preferred term and use it consistently.

An "Insufficient/Inadequate/Non-diagnostic" categorization may result from a variety of technical, preparation, and sampling issues and is defined in relation to the clinical history, physical examination and imaging findings, and ultimately the material for assessment on the direct smears or in LBC preparation. This is why a descriptive definition of this category is preferred over a definition based on the number of cells.

Any specimen is regarded as adequate if it demonstrates a pathological process consistent with the clinical setting and imaging findings. If there are any atypical features in the cells or the background, even if there is suboptimal preparation or degenerative limitations, the case is categorized as "Atypical" rather than "Insufficient". When only benign cells, such as adipocytes or skeletal muscle fibres, are present, some cytopathologists regard this as "Non-diagnostic" if the FNAB target was regarded as a suspicious mass or lesion; others describe and categorize the material on the smears as "Benign" and add a mandatory caveat that "the material may not represent the targeted lesion". In this first edition of the WHO Reporting System for Soft Tissue Cytopathology (WHO System), both approaches are acceptable; an institution should choose which approach to take, stick to it, and clearly communicate this approach to their clinicians. In both scenarios, a repeat biopsy, most commonly a repeat FNAB or a CNB, is required.

The FNAB sample may be "Insufficient", but a later cell block or other ancillary test may provide sufficient material for a diagnosis. An institution or cytopathologist can decide whether to issue the FNAB report and then later a supplementary report where the diagnostic category is changed, or to report the FNAB only once all cell block and ancillary tests are available.

The reasons why the FNAB is categorized as "Insufficient" should be stated in the report, such as because of obscuring blood or ultrasound gel, poor smearing of the material on the slides, slow air-drying artefact in Giemsa stains, air-drying artefact in alcohol-fixed Pap-stained slides, crush artefact, lysis of cells due to contamination with local anaesthetic, formalin vapour effect, or low cellularity of the sample due to technical difficulties in obtaining material. The nature of the specimen and poor FNAB technique by the proceduralist also have an effect on adequacy.

Definition

Bode-Lesniewska B
Field AS
Monaco SE
Raymond WA
Rekhi B
Teot LA

A specimen categorized as "Inadequate/Insufficient/Non-diagnostic" lacks sufficient material, in quantity or quality, for a reliable diagnosis.

Discussion and background

Bode-Lesniewska B
Field AS
Monaco SE
Raymond WA
Rekhi B
Teot LA

Reported rates of the "Insufficient/Inadequate/Non-diagnostic" category vary widely {1001,753,720,188}, influenced by the criteria used to define adequacy, the type of procedure, imaging and clinical findings, and the skills of the person performing the procedure. The definition is not based on the number of cells, because no strictly numerical cut-off value can adequately reflect the wide variety of tissues sampled; the broad differential diagnosis of inflammatory, degenerative, and neoplastic lesions; and the need for correlation of the cytopathological material findings with the clinical and imaging features of the lesion. Using a definition of "no or too few cells", the "Insufficient" frequency rate for soft tissue lesions has been reported as about 3% {705}. The rate was 4% with a definition of "when the quality or quantity of the diagnostic material was insufficient for evaluation" or if there was a discrepancy in the triple test of the cytomorphological, clinical, and imaging provisional diagnoses {753}. One recent study suggested a definition of adequacy as "5 clusters of 10 unobscured cells on all slides", but no rationale for this number was provided {1068}. In a meta-analysis of 13 reports on the adequacy of bone and soft tissue FNAB, the range of adequate specimens for soft tissue lesions was 39–95% {188}, somewhat lower, but not statistically significantly so, than for bone samples at 83–95%.

FNAB samples of soft tissue lesions may be hypocellular, particularly vascular lesions, lipomas, or ganglion cysts, and the background material and clinical correlation may imply an adequate preparation even though there are very few cells, as for a typical lipoma. But in the imaging setting of a clearly defined mass, rather than a lipoma, low cellularity suggests an inadequate sample. Site also influences concepts of adequacy; for example, the differential diagnosis of deeply located, intramuscular, and especially large fatty tumours includes lipoma-like atypical lipomatous tumour / well-differentiated liposarcoma, and the requirement for adequate material shifts not only in regard to the amount and features of the material on the FNAB smears, but also as to the availability of material for studies to determine *MDM2* amplification status {753}.

FNAB smears consisting exclusively of blood cannot be considered diagnostic. So the diagnosis of haemangioma requires correlation with imaging {1001}, although tissue fragments containing blood vessels may occasionally be diagnostic of haemangioma and can exclude other well-vascularised lesions such as solitary fibrous tumour {787}.

Among other mesenchymal tumours, the high content of collagen-rich sclerotic, extracellular matrix, as found for example in desmoid fibromatosis or low-grade fibromyxoid sarcoma, is often associated with low cellularity due to the inherent properties of the tumour {282,1058}, and CNB is often required {80,344}.

Risk of malignancy and diagnostic management recommendations

Bode-Lesniewska B
Field AS
Monaco SE
Raymond WA
Rekhi B
Teot LA

Published reports on the ROM for soft tissue FNAB are limited, but the ROM for the "Insufficient/Inadequate/Non-diagnostic" category is often reported as high, most likely due to sampling error.

In a systematic review with meta-analysis of 13 articles on FNAB of bone and soft tissue lesions, there were 7.7% inadequate samples, with adequacy rates for soft tissue lesions ranging from 38.6% to 94.8% {188}. In a recent report of 828 patients, with a 4% inadequate rate, the ROM was 42%, but this included a CNB with each FNAB for all but 2 patients {753}. Another study analysed 1114 soft tissue and bone FNAB specimens, most of which had ROSE, with 51% of the FNAB procedures performed without image guidance; the inadequate rate was 3%, and more than half of the 37 inadequate cases were found to be malignant at follow-up {696}. A retrospective study of FNAB samples of 301 soft tissue lesions {1001} found that 22 cases (7%) were inadequate samples, including 9 haemangiomas and 2 malignant tumours, yielding a ROM of 9%. A recent large single-institution retrospective study of 2214 cases showed a ROM of 29.87% for the "Insufficient" category, but it also showed, interestingly, that the ROM for all categories varied with the FNAB cytopathological pattern, from low for lipomatous tumours; to higher for spindle cell, epithelioid, and myxoid tumours; to very high for pleomorphic and round cell tumours {460}.

An "Insufficient" categorization should initiate correlation with the clinical and imaging findings. Whenever there is discordance between the clinical, imaging, and cytomorphological findings, a repeat specimen should be requested. If a lesion is suspicious clinically and/or on imaging and the diagnosis remains unresolved after FNAB sampling, CNB or incisional or excisional biopsy should be recommended. The application of guidance to the FNAB decreases the sampling error and is recommended for a lesion that is difficult to distinctly locate by palpation or is deep-seated, and ROSE is recommended to enable immediate progression to CNB at the same patient visit if the FNAB is "Insufficient" {80}.

Sample reports: Insufficient/Inadequate/ Non-diagnostic

Rekhi B
Field AS
Qian X

The sample reports provided here are based on the standardized cytopathology report in the *Diagnostic categories and report structure* section of the first chapter. See that section for a discussion on the structure and components.

These are sample reports that include the components required in one possible format; the final report format depends on local practice and local laboratory information system requirements. For brevity, demographics and ROSE are not presented here.

For consistency, the term "Insufficient" has been selected for these three sample reports. Cytopathologists and their institutions should decide whether their laboratory will use "Insufficient", "Inadequate", or "Non-diagnostic" for this category, and use it consistently and not in an ad hoc way. See the introduction at the beginning of this chapter for a discussion regarding the use of the term "Non-diagnostic".

Each institution should select a term for the main heading of the diagnostic summary, such as "Diagnostic summary" (as used in the examples below), "Diagnosis", or "Final diagnosis", and use it consistently.

Sample report 1

Specimen type:
CT-guided FNAB
Clinical and imaging information:
14-year-old male, lump over his left sinonasal region. MRI: 90 mm, well-defined, lobulated right sphenopalatine region. PET-CT: avid soft tissue mass. ? juvenile nasal angiofibroma.

Diagnostic summary:
Site: Left sinonasal
Category: Insufficient
Diagnosis: Insufficient material for diagnostic assessment

Material received:
Five air-dried slides and two alcohol-fixed slides. 3 mL bloodstained fluid prepared for cell block.

Microscopic description:
Blood with very occasional spindle, possible endothelial, cells present. Only blood is seen in the cell block.

Comment: Repeat FNAB is recommended.

Sample report 2

Specimen type:
FNAB
Clinical and imaging information:
35-year-old female, 56 mm soft tissue mass right side of neck. MRI shows infiltrative 55 mm lesion within sternocleidomastoid muscle, isointense on T1-weighted and heterogeneously hyperintense on T2-weighted images.

Diagnostic summary:
Site: Right sternocleidomastoid muscle
Category: Insufficient
Diagnosis: Insufficient material for diagnostic assessment

Material received:
Four air-dried slides, two alcohol-fixed slides. 1 mL bloody fluid for cell block.

Microscopic description:
One paucicellular air-dried Giemsa-stained smear shows a minute stromal fragment consisting of several spindle cells with a few single spindle cells in a bloody background. The other smears show blood. The cell block shows blood only.

Comment: There is insufficient material for diagnostic assessment. Correlation with clinical and imaging findings is required, and repeat study is recommended.

Sample report 3

Specimen type:
CT-guided FNAB
Clinical and imaging information:
55-year-old male with a slow-growing left thigh mass. MRI shows a 50 × 45 × 60 mm heterogeneously enhancing solid mass in the vastus medialis muscle, suspicious for sarcoma.

Diagnostic summary:
Site: Left vastus medialis
Category: Insufficient
Diagnosis: Blood with fibrin clot (see comment below)

Microscopic description:
Blood is present with a fibrin clot.

Material received:
Four air-dried slides and a container that includes a blood clot

Comment: There is insufficient material for diagnostic assessment. Correlation with imaging findings and repeat FNAB with ROSE and/or CNB is recommended.

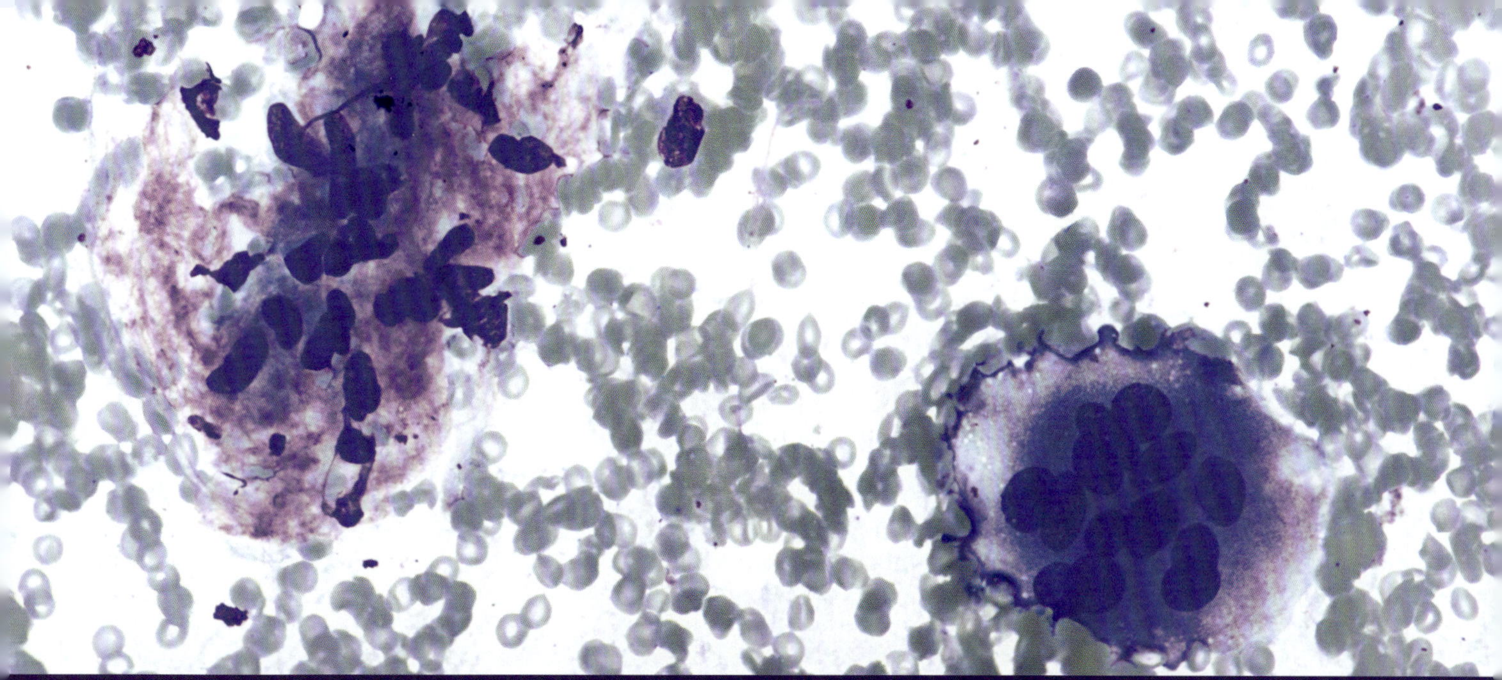

4

Diagnostic category: Benign

Edited by: Bode-Lesniewska B, Chebib I, Domanski HA, Field AS, Jo VY, Klijanienko J, Mehrotra R, Pitman MB, Qian X, Schmitt F, Teot LA

(Continued on next page)

4

Diagnostic category: Benign (continued)

Introduction

Dodd LG
Kerr DA

A "Benign" categorization is applied when a sample is adequate for interpretation and shows unequivocal features of a benign lesion. This may represent a specific benign neoplasm or inflammation process.

The "Benign" category of soft tissue tumours includes an assortment of neoplasms that are further subclassified based on distinctive cytomorphological features that manifest as an identifiable "pattern", including specific types of stroma or matrix constituting adipocytic, myxoid, and chondro-osseous patterns; a prominent cellular feature such as inflammation or multinucleate giant cells; or a specific cell shape, as in spindle or epithelioid patterns.

The fifth-edition WHO classification of soft tissue tumours recognizes an "intermediate" category of soft tissue lesions based on their biological potential {1503}, and this is further subdivided into "locally aggressive" neoplasms such as deep or aggressive fibromatosis, a neoplasm that is locally aggressive but will not metastasize, and "rarely metastasizing" neoplasms that are occasionally aggressive or have a very low but nevertheless real and documented propensity for metastasis. In this first WHO Reporting System for Soft Tissue Cytopathology (WHO System), the "intermediate" lesions of the WHO classification are divided and categorized into two distinct categories: "locally aggressive" lesions such as fibromatosis into the "Benign" category, and "rarely metastasizing" tumours such as angiomatoid fibrous histiocytoma into the "Soft tissue neoplasm of uncertain malignant potential" ("STNUMP") category. The "STNUMP" category acknowledges that with selected neoplasms, the cytopathological and often the histopathological and ICC features are

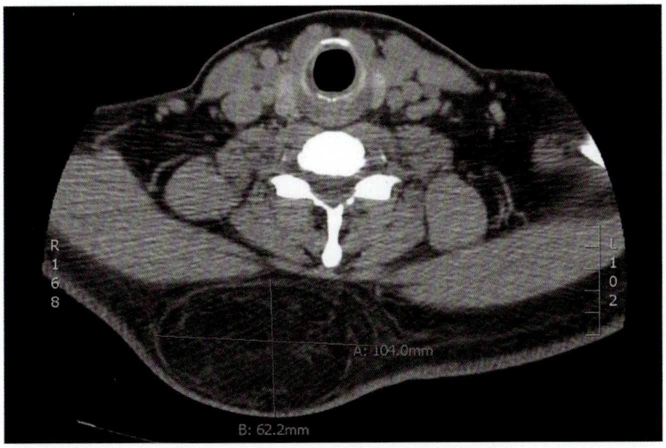

Fig. 4.01 Spindle cell lipoma imaging. A benign lesion (spindle cell lipoma) of the posterior thorax. The lesion is circumscribed and sharply demarcated.

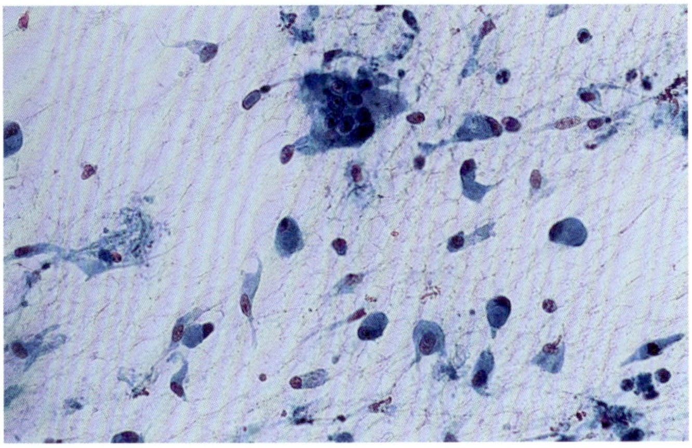

Fig. 4.02 Myositis ossificans. An FNAB from myositis ossificans shows a dispersed population of moderately pleomorphic cells, as well as a multinucleate giant cell (Pap).

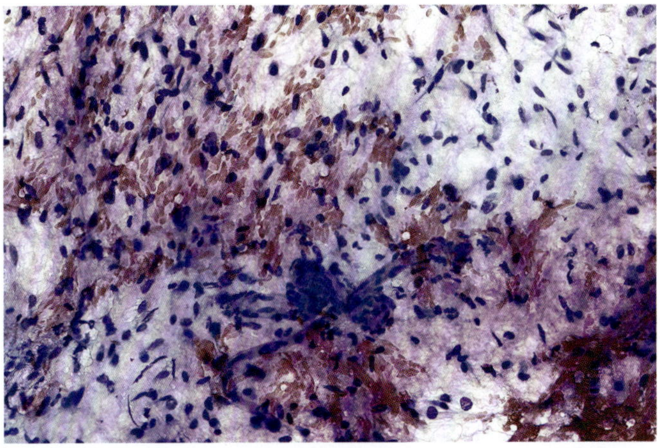

Fig. 4.03 Intramuscular myxoma. In intramuscular myxoma, bland spindle to stellate cells are enmeshed in a myxoid stroma (Giemsa).

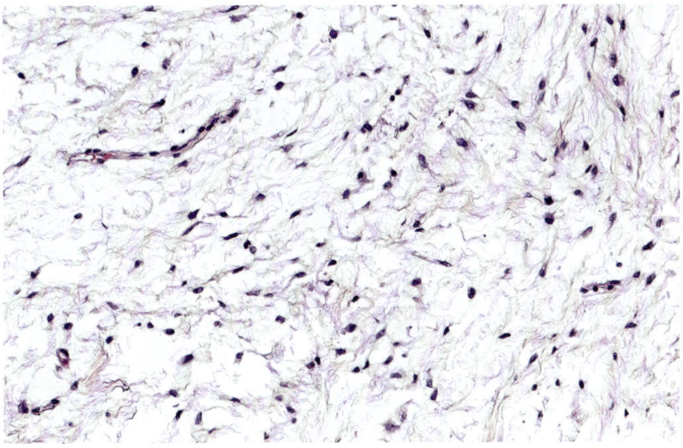

Fig. 4.04 Intramuscular myxoma. Corresponding cell block sections of an intramuscular myxoma show cytologically bland spindle to stellate cells in a pale myxoid stroma with scant vasculature (H&E).

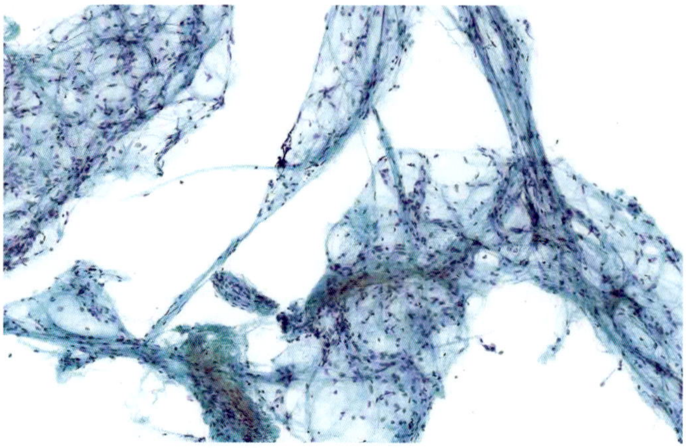

Fig. 4.05 Lipoma. An FNAB of a lipoma is composed predominantly of mature adipose tissue without cytopathological atypia (Pap).

not always a reliable predictor of the behaviour of the neoplasm, and that some unpredictable neoplasms, although most commonly behaving in a benign fashion, may have a small potential for malignant behaviour.

Definition

Dodd LG
Kerr DA

A specimen categorized as "Benign" demonstrates unequivocal benign cytopathological features, which may or may not be diagnostic of a specific process or benign neoplasm.

Discussion and background

Dodd LG
Kerr DA

Benign soft tissue lesions greatly outnumber aggressive or malignant tumours, including sarcomas, by an estimated factor of 100 to 1 {1214}. For the most part, benign soft tissue tumours mimic their associated normal tissue counterparts. Lipoma, for example, bears such a similar appearance to normal fat that it is often almost impossible to distinguish the two on cytomorphology. Objective cytopathology features such as uniformity, homogeneity, monomorphic features, and mitotic inactivity are generally descriptors associated with benign or very low risk neoplasms. Many of the lesions included in this FNAB category are not neoplastic, such as focal fat necrosis, mass-forming inflammatory processes, and ganglion cysts, but they are included because they fall into the differential diagnosis of neoplastic lesions clinically and on imaging, and they are frequently sampled by FNAB.

Many benign lesions are easily recognizable on FNAB and often produce low to modest cellularity with a uniform population of individual cells without significant pleomorphism or atypia. There are notable exceptions such as nodular fasciitis, which can be alarmingly cellular and show extensive cellular pleomorphism; myositis ossificans with marked nuclear pleomorphism; and nerve sheath tumours and leiomyomas that can show focal nuclear atypia.

Benign does not necessarily mean inconsequential, because benign tumours can cause significant morbidity by obstruction, impingement, or other physical mechanisms. In addition, not all benign tumours are easily removed. For example, vascular neoplasms and malformations can be large and infiltrative, necessitating difficult and often multistage removal. Fibromatosis, a locally aggressive tumour, has historically been treated surgically but is difficult to eradicate, with patients often enduring multiple excisions, deformities, and even limb loss, and the treatment paradigm for this entity has largely shifted to a wait-and-see approach, with consideration of medical therapies {884}. In addition, some benign lesions may be transient or self-limited, such as nodular fasciitis {385}.

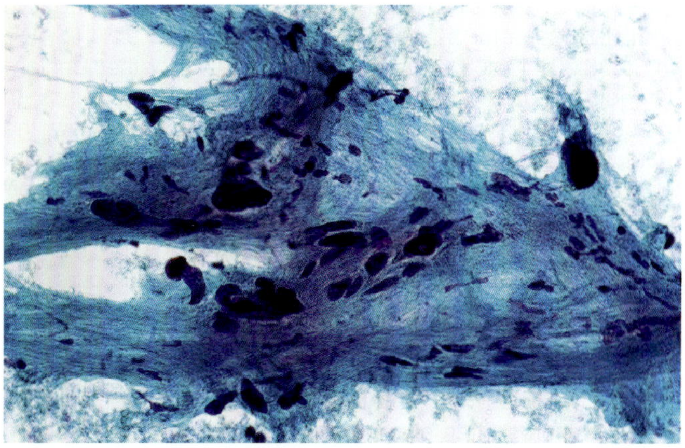

Fig. 4.06 Schwannoma with atypia. An example of cellular atypia in a benign neoplasm: degenerative change (so-called "ancient change") in a benign schwannoma (Pap).

Risk of malignancy and diagnostic management recommendations

Dodd LG
Kerr DA

The ROM for the "Benign" category of soft tissue neoplasms is very low. Overall accuracy in FNAB of soft tissue is affected by individual cytopathologists' experience, which can be limited other than in specialist orthopaedic and oncological institutions where relatively rare soft tissue neoplasms tend to be seen more frequently, and by the availability and use of a multidisciplinary approach {832}.

The sensitivity and specificity of FNAB for separating benign from malignant soft tissue lesions ranges depending on various study parameters, with an overall sensitivity of 97.4% and specificity of 98.2% in a large meta-analysis {188}. The negative predictive value for a benign lesion ranges from 94% to 98% {763,696,33,1470,681,1017,753}, and the ROM for the "Benign" category can be conservatively estimated to be 5% or less. In a recently published single-institution retrospective review, the ROM was 2.49% {460}, although this same review showed that the overall ROM across the categories varied with the cytomorphological pattern, from 3% for lipomatous tumours to 62.78% for spindle cell, 78.15% for epithelioid, 84.58% for myxoid, 94.26% for pleomorphic, and 100% for round cell tumours.

One of the difficulties with diagnostic accuracy in the "Benign" category is the subset of lesions that show significant cytopathological atypia or pleomorphism despite their benign behaviour; for example, benign peripheral nerve sheath tumours often show extensive nuclear pleomorphism and atypia, so-called "ancient change", despite their benign nature, potentially leading to a misdiagnosis of malignancy {320}. The other cytomorphological features of malignancy, such as mitotic activity, necrosis, and hypercellularity, should be present and commensurate with the degree of atypia before categorization as an indeterminate or "Malignant" lesion. Likewise, the cytopathological appearances of the so-called "pseudosarcomas", including nodular fasciitis and myositis ossificans, can result in false positive diagnoses {333}.

A "Benign" soft tissue FNAB should be correlated with the clinical and imaging findings and with ancillary testing, such as ICC for MDM2 in fat neoplasms. The management of soft tissue lesions categorized as "Benign" depends on many factors, including lesion size, depth, and location, as well as patient comfort and preference. Some benign lesions are removed for cosmetic purposes only, and some can be monitored clinically for signs of growth or change. Surgical removal is best accomplished with thoughtful preoperative planning and assessment. With some benign or locally aggressive lesions, such as desmoid fibromatosis, active surveillance is the current preferred approach in most clinical scenarios {884}.

Evaluation of any soft tissue lesion, including those that are suspected to be benign, should begin with a detailed patient history and physical examination. In superficial locations, the lesion size, location, depth, mobility, and consistency often provide invaluable information that can direct additional study. Patients should be asked about the duration and growth of the lesion, as well as factors such as pain or sensitivity to touch and pressure. Radiating pain, a phenomenon known as Tinel's sign, is a characteristic feature of peripheral nerve sheath tumour. Likewise, detection of pulsation is typical of a vascular lesion {387}.

Further evaluation of a suspected soft tissue tumour often includes imaging studies. Although MRI is the modality of choice, plain radiographs and ultrasound evaluation are often useful and can be a cost-effective means of evaluating lesions that do not need further imaging evaluation, and ultrasound is often very useful to direct the FNAB {471,1016}. Further evaluation of a lesion with MRI can be particularly useful in the evaluation of tumour size, borders, and relationships to adjacent structures, as well as the presence or absence of tumour heterogeneity or homogeneity. Cystic change and necrosis are other features that can influence the tumour subtype differential diagnosis.

Acute inflammation

Michelow P
Silverman J

Definition

Acute inflammation yields a purulent material consisting of neutrophils and variable numbers of histiocytes with cellular debris in a fibrinous background.

Clinical features and imaging

Soft tissue infections include a range of clinical lesions, from mild infections such as impetigo and uncomplicated cellulitis to life-threatening conditions, including necrotizing fasciitis. Clinically, soft tissue infections present as tender, oedematous, warm and erythematous swellings. Systemic signs and symptoms that can be seen in more severe infections include fever, hypothermia, tachycardia, and hypotension. The most common causes are bacteria such as *Staphylococcus aureus* and *Streptococcus* spp. Other etiological agents, especially in immunosuppressed individuals, can also cause soft tissue infections. These include infections by bacteria such as *Bartonella* spp., *Vibrio vulnificus*, non-tuberculous mycobacteria, and the bacteria that cause leprosy; fungal infections such as candidiasis, aspergillosis, and zygomycosis; viral infections such as herpes zoster and herpes simplex infection; and parasitic infections including leishmaniasis {167,1093,962,1238,522,501,389,1348}. Non-infectious causes of inflammation include a foreign body such as a splinter. MRI is the most sensitive diagnostic imaging modality, although CT is more widely available and can detect many necrotizing infections and foreign bodies. Ultrasound is useful for diagnosing soft tissue collections and can be used to direct the FNAB for diagnostic purposes. Plain X-rays are rarely helpful {55,550}.

Histopathology

An abscess is a cavity filled with acute inflammatory cells and necrotic debris. Granulation tissue and later fibrosis surround the abscess cavity. Marked acute inflammation, involving subcutaneous fat with extensive necrosis, is seen in necrotizing fasciitis, with ulceration of overlying tissue, thrombosis, vasculitis, and extension of inflammation into skeletal muscle. The causative organism may be seen microscopically, although in many cases ancillary tests are required.

Key diagnostic cytopathological features

- Large numbers of neutrophils
- Necrotic debris and fibrin in background
- In the later stages, chronic inflammatory cells such as lymphocytes and histiocytes, as well as granulation tissue
- Reparative changes in non-inflammatory cells
- Specific infectious organisms may be seen on routine and special stains

Reference(s): {411}

Discussion and differential diagnosis

FNAB is a rapid, virtually pain-free, and simple procedure to procure a sample for cytopathology and microbiological investigation, especially because contamination is minimized {477,50}.

Benign entities in the differential diagnosis include epidermoid inclusion cyst, where numerous anucleate squamous cells and a small number of nucleated squamous cells, keratinous debris, and multinucleated histiocytes are seen, along with pus. Acute inflammatory cells may be seen in inflamed branchial cysts, where squamous cells make the diagnosis, and in thyroglossal duct cysts, where variable often scant numbers of squamous cells and respiratory type epithelium are seen with the possible inclusion of thyroid follicular cells and colloid. Clinical and imaging correlation is required {189}. In an immunosuppressed host, mycobacterial infection may present as acute suppurative necrosis.

Acute inflammatory cells may be seen in Hodgkin lymphoma, myeloid leukaemias, and non-Hodgkin lymphomas, especially T-cell lymphoma {365,424}. Marked, mainly acute inflammation is also a feature of metastatic squamous cell carcinoma; in a soft tissue FNAB showing acute inflammation, the slides should be carefully screened to ensure that underlying malignant cells are not missed.

Ancillary testing

Microbiological investigations on FNAB purulent material should include Gram staining, an acid-fast stain such as Ziehl–Neelsen or similar, and fungal stains such as a methenamine silver stain, in addition to culture and sensitivity. Microbiological culture and sensitivity are virtually mandatory, and ICC, in situ hybridization, and PCR can be added when appropriate and available. Blood tests include full blood counts, inflammatory markers, and serology. Ancillary tests may also be used to exclude an underlying neoplastic process {962,969,1057,444,50}.

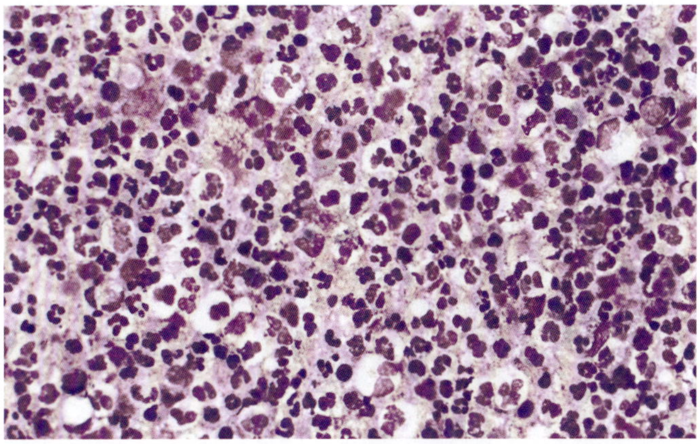

Fig. 4.07 Acute inflammation. Acute inflammation due to *Staphylococcus aureus* (Giemsa).

Granulomatous and suppurative granulomatous inflammation

Carrilho C
Lokuhetty D
Michelow P

Definition

Granulomatous inflammation is characterized by epithelioid granulomas with or without necrosis and multinucleated giant cells. Suppurative granulomatous inflammation additionally includes a suppurative component of neutrophils and cellular debris.

Clinical features and imaging

Granulomatous lesions in soft tissue usually present as a mass or swelling and can mimic a soft tissue tumour. Heat and erythema are usually less pronounced than in purely acute inflammation, and ulcers can be present in the skin overlying the site of infection, along with sinus formation with serosanguinous or suppurative discharge. Depending on the etiological agent, the lesions can be solitary, multifocal, or disseminated. Systemic signs can be present, including weight loss, fever, and night sweats. Patient history, such as contact with pulmonary tuberculosis, HIV status, migration, travel, and country of residence can be useful for diagnosis {147,60,371}.

Histopathology

Granulomas are composed of epithelioid histiocytes, along with multinucleated histiocytes as giant cells. Central necrosis, caseous or non-caseous, can be present or absent, as can suppuration. The etiological agent can sometimes be identified with routine and/or special stains and other investigations.

Key diagnostic cytopathological features

- Epithelioid granulomas, which can include multinucleated giant cells, in a background that can include necrosis and/or suppuration
- Epithelioid histiocytes with elongated, "footprint" or oval nuclei, with fine chromatin and inconspicuous nucleoli
- The cytoplasm of histiocytes is eccentric and abundant, sometimes syncytial and pale
- Depending on the etiology, inflammatory cells (mainly lymphocytes, histiocytes, multinucleated histiocytes, neutrophils, and eosinophils) can be present in the background, mixed with a variable amount of necrosis
- Infectious microorganisms can be identified with special stains for mycobacteria, including acid-fast stains (e.g. Ziehl–Neelsen, rhodamine–auramine, and autofluorescence of Pap stains) and fungal stains (e.g. methenamine silver and DPAS stains)

Reference(s): {937,1123,411}

Discussion and differential diagnosis

Granulomatous and suppurative granulomatous lesions can involve soft tissues in the setting of *Mycobacterium tuberculosis* infection, atypical mycobacterial infections, other non-tuberculous

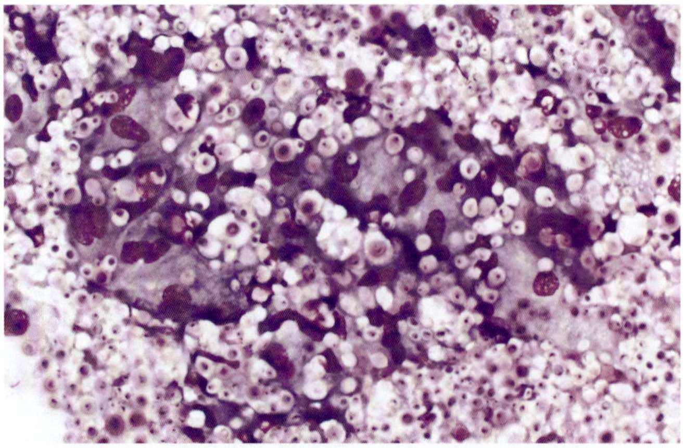

Fig. 4.08 Granulomatous inflammation and cryptococcosis. Poorly formed granulomas in the centre of the field, within a background with *Cryptococcus* (Giemsa).

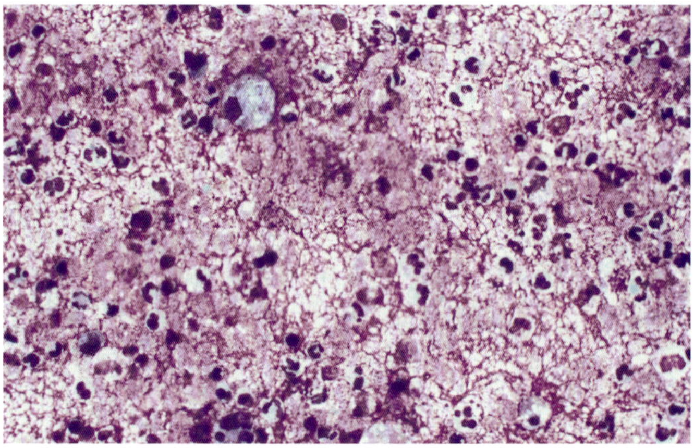

Fig. 4.09 Tuberculosis with suppurative inflammation. Background with acute suppurative necrosis and foamy histiocytes (Giemsa).

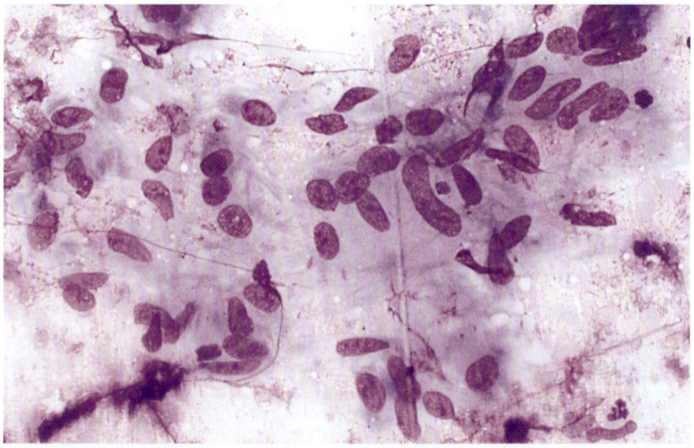

Fig. 4.10 Tuberculous suppurative necrotizing inflammation. Epithelioid granuloma in a background of suppurative necrosis (Giemsa).

mycobacterial diseases (e.g. Buruli ulcers, leprosy), and actinomycosis. Granulomas associated with caseous necrosis in the background or suppuration with neutrophils can be found in tuberculosis and are associated with variable numbers of mycobacteria as observed in the Ziehl–Neelsen stain and its variants {937}. Atypical mycobacterioses tend to have a greater number of mycobacteria in the foamy cytoplasm of histiocytes and negative curved bacilli in the background serum in Giemsa stains.

Fungal infections include cryptococcosis, histoplasmosis, aspergillosis, candidiasis, blastomycosis, coccidioidomycosis, sporotrichosis, and mycetomas. Granulomatous and suppurative granulomatous patterns with or without non-caseous necrosis admixed with eosinophils can be found in fungal infections. In some cases, identification of the etiological agent is possible in the routine stain on the basic morphological features, but this must be complemented with specific special stains if available {1123}.

Parasitic infections including filariasis and cysticercosis can also elicit granulomatous and granulomatous suppurative inflammation {985,25,147,494,60,371,1148,372}.

The causes of non-infectious granulomatous conditions are multiple and include foreign-body reactions (e.g. to cosmetic soft tissue fillers), sarcoidosis, autoimmune and allergic conditions, drug reactions, and neoplasia. In these conditions, granulomas present without necrosis. Giant multinucleated cells can be numerous in the response to foreign bodies {507,1123}.

Some tumours are granulomatous, include a reactive granulomatous component, or resemble granulomas and should be considered in the differential diagnoses of epithelioid granulomas. These include Kaposi sarcoma, epithelioid sarcoma (usual type), Hodgkin and non-Hodgkin lymphomas, metastatic germ cell tumour, and nasopharyngeal carcinoma {666,175, 1063,749,212,1307,1242}. Metastatic squamous cell carcinoma is the most notable to elicit a granulomatous response. Careful examination of smears for scattered malignant cells and the use of appropriate ancillary testing are required.

Ancillary testing

Special stains such as the Ziehl–Neelsen are useful for mycobacterial infections, and methenamine silver and DPAS are useful for fungal infections. Fluorescence microscopy is also used in mycobacterial infections. Polarization helps to identify foreign bodies in foreign-body granulomas. Mucicarmine stains the cryptococcal capsule, which is also seen as a negative image between the positive yeast body and the surrounding serum in the Giemsa stain, highlighting the diagnostic narrow neck budding. Correlation with culture and PCR is helpful when available. ICC with appropriate markers is useful to distinguish tumours presenting with granulomas {1123,937,714,1063,749,212,1307,1242,1178}.

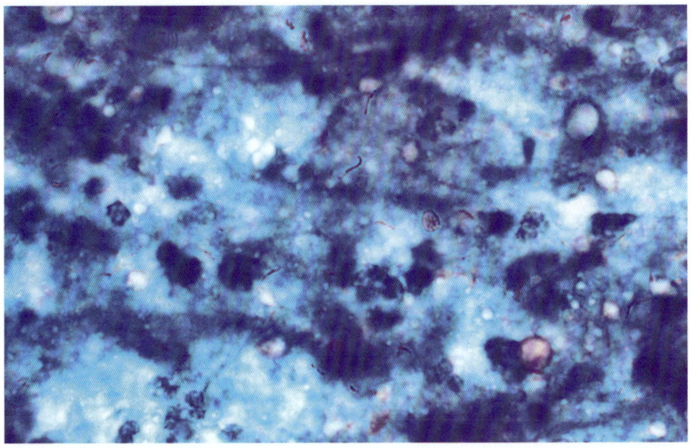

Fig. 4.11 Tuberculosis. Presence of mycobacteria bacilli stained in red on Ziehl–Neelsen stain.

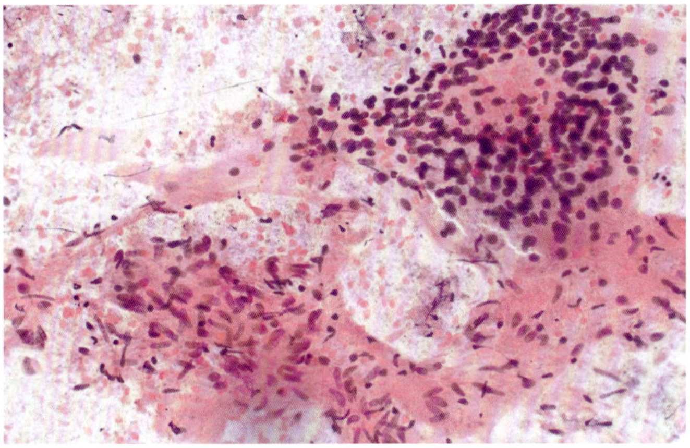

Fig. 4.12 Granulomatous inflammation in tuberculosis. Epithelioid granuloma with a giant/multinucleated cell (Pap).

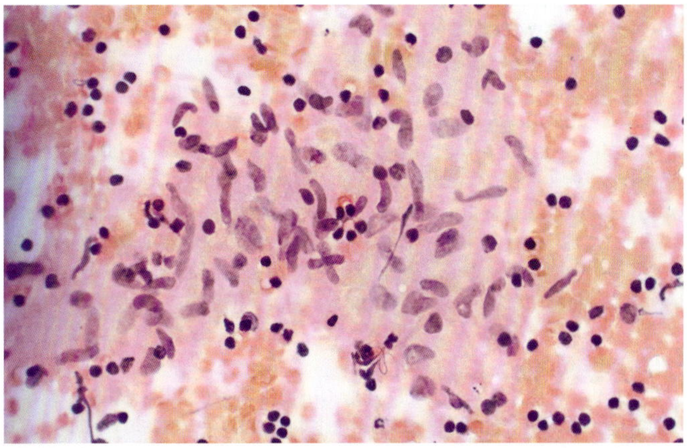

Fig. 4.13 Granulomatous inflammation in tuberculosis. Epithelioid granuloma: epithelioid histiocytes with elongated nuclei and abundant and vaguely syncytial cytoplasm (Pap).

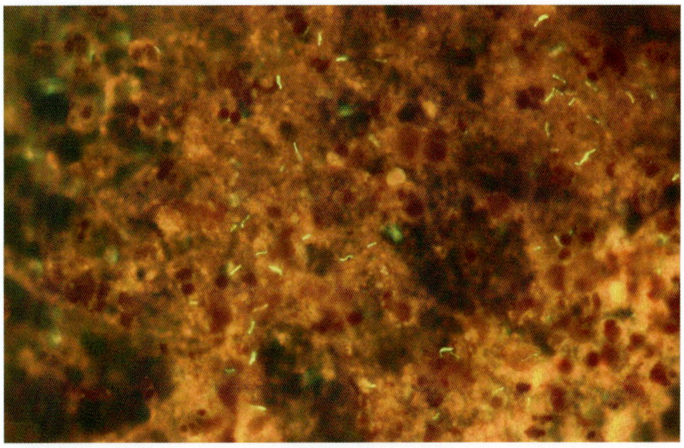

Fig. 4.14 Tuberculosis autofluorescence. Brilliant green autofluorescence of mycobacterial infection in a Pap-stained direct smear.

Fat necrosis

Silverman J
Chebib I
Kerr DA

Definition

Fat necrosis is a non-neoplastic inflammatory lesion characterized by necrotic adipose tissue often accompanied by acute and chronic inflammatory cells and foamy vacuolated histiocytes.

Clinical features and imaging

Fat necrosis is commonly secondary to trauma, operative procedures, or acute pancreatitis. Fat necrosis presents as a painless, solitary mass, which when superficial can be relatively firm and circumscribed on palpation. When involving the breast, it is most often seen in perimenopausal women after trauma, surgery, irradiation, or CNB, or it can occur without apparent cause {1376,1446}. Similarly, in extramammary sites, there is often a history of trauma or an operative procedure, although the etiology may be unknown. Fat necrosis can occur in both normal and neoplastic fat and can clinically simulate malignancy. An uncommon disorder of infants is subcutaneous fat necrosis of the newborn, which is a transient panniculitis.

With mammography, fat necrosis can have varying appearances, including discrete, circumscribed, or oval radiolucent cysts; focal mass-like structures; and occasionally an ill-defined spiculated mass, which can simulate a carcinoma. Ultrasound shows a well-circumscribed to ill-defined solid or cystic nodule, often associated with distortion of the breast parenchyma. The findings can vary depending on the stage of evolution of the process, including the degree of fibrosis that causes the architectural distortion simulating malignancy {695}.

Histopathology

The features of fat necrosis vary depending on this stage of the lesion. Early fat necrosis is characterized by necrosis of adipose tissue with fine vacuolization of adipocytes and nuclear dropout, with or without haemorrhage and cystic degeneration. In the intermediate stage, a mixed inflammatory cell infiltrate of histiocytes, lymphocytes, plasma cells, and occasional eosinophils can be seen, along with early fibrosis and haemosiderin deposition. Histiocytes surrounding fat vacuoles can be present, and occasional multinucleated histiocytes are noted. Late-stage fat necrosis demonstrates increased amounts of fibrosis, with or without calcification. Loculated foci of necrotic adipose tissue can be surrounded by fibrosis, forming an oil cyst, which can also contain calcification in its wall. Occasionally, a cellular proliferation of histiocytes can occur in mammary, omental, and mesenteric fat necrosis. The histiocytes can become spindle, arranged in a fascicular pattern admixed with chronic inflammatory cells and multinucleated giant cells. This cellular spindle cell histiocytic proliferation can form a mass, which can simulate a malignancy.

Key diagnostic cytopathological features

- Tissue fragments of degenerating and necrotic anuclear fat
- Foamy histiocytes and multinucleated histiocytes
- Occasional inflammatory cells
- Free lipid droplets in background, seen best at ROSE in the Giemsa stain
- Granular necrotic debris showing variable staining (Giemsa)
- Radially oriented refractile needle-shaped crystals are seen in subcutaneous fat necrosis of newborn

Reference(s): {19,1266,530,851}

Discussion and differential diagnosis

Fat necrosis, when occurring in the breast, can simulate malignancy, especially when skin retraction and thickened skin are present and imaging demonstrates a stellate lesion. Helpful features for a definitive diagnosis of fat necrosis are the bland appearance of the histiocytes and the lack of definite epithelial

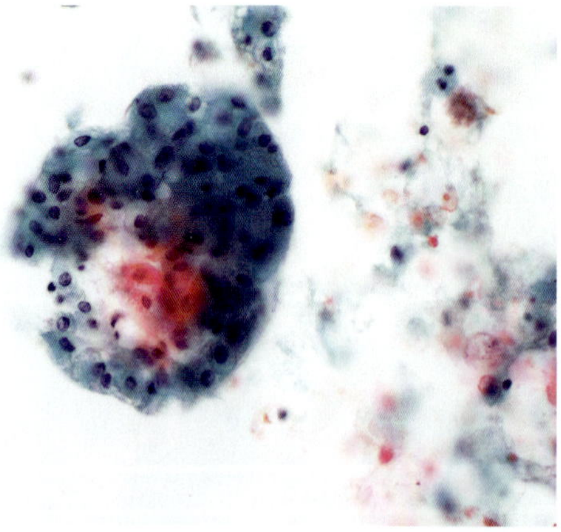

Fig. 4.15 Fat necrosis. Fat necrosis showing aggregates of foamy macrophages (Pap).

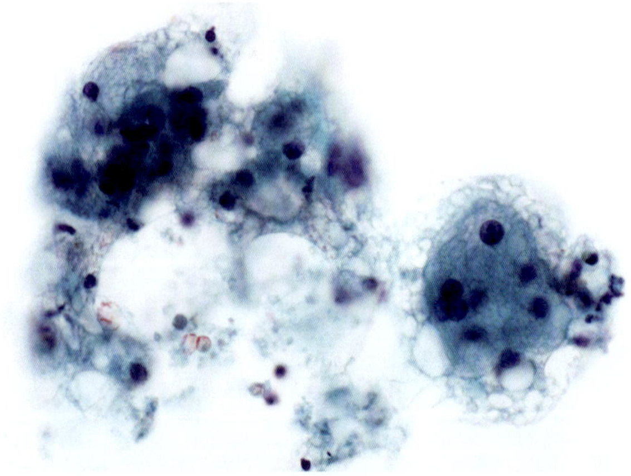

Fig. 4.16 Fat necrosis. Fat necrosis showing foamy macrophages and multinucleated giant cells (Pap).

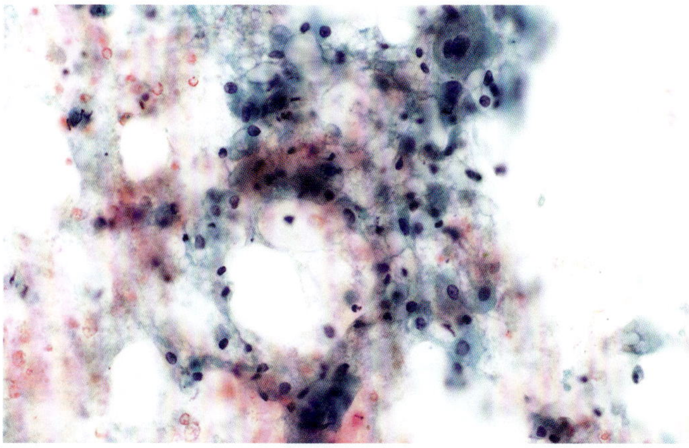

Fig. 4.17 Fat necrosis. Fat necrosis showing degenerated fat, blood, and foamy macrophages (Pap).

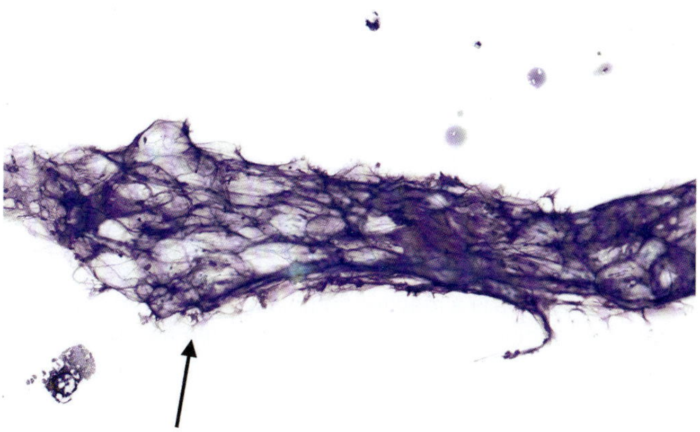

Fig. 4.18 Fat necrosis involving an intra-abdominal lipoma. Early fat necrosis involving an intra-abdominal lipoma shows vacuolization of adipocytes (arrow), many of which are anucleate. FISH was negative for *MDM2* amplification, helping to exclude a well-differentiated liposarcoma (Giemsa).

cells showing any nuclear atypia. Fat necrosis can occur in a lipoma, and it lacks the atypical nuclei, lipoblasts, and confirmatory molecular abnormalities of liposarcoma.

Ancillary testing

The histiocytes in fat necrosis are positive for CD68 and CD163, and CK7 is negative in cases where FNAB has been performed to assess recurrent breast carcinoma in the postsurgical setting. Fat necrosis in the omentum and other deep sites raises a differential diagnosis of liposarcoma, and MDM2 by ICC is negative in fat necrosis.

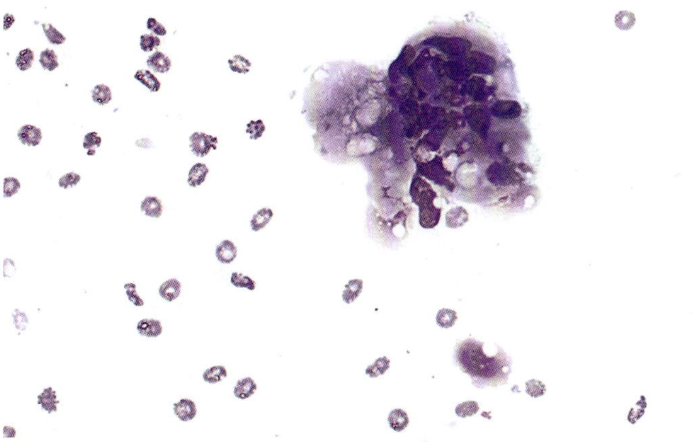

Fig. 4.19 Fat necrosis. Fat necrosis showing histiocytes with foamy cytoplasm and a multinucleated giant cell (Giemsa).

Ischaemic fasciitis

Qian X
Holmes BJ

Definition

Ischaemic fasciitis is a reactive fibroblastic/myofibroblastic proliferation occurring in the deep subcutis, often associated with chronic pressure and consequent ischaemia of tissue overlying bone.

Clinical features and imaging

Ischaemic fasciitis has a marked predilection for elderly patients in their eighth and ninth decades of life who are physically debilitated or immobilized. It usually arises around the limb girdles, sacral region, and greater trochanter. Ischaemic fasciitis forms an ill-defined lesion, usually 30–40 mm but as large as 100 mm, located in the deep subcutis, with or without extension into skeletal muscle. It demonstrates characteristic zonation, with a circumscribed low-signal centre surrounded by peripheral enhancement on MRI with contrast {975,808,823,609}.

Histopathology

Ischaemic fasciitis is characterized by a distinct zonal appearance, with a central hypocellular and avascular area showing fibrinoid, pseudocystic degeneration and/or fat necrosis. The peripheral cellular area contains a granulation tissue vascular proliferation admixed with fibroblasts and myofibroblasts of varying sizes and shapes, some with a ganglion cell–like appearance. Myxoid stroma, hyalinosis of vessel walls, an inflammatory infiltrate, and extravasated erythrocytes may be present. Mitotic figures are variable, but atypical forms are absent {975,1098,823}.

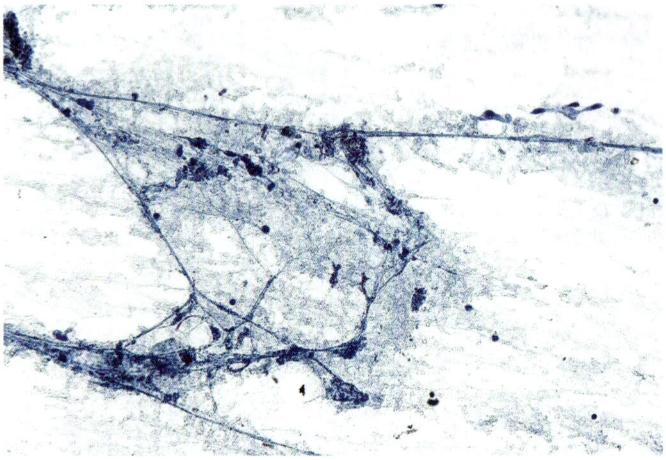

Fig. 4.21 Ischaemic fasciitis. Scattered aggregates and singly dispersed spindle cells with round to ovoid nuclei in a background of blood and granular debris (Pap).

Key diagnostic cytopathological features

- Mild to moderate cellularity
- Tissue fragments and single cells of varying sizes
- Spindle to stellate cells with round to oval nuclei with smooth nuclear contours and varying chromatin ranging from open to smudged and hyperchromatic (Pap)
- Ample granular and vacuolated cytoplasm, staining light blue-green (Pap) and blue-grey (Giemsa)

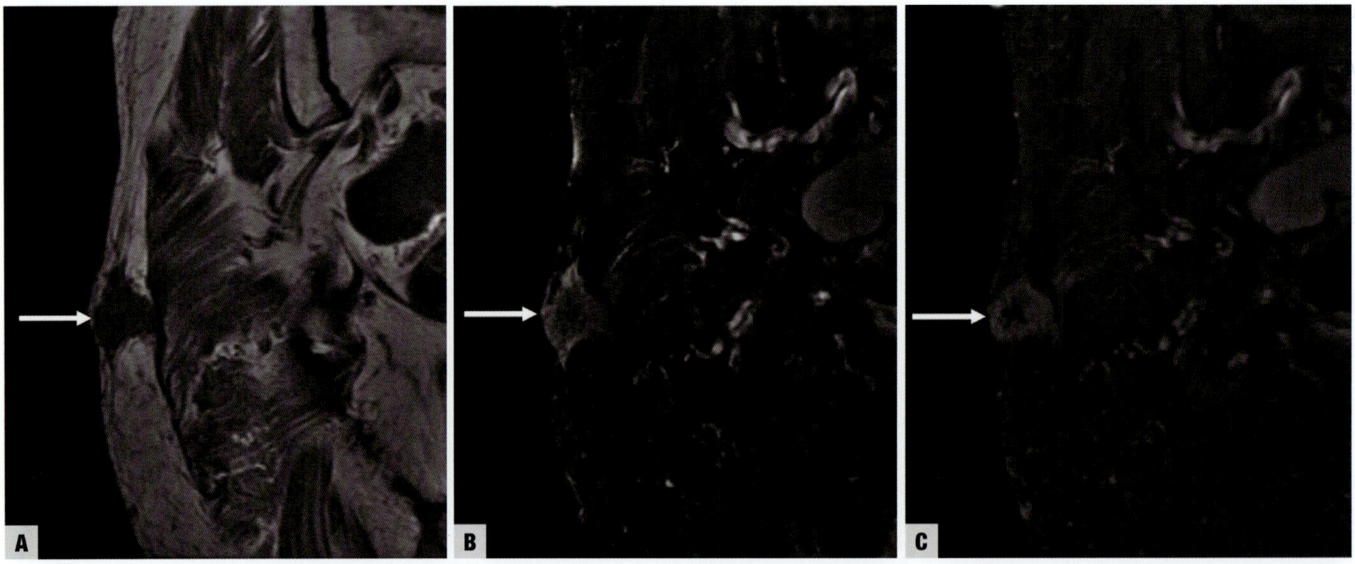

Fig. 4.20 Ischaemic fasciitis. MRI of ischaemic fasciitis in a 91-year-old man with tender palpable mass on lateral aspect of right hip. An irregular mass is seen in the subcutaneous tissues over the right lateral hip abutting the underlying fascia (arrows), with low signal on the coronal T1-weighted image (**A**), intermediate T2 signal intensity on the coronal fat-saturated proton density–weighted image (**B**), and corresponding enhancement with a central area of non-enhancing necrosis on the fat-saturated coronal T1-weighted image after gadolinium administration (**C**). Biopsy confirmed ischaemic fasciitis.

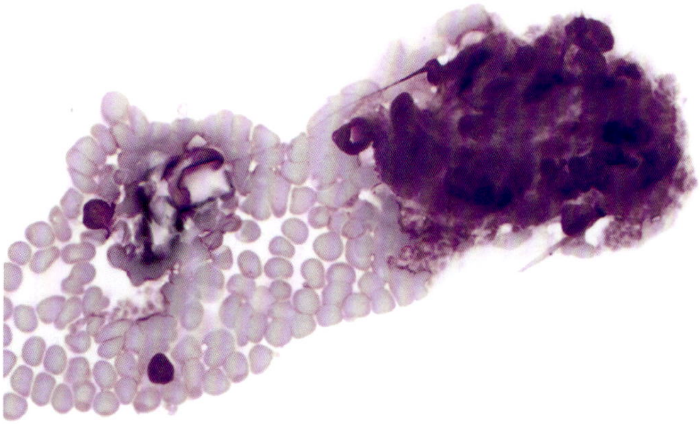

Fig. 4.22 Ischaemic fasciitis. Occasional aggregates of spindle and histiocytic cells, some with degenerative, dark, smudged nuclei (Giemsa).

- Occasional ganglion-like cells and inflammatory cells
- Myxoid matrix, blood, and granular debris in background, particularly in Giemsa

Reference(s): {688,333}

Discussion and differential diagnosis

Proliferative fasciitis and proliferative myositis share many morphological features with ischaemic fasciitis, but these lesions occur in younger patients, are not associated with chronic pressure, and lack the central necrosis and granulation tissue–like capillaries that are characteristic of ischaemic fasciitis. Because of the presence of necrotic debris, large ganglion-like cells, and ischaemic and degenerative nuclear hyperchromasia, ischaemic fasciitis can be easily mistaken for spindle cell sarcomas, such as myxofibrosarcoma and myxoinflammatory fibroblastic sarcoma, both of which show more cellular smears and more prominent nuclear pleomorphism. Multinucleated tumour giant cells and atypical mitotic figures are more commonly seen in the sarcomas {1199,839}.

Ancillary testing

Ischaemic fasciitis may show focal positivity for SMA, desmin, and CD34, supporting its fibroblastic or myofibroblastic nature. The spindle cells in a subset of cases may show MDM2, CDK4, and p16 expression by ICC, without evidence of *MDM2* gene amplification {1526}.

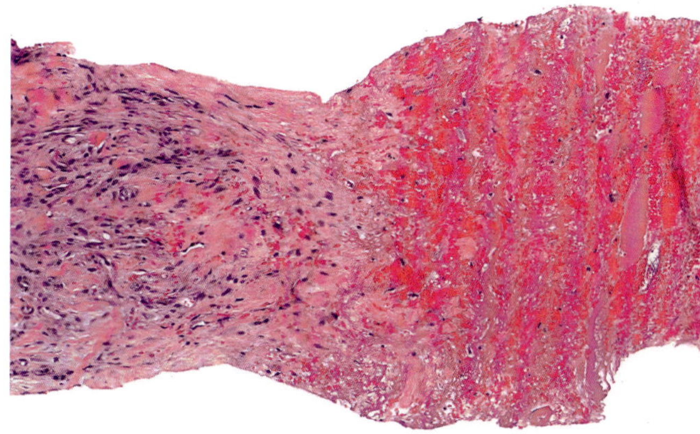

Fig. 4.23 Ischaemic fasciitis. CNB showing a zonal pattern, with a granulation tissue–like vascular proliferation that abruptly transitions to avascular fibrinoid necrosis (H&E).

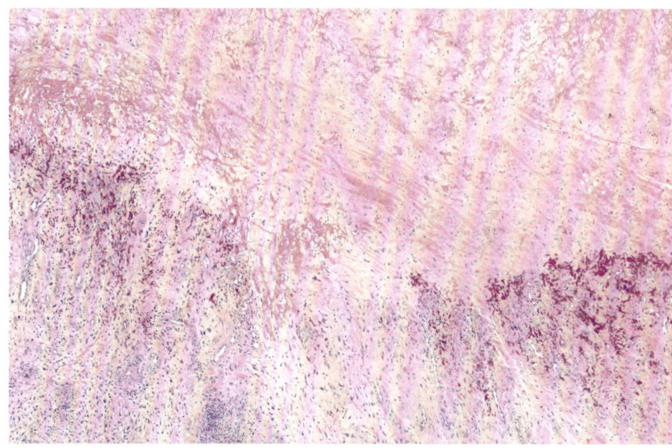

Fig. 4.24 Ischaemic fasciitis. Excisional biopsy demonstrating distinct zonation. The cellular region contains myxoid stroma with fibroblasts, myofibroblasts, vascular proliferation with hyalinosis of vessel walls, and extravasated erythrocytes. There is an adjacent region of hypocellular necrosis (H&E).

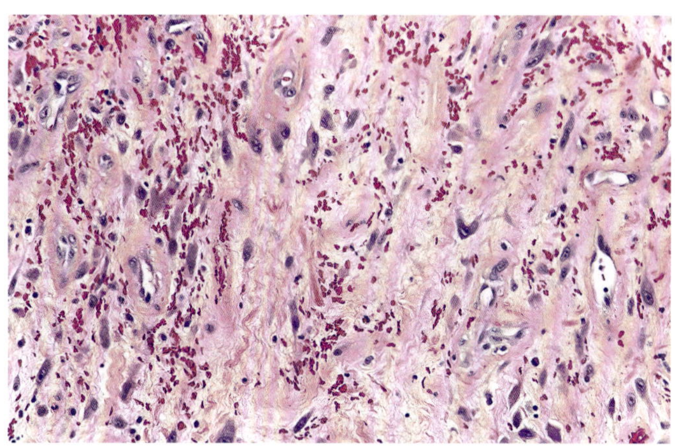

Fig. 4.25 Ischaemic fasciitis. The cellular region demonstrates myofibroblasts with morphology ranging from spindle to stellate or ganglion-like (H&E).

IgG4-related disease

Bongiovanni M

Definition

Immunoglobulin G4 (IgG4)-related disease (IgG4-RD) or IgG4-related sclerosing disease (IgG4-RSD) is a clinicopathological entity marked by IgG4-positive plasma cell infiltration and fibrosis in one or more organs.

Clinical features and imaging

Diagnosis of IgG4-RD requires the characteristic microscopic appearance along with an increased number of IgG4-positive plasma cells and an elevated IgG4:IgG plasma cell ratio in tissue {317}. IgG4-RD or IgG4-RSD most commonly affects middle-aged and elderly men. In FNAB, IgG4-RD is mostly encountered in the head and neck region, including the salivary glands, as well as in the lung, the pancreatobiliary tract, and the liver.

Patients generally present with symptoms referable to the formation of a mass that is increasing in volume and that is visible if superficial (e.g. in salivary gland) or that causes organ compression if deeply located (e.g. in the pancreas or in the hepatobiliary region). Fever and constitutional symptoms are uncommon {317,1137}.

Histopathology

Three major histopathological features are present: a dense lymphoplasmacytic infiltrate, fibrosis arranged at least focally in a storiform pattern, and obliterative phlebitis. The presence of two of these three features supports the diagnosis, and the dense lymphoplasmacytic infiltrate and storiform-type fibrosis are usually present. Phlebitis without obliteration of the lumen and an increased number of eosinophils may also be present {317}.

Key diagnostic cytopathological features

- Predominance of small lymphocytes with abundant plasma cells, a variable number of eosinophils, and sometimes macrophages
- Fibroblasts and myofibroblasts are intermingled with the inflammatory infiltrate
- Occasional tissue fragments showing irregularly arranged spindle cells may be present

Reference(s): {828,1137,142}

Discussion and differential diagnosis

A firm cytopathological diagnosis of IGg4-RD is not possible on cytomorphology and always requires ICC assessment of IgG and IgG4 positivity in the plasma cells and careful correlation with all clinical and imaging findings. FNAB of patients with IgG4-RD shows a prominent lymphoplasmacytic infiltrate. Smears almost never display storiform-type fibrosis or obliterative phlebitis, but these features may be present in cell blocks.

The differential diagnosis includes all other inflammatory processes that can develop with pseudonodular masses in superficial and deep locations. The presence of granulomas, giant cells, and abundant neutrophils suggests an inflammatory or infectious process and not IgG4-RD.

Ancillary testing

ICC to assess the number of IgG4-positive plasma cells and the IgG4:IgG plasma cell ratio is absolutely essential to support the diagnosis of IgG4-RD. The cut-off point for the number of IgG4-positive plasma cells per mm^2 varies between different organs; in small specimens, a cut-off point of > 4 IgG4-positive plasma cells per mm^2 has been proposed. In addition, an IgG4:IgG plasma cell ratio of > 40% has been proposed as a cut-off value in any organ. However, even if both cut-off values are exceeded, the diagnosis of IgG4-RD always requires careful correlation with all clinical and imaging findings {317}.

Lipoma

Monaco SE
Pantanowitz L

Definition
Lipomas are benign tumours composed of mature adipocytes.

Clinical features and imaging
Lipomas are the most common mesenchymal tumours. They present as painless lesions of variable size in the superficial soft tissue, within skeletal muscle, or rarely within visceral organs and bone. In large lesions or those in the deep retroperitoneum, an atypical lipomatous tumour / well-differentiated liposarcoma (ALT/WDLPS) must be excluded {192,1402}. Lipomas occur most commonly in adults aged 40–60 years and rarely in children, in whom lipomas and lipoblastoma represent < 10% of soft tissue tumours {1402}. Some lipoma subtypes are associated with characteristic findings or locations, such as spindle cell / pleomorphic lipomas, with a predilection for the posterior shoulder and neck {1538}, and angiolipomas, which are commonly painful and arise on the extremities {1286}. Rare familial cases or cases in genetic syndromes associated with lipomas or lipomatosis have been described, such as in Gardner syndrome and Madelung disease, in addition to cases associated with medications such as HAART for the treatment of HIV infection {397,99}. Patients with Dercum disease or adiposis dolorosa typically have multiple painful lipomas. On imaging, lipomas typically show a well-circumscribed uniform lesion outlined by a greater density of the soft tissue around the lesion. On CT, hypodense areas are typically indicative of a lipomatous tumour.

Histopathology
Lipomas are well-circumscribed lesions with uniform mature adipocytes displaying univacuolated clear cytoplasm and bland nuclei without appreciable nucleoli. Small thin- and thick-walled blood vessels can be identified, in addition to relatively thin fibrous septa. Various histopathological subtypes have been described, including spindle cell / pleomorphic, chondroid, angiolipoma, myolipoma, angiomyolipoma, myelolipoma, fibrolipoma, adenolipoma, ossifying, and myxolipoma. Lipoma subtype can also be defined by anatomical location, such as intramuscular lipoma.

Key diagnostic cytopathological features
- Variable cellularity
- Tissue fragments of mature adipocytes
- Uniform adipocytes contain a single large cytoplasmic clear vacuole and small nuclei with inconspicuous nucleoli
- Occasional histiocytes with multivacuolated cytoplasm (lipophages) may be seen with trauma or fat necrosis
- Floret-like giant cells can be seen in spindle cell / pleomorphic lipomas
- Metachromatic or myxoid matrix can be seen, especially in fibrolipomas or myxolipomas
- Blood vessel fibrin thrombi may be observed in angiolipomas, best seen in cell blocks
- Often have a bloody background with evidence of fat globules as small round open spaces in the stained background (Giemsa stain)

Reference(s): {675,1396,1398,1407,467}

Discussion and differential diagnosis
Although the diagnosis of a benign lipoma can be made on cytopathology, there should be careful investigation for atypical features, in addition to correlation with clinical and imaging features, before rendering such a diagnosis {675}.

The main differential diagnosis is fibroadipose tissue near another lesion of interest that has not been sampled, and

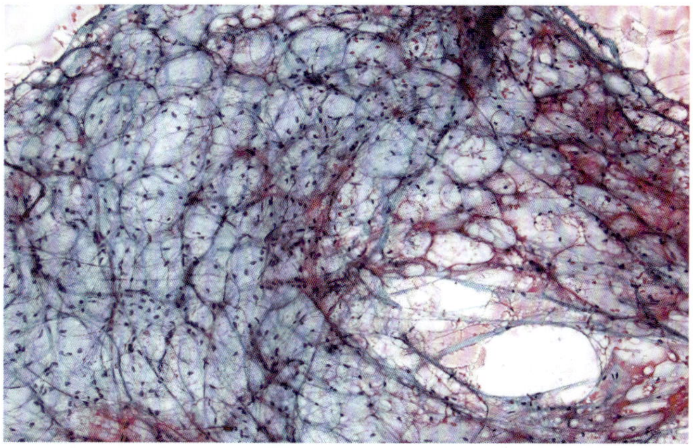

Fig. 4.26 Lipoma. A tissue fragment of mature fat consistent with a lipoma (Pap).

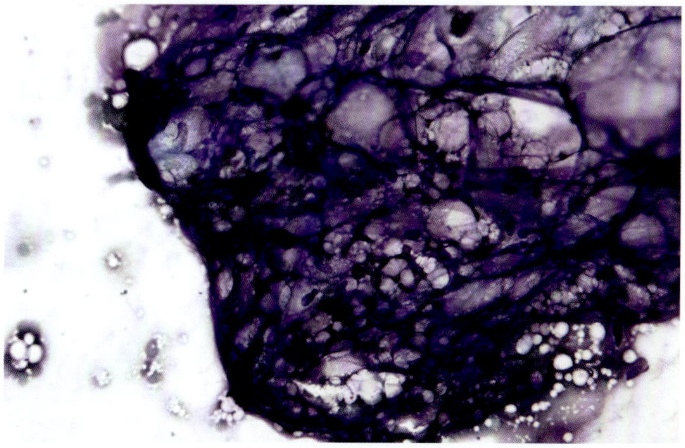

Fig. 4.27 Lipoma. A tissue fragment of fat from a lipoma, with some evidence of a degree of fat necrosis (Giemsa).

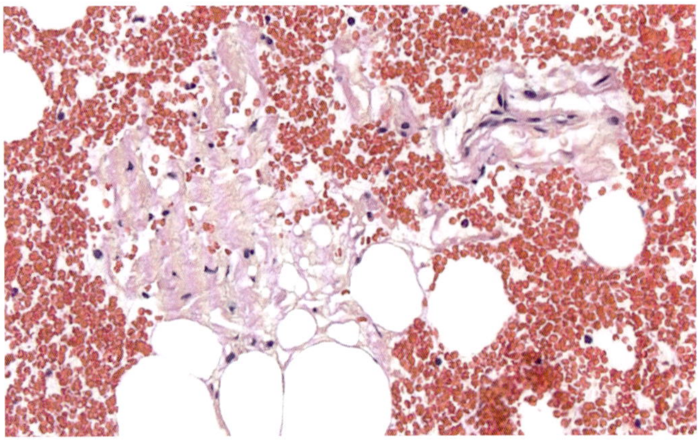

Fig. 4.28 Lipoma. Fragments of fat with small capillaries (cell block, H&E).

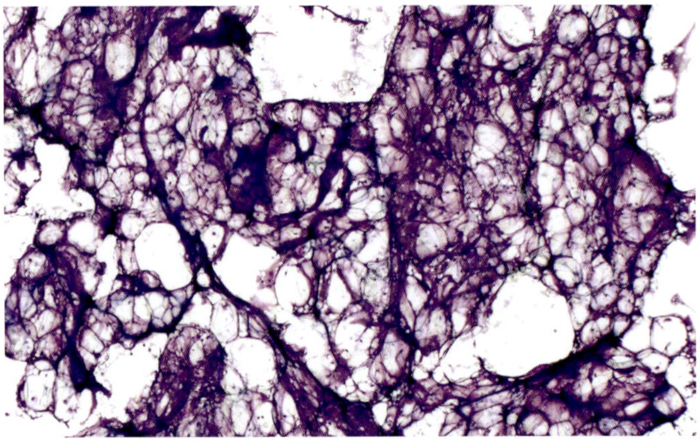

Fig. 4.29 Angiolipoma. Tissue fragments of mature adipocytes with prominent thin-walled branching vessels (Giemsa).

clinical and imaging correlation is mandatory. Fat necrosis, lipoblastoma, lipogranuloma, and hibernoma are other benign fat lesions to exclude. Fat necrosis shows tissue fragments of dead adipocytes lacking nuclei, with punctate debris and occasional histiocytes. Lipoblastoma often contains mature adipocytes and lipoblasts, and it is associated with myxoid stroma. Lipogranulomas consist of epithelioid histiocytes and vacuolated histiocytes containing fat, some multinucleated, with occasional lymphocytes. Histiocytic lesions such as xanthoma and xanthelasma and neoplasms and disorders such as Erdheim–Chester disease can also mimic lipomas, given they may exhibit only mild nuclear atypia and contain vacuolated cells {1136}. The distinction between lipomas and ALT/WDLPS relies on the site and imaging findings, although ALT/WDLPS may show a more

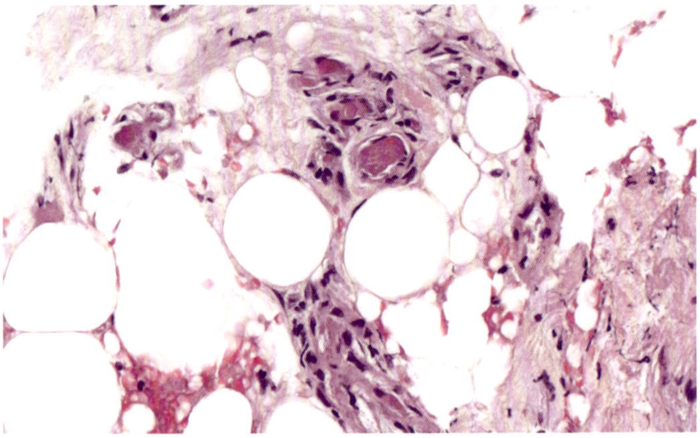

Fig. 4.30 Angiolipoma. Fat containing small blood vessels containing microthrombi (tissue section, H&E).

prominent fibrovascular pattern in tissue fragments and potentially multivacuolated and univacuolated lipoblasts with variably hyperchromatic nuclei. Spindle cell lipomas overlap with other spindle cell lesions of the soft tissue (e.g. myofibroblastoma and desmoid-type fibromatosis {1444,1402,1564}) and fat-forming or "lipomatous" solitary fibrous tumour {516}. Less common entities included in the differential diagnosis are silicon granuloma and neoplasms with clear cell features, such as signet-ring cell carcinoma, balloon cell melanoma, and perivascular epithelioid cell tumour (PEComa).

Ancillary testing

By ICC, lipomas are positive for S100. CD34 can be positive in spindle cell / pleomorphic lipomas, and it may highlight the thin-walled vasculature in routine lipomas. Most lipomas show abnormalities of chromosome 12, including trisomy 12, or structural rearrangements of *HMGA1* (chromosome 6p21-p23) or *HMGA2* (chromosome 12q13-q15). Less common alterations of chromosome 13 have been reported, including rearrangements in angiolipomas and deletions of chromosome 13q, which is more common in spindle cell lipomas. ICC showing nuclear PLAG1 positivity or *PLAG1* FISH studies can be helpful in the diagnosis of lipoblastomas, seen more commonly in children {841}. *MDM2* amplification is a feature of atypical lipomatous lesions, such as ALT/WDLPS and dedifferentiated liposarcoma, and it should be negative in lipomas {235}. Rare examples of MDM2 positivity in hibernomas have been reported {1427}. Specific markers such as STAT6 for solitary fibrous tumour can help exclude other tumours with lipoma-like features.

Hibernoma

Domanski HA
Bui M

Definition

Hibernoma is a rare, benign lipomatous tumour showing brown fat differentiation.

Clinical features and imaging

Hibernomas account for 1% of all adipocytic tumours and typically occur in young adults. Most cases present as a slow-growing, well-defined, painless subcutaneous mass in the thigh, back, upper trunk, head and neck, or upper extremities. Deep-seated hibernomas account for fewer than 10% of cases and occur in intra-abdominal, retroperitoneal, and intrathoracic locations {454,117,896}.

On MRI, classic hibernomas are slightly hypointense, and lipoma-like hibernomas are isointense to subcutaneous fat on T1-weighted images. On T2-weighted MRI, high signal intensity is typical. Hibernomas display marked or moderate lack of homogeneity, with prominent septa and vascular structures {1186,723,833}. Hibernomas are easily detectable on PET because they contain abundant mitochondria and are highly metabolically active {89,723}.

Histopathology

Classic hibernomas are composed of three cell types in varying proportions: large brown fat cells with finely vacuolated and eosinophilic granular cytoplasm and small bland central nuclei, mature adipocytes, and vacuolated lipoblast-like cells. Most hibernomas have a prominent capillary network. Subtypes include the lipoma-like and rare myxoid and spindle cell subtypes {454,117}. Hibernomas mimicking atypical lipomatous tumour have been reported, but nuclear atypia and mitoses are absent {46}.

Key diagnostic cytopathological features

- Moderate to high cellularity
- Tissue fragments and sheets of polygonal and oval cells with abundant cytoplasm
- Brown fat hibernoma cells with microvacuolated and granular cytoplasm and small, uniform central nuclei
- Mix of areas of regular adipocytes and areas of round brown fat cells
- Numerous capillaries
- Rare lipoblast-like cells with univacuolated or multivacuolated clear cytoplasm

Discussion and differential diagnosis

The differential diagnosis includes atypical lipomatous tumour / well-differentiated liposarcoma, lipoma with regressive changes, adult rhabdomyoma, granular cell tumour, and fat necrosis. The centrally located, small, bland nucleus helps to distinguish multivacuolated brown fat cells from atypical lipoblasts containing hyperchromatic, irregular, and scalloped nuclei {812,1394, 1235,352,1476}. Hibernomas with a large proportion of mature

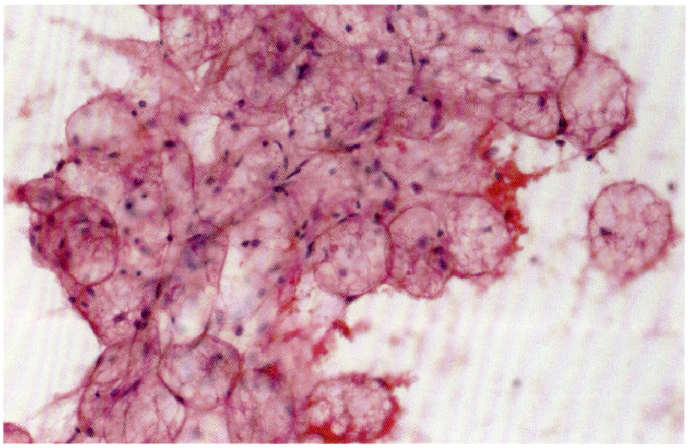

Fig. 4.31 Hibernoma. A tissue fragment of polygonal brown fat cells with vacuolated cytoplasm and centrally placed small uniform nuclei, along with delicate capillaries (H&E).

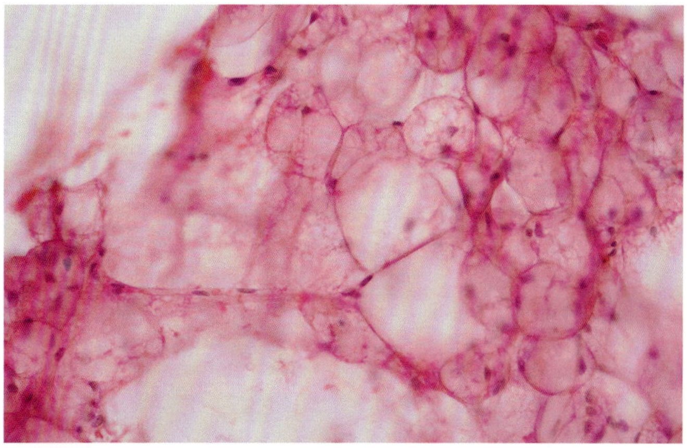

Fig. 4.32 Hibernoma. Hibernoma cells intermingled with mature adipocytes, which is commonly seen (H&E).

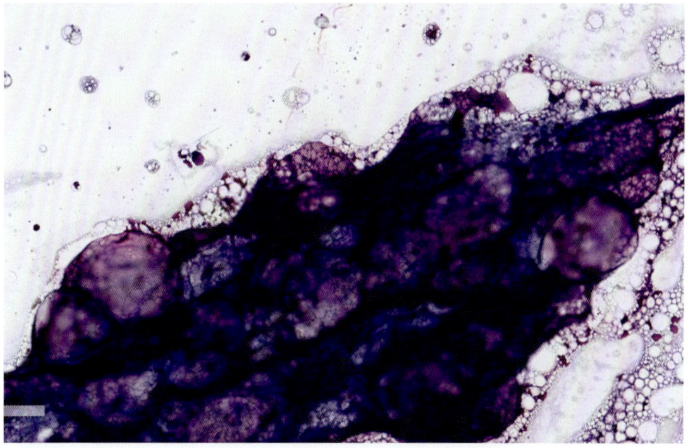

Fig. 4.33 Hibernoma. A tissue fragment of polygonal brown fat cells with abundant vacuolated cytoplasm (Giemsa).

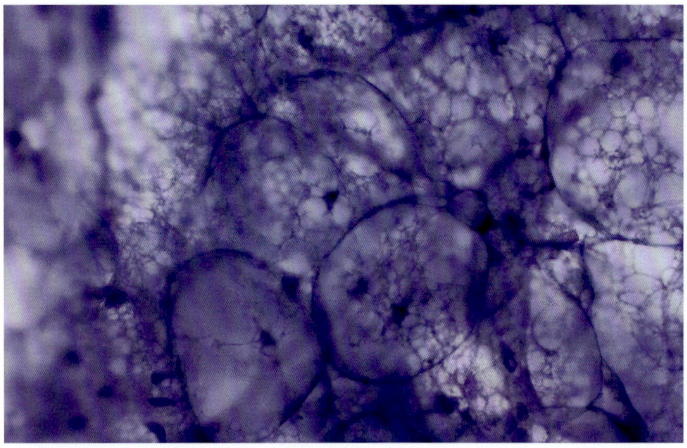

Fig. 4.34 Hibernoma. Brown fat cells with abundant vacuolated cytoplasm and centrally placed small uniform nuclei (Giemsa).

adipocytes, histiocytes, and lipophages resembling brown fat can be wrongly diagnosed as common lipoma {812,352}. Granular cell tumour and adult rhabdomyoma display a granular rather than microvacuolated cytoplasm and lack adipocytic differentiation {352}.

Ancillary testing

There is no distinctive ICC for hibernomas. Most hibernomas are characterized by recurrent genetic changes involving structural rearrangements of 11q13 {860,1031} resulting in *MEN1* and *AIP* codeletion {1031}.

Lipoblastoma

Teot LA

Definition

Lipoblastoma is a benign neoplasm of embryonal white fat, which may be a localized or diffuse tumour, with a tendency for local recurrence if incompletely excised.

Clinical features and imaging

More than 90% of lipoblastomas occur in children aged < 5 years {226,241}. Tumours vary from superficial and circumscribed to deep and infiltrative, and they most often arise in the trunk and extremities. Ultrasonography of superficial lipoblastoma reveals a septate, hyperechoic mass. On T1-weighted images, MRI demonstrates a lobular, septate mass comprising fat similar to or lower than mature fat in intensity, as well as non-adipose soft tissue elements, with or without compartmental invasion {1156,965,301}.

Histopathology

Lipoblastoma is made up of adipocytes arrayed in lobules, separated by fibrovascular septa, and myxoid areas with primitive mesenchymal cells and plexiform vasculature {226,252,561, 241}. The neoplastic cells span a continuum from primitive stellate or spindle cells, to multivacuolated or signet-ring lipoblasts, to mature adipocytes {226,252,561,241}.

Key diagnostic cytopathological features

- Hypocellular to moderate cellularity
- Fragments of fat with delicate branching vessels
- Variable proportions of mature adipocytes admixed with multivacuolated and signet-ring lipoblasts
- Variably prominent myxoid matrix with spindle cells and naked oval nuclei
- Spindle cells with moderate, pale, basophilic cytoplasm and monomorphic ovoid nuclei with fine chromatin and distinct nucleoli
- Absent or minimal atypia among spindle cells
- No mitoses or necrosis

Reference(s): {741,407,21}

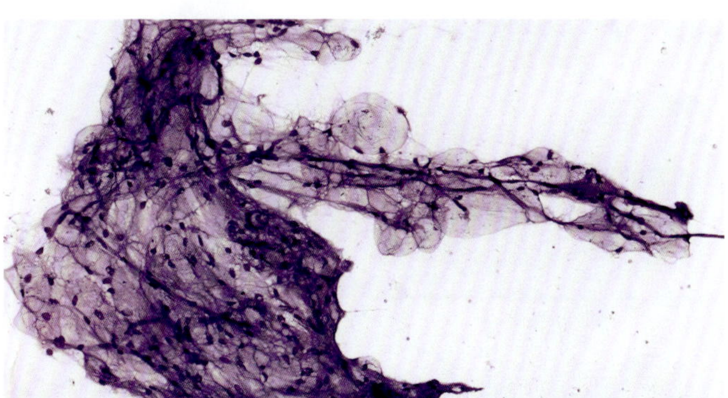

Fig. 4.35 Lipoblastoma. A tissue fragment with delicate branching vessels and multivacuolated lipoblasts admixed with mature adipocytes (Giemsa).

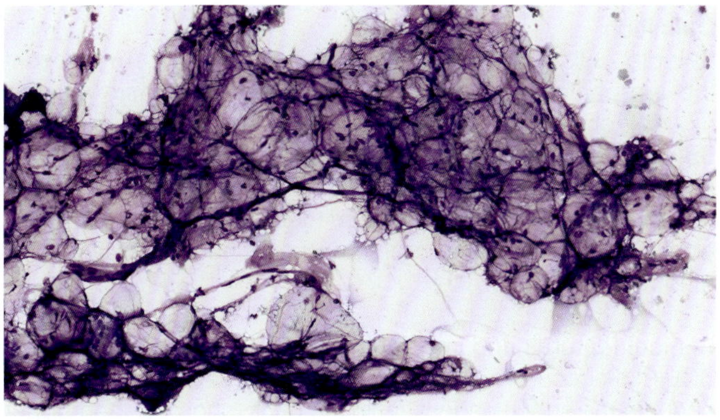

Fig. 4.36 Lipoblastoma. A tissue fragment consisting of multivacuolated lipoblasts, mature adipocytes, and scattered spindle cells. Scant myxoid matrix is present in the background (Giemsa).

Discussion and differential diagnosis

Mature lipoblastoma can mimic lipoma, but the myxoid matrix, spindle cells, and delicate vessels are clues to the correct diagnosis {741,407,21}. Predominantly myxoid lipoblastoma can be confused with myxoid liposarcoma, although that entity is exceedingly rare in the first decade of life. In contrast to myxoid liposarcoma, lipoblastoma lacks primitive small round cells, nuclear atypia, mitoses, and necrosis {741,407,21}. The new entity "lipoblastoma-like tumour" has been added in the forthcoming sixth-edition WHO classification of soft tissue and bone tumours, and its FNAB cytopathology awaits further studies.

Ancillary testing

Approximately 70% of lipoblastomas harbour *PLAG1* gene rearrangements detectable by FISH or other molecular methods {559,488,273}. Tumours show nuclear staining of spindle and some fat cells for PLAG1 {890}, as well as cytoplasmic staining of spindle cells for desmin {759}. These features help to distinguish lipoblastoma from lipoma and myxoid liposarcoma.

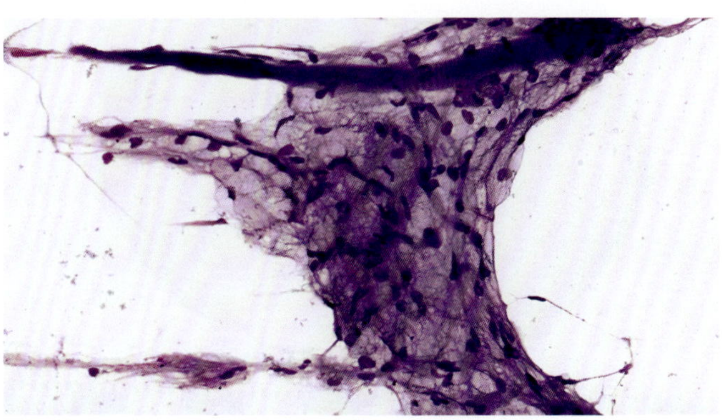

Fig. 4.37 Lipoblastoma. A tissue fragment showing occasional multivacuolated lipoblasts with small vacuoles of various sizes, some indenting the nuclei (Giemsa).

Spindle cell / pleomorphic lipoma

Domanski HA
Qian X

Definition

Spindle cell and pleomorphic lipomas (SCL/PLs) represent the morphological spectrum of a single neoplasm sharing distinct clinical, ICC, molecular, and prognostic features. Spindle cell lipoma (SCL) is a benign adipocytic tumour composed of variable amounts of mature adipocytes, bland spindle cells, and ropy collagen. Pleomorphic lipoma (PL) in addition contains pleomorphic and multinucleated floret-like giant cells.

Clinical features and imaging

SCL/PLs account for 1.5% of adipocytic neoplasms {423}. Most occur in the subcutaneous fat in the neck, shoulder, and upper back of middle-aged to elderly patients, particularly men {383, 1301,64,423}. Less common locations include the face, scalp, orbit, oral cavity, tongue, limbs, and trunk {383,64,423,195, 1432}. Rarely, dermal and intramuscular locations have been reported {1432,443}.

SCL/PLs present as a well-circumscribed, subcutaneous mass with variable imaging appearances depending on the proportions of adipose and non-adipose components {700}. Occasionally, the presence of minimal or no intralesional macroscopic fat may make them difficult to recognize on imaging {632,718,1543}.

Histopathology

SCL/PLs are composed of variable amounts of bland spindle cells, mature adipose tissue, and ropy collagen bundles in a fibrotic or fibromyxoid stroma {383,64,423}. PLs contain a component of pleomorphic spindle cells and multinucleated

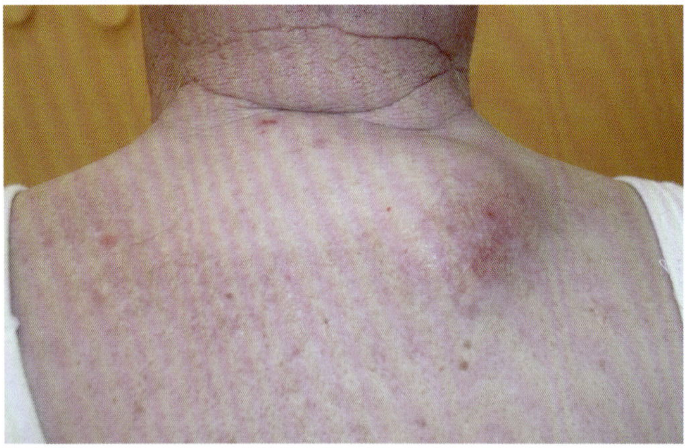

Fig. 4.38 Spindle cell lipoma. Spindle cell lipoma presenting as a subcutaneous mass in the posterior neck.

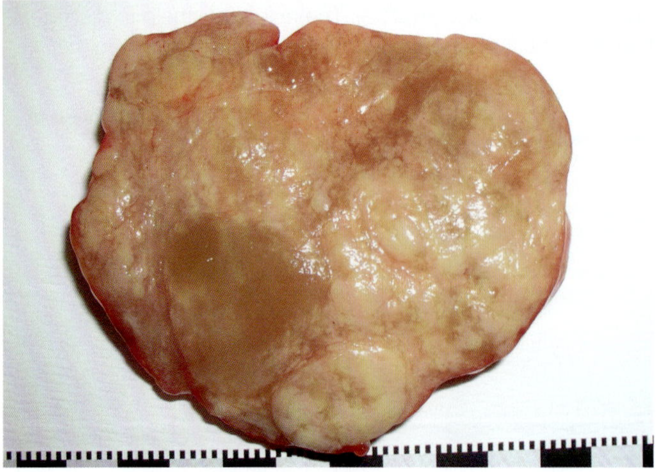

Fig. 4.39 Spindle cell lipoma. A resection specimen with a variable yellow, greyish-brown, and myxoid cut surface.

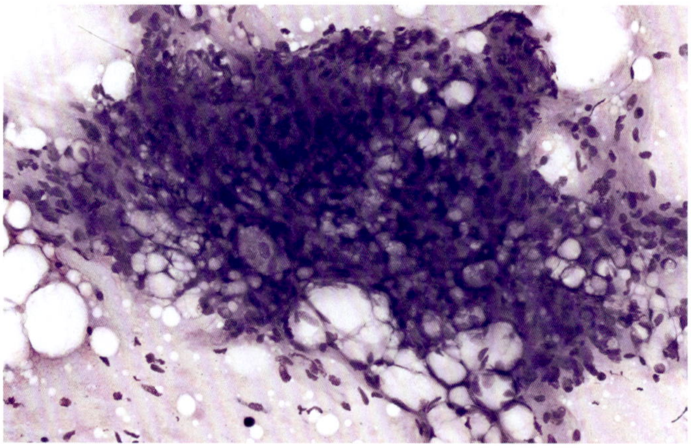

Fig. 4.40 Spindle cell lipoma. A tissue fragment consisting of adipocytes separated by spindle cell regions. There is a suggestion of a finely granular background (Giemsa).

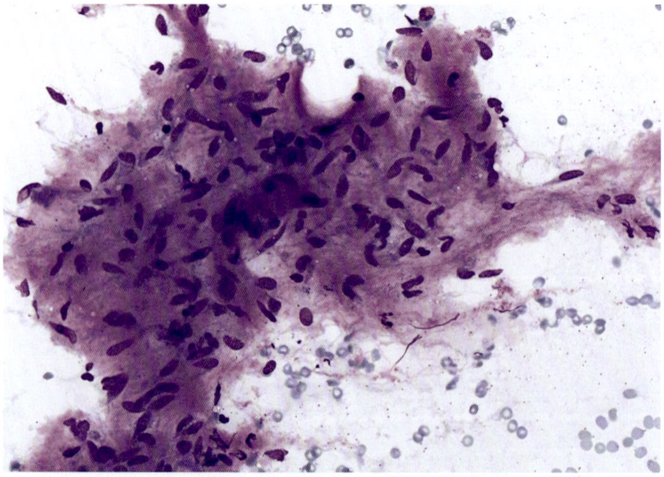

Fig. 4.41 Spindle cell lipoma. A tissue fragment consisting of spindle cells having bland spindle and wavy nuclei (Giemsa).

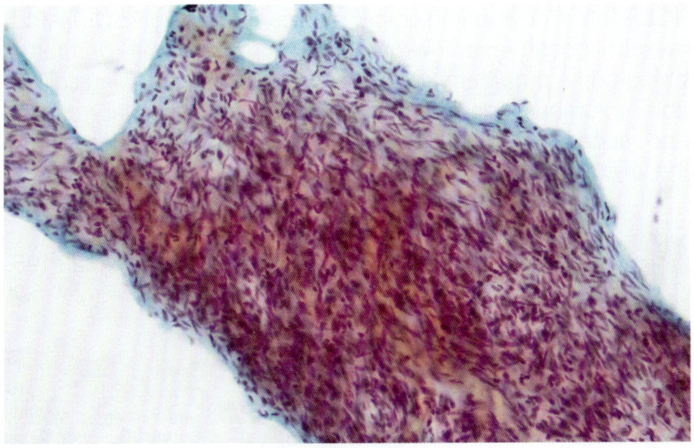

Fig. 4.42 Spindle cell lipoma. A tissue fragment of the fat-poor subtype of spindle cell lipoma, consisting of uniform spindle cells (LBC, Pap).

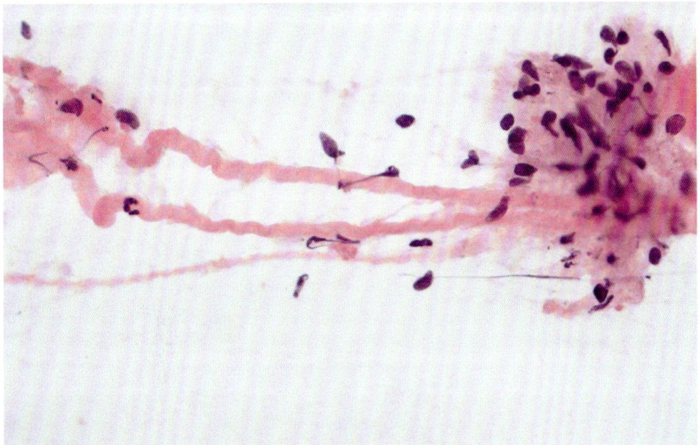

Fig. 4.43 Spindle cell lipoma. Long and narrow collagen fibres attached to a tissue fragment of spindle cells (H&E).

floret-like giant cells. Mast cells are common findings, and lipoblasts may be seen in a subset of cases, while mitoses are very rare and necrosis absent. Histopathological subtypes include fat-poor {135,1218}, myxoid {1515,206}, (pseudo)angiomatous {548,206}, and plexiform {1552} SCL/PLs. Focal cartilaginous and/or osseous metaplasia {423} and/or extramedullary haematopoiesis {1269} can be present.

Key diagnostic cytopathological features

- Cellularity varies, from scant to moderate to occasionally high
- Mix of mature fat tissue fragments and bland spindle cells seen in small tissue fragments or singly
- Fragments of brightly eosinophilic (on H&E staining) hyaline collagen fibres
- Occasional myxoid background
- Occasional fragments of capillaries or capillary network
- Mast cells, particularly in smears with myxoid background
- Variable number of floret cells and pleomorphic epithelioid / polygonal / spindle cells with smudged chromatin in pleomorphic lipoma
- Rarely lipoblasts

Reference(s): {347,341,20,284,701,1046,816,531,524,95,684,18,842,1538,207,1396,97,1222}

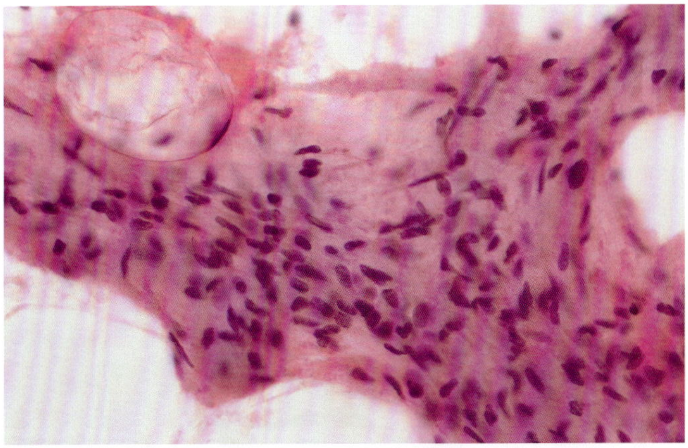

Fig. 4.44 Spindle cell lipoma. A tissue fragment showing a small number of adipocytes and predominantly spindle cells (H&E).

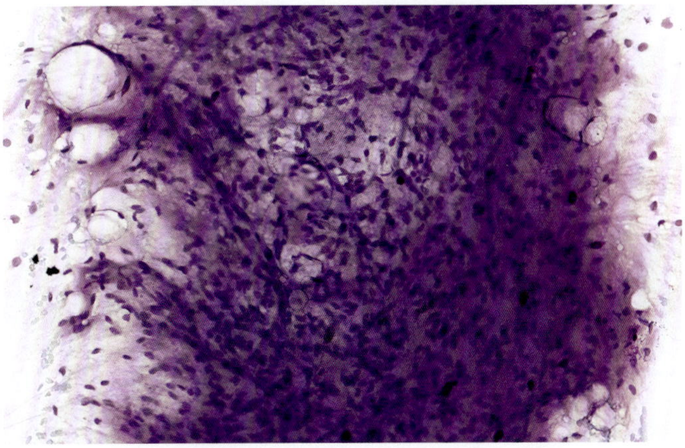

Fig. 4.45 Spindle cell lipoma. A tissue fragment of myxoid spindle cell lipoma resembling myxoid liposarcoma, with myxoid background matrix and small capillaries (Giemsa).

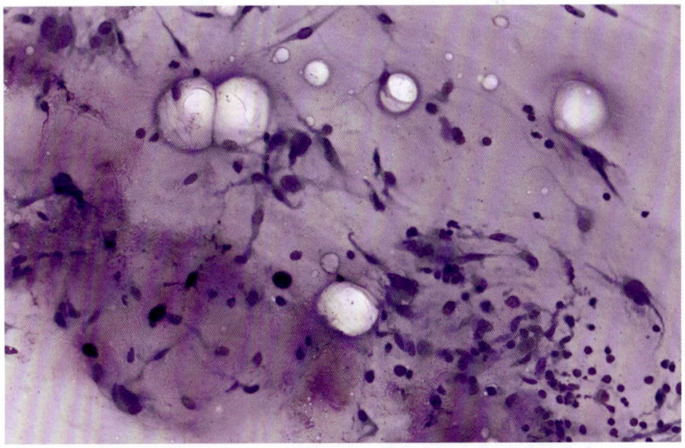

Fig. 4.46 Pleomorphic lipoma. A mixture of mature fat, floret cells, and spindle cells with bland elongated nuclei, in a prominent myxoid background matrix (Giemsa).

Discussion and differential diagnosis

The differential diagnosis of SCL/PL includes a variety of spindle cell, pleomorphic, and myxoid soft tissue tumours, because of the variable proportions of spindle cells, fat, and collagen; the presence of a myxoid background and floret cells; and the occasional presence of pleomorphic epithelioid or polygonal or spindle cells and lipoblasts. Atypical spindle cell / pleomorphic lipomatous tumours (ASCLT/APLTs) share most histopathological features with SCL and PL {798,878,926,266,899}, and they appear indistinguishable in cytopathological smears, but increased cytopathological atypia of nuclei on smears should prompt consideration of ASCLT/APLT. The differentiation of SCL/PL from cytopathological mimics, including ASCLT/APLT, myxoid liposarcoma, low-grade myxofibrosarcoma, dermatofibrosarcoma protuberans, schwannoma, and fat-forming solitary fibrous tumour, generally requires the use of ancillary studies and access to clinical and imaging findings. Smears from the myxoid variant of SCL/PL lack the thick-walled vessels of

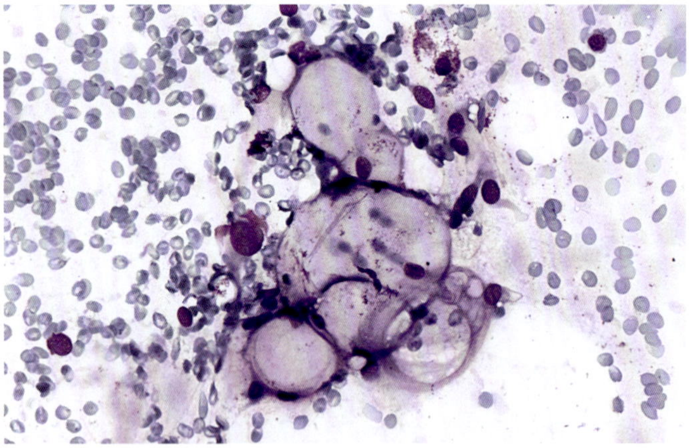

Fig. 4.47 Pleomorphic lipoma. Adipocytes and occasional mononuclear cells showing enlarged nuclei with smudged chromatin (Giemsa).

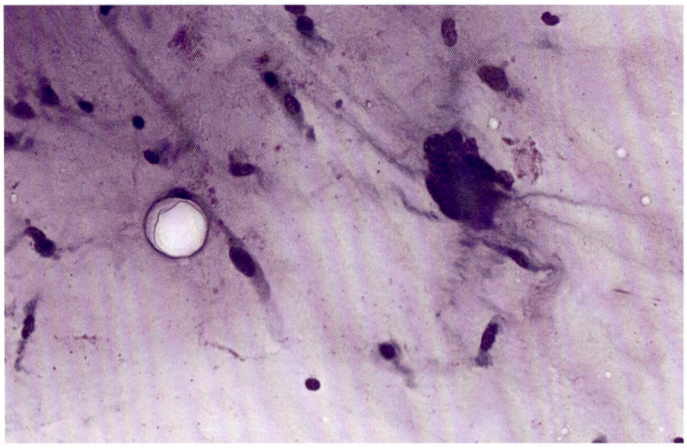

Fig. 4.48 Pleomorphic lipoma. Spindle cells with elongated nuclei and a floret cell in a prominent myxoid matrix (Giemsa).

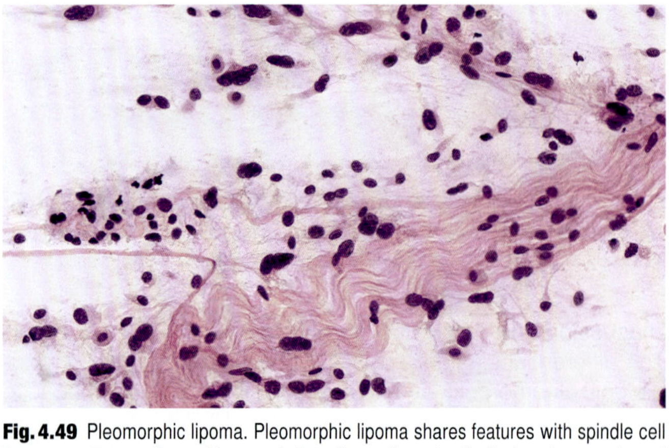

Fig. 4.49 Pleomorphic lipoma. Pleomorphic lipoma shares features with spindle cell lipoma, such as collagen fibres, spindle cells, and mast cells; it also shows enlarged nuclei and floret cells (at 12 o'clock in this image) (H&E).

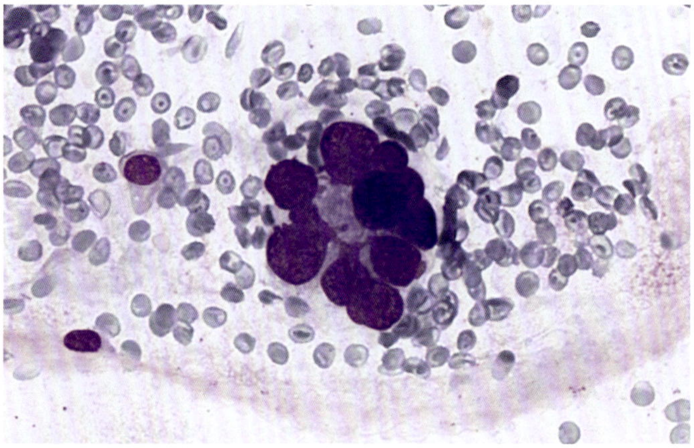

Fig. 4.50 Pleomorphic lipoma. A floret cell with multiple, relatively uniform nuclei (Giemsa).

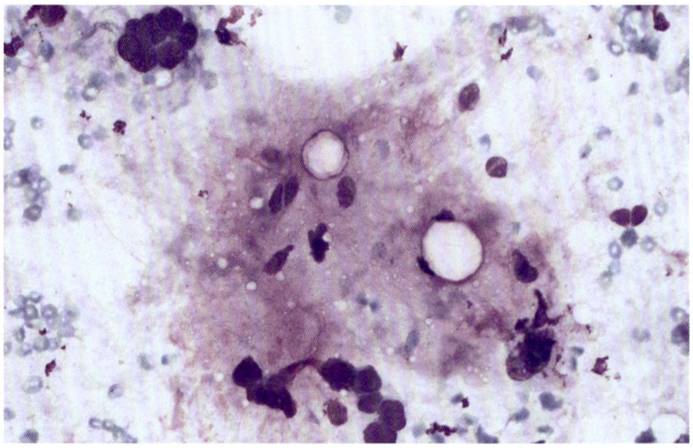

Fig. 4.51 Atypical spindle cell / pleomorphic lipomatous tumour. Occasional mature fat cells mixed with floret cells and single spindle or epithelioid cells with enlarged nuclei resembling smears of pleomorphic lipoma (Giemsa).

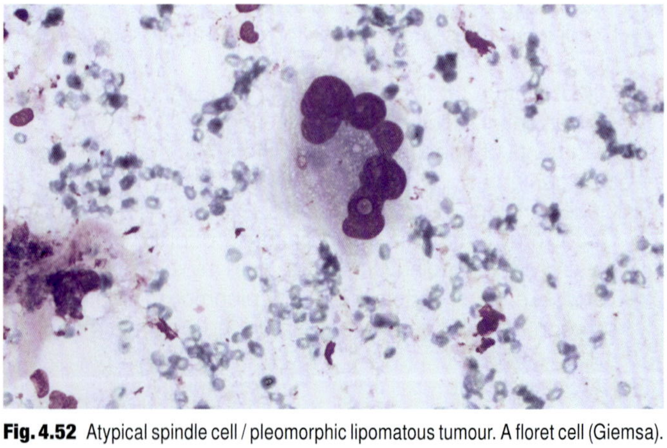

Fig. 4.52 Atypical spindle cell / pleomorphic lipomatous tumour. A floret cell (Giemsa).

myxofibrosarcoma. The presence of hyaline collagen fibres, in variable amounts from case to case, is an important clue for the diagnosis of SCL/PL {347}. The clinical presentation of dermatofibrosarcoma protuberans differs from that of SCL/PL, and there is a lack of collagen fibres in smears.

Ancillary testing

By ICC, the spindle cells are positive for CD34 and often BCL2. Demonstration of loss of the *RB1* locus and/or RB1 protein expression can support the diagnosis in selected cases {278, 113,206,820}. Detection of *DDIT3* rearrangement in myxoid liposarcoma and presence of cytopathological atypia in ASCLT/APLT help distinguish them from SCL/PL. Positivity for CD34 and negativity for S100 helps to exclude schwannoma, and negativity for STAT6 helps to exclude fat-forming solitary fibrous tumour.

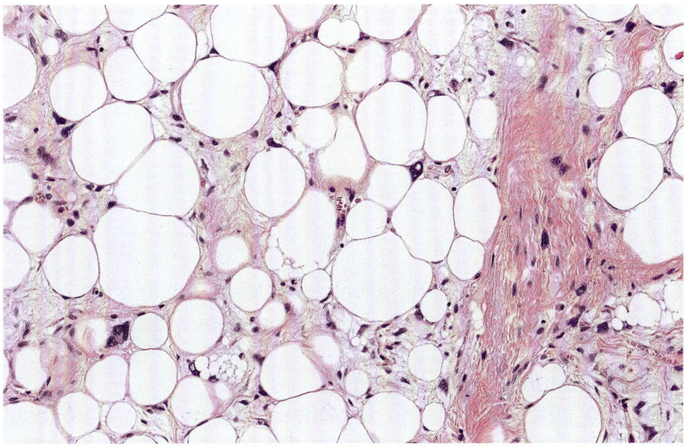

Fig. 4.53 Atypical spindle cell / pleomorphic lipomatous tumour. Adipocytes, atypical spindle cells, multinucleated floret cells, and a collagenous region (H&E).

Chapter 4

Ganglion cyst

Qian X

Definition
Ganglion cyst is a degenerative cystic lesion most often occurring in the periarticular fibrous tissue or synovium.

Clinical features and imaging
Ganglion cysts present as a palpable lesion, with or without associated pain, and occur most commonly in the hands, wrists, knees, ankles, and feet. They have a predilection for females and often occur between the ages of 20 and 40 years, but they have also been described in paediatric patients and in the elderly. On MRI, ganglion cysts appear as homogeneous, lobulated masses originating from tendons, ligaments, tendon sheaths, menisci, or joint capsules. Ultrasound shows a hypoechoic mass showing continuity with the adjacent joint capsule or adjacent soft tissue, without significant vascularity on colour Doppler {931,1479,1388}.

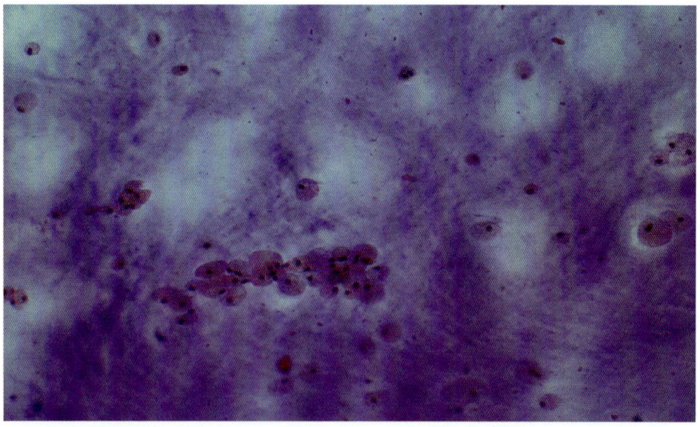

Fig. 4.54 Ganglion cyst. Hypocellular smears contain scattered histiocytes, some in small loose clusters, in a background of abundant granular myxoid matrix (Giemsa).

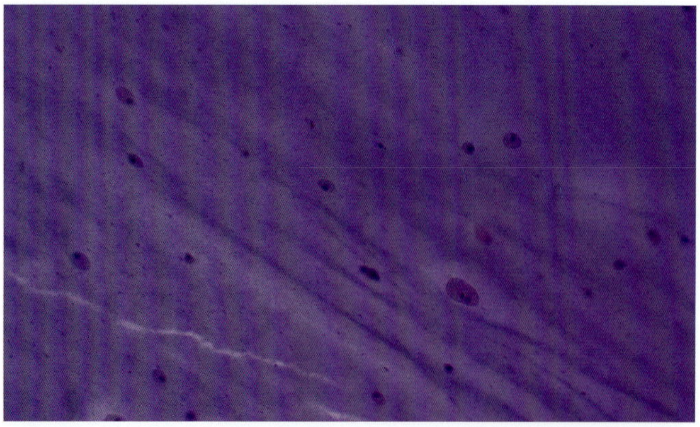

Fig. 4.55 Ganglion cyst. The copious myxoid matrix material stains a striking blue-violet on Giemsa.

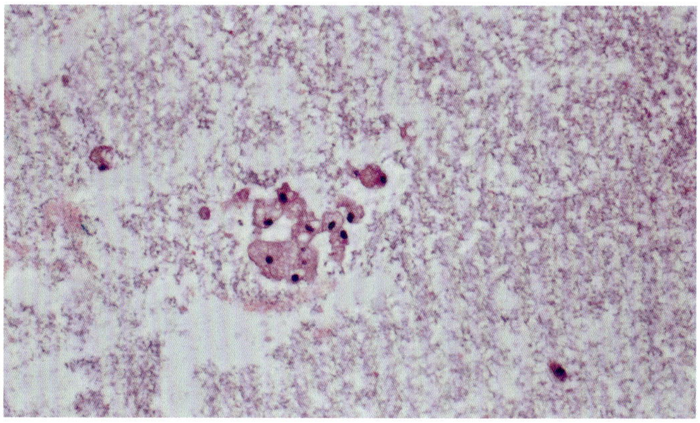

Fig. 4.56 Ganglion cyst. Cell block sections show similar histiocytes with abundant vacuolated cytoplasm in a background of granular amorphous matrix material (H&E).

Histopathology
Ganglion cysts are characteristically unilocular or multilocular cysts or clefts within degenerative capsular or tendinous tissue. No cyst-lining cells are present. The cystic mucoid material is usually not apparent in postfixation, embedded, and sectioned slides {331,1080}.

Key diagnostic cytopathological features
- Extremely low cellularity
- Abundant granular myxoid background material with variable consistency
- Isolated bland histiocytes with oval nuclei and granular to foamy cytoplasm
- Lack of any vasculature

Reference(s): {330,331,785,1241}

Discussion and differential diagnosis
FNAB produces viscous mucoid material, which is often difficult to expel from the FNAB needle.

Given their periarticular location, ganglion cysts closely resemble synovial cysts and juxta-articular myxoma on imaging. Synovial cysts represent true herniation of the synovial membrane through the joint capsule; they more commonly occur in association with cranial and lumbar spine joints, and smears may contain synovial cells. In addition to abundant myxoid material on smears, juxta-articular myxomas show scattered loose tissue fragments of bland spindle cells with long cytoplasmic processes, which are absent in ganglion cysts {1080,785}.

Ancillary testing
Synovial cells can be highlighted by D2-40 ICC; they are also positive for CD163, as are histiocytes.

Intramuscular myxoma and juxta-articular myxoma

Qian X
Bui M

Definition

Intramuscular myxoma is a benign hypocellular soft tissue neoplasm composed of bland spindle cells embedded in a usually abundant myxoid and hypovascular stroma. Juxta-articular myxoma typically arises in the vicinity of a large joint and lacks *GNAS* mutation.

Clinical features and imaging

Patients usually present with a painless, slowly growing soft tissue mass involving the muscles of the thigh, shoulder, buttocks, and upper arm, typically in adults aged 40–70 years, with a female predominance {381,546}. On MRI, the tumours are well circumscribed with slightly lobulated edges, and they are homogeneously hypointense on T1-weighted images and extremely hyperintense on T2-weighted images {91,1103}. Most intramuscular myxomas are sporadic, but a minority present as multiple lesions and are associated with fibrous dysplasia of bone, a condition called Mazabraud syndrome {616,861}.

Histopathology

Intramuscular myxoma is composed of uniform, bland spindle to stellate cells separated by abundant extracellular, hypovascular myxoid stroma. At the periphery, infiltration of tumour cells into surrounding skeletal muscle fibres is often present, which should not be mistaken for a sign of malignancy. Areas may show increased cellularity and slightly conspicuous capillary to occasional thick-walled, poorly formed short "stubby" vessels; if this pattern is predominant, the diagnosis of "cellular myxoma" may be rendered. Cytopathological atypia such as nuclear pleomorphism and hyperchromasia, mitoses, and necrosis are absent {943,1021,1443}.

Key diagnostic cytopathological features

- Low cellularity
- Abundant smooth or granular myxoid matrix, best seen on Giemsa smears
- Absent or very scant vascular component
- Uniform cells with long fibrillary cytoplasmic processes and single oval nuclei with uniform chromatin and inconspicuous nucleoli
- Loose tissue fragments of spindle cells and occasional short stubby vessels in cellular myxoma
- Absence of cytopathological atypia, mitoses, or necrosis

Reference(s): {1532,1465,785}

Discussion and differential diagnosis

The differential diagnosis of intramuscular myxoma is broad and includes any soft tissue tumour that may show hypocellular myxoid material and low-grade spindle cells, including ganglion cyst, juxta-articular myxoma, nodular fasciitis, soft tissue perineurioma with prominent myxoid stroma, low-grade myxofibrosarcoma, low-grade fibromyxoid sarcoma, and myxoid liposarcoma with pulmonary oedema-like areas {1532,1465,785}.

Ganglion cyst is a degenerative soft tissue lesion that commonly occurs in the hands and wrists as a result of trauma. It contains only abundant granular myxoid material and occasional histiocytes, and it lacks the spindle, stellate, myxoma cells {330, 331}. Juxta-articular myxoma is a benign myxoid lesion arising adjacent to large joints. Although morphologically resembling intramuscular or cellular myxoma, juxta-articular myxoma appears to occur commonly in men and lacks *GNAS* mutations {1045}. The distinction between soft tissue perineurioma with its slenderer perineural cells and intramuscular/cellular myxoma is difficult and relies on ICC. Both myxofibrosarcoma and myxoid liposarcoma have a more complex vascular component, and low-grade myxofibrosarcoma and low-grade fibromyxoid sarcoma have more notable nuclear atypia.

Ancillary testing

ICC is not helpful to establish the diagnosis of intramuscular myxoma, but it is essential to exclude its mimics. Tumour cells are consistently negative for MUC4 and may be positive for CD34, EMA, and rarely SMA {1532,785}. Soft tissue perineurioma expresses EMA and claudin-1, allowing distinction from intramuscular myxomas. Many intramuscular myxomas harbour activating mutations in codon 201 of *GNAS*, which can be detected by NGS and can be diagnostically helpful in distinguishing cellular myxoma from low-grade myxofibrosarcoma {303,1508,1362}.

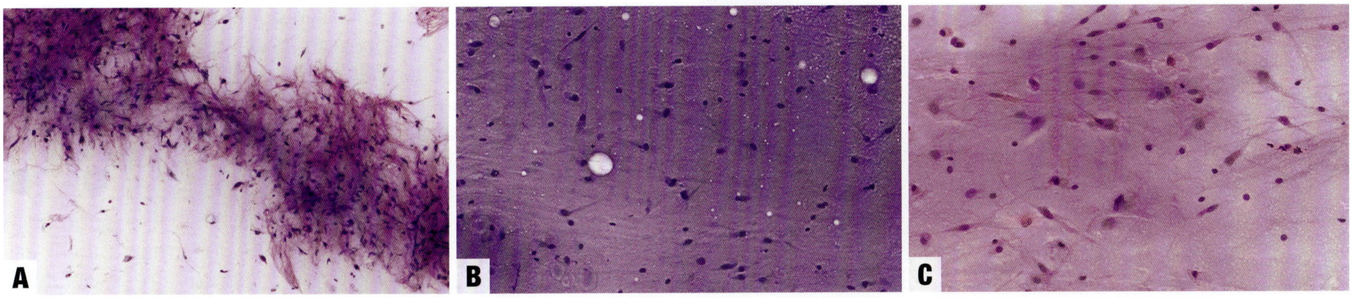

Fig. 4.57 Intramuscular myxoma. **A** Spindle cells with fine, delicate, elongated cytoplasm in a myxoid background (Pap). **B** Spindle cells with fine, elongated cytoplasm and oval nuclei in a myxoid background (Giemsa). **C** Spindle cells with elongated, thin cytoplasm and oval nuclei with fine, even chromatin in a myxoid background (H&E).

Fibromatosis

Domanski HA
Dodd LG

Definition

Fibromatosis is a locally aggressive but non-metastasizing fibroblastic and myofibroblastic neoplasm with an infiltrative growth pattern and propensity for local recurrence.

Clinical features and imaging

Superficial fibromatoses, such as palmar and plantar fibromatoses, occur in the hands and feet {1350}. Deep desmoid-type fibromatoses commonly arise in the deep soft tissues of the extremities, abdominal and chest walls, breast, retroperitoneum, and abdominal cavity, and less commonly in the head and neck and paraspinal regions {1023,1224,261}. The FNAB findings in these lesions are the same, and therefore they are presented together in this section.

Palmar fibromatosis, also known as Dupuytren contracture, tends to grow slowly and to manifest as one or more nodules of firm tissue leading to induration and in some instances contracture of the volar aspect of the hand and fingers. Plantar fibromatosis causes deformation of the plantar aspect of the feet; the changes are relatively less severe than those associated with palmar fibromatosis, but they can cause significant pain. Abdominal wall lesions referred to as desmoid tumours are typically centred on the rectus musculature and often develop in peripartum women. Intra-abdominal forms of fibromatosis occur within the pelvis, in the mesentery, and very rarely in the pancreas {478,930,1353}.

Both forms of fibromatosis occur in a wide age range, predominantly in young and middle-aged adults, although they can also occur in infants and children {163,910,238}. Women are twice as likely to be affected as men {1157}. Paediatric patients presenting with a desmoid tumour should be evaluated for adenomatous polyposis coli, because this is often the first sign of an inherited syndrome involving mutation of the *APC* gene.

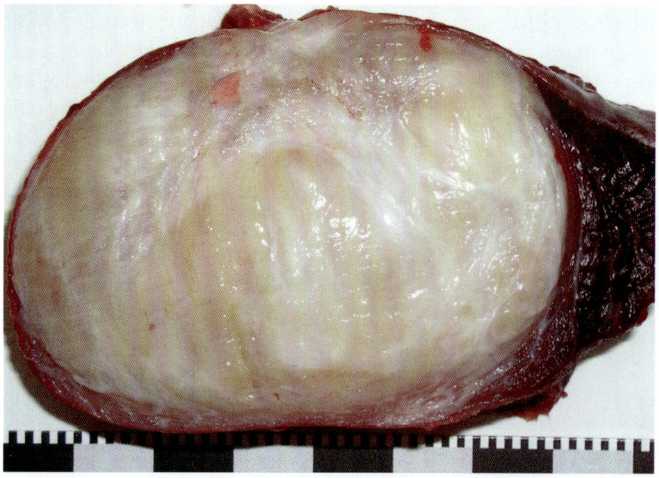

Fig. 4.58 Desmoid fibromatosis. Gross examination reveals a firm, glistening greyish-white and yellowish cut surface, with infiltration into surrounding skeletal muscle.

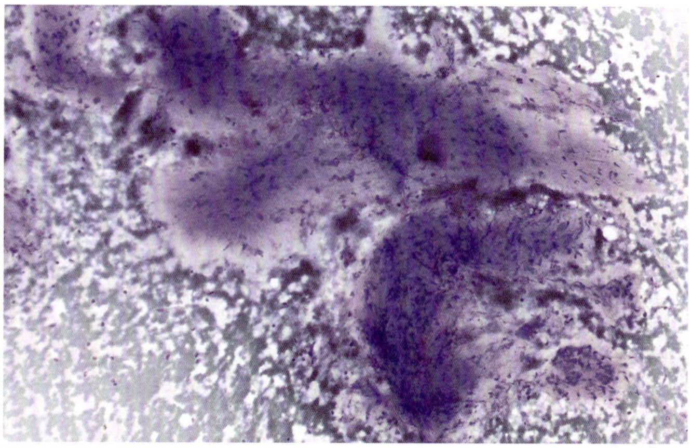

Fig. 4.59 Desmoid fibromatosis. Tissue fragments of metachromatic matrix with scattered, embedded, poorly visualized spindle cells (Giemsa).

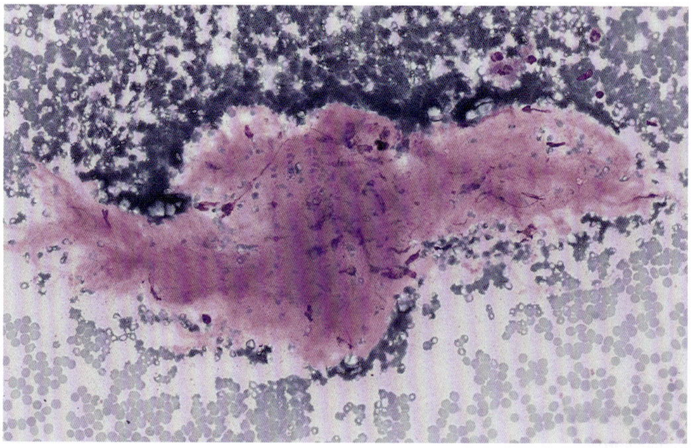

Fig. 4.60 Desmoid fibromatosis. A tissue fragment of nonspecific hypocellular connective tissue and scant spindle cells (Giemsa).

Desmoid fibromatoses may occur sporadically or in association with familial adenomatous polyposis, a variant of which is known as Gardner syndrome. An estimated 10–20% of desmoid tumours occur in association with familial adenomatous polyposis {395}. Patients with Gardner syndrome have germline mutations of the *APC* tumour suppressor gene, whereas patients with sporadic cases most often have point mutations of the gene that encodes for β-catenin (*CTNNB1*). Dysregulation of the β-catenin/WNT regulation pathway results in abnormal β-catenin accumulation in both the cytoplasm and nucleus of the tumours cells, as well as increased cellular proliferation {829,636}.

The imaging features of fibromatosis, both the superficial and deep subtypes, are nonspecific. Lesions may appear circumscribed or ill defined. MRI signal intensity on T2-weighted imaging varies depending on the relative overall cellularity of the lesion {1299,801,1016}.

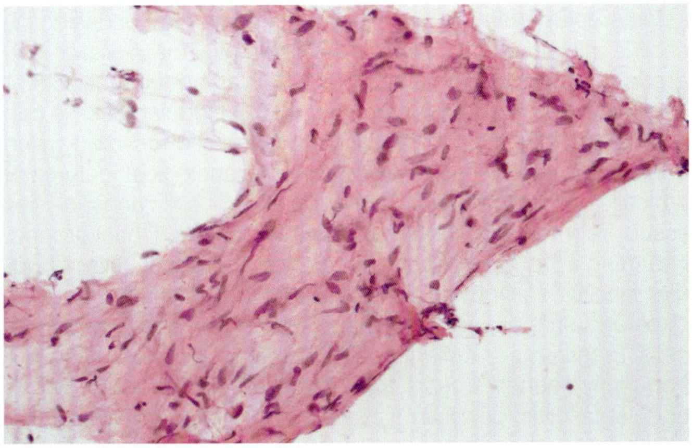

Fig. 4.61 Desmoid fibromatosis. Fragment of collagenous matrix with scattered, embedded spindle cells, separated by fibrillary collagen strands (H&E).

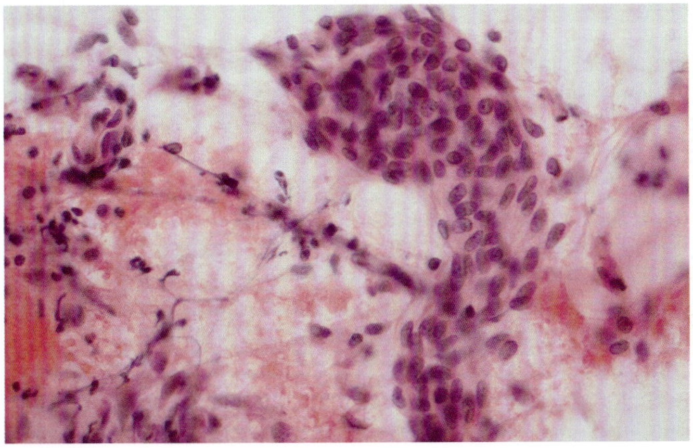

Fig. 4.62 Desmoid fibromatosis. A cohesive tissue fragment composed predominantly of bland spindle cells and poorly cohesive spindle cells, some with crush artefacts (H&E).

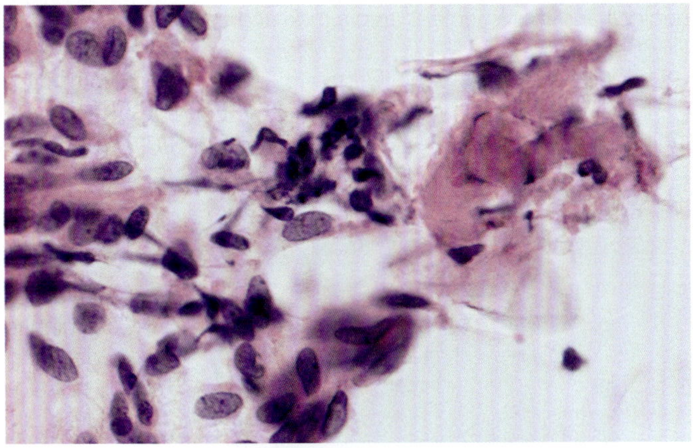

Fig. 4.63 Desmoid fibromatosis. Loosely cohesive bland spindle cells with oval nuclei and an admixture of small fragments of collagenous tissue (H&E).

Histopathology

Fibromatosis is characterized by long, intersecting fascicles of cells that can span an entire low-power field of view. The tumour contains small to medium-sized vessels, occasionally in irregular or staghorn shapes. Other findings include occasional areas of oedema, areas of keloid-like collagen deposition, chronic inflammation, and focal nodular fasciitis–like regions. Individual tumour cells have thin and long eosinophilic cytoplasm but indistinct cytoplasmic borders. Nuclei tend to be fusiform or oval and fairly uniform in size and shape. Mitoses are very rare. As mentioned elsewhere, fibromatosis tends to infiltrate adjacent soft tissues. In skeletal muscle, fibromatosis often insinuates in and surrounds individual muscle bands.

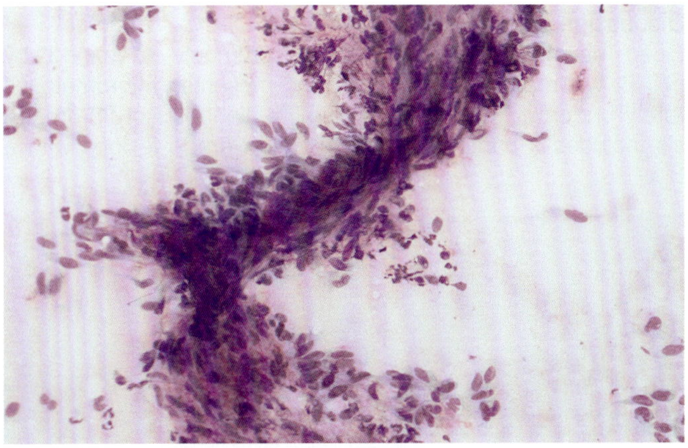

Fig. 4.64 Desmoid fibromatosis. Bland spindle cells in long fascicles separated by fibrillary collagen, a useful clue in the diagnosis of desmoid fibromatosis (Giemsa).

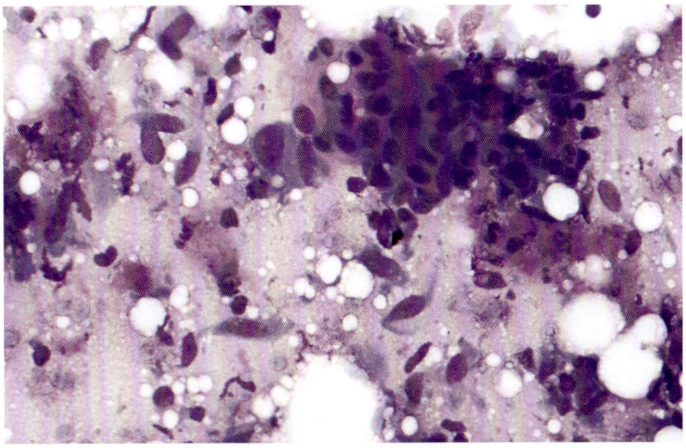

Fig. 4.65 Desmoid fibromatosis. Small tissue fragments with metachromatic myxoid stroma and separate single cells with slightly pleomorphic nuclei with inconspicuous nucleoli (Giemsa).

Key diagnostic cytopathological features

- Scant to moderate cellularity
- Tissue fragments of bland spindle cells separated by finely fibrillary collagen arranged in long fascicles
- Single or loosely cohesive, bland spindle cells without nuclear atypia
- Oval to elongate nuclei with finely granular chromatin and indistinct cytoplasm
- Crush artefact and stripped nuclei
- Occasionally mild anisokaryosis
- Fragments of collagenous and metachromatic (Giemsa) matrix material
- Fragments of degenerating skeletal muscle when lesion adjacent to or within muscle

Reference(s): {1141,1058,1381,213,1106,1382,936,1546,1353}

Discussion and differential diagnosis

Deep desmoid fibromatoses are commonly examined by FNAB, whereas plantar, palmar, and mesenteric fibromatoses rarely undergo FNAB. The differential diagnosis of fibromatosis includes a number of benign to low-grade lesions with a spindle cell pattern. Smears from desmoids may occasionally show a myxoid matrix, evoking the differential diagnosis of low-grade myxoid spindle cell lesions, such as nodular fasciitis or low-grade fibromyxoid sarcoma (LGFMS). Nodular fasciitis can simulate fibromatosis in its clinical presentation involving skin and shows substantial overlap in cytomorphological features. It typically has a more dispersed population of cells and includes tissue fragments of these cells within a myxoid background, imparting a "tissue culture" appearance. Individual cells of nodular fasciitis show more variability and can display a range of sizes and shapes, with polygonal, epithelioid, or plasmacytoid cells. Fragments of collagenous and metachromatic stroma are frequently seen in smears from desmoids and are very rare in nodular fasciitis; ganglion-type cells and prominent nucleoli are a frequent and distinctive feature in samples of nodular fasciitis but are usually absent in fibromatoses {276,52}.

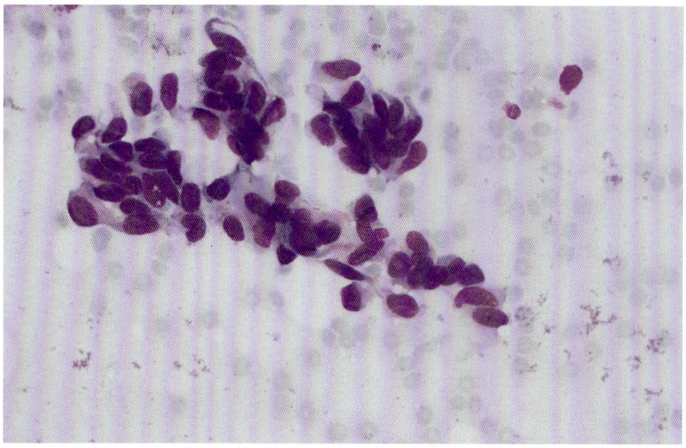

Fig. 4.66 Desmoid fibromatosis. Loosely cohesive uniform spindle cells with oval to elongated nuclei with evenly distributed chromatin. Some cells have cytoplasmic processes (Giemsa).

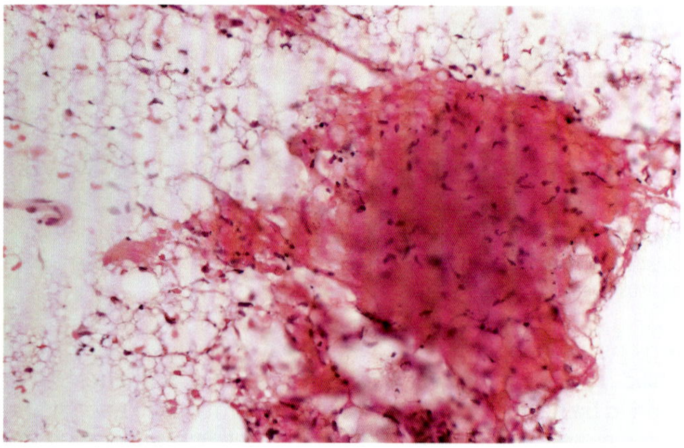

Fig. 4.67 Fibromatosis. A large hypocellular fragment of dense stroma and associated small spindle cells (H&E).

Benign peripheral nerve sheath tumours, including schwannoma and neurofibroma, can also cause considerable diagnostic confusion. Both of these lesions are characterized by moderately cellular smears, often with fragments of metachromatic stromal material. Unlike in fibromatosis, however, the spindle cells of nerve sheath tumours have distinctive nuclear features of a marked curved or comma shape and tapered or pointed ends. In addition, many of the nuclei of nerve sheath tumours show distinctive intranuclear pseudoinclusions {346,332}.

Myofibroblastoma also shows extensive overlap with fibromatosis, but it tends to be more superficially located and occurs preferentially in the breast, inguinal/pelvic regions, and gynaecological tract.

Another soft tissue lesion that can be difficult to distinguish from fibromatosis is low-grade myofibroblastic sarcoma, a rare neoplasm with wide anatomical site and age distributions and fibromatosis-like histopathological features {922,418}. Smears of low-grade myofibroblastic sarcoma show spindle cells with elongated, fusiform, occasionally angulated nuclei with small nucleoli and more nuclear atypia than seen in desmoid tumours {1386}.

One of the most difficult lesions to separate from fibromatosis is LGFMS. These two neoplasms share numerous features, including bland spindle cells, fragments of stroma and dispersed spindle cells or naked nuclei in the background, and

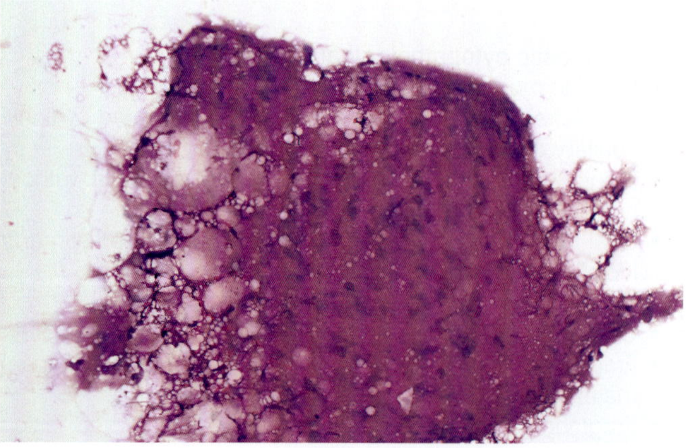

Fig. 4.68 Fibromatosis. A large hypocellular dense stromal tissue fragment with poorly seen nuclei and abundant collagen from a recurrent "deep" fibromatosis, which has infiltrated fat (6 to 9 o'clock) (Giemsa).

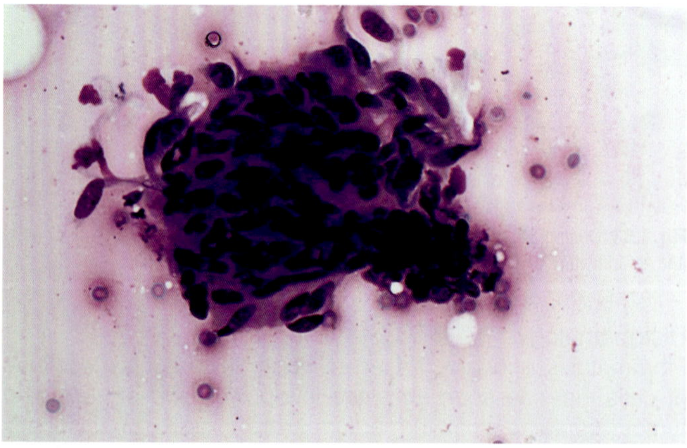

Fig. 4.69 Fibromatosis. Small bland spindle cells making up a cellular tissue fragment (Giemsa).

finely granular nuclear chromatin that can show perinucleolar clearing ("vesicular" chromatin on Pap), although desmoid fibromatoses are less cellular {351}. ICC is very useful in this differential diagnosis.

Ancillary testing

Nuclear β-catenin staining is often used to confirm a fibromatosis and separate this entity from its look-alikes {132}, but this is not entirely specific: up to 20% of tumours either fail to stain or show a nonspecific cytoplasmic staining pattern {177}. Fibromatosis also expresses markers of myofibroblastic differentiation, including MSA and SMA. Desmin is usually negative but may show focal positivity. Helpful negative stains include EMA, CD34, S100, and KIT (CD117). S100 is strongly positive in nerve sheath tumours but negative in fibromatosis. Positive staining for CD34 is helpful in confirming a diagnosis of myofibroblastoma and excluding fibromatosis. Low-grade myofibroblastic sarcomas do not express nuclear β-catenin. LGFMS shows diffuse immunoreactivity for MUC4, a feature not identified in fibromatosis {359}, and LGFMS can also be confirmed by demonstrating the *FUS*::*CREB3L2* or *FUS*::*CREB3L1* fusion that characterizes this neoplasm.

Nodular fasciitis

Domanski HA
Gajdzis P

Definition

Nodular fasciitis is a self-limited mesenchymal neoplasm that usually occurs in subcutaneous tissue composed of plump fibroblastic/myofibroblastic cells and usually harbours *USP6* rearrangement.

Clinical features and imaging

Nodular fasciitis arises commonly in the subcutaneous tissues in conjunction with the fascial surface of the upper extremities, trunk, and head and neck in young adults, although it can occur at almost any anatomical location and in any age group {916,1297,974,127}. Occasional cases arise in intramuscular and rarely intra-articular sites {578} or in the dermis {300,1128, 1025}. Nodular fasciitis grows rapidly over a period of weeks or a few months and usually presents as a small, often tender nodule, rarely exceeding 50 mm {1297,974}. Uncommon subtypes of nodular fasciitis include intravascular fasciitis, arising in small and medium-sized blood vessels {1128,1084, 204}, and cranial fasciitis, occurring commonly in the temporal and parietal deep layers of the scalp of young children (mostly infants), with common involvement of the underlying bone {781,1460}. The MRI features of nodular fasciitis are non-specific, with a wide variety of imaging differential diagnoses {587,813,260}.

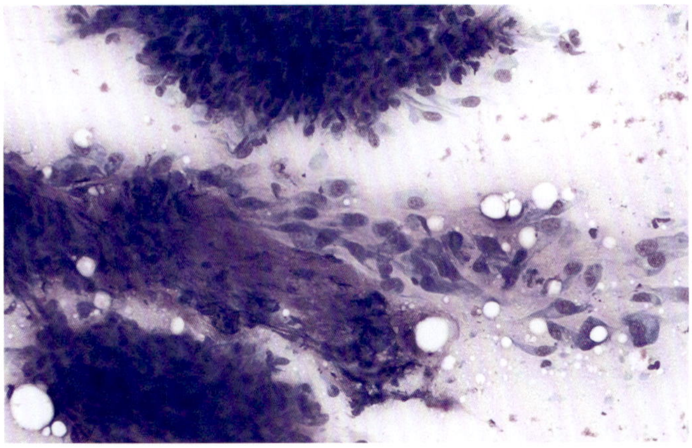

Fig. 4.72 Nodular fasciitis. Cellular tissue fragments composed of spindle cells and single myofibroblasts in a collagenous and myxoid background, with some dispersal of similar intact single cells (Giemsa).

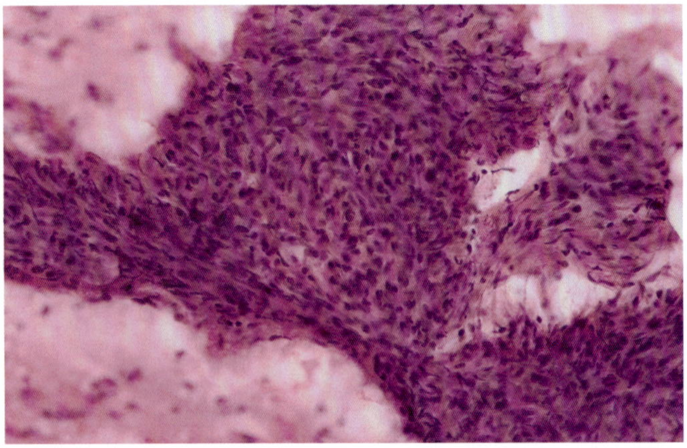

Fig. 4.70 Nodular fasciitis. Cohesive cellular 3D tissue fragments of spindle cells with collagenous stroma (H&E).

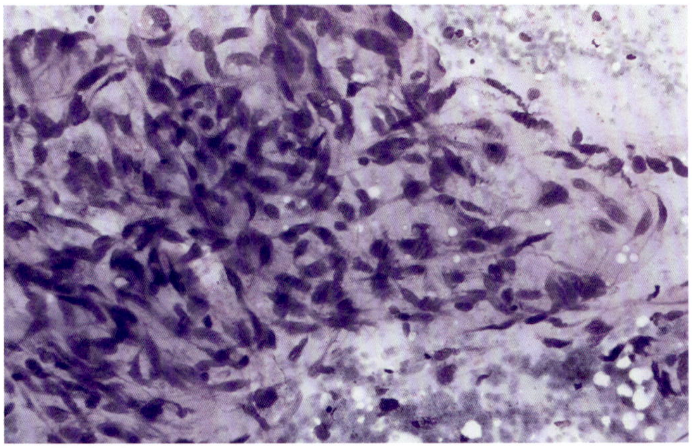

Fig. 4.73 Nodular fasciitis. Poorly cohesive myofibroblasts within a myxoid stroma (Giemsa).

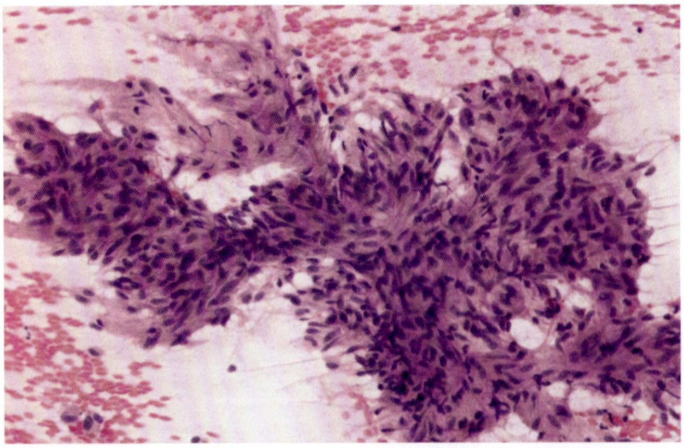

Fig. 4.71 Nodular fasciitis. Tissue fragments of irregularly arranged spindle cells with a "cell culture" appearance (H&E).

Histopathology

Nodular fasciitis is usually a cellular neoplasm composed of plump spindle to stellate cells with bland ovoid, vesicular nuclei with small nucleoli. Tumour cells are arranged in loose fascicles with a "tissue culture"–like growth pattern in fibromyxoid stroma. Storiform or whorled growth patterns may be observed in cellular areas. Stroma may be scant to abundant, with stromal matrix ranging from myxoid to densely collagenized, and often keloid-like in older lesions. Areas of cystic degeneration, mitoses, scattered lymphocytes, histiocytes, osteoclast-type giant cells, and extravasated erythrocytes are relatively common {1297,974,127}. Osseous metaplasia may be seen in nodular and cranial fasciitis {285,781}.

Key diagnostic cytopathological features

- High cellularity
- Tissue fragments and dispersed single cells in variable proportions
- Loosely cohesive tissue fragments of spindle cells within a myxoid background producing a "tissue culture" appearance
- Predominant spindle cells, with less common polygonal, epithelioid, and plasmacytoid cells
- Plump polyhedral or triangular cells resembling ganglion cells with abundant eccentric cytoplasm and one or two nuclei and prominent nucleoli, occasionally as multinucleated cells
- Rarely, osteoclast-like multinucleated giant cells
- Eccentric sparse to abundant cytoplasm that can have bipolar or unipolar cytoplasmic tails, often curved or elongated
- Nuclei of variable size and shape, round to ovoid or more elongated
- Variably prominent nucleoli
- Mitoses, occasionally frequent, with no atypical mitoses
- Admixture of inflammatory cells
- No necrosis

Reference(s): {485,51,333,627,1146,1514,785,1096,1124,1115,1217, 750,128,1312,1343,1223,764,894,52,276}

Discussion and differential diagnosis

The main differential diagnoses of nodular fasciitis include pleomorphic, spindle cell, and myxoid sarcomas and desmoid fibromatosis. In contrast to nodular fasciitis, most high-grade sarcomas are composed of pleomorphic tumour cells containing irregular hyperchromatic nuclei with coarse chromatin and often prominent nucleoli, and atypical mitotic figures and necrosis are common. Synovial sarcomas may show bland cytopathological features {32}, but these neoplasms usually present as slowly growing, deep soft tissue masses and display characteristic ICC and molecular profiles {1559} that distinguish them from nodular fasciitis. Smears of dermatofibrosarcoma protuberans may mimic those of nodular fasciitis {350}, but the slow-growing and superficial dermal presentation, with bluish, red, or brown discolouration of the skin, is different from the subcutaneous location and rapid growth of nodular fasciitis.

Desmoid fibromatosis arises deeply, and it commonly infiltrates skeletal muscle. It produces less cellular smears and bland spindle cells separated by hyalinized collagenous and rarely myxoid stroma {1058,282}. Other soft tissue lesions sharing at least some cytopathological features with nodular fasciitis are granulomatous lesions, inflammatory myofibroblastic tumour, schwannoma, and neurofibroma. All of these lesions show clinical features and ICC profiles distinct from those of nodular fasciitis. Smears of nodular fasciitis in the head and neck region can be confused with pleomorphic adenoma due to the myxoid stroma and spindle myoepithelial cells, but features such as a predominance of spindle cells with cytoplasmic processes, prominent nucleoli, and occasional mitoses favour a diagnosis of nodular fasciitis over pleomorphic adenoma {485, 51,1096,1217}.

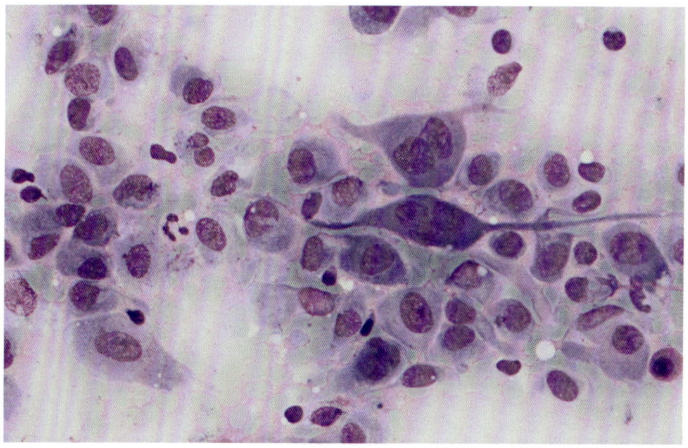

Fig. 4.74 Nodular fasciitis. Single fibroblasts/myofibroblasts varying in size, with abundant, often eccentric cytoplasm, as well as occasional cytoplasmic processes and occasional binucleates; there are occasional inflammatory cells in the background (Giemsa).

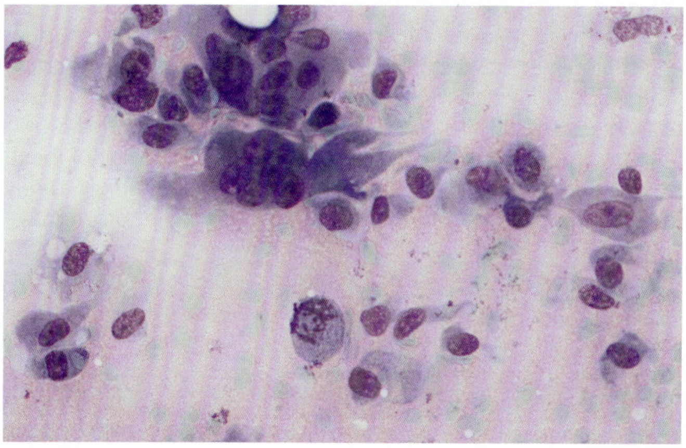

Fig. 4.75 Nodular fasciitis. Larger, often multinucleated fibroblastic/myofibroblastic cells with oval nuclei and abundant cytoplasm, along with single intact plump spindle cells. A single typical mitosis is present (Giemsa).

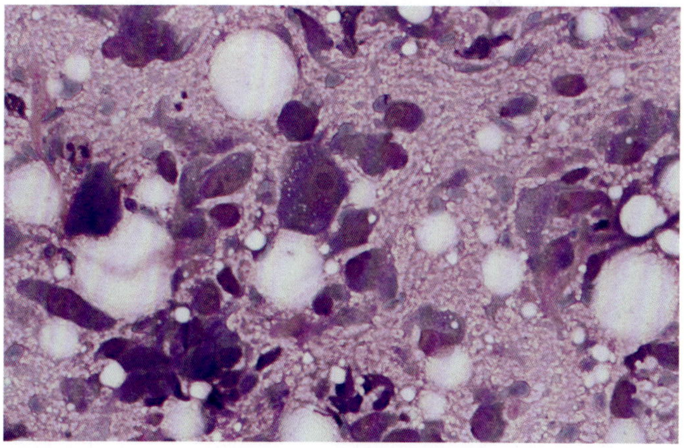

Fig. 4.76 Nodular fasciitis. Single cells, which are large, polygonal, plump spindle in type, with abundant, often eccentric cytoplasm, showing moderate anisonucleosis and occasional prominent nucleoli, in a proteinaceous background (Giemsa).

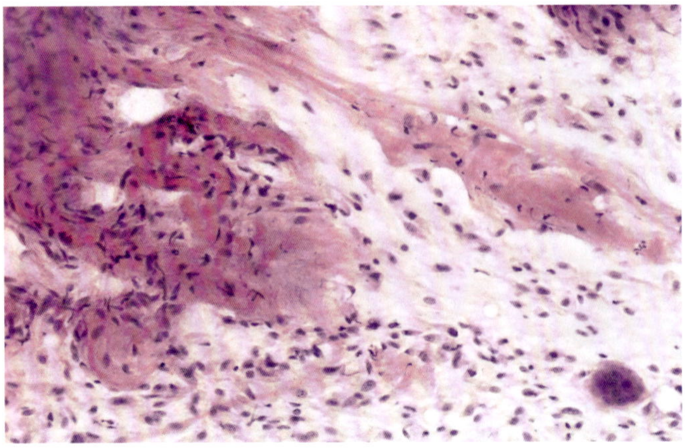

Fig. 4.77 Nodular fasciitis. Loosely cohesive tissue fragments of spindle cells with abundant collagenous stroma, as well as plentiful small spindle cells and a single osteoclast-like giant cell in the background (H&E).

Proliferative fasciitis and proliferative myositis are pseudosarcomatous lesions closely related to, but much less common than, nodular fasciitis. Both occur predominantly in middle-aged or older adults {231,382,693}, with a rare subtype of proliferative fasciitis described in children {912}. The clinical course of these lesions mimics that of nodular fasciitis; they grow rapidly, rarely exceeding 50 mm, and are often tender or painful. Proliferative fasciitis most commonly develops in the subcutaneous tissue of the upper extremities, followed by the lower extremities and trunk, whereas proliferative myositis arises intramuscularly, most commonly in the trunk, followed by the shoulder girdles, upper arms, and less often thighs. Both proliferative fasciitis and proliferative myositis share many FNAB features with nodular fasciitis, such as spindle cells with cytoplasmic processes and round or oval nuclei in addition to plump polygonal, epithelioid cells and a variable number of ganglion-like cells with prominent nucleoli {852,223,721,1239}. The myxoid background matrix is less prominent and the ganglion-like cells are usually numerous and often exhibit large nucleoli in proliferative fasciitis. In proliferative myositis, smears contain multinucleated regenerating muscle fibres in addition to the fibroblastic/myofibroblastic cells {1513}. Mitotic figures can be found in both lesions. The ICC profile is similar to that of nodular fasciitis {378,852,223}, but unlike in nodular fasciitis, neither a recurrent genomic abnormality nor translocation has been found in these lesions.

Ancillary testing

Nodular fasciitis expresses SMA, calponin, and CD10. Desmin, h-caldesmon, S100, and CD34 are negative. CD68 is positive in intralesional osteoclast-like multinucleated cells {974,847}. β-catenin expression can be positive in some cranial fasciitis cases {1143}. Dermatofibrosarcoma protuberans demonstrates positivity for CD34.

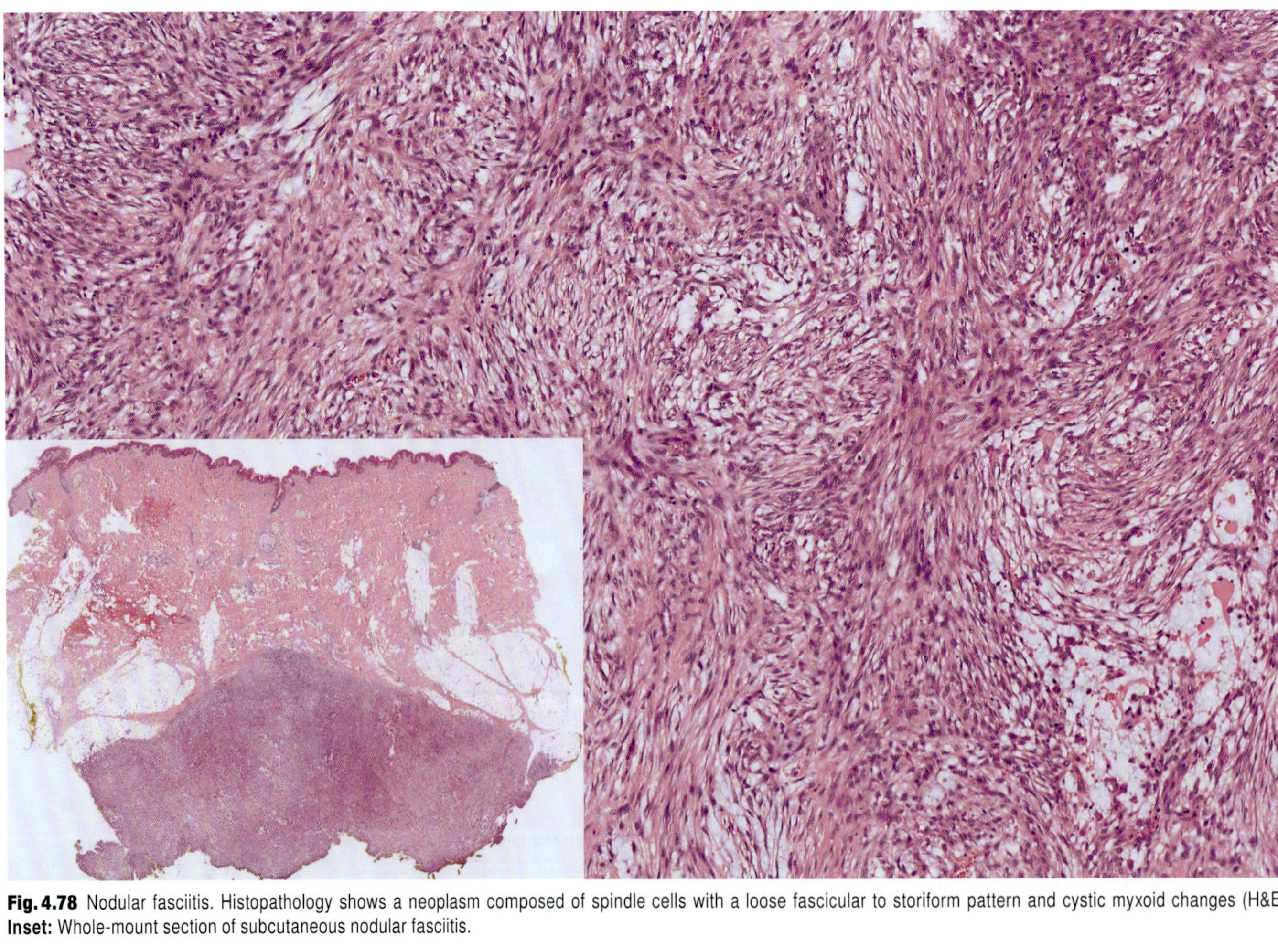

Fig. 4.78 Nodular fasciitis. Histopathology shows a neoplasm composed of spindle cells with a loose fascicular to storiform pattern and cystic myxoid changes (H&E). **Inset:** Whole-mount section of subcutaneous nodular fasciitis.

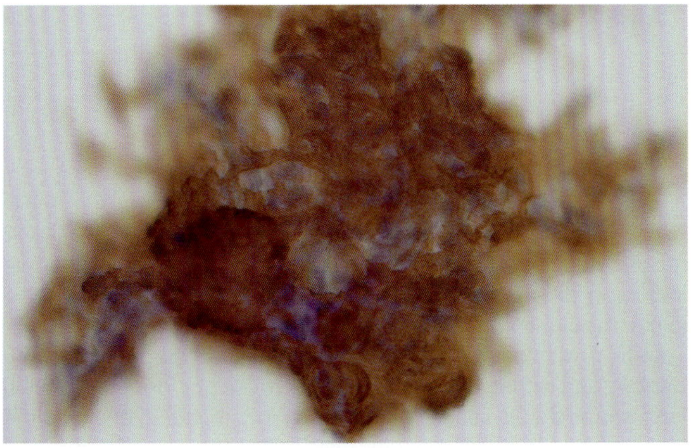

Fig. 4.79 Nodular fasciitis. The neoplastic cells express SMA (LBC, ICC SMA).

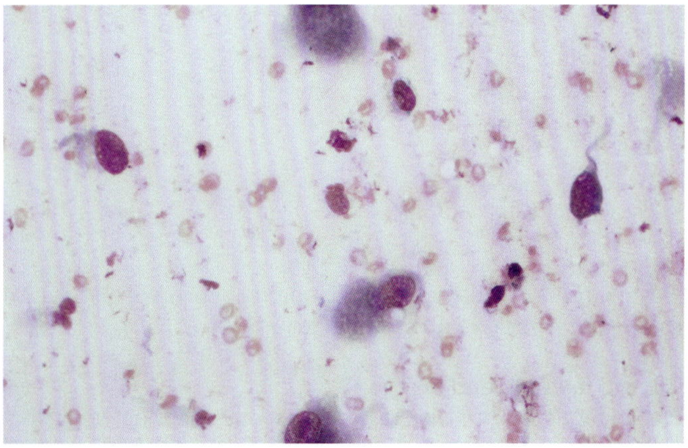

Fig. 4.81 Proliferative myositis. Scattered ganglion-like cells and occasional plump spindle cells (Giemsa).

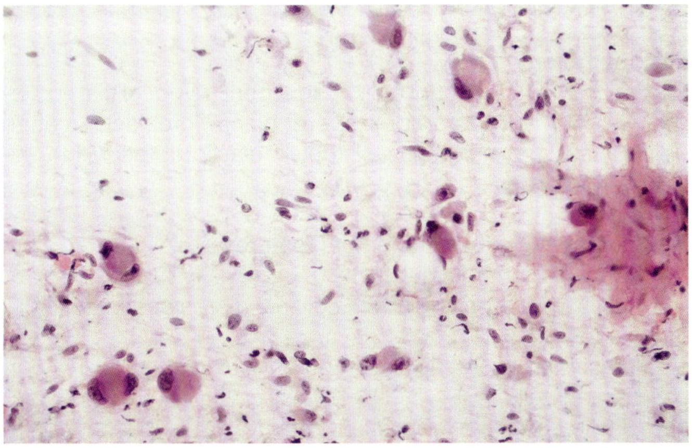

Fig. 4.80 Proliferative fasciitis. Cellular heterogeneity, with single small spindle fibroblasts/myofibroblasts and mononucleated or binucleated large ganglion-like cells and fragment of collagenous stroma (H&E).

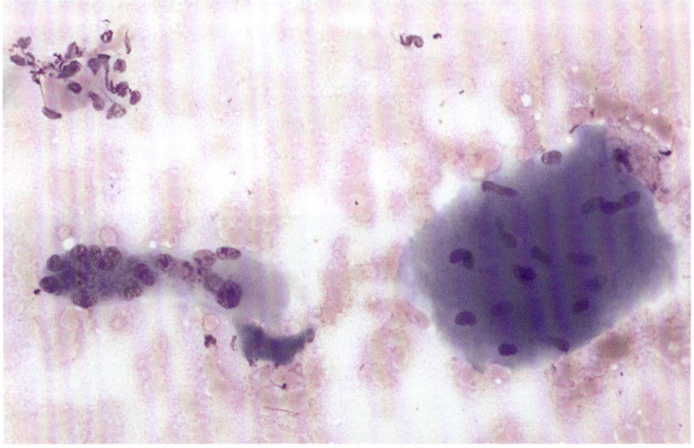

Fig. 4.82 Proliferative myositis. Muscle fragments and multinucleated regenerating muscle fibre (central) are occasional findings in smears (Giemsa).

The majority of nodular fasciitis cases are characterized by recurrent translocations involving *USP6*, and the *MYH9*::*USP6* fusion product is the most common, found in two thirds of cases {385,1086}. Other *USP6* gene fusion partners have also been described {1086}. *USP6* rearrangements are not specific to nodular fasciitis; they can also be found in other benign soft tissue and bone tumours, such as myositis ossificans and aneurysmal bone cyst {1298,118,1048}. *USP6* rearrangements can be identified by FISH, PCR, or NGS {1086,1298,1233}. The percentage of break-apart FISH signals decreases during ageing of nodular fasciitis, which can be a potential source of false negative results in older lesions {1233}.

Elastofibroma

Domanski HA
Dodd LG
Gajdzis P

Definition

Elastofibroma is a benign, ill-defined proliferation of fibroelastic tissue with excessive abnormal elastic fibres.

Clinical features and imaging

Elastofibroma is a soft tissue proliferation of uncertain origin that occurs predominantly in elderly individuals about 70 years of age, particularly women {998,1028,1047,533,279}. Although the exact prevalence of elastofibroma is unknown, in larger studies, the lesions were reported in 0.8–2.73% of elderly individuals by CT, and an incidence rate of 13–17% has been reported in autopsy studies {1389,155,45,630}. The lesion commonly presents as a slowly growing unilateral or occasionally bilateral mass, ranging from 20 to 150 mm, located between the subscapular area and the chest wall {1028,1047}. There have been reports of rare multiple lesions and lesions in atypical locations, including different parts of the thoracic wall, extremities, neck, joints, mediastinum, and viscera {1047,279,39}.

MRI of elastofibroma, which has a higher diagnostic confidence than either ultrasound or CT, reveals a double-convex, lens-shaped soft tissue mass with a low signal intensity, similar to that of skeletal muscle, interlaced with strands of fat on both T1-weighted and T2-weighted sequences {1028,1426,115}. Elastofibromas are easily detectable on PET-CT due to their hypermetabolic nature {1422,1135}.

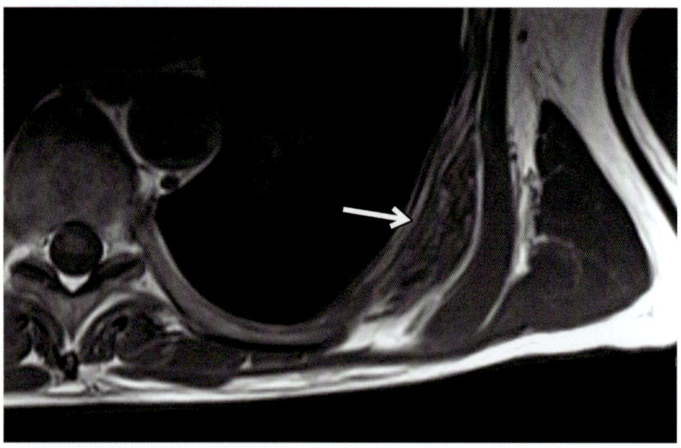

Fig. 4.83 Elastofibroma. MRI shows a heterogeneous soft tissue mass (arrow) with a signal intensity equal to that of skeletal muscle, interlaced with areas showing the signal intensity of fat.

Histopathology

Elastofibroma is composed of abundant hypocellular collagenous stroma with an admixture of bland fibroblasts, mature adipocytes, and numerous disrupted elastic fibres within the collagenous stroma.

Key diagnostic cytopathological features

- Scant to moderate cellularity
- Fat tissue intermingled with collagen fibres and bland spindle cells
- Loosely cohesive tissue fragments or dispersed uniform spindle cells
- Elastic fibres are present as linear (braid-like) and globular bodies with a shell-like and stellate appearance and serrated "moth-eaten" edges, best seen in the Pap stain

Reference(s): {540,1004,1002,337,1453,348,967,1113,1448,989,556}

Discussion and differential diagnosis

The pathogenesis of elastofibroma is still unclear and a matter of debate {452,1047,664,765,325,1029,1384}. The main diagnostic feature is the presence of elastic fibres with serrated borders,

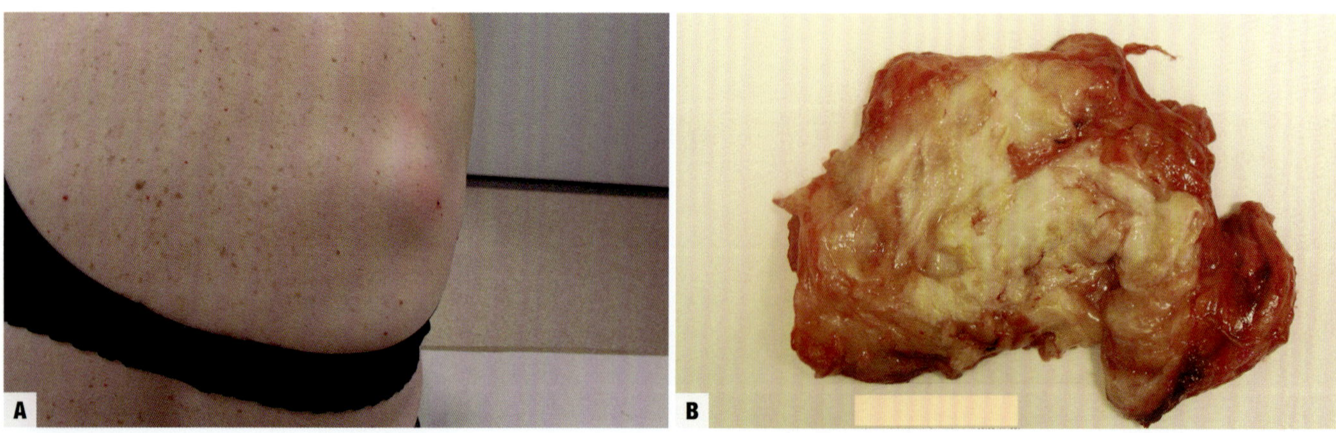

Fig. 4.84 Elastofibroma. **A** Clinical presentation of elastofibroma. **B** A poorly circumscribed rubbery mass with greyish-white cut surface and intervening fat.

corresponding to faulty elastin fibrillogenesis. These structures are usually easy to find in alcohol-fixed Pap-stained smears but are very subtle or invisible in air-dried Giemsa-stained smears {337,348}. The differential diagnosis includes extra-abdominal desmoid fibromatosis, spindle cell lipoma, and nuchal fibroma.

Ancillary testing

The elastin Verhoeff–Van Gieson stain is positive in cell block material, showing fragmented abnormal elastic fibres.

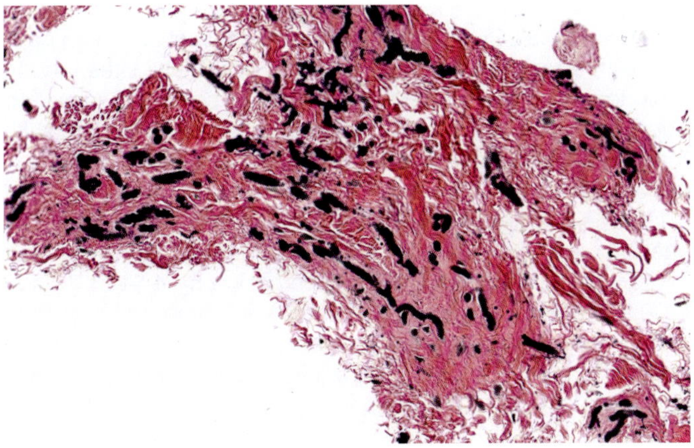

Fig. 4.85 Elastofibroma. Abnormal elastic fibres in a histopathological section of elastofibroma (Verhoeff–Van Gieson stain).

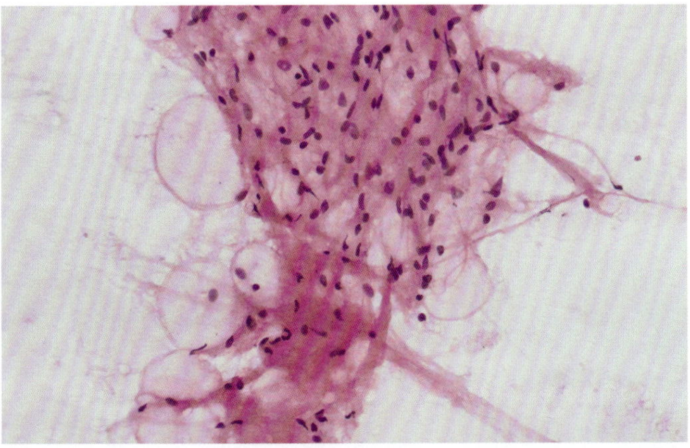

Fig. 4.86 Elastofibroma. Mature adipocytes mixed with hypocellular collagenous stroma and spindle cells in a tissue fragment (H&E).

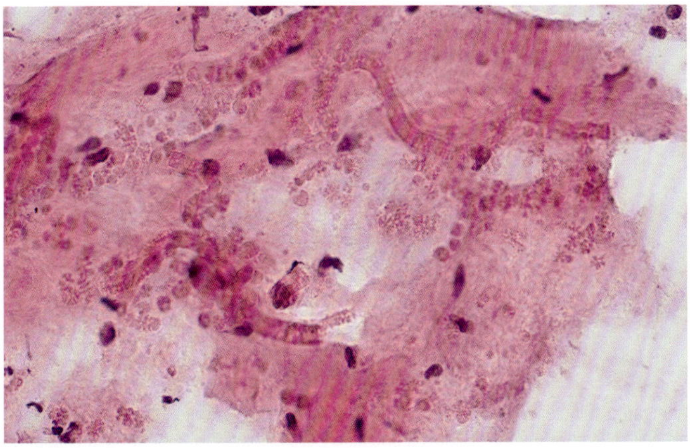

Fig. 4.87 Elastofibroma. Abnormal elastic fibres that appear as linear (braid-like), globular, and stellate structures with serrated edges (H&E).

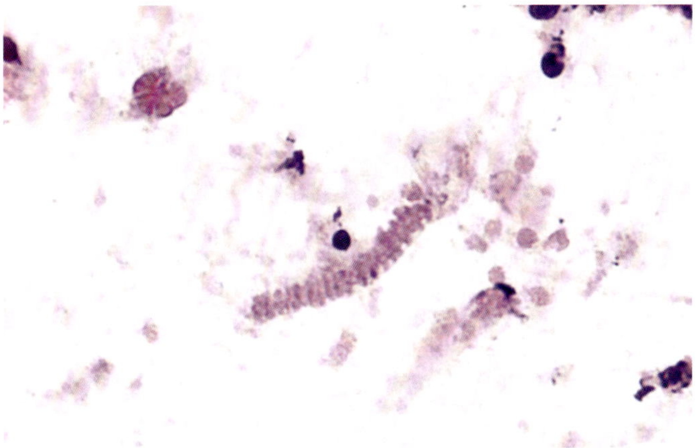

Fig. 4.88 Elastofibroma. Elastic fibres that appear as linear (braid-like), globular, and stellate structures with serrated edges (H&E).

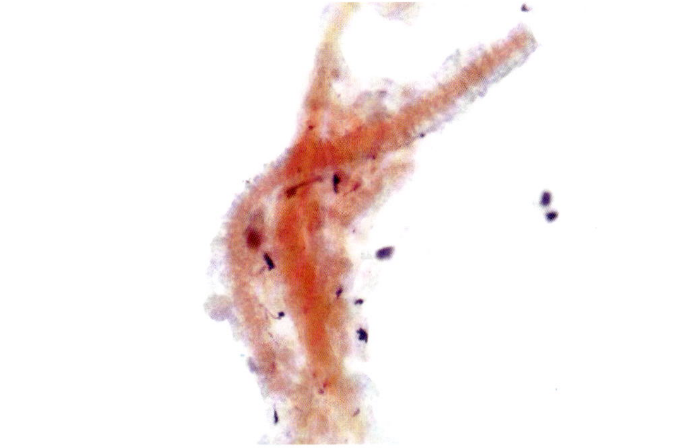

Fig. 4.89 Elastofibroma. Elastic fibres are linear (braid-like), globular, and stellate structures with serrated edges (Pap).

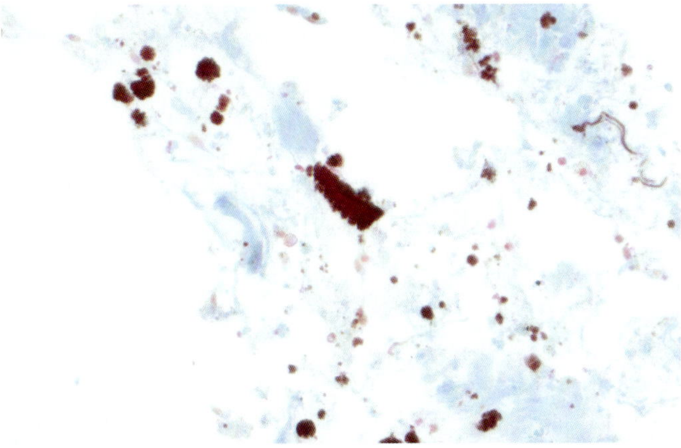

Fig. 4.90 Elastofibroma. Abnormal elastic fibres (cell block, Verhoeff–Van Gieson stain).

Haemangiomas

Monaco SE
Bode-Lesniewska B
Domanski HA
Jo VY

Definition

Haemangiomas are benign tumours consisting of a small blood vessel proliferation.

Clinical features and imaging

Haemangiomas are benign vascular tumours that occur more commonly in children than in adults, and predominantly in superficial locations of the head and neck region. Deep tumours involving the bones, liver, and other visceral sites can also occur {1033,1032}. The International Society for the Study of Vascular Anomalies (ISSVA) classifies vascular anomalies as tumours that can be benign, locally aggressive or borderline, or malignant, or as malformations that are simple, combined, or "other" {614}. Some subtypes of haemangioma are based on the type of vessels involved, such as capillary, venous, arteriovenous, lymphatic, or littoral cell; others are based on the morphology, including hobnail, papillary, and glomeruloid, or on the location, such as synovial haemangioma and intramuscular angioma {1033}. Clinically, these lesions present as raised papules with a red or violaceous colour in superficial sites, and in deep locations they present with haemoptysis and pressure on adjacent structures or as incidental findings on imaging. With rapid growth, these lesions may cause thrombocytopenia due to consumption {376}.

Infantile haemangiomas represent the most common soft tissue tumours in the first months of life, with growth until about 1 year of age and spontaneous regression by 4 years of age {200}, whereas congenital haemangiomas are largest at birth and usually show partial or complete regression {156}. Synovial haemangiomas occur within the joint space of young patients and may be associated with pain or osteoarthritis.

Benign vascular tumours show vascular flow on Doppler ultrasound imaging or postcontrast enhancement peripherally on CT {1500}. They are thought to arise due to endothelial proliferation with uncontrolled angiogenesis due to abnormalities in the HIF1α, VEGF, or PI3K/AKT pathways. There is an

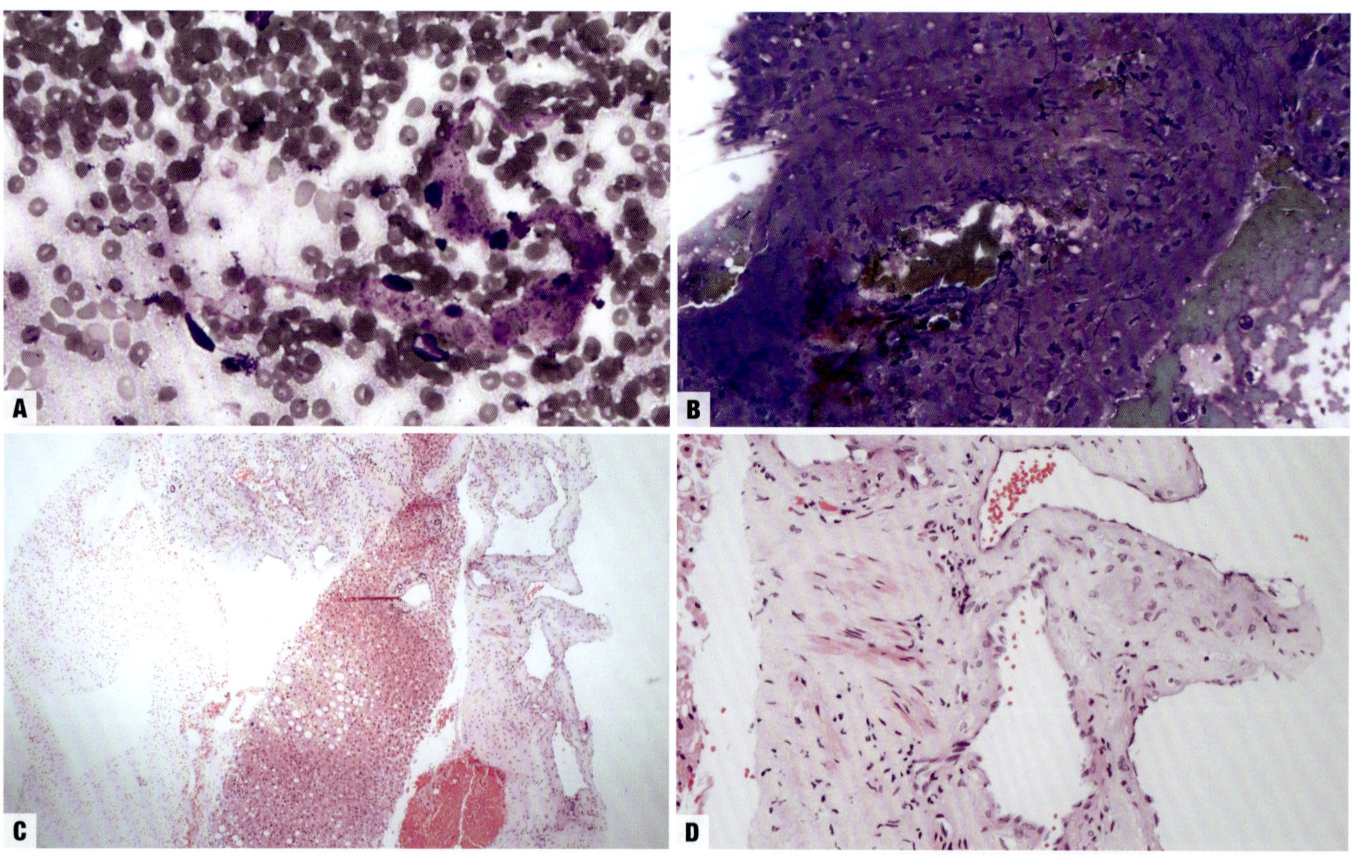

Fig. 4.91 Haemangioma of liver. Four images from the same case. **A** Occasional stripped, elongated spindle nuclei and a platelet clot in bloody background that requires imaging correlation to suggest a haemangioma (Giemsa). **B** A tissue fragment of poorly defined spindle cells and collagenous stroma (Giemsa). **C** Core biopsy of liver showing fatty change (12 to 6 o'clock) and cores of vascular tumour with irregular, often dilated, thin-walled vessels separated by collagenous stroma with spindle cells (core biopsy, H&E). **D** Irregular, thin-walled, variably dilated blood vessels separated by paucicellular collagen tissue of haemangioma (core biopsy, H&E).

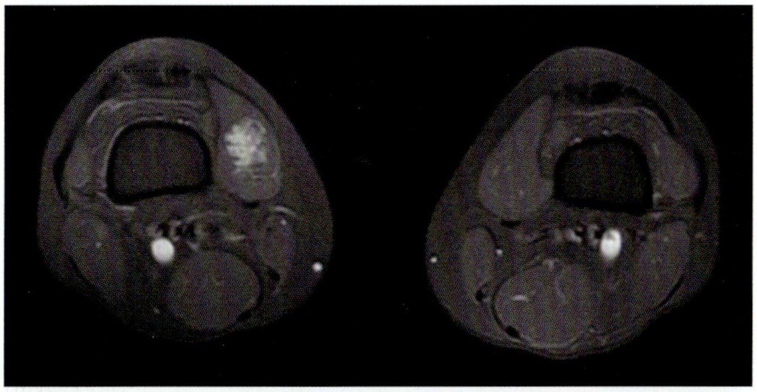

Fig. 4.92 Intramuscular haemangioma. MRI of a mass in the right vastus medialis.

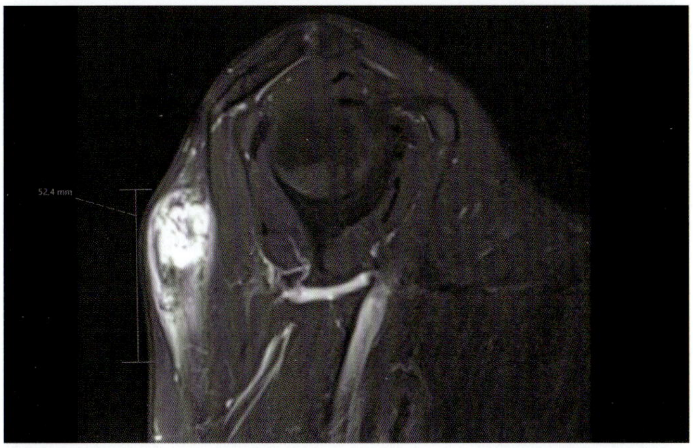

Fig. 4.93 Intramuscular haemangioma. MRI of a mass in the soft tissue of the shoulder.

association between vascular tumours and malformations such as in Sturge–Weber syndrome, von Hippel–Lindau syndrome, and *PIK3CA*-related overgrowth syndromes (e.g. Klippel–Trénaunay syndrome) {84,1097,979,902}. Treatment decisions depend on the age of the patient, rate of tumour growth or regression, potential complications of the lesion (e.g. scarring), tumour location, risks and benefits of treatment, and availability of medical expertise. Some treatments include steroids, other systemic medications, laser therapy or sclerotherapy, embolization, and/or surgical resection {76,88,302}. The lesions can recur if incompletely excised, but malignant transformation to angiosarcoma is rare and primarily reported in adults with deep lesions {1201}.

Histopathology

Haemangiomas are well-circumscribed, lobular proliferations of capillary-sized blood vessels with a single layer of endothelium, usually arising from a larger feeding vessel. Epithelioid haemangiomas tend to have plump and rounded endothelial cells, and not the standard spindle cell. Cavernous haemangiomas show dilated vascular channels. Congenital haemangiomas show a solid pattern with increased mitoses in the rapid growth phase, and more well-defined vascular channels as they mature. Infantile haemangioma has an early proliferative phase with immature dendritic-type cells, then an early regressive phase where capillaries dilate and start to show apoptotic debris in the basement membrane, followed by late regression with ghosts of capillaries {376}. Phleboliths may be seen in vascular channels of spindle cell haemangiomas.

Key diagnostic cytopathological features

- Variable, usually scant cellularity due to blood dilution
- Rare bland spindle cells with cytoplasmic tapering within a bloody background
- Tissue fragments of spindle cells within fibrous stroma with vague vasoformation
- Cell blocks may show tissue fragments with vascular spaces with red blood cells within fibrous stroma
- Scant inflammatory cells, which are more common in granulation tissue

Reference(s): {1215,170,1374}

Discussion and differential diagnosis

FNAB is not typically performed, because of the characteristic imaging findings, a high "Insufficient" rate, and a potential increased risk of bleeding complications. Subclassification into the type of vascular proliferation can be challenging based on the limited material, leading to a somewhat vague diagnosis of a "benign vascular tumour or proliferation favouring a haemangioma".

Benign vascular tumours, such as haemangiomas, can be challenging to diagnose on small biopsies and require clinical and imaging correlation. They can mimic vascular

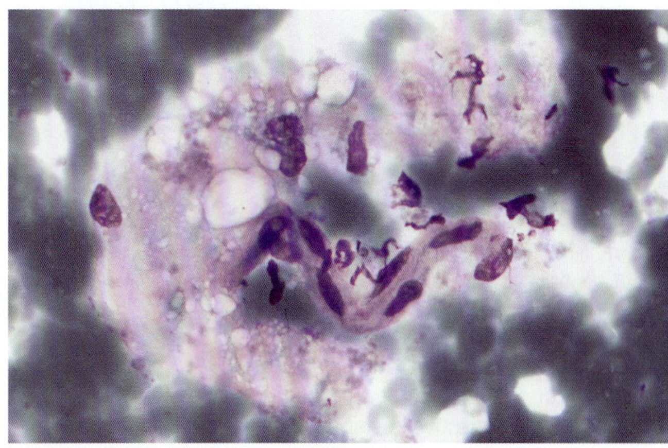

Fig. 4.94 Intramuscular haemangioma. A minute tissue fragment suggestive of a thin vessel, consisting of bland spindle cells (Giemsa).

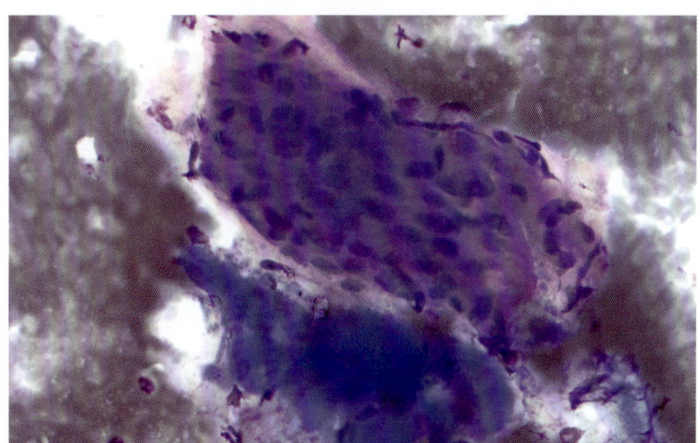

Fig. 4.95 Intramuscular haemangioma. A moderately cellular tissue fragment of spindle cells, with no definite vessel formation (Giemsa).

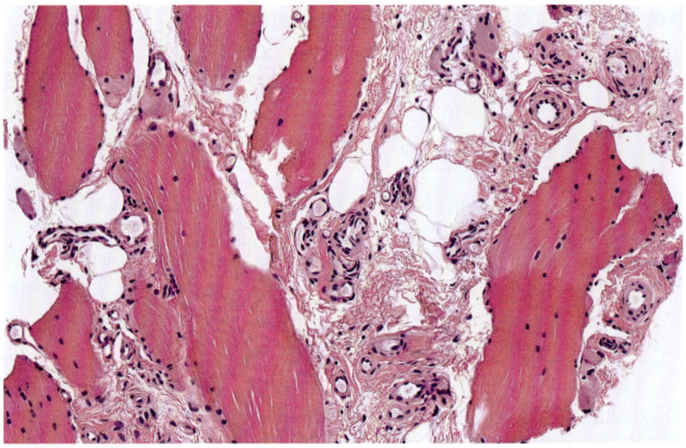

Fig. 4.96 Intramuscular haemangioma. Collections of capillaries and slightly more open small vessels in the interstitium between skeletal muscle fibres and occasional degenerate small muscle fibres (H&E).

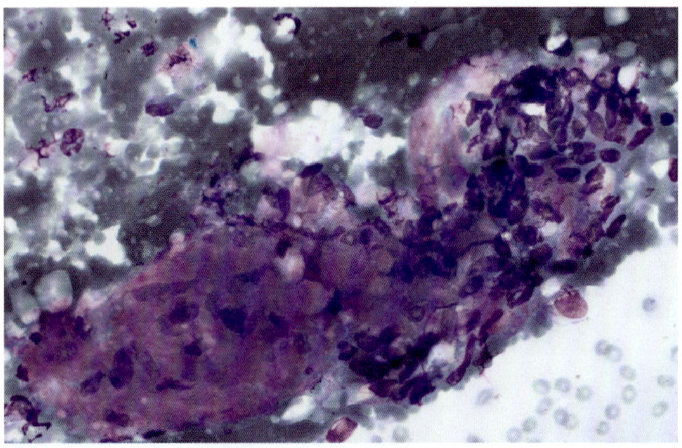

Fig. 4.97 Intramuscular haemangioma. A tissue fragment of collagen and spindle cells, as well as a more cellular area where the orientation of the spindle cells suggests small vessels (Giemsa).

malformations and granulation tissue with angiogenesis, and the history can be critical, because a history of trauma raises the possibility of reactive granulation tissue. Haemangioendotheliomas are typically more epithelioid (with intracellular vascular lumina containing red blood cells) and infiltrative, with an indeterminate biological behaviour ranging between that of haemangiomas and angiosarcomas {662,1415}. Pulmonary sclerosing pneumocytoma, which was previously referred to as sclerosing haemangioma of the lung, shows positivity for

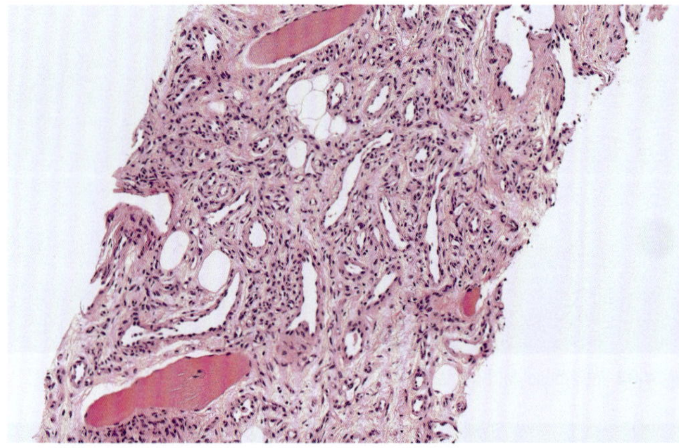

Fig. 4.98 Intramuscular haemangioma. Collection of small vessels, some resembling capillaries, with a range of more dilated, irregular, thin-walled vessels separated by paucicellular collagen and occasional residual skeletal muscle strands (CNB, H&E).

TTF1, EMA, and cytokeratin in the surface cells {599}. Kaposi sarcoma tends to have more pointed slit-like spaces with cytoplasmic eosinophilic globules, occurs most commonly in HIV-positive patients, and has KSHV/HHV8 positivity that is not seen in haemangiomas.

Ancillary testing

Haemangiomas are positive for vascular ICC markers, which include CD31, CD34, von Willebrand factor, thrombomodulin, FLI1, and ERG, and they are usually negative for cytokeratins. GLUT1 is positive in infantile haemangioma and negative in congenital haemangioma. D2-40 (podoplanin) is positive in lymphatic proliferations {453}. The key negative stains in these lesions include KSHV/HHV8 to exclude Kaposi sarcoma and TFE3, which is seen in epithelioid haemangioendothelioma. Cytokeratin can show some weak staining in vascular tumours, but this is more common in epithelioid angiosarcoma {11}.

Molecular studies are increasingly being used, particularly in challenging cases; mutations in *RASA1*, *GNAQ*, and *PDGFRB* have been reported in haemangiomas {1300}, but molecular abnormalities become more important in supporting the diagnosis of an intermediate to malignant vascular lesion. The recent discovery of *YAP1*, *TFE3*, *CAMTA1*, and *MAML2* rearrangements in epithelioid haemangioendotheliomas has made the definitive diagnosis of these neoplasms easier on small biopsies {68,312,357}.

Leiomyoma

Domanski HA
Qian X

Definition
Leiomyomas are benign smooth muscle tumours that occur in the deep soft tissue or the abdominal-retroperitoneal cavity or in various viscera.

Clinical features and imaging
Leiomyomas commonly occur in deep dermis or skeletal muscle in extremities, or they arise in the muscularis propria of the gastrointestinal tract or the urinary tract. ER-positive leiomyomas in women can occur in the abdominal-retroperitoneal cavity or abdominal wall. Leiomyomas are typically detected radiologically as a well-circumscribed mass {136,1060,947,942,805,592}. The tumour size ranges widely, from < 10 mm for a submucosal leiomyoma in the gastrointestinal tract up to > 300 mm for a retroperitoneal leiomyoma {639,1060,938}. Leiomyomas in the gastrointestinal tract are much more commonly seen in the oesophagus than in the stomach. These submucosal leiomyomas can be successfully sampled by endoscopic FNAB {639,1435,966}.

Histopathology
Most tumours show a circumscribed bland spindle cell proliferation arranged in intersecting fascicles. The spindle cells have eosinophilic cytoplasm and slender nuclei with blunt ends, without cytopathological atypia such as nuclear enlargement, pleomorphism, or hyperchromasia. Mitoses are exceedingly rare, and necrosis is absent. Degenerative changes such as hyalinization, calcifications, and myxoid or cystic change are not uncommon {938}.

Key diagnostic cytopathological features
- Typically low, occasionally high, cellularity
- Large cohesive tissue fragments with smooth edges and variable cellularity, consisting of spindle cells
- Bland slender spindle cells with blunt-ended nuclei showing vesicular chromatin and without cell borders (Pap)
- Extremely clean background without stroma or single cells
- Lack of nuclear atypia, mitotic figures, or necrosis

Reference(s): {1345,1346,966,1383,639}

Discussion and differential diagnosis
Leiomyoma can be suspected based on cytopathology and unequivocally diagnosed with confirming ICC on cell blocks.

The differential diagnosis depends partly on the tumour location and includes most bland spindle cell neoplasms. For subepithelial intramural leiomyomas in the gastrointestinal tract, common considerations include gastrointestinal stromal tumour, peripheral nerve sheath tumour, solitary fibrous tumour, glomus tumour, desmoid fibromatosis, perivascular epithelioid cell tumour (PEComa), and even normal muscular propria. For superficial cutaneous lesions, angioleiomyoma and smooth muscle hamartoma enter the differential diagnosis. Ancillary ICC is necessary to distinguish leiomyoma from its mimics.

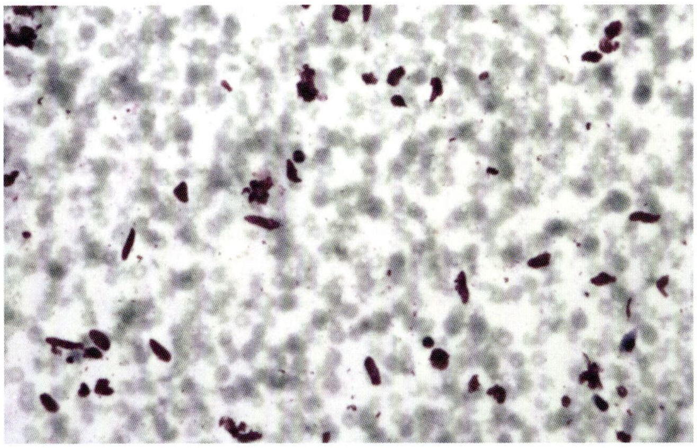

Fig. 4.99 Leiomyoma. Stripped spindle and occasionally more round nuclei are present with very occasional intact single spindle cells in a bloody background (Giemsa).

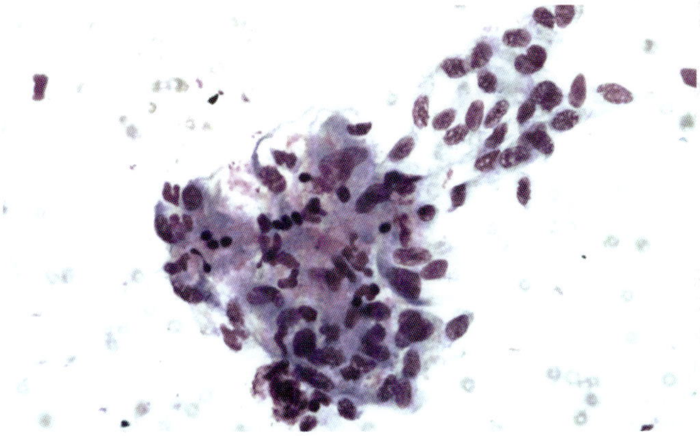

Fig. 4.100 Leiomyoma. A tissue fragment showing solid and less cohesive regions of spindle cells with elongated oval to round-ended nuclei and wispy spindle cytoplasm, seen best in the discohesive region, with some collagenous stroma in the solid region (Giemsa).

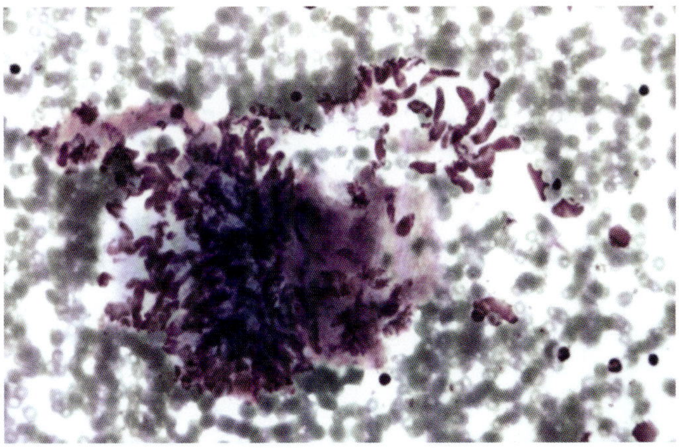

Fig. 4.101 Leiomyoma. Stripped and mildly distorted elongated nuclei with rounded ends adjacent to a dense tissue fragment showing a more collagenous region and a more crowded cellular region of spindle nuclei (Giemsa).

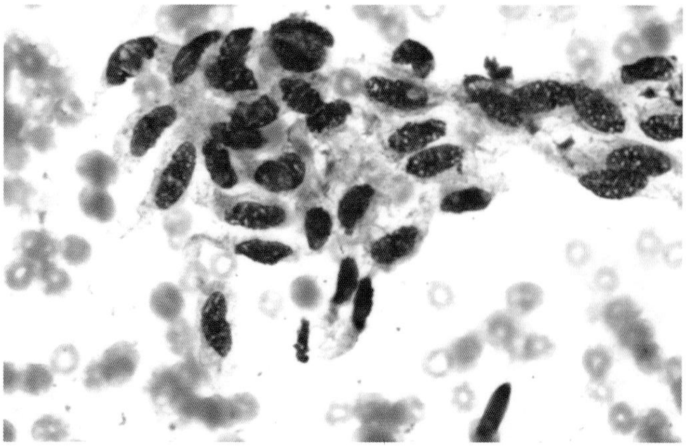

Fig. 4.102 Leiomyoma. Spindle cells with elongated mildly pleomorphic oval to spindle nuclei and wispy spindle cytoplasm (Giemsa).

Sharing identical ICC, well-differentiated leiomyosarcoma is the most important differential diagnosis. Although the presence of nuclear pleomorphism, conspicuous mitoses, and increased single cells in the background suggest leiomyosarcoma, the distinction between leiomyoma with degenerative nuclear atypia and low-grade leiomyosarcoma is extremely difficult {1383,105,346,732}. Therefore, the term "smooth muscle neoplasm of uncertain malignant potential" may be used when the distinction between the two entities is not possible on needle biopsy {938}.

Ancillary testing

By ICC, leiomyomas express desmin, SMA, and/or h-caldesmon. In addition, leiomyomas (especially in distal oesophagus and rectum) may contain scattered increased numbers of interstitial cells of Cajal, which are usually highlighted by DOG1 and KIT (CD117) ICC {947,942}. ER and PR are typically positive in retroperitoneal abdominal leiomyomas, especially in women {1060}. In situ hybridization for EBV-encoded small RNA (EBER) can be diagnostically helpful in identifying EBV-associated smooth muscle tumours in immunocompromised patients {938}.

Schwannoma

Jo VY
Domanski HA
Gajdzis P
Zarka MA

Definition

Schwannoma is a nerve sheath tumour composed entirely or nearly entirely of differentiated neoplastic Schwann cells.

Clinical features and imaging

Schwannomas arise most commonly in the 20–50 years age range, but they can occur at any age, with no sex predilection. They most commonly present as a slow-growing, superficial soft mass within the head and neck region and upper and lower extremities, often associated with a peripheral nerve. Pain may be elicited by FNAB. They can also arise within the paravertebral area, retroperitoneum, posterior mediastinum, visceral regions (including gastrointestinal tract), and bone {1457}. Schwannomas may be clinically confused with a lymph node, particularly within the head and neck region.

Most cases are sporadic, but multiple schwannomas are a feature of neurofibromatosis type 2 and schwannomatosis. Bilateral cerebellopontine angle tumours arising from the vestibular division of the eighth cranial nerve are a definitional criterion for neurofibromatosis type 2 {391}. Among sporadic cases, there is an established increased incidence associated with prior irradiation.

Schwannomas are usually isointense to hyperintense when compared to skeletal muscle on T1-weighted MRI. They are hyperintense on fluid-sensitive images and diffusely enhancing on contrast-enhanced imaging {267}.

Schwannomas follow a benign course {145}. Malignant transformation is extremely rare, and reported examples include epithelioid malignant peripheral nerve sheath tumour (MPNST) and epithelioid angiosarcoma {908}.

Histopathology

Conventional schwannomas are a well-circumscribed mass surrounded by a perineural capsule. They are characteristically composed of uniform spindle cells arranged in variable proportions of cellular fascicular arrays, often with nuclear palisading (Antoni A), and hypocellular, less organized areas (Antoni B). Compact rows of palisaded nuclei separated by fibrillary processes known as Verocay bodies are often present in the Antoni A areas. Oedematous, myxoid stromal, and cystic change are seen in Antoni B areas. The tumour cell nuclei can be spindle, tapered, elongated, buckled, or ovoid. Nuclear inclusions, nuclear atypia, and mitotic figures may be present. Vessels with hyalinized walls and foamy macrophages are common in Antoni B areas. Lymphoid aggregates are often present in a subcapsular distribution, or at the periphery in unencapsulated tumours, which is especially common in visceral sites.

Subtypes include ancient schwannoma, cellular schwannoma, plexiform schwannoma, epithelioid schwannoma, and

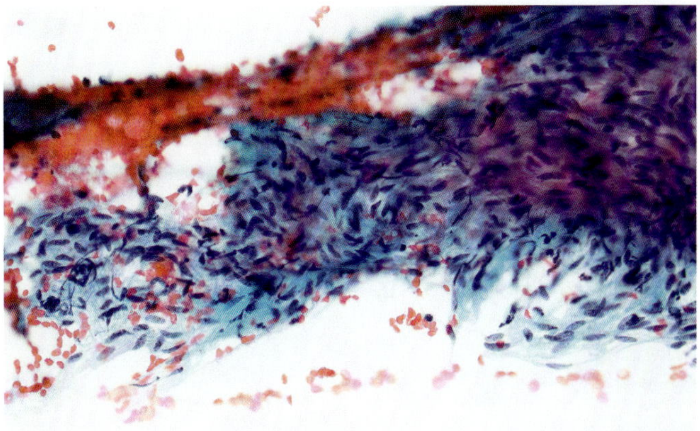

Fig. 4.104 Schwannoma. A syncytial tissue fragment made up of spindle cells with ovoid and buckled nuclei with tapered tips and ill-defined, fibrillary cytoplasm (Pap).

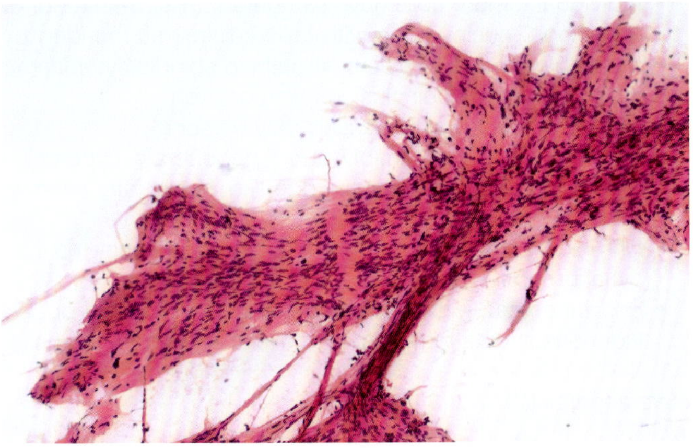

Fig. 4.103 Schwannoma. A tissue fragment composed of uniform spindle cells with nuclear palisading and areas without nuclei, creating Verocay bodies (in particular centrally) (H&E).

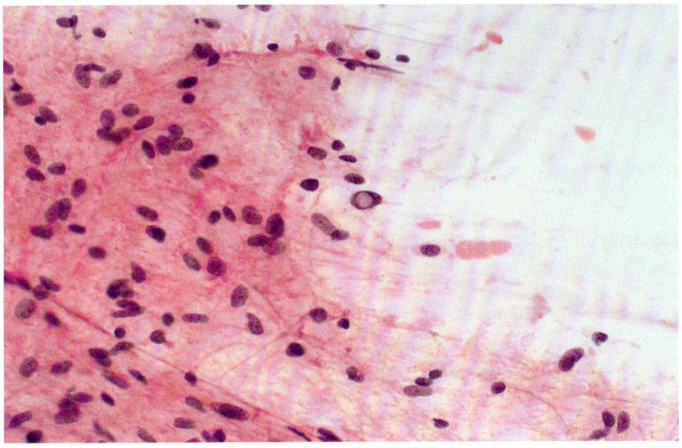

Fig. 4.105 Schwannoma. A tissue fragment with spindle cells with elongate, sometimes wavy nuclei in a fibrillary stroma. Nuclear inclusions are a common finding (H&E).

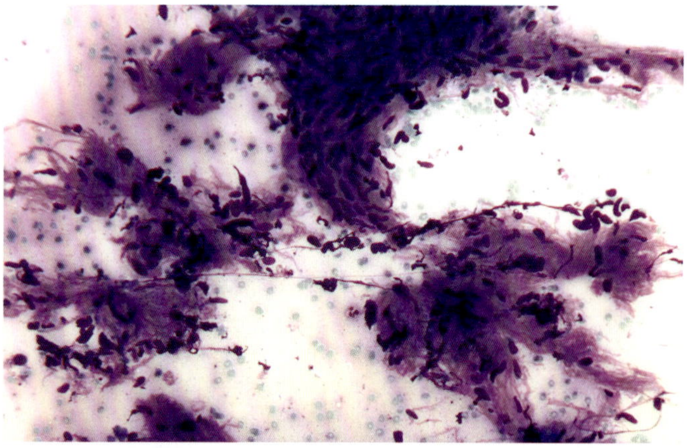

Fig. 4.106 Schwannoma. Tissue fragments showing intertwining spindle cells in a net-like pattern with fibrillary stroma (Giemsa).

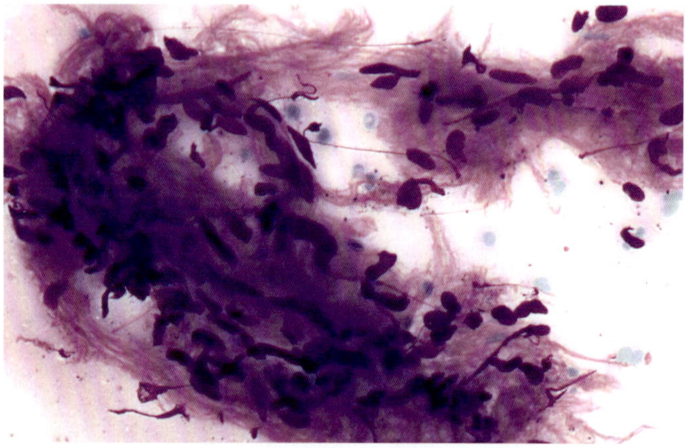

Fig. 4.107 Schwannoma. Boomerang, wavy nuclei in a fibrillary stroma with a vaguely formed Verocay body (Giemsa).

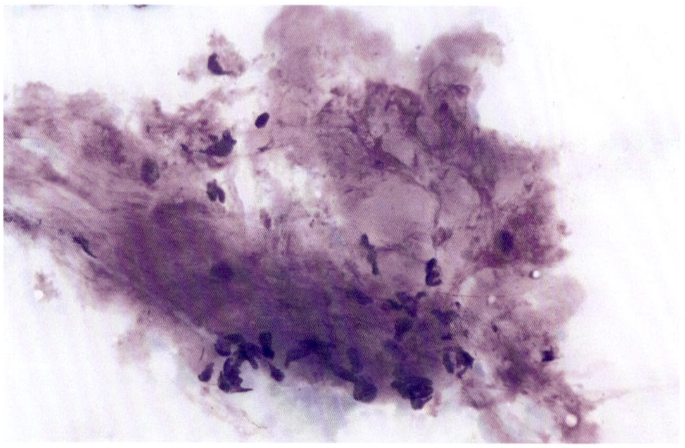

Fig. 4.108 Schwannoma. A hypocellular tissue fragment with delicate fibrillary stroma and focal elongated nuclei (Giemsa).

microcystic/reticular schwannoma. The ancient subtype shows marked, degenerative nuclear atypia. Cystic or ischaemic change, extensive hyalinization, haemorrhage, and microcalcifications are often present.

Cellular schwannomas are exclusively or predominantly composed of Antoni A areas without Verocay bodies {1518}. They show hypercellularity, as well as hyperchromatic nuclei, mitotic activity, and microscopic necrosis suggesting MPNST; however, the presence of typical features, including encapsulation, hyalinized blood vessels, and whorls of Schwann cells, makes the diagnosis {1518,1519}.

Plexiform schwannomas involve multiple nerve fascicles and show a prominent multinodular or plexiform architecture, appearing as conventional or cellular schwannoma {124}. Tumours often arise at younger ages and are common in the head and neck region. Traditional well-formed capsules and hyalinized vessels are absent.

Epithelioid schwannomas are rare; most cases are sporadic but some may be associated with schwannomatosis {543, 650}. Tumours are multilobular and predominantly epithelioid, with tumour cells in nests or linear arrays within a myxoid or hyalinized stroma. The tumour cells have pale cytoplasm and round uniform nuclei with small or inconspicuous nucleoli and occasional pseudoinclusions. Cytopathological atypia is not present. Areas of conventional schwannoma may be present. Loss of SMARCB1 is common, seen in approximately 40% of cases, and is associated with *SMARCB1* inactivation {650, 1251}. Rarely, epithelioid schwannoma undergoes malignant transformation to epithelioid MPNST.

Microcystic or reticular schwannomas are extremely rare and occur most commonly in the visceral organs, most frequently in the gastrointestinal tract {822}). These tumours show a reticular arrangement of spindle cells in a myxoid or hyalinized background, with frequent microcyst formation. The presence of Antoni A tissue is helpful in making the diagnosis.

Key diagnostic cytopathological features

- Moderate to high cellularity
- Fascicular and/or syncytial tissue fragments of spindle cells
- Syncytial tissue fragments, often made up of 3D arrays of intertwining spindle cells in a net-like or "twisted-rope" pattern
- Antoni A and B regions are usually not distinguishable, but tissue fragments may range from hypercellular to sparsely cellular
- Variably sized syncytial tissue fragments of spindle cells show occasional nuclear palisades and ill-defined cytoplasm in a fibrillary, collagenous, and/or myxoid matrix
- Single spindle cells in the background may be seen
- Individual tumour cells have elongated, oval, S-shaped, or "fish-hook" nuclei, often with tapered tips, surrounded by a variable amount of pale or ill-defined spindle cytoplasm
- Intranuclear pseudoinclusions are common
- Hyalinized thick-walled vessels may be seen
- Scattered atypical variably sized degenerate hyperchromatic and pleomorphic smudge-like nuclei are seen in "ancient" variants
- Chronic inflammatory cell infiltrate may accompany the syncytial groups
- Schwannomas with cystic degeneration or myxoid or collagenous stroma may be paucicellular and non-diagnostic

Reference(s): {197,724,345,332}

Discussion and differential diagnosis

Although schwannomas usually provide diagnostic material, they may be difficult to distinguish from both benign and malignant spindle cell neoplasms on cytomorphological grounds, but most differential diagnoses can be resolved by ICC.

Schwannoma may overlap with spindle cell lipoma with large syncytial tissue fragments of bland spindle cells; however, the spindle cell lipoma characteristically shows extensive myxoid stroma, mature adipose tissue, and collagen fibres.

Neurofibroma may be confused with schwannoma; however, neurofibromas show an extensive myxoid background, with Schwann cells admixed with perineural cells, fibroblasts, and axons.

Focal "ancient" degenerative nuclear atypia in conventional or ancient schwannoma should not be misinterpreted as evidence of malignancy, especially when mitotic activity and necrosis are absent {332,345}.

An important differential diagnosis to consider is a low-grade MPNST, especially with cellular schwannoma {554}. The distinction between these two entities can be difficult. Cellular schwannomas are often devoid of Antoni B areas, and FNAB shows tissue fragments of tumour cells with greater cellularity, scattered single cells, and stripped nuclei. Some cases demonstrate more marked degrees of nuclear atypia, including pleomorphic cells, than conventional schwannomas, and mitotic figures can be present. Similar features can be present in MPNST, but cellular schwannomas often maintain a fish-net architecture containing uniform spindle nuclei, whereas MPNSTs generally show a greater degree of disorganization, single cells, stripped nuclei, and more plentiful mitoses (including atypical forms). ICC is helpful.

At gastrointestinal sites, schwannoma should be distinguished from gastrointestinal stromal tumour and leiomyoma, because all three entities show overlapping features of uniform spindle cells and fascicular and/or syncytial tissue fragments. ICC makes this possible on FNAB material

Ancillary testing

Schwannomas, including cellular schwannomas and the epithelioid and reticular subtypes, demonstrate strong diffuse positivity for S100 and SOX10 {1030,677}, and perineural cells in the capsule are positive for EMA. Some tumours in the mediastinum may show staining for keratin {399}. Spindle cell lipoma is positive for CD34 and characterized by loss of RB1 expression. S100 is positive in neurofibroma, but the extent of staining is much less than that seen in schwannoma, because in neurofibroma the Schwann cells make up a smaller proportion of the neoplastic cells. MPNSTs frequently show lack of or only focal weak staining for S100 and SOX10 {1092}. Loss of H3 p.K28me3 (K27me3) occurs in MPNST, although it is more frequent in high-grade tumours, whereas all schwannomas show retained expression of H3 p.K28me3 (K27me3) {957}.

Gastrointestinal stromal tumour is consistently positive for DOG1 and KIT (CD117), and leiomyoma can be identified by the smooth muscle markers SMA, desmin, and caldesmon.

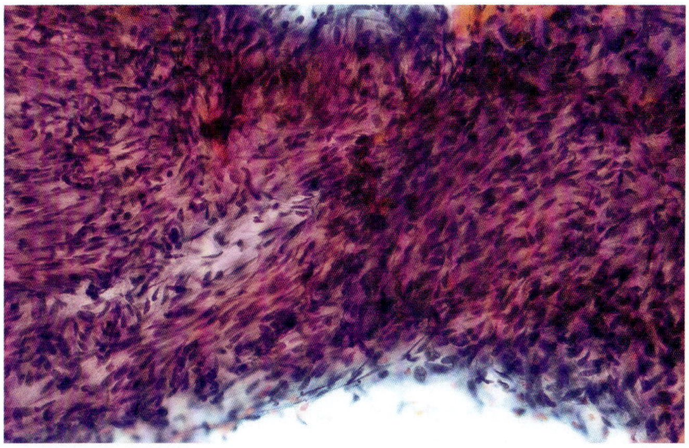

Fig. 4.109 Cellular schwannoma. A dense tissue fragment with spindle cells showing increased cellularity, with overlapping nuclei and fascicular growth (Pap).

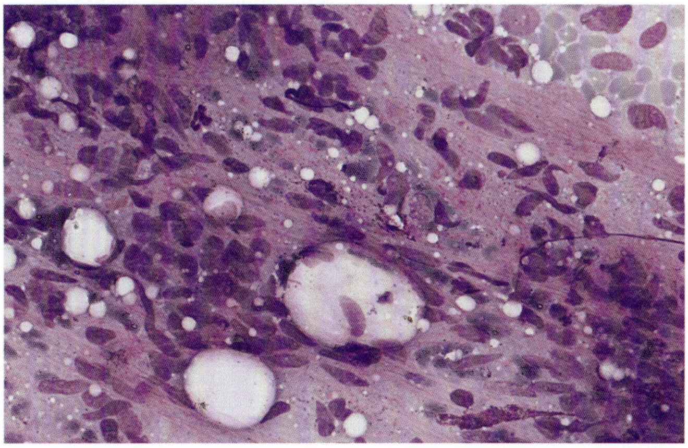

Fig. 4.110 Ancient schwannoma. Mildly atypical elongated and occasionally bent nuclei and fibrillary background, which needs to be differentiated from low-grade malignant peripheral nerve sheath tumour by lack of mitoses and necrosis (Giemsa).

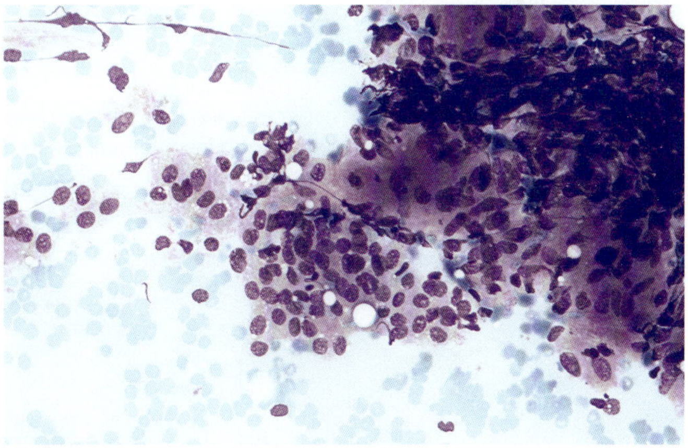

Fig. 4.111 Epithelioid schwannoma. Typical spindle cell schwannoma (12 to 4 o'clock) associated with a population of discohesive round epithelioid cells with round nuclei (Giemsa).

Neurofibroma

Chebib I
Domanski HA
Jo VY

Definition

Neurofibroma is a benign peripheral nerve sheath tumour consisting of differentiated Schwann cells, perineurial/perineurial-like cells, fibroblasts, mast cells, and residual interspersed myelinated and non-myelinated axons embedded in a myxoid and collagenous extracellular matrix.

Clinical features and imaging

Sporadic neurofibromas present as superficial tumours of skin and subcutaneous tissue associated with small superficial nerves or less commonly involving medium to major nerve trunks as deep-seated neoplasms. Cutaneous neurofibromas are typically asymptomatic, mobile, and without specific anatomical distribution. Larger or deep-seated tumours present with neuropathic changes including motor and/or sensory deficits in the nerve distribution. Patients with neurofibromatosis type 1 (NF1) present with multiple cutaneous and deep-seated neurofibromas that often involve paraspinal nerve trunks and are large and plexiform. Patients with NF1 also present with other cutaneous findings, including café-au-lait spots and axillary and inguinal freckling, as well as Lisch nodules (pigmented nodules of the iris), optic gliomas, and dysplastic lesions of bone such as sphenoid dysplasia and cortical thinning. Sporadic neurofibromas present after the second decade of life and without sex predilection. Diffuse and plexiform neurofibromatosis in patients with NF1 may present congenitally.

The imaging features of neurofibroma are dependent on the morphological subtype. Nodular neurofibroma shows superficial tumours that may be multiple in patients with NF1 {164,994, 1392,702}. Diffuse-type neurofibromas show infiltration of subcutaneous tissues on cross-sectional imaging. Plexiform neurofibromas have characteristic long, multinodular enlargement of large nerves and nerve roots, especially the lumbosacral and brachial plexus. They are often bilateral and involve multiple levels. They may cause bone remodelling of the vertebrae when arising in nerve roots. They are isointense to hyperintense on T2-weighted MRI. The target sign of peripheral hyperintensity and central hypointensity/isointensity is suggestive of a peripheral nerve sheath tumour.

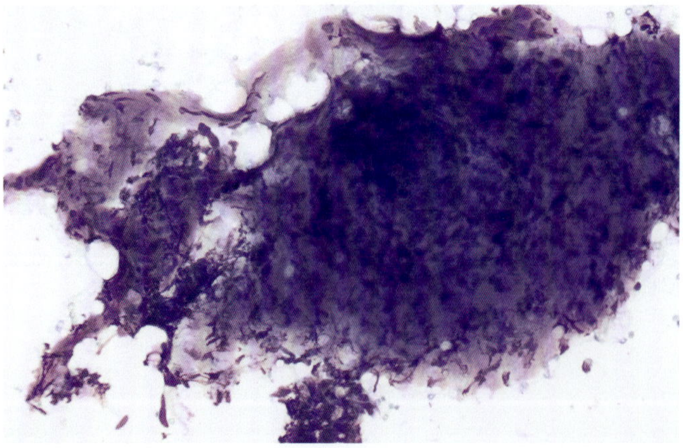

Fig. 4.112 Neurofibroma. A cohesive, thick tissue fragment with poorly seen spindle cells in a myxoid background (Giemsa).

Histopathology

Neurofibromas can show nodular, diffuse, or plexiform growth patterns {911}. Nodular neurofibromas show a well-circumscribed but unencapsulated tumour with uniform distribution of bland-appearing spindle cells, with a combination of Schwann cells and fibroblasts in a background of myxoid to fibrotic stroma. The collagen shows wiry strands, imparting a fragmented or "shredded carrot" appearance. There is often an intermixed population of mast cells. By ICC, neurofibromas contain a mixture of perineurial/perineurial-like cells and small axons.

Diffuse-type neurofibromas have similar histomorphology but lack circumscription, are often large, and infiltrate into the surrounding dermis and subcutaneous tissue. Plexiform neurofibromas are typically large and multinodular, with each nodule surrounded by perineurium. They often involve larger nerves or a nerve plexus and have a "bag of worms" or "ropy" gross appearance.

Alternative morphology is rarely seen in neurofibromas and includes pseudomeissnerian corpuscles, melanin deposition, sclerosis, metaplastic bone, and rarely epithelioid change.

Cytopathological atypia may be seen, such as degenerative atypia showing nuclear enlargement and hyperchromasia. Atypical neurofibromatous neoplasm of uncertain biological potential is a histopathological diagnosis that requires the presence of at least two of the following features: cytopathological atypia, hypercellularity, loss of classic neurofibroma architecture, and mitotic activity.

Key diagnostic cytopathological features

- Low cellularity
- Small tissue fragments of cohesive spindle cells with curved, comma, bent, or wavy nuclei
- May have occasional stripped nuclei
- Myxoid or fibromyxoid collagenous matrix

Reference(s): {1184,1465}

Discussion and differential diagnosis

The cytopathological differential diagnosis of neurofibroma includes schwannoma, spindle cell lipoma, solitary fibrous tumour, intramuscular myxoma, and low-grade malignant peripheral nerve sheath tumours. Schwannomas usually produce more cellular smears than do neurofibromas, but distinguishing schwannomas from neurofibromas requires clinical correlation because the spindle cells of these tumours may be indistinguishable, and the Schwann cells of each stain with S100 and SOX10. Neurofibromas may contain intermixed perineurial/perineurial-like cells; these may also be present at the periphery of schwannomas.

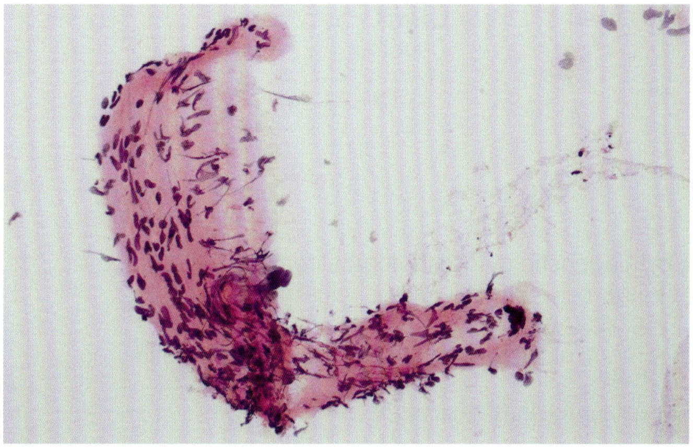

Fig. 4.113 Neurofibroma. Spindle cells with ill-defined cytoplasm embedded in collagenous stroma (H&E).

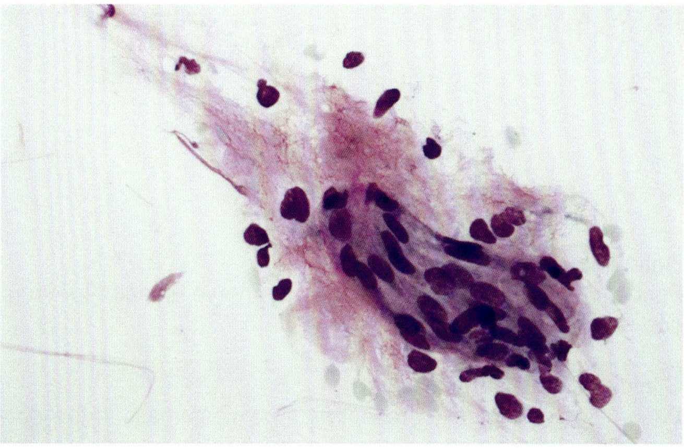

Fig. 4.114 Neurofibroma. A minute tissue fragment of spindle cells with pale blue spindle cytoplasm aligned in a background of myxoid-fibrillary matrix (Giemsa).

Spindle cell lipomas typically occur in the neck and upper back and show more-cellular smears composed of blunt spindle cells arranged in cohesive tissue fragments and as single cells with intermixed adipocytes.

Solitary fibrous tumours show well-circumscribed neoplasms with variably cellular smears, often with prominent single cells in a bloody background.

Intramuscular myxomas produce very hypocellular smears with prominent myxoid matrix, and any cellular component is negative for S100 and SOX10.

Low-grade variants of malignant peripheral nerve sheath tumour are very difficult to distinguish from neurofibromas showing cytopathological atypia due to ancient change.

Ancillary testing

In neurofibromas, the Schwann cells are positive for S100 and SOX10, and perineurial/perineurial-like cells are positive for EMA, GLUT1, claudin-1, and CD34 (which also highlights intermixed fibroblasts). Axons can be seen with neurofilament ICC. CD34 is positive in both spindle cell lipomas and neurofibroma, as well as in solitary fibrous tumours, which are characteristically positive for nuclear STAT6.

Staining for S100 and SOX10 is often strong in neurofibromas, whereas expression is focal or absent in malignant peripheral nerve sheath tumour. Loss of H3 p.K28me3 (K27me3) by ICC is extremely helpful in the interpretation of malignant peripheral nerve sheath tumour but occurs only rarely in low-grade variants.

Molecular testing is only rarely used. NGS to identify underlying mutations in *NF1* may be performed, but the large number of exons, presence of several pseudogenes, and lack of mutation hotspots with many pathogenic mutations and deletions pose challenges {1082}.

Perineurioma

Qian X
Chebib I

Definition

Perineuriomas are benign peripheral nerve sheath tumours composed entirely of perineurial cells.

Clinical features and imaging

Perineuriomas typically present as a painless mass in the dermis or the subcutaneous or deep soft tissue, or they can be intraneural or intramucosal {409,1190,1147,581}. They typically occur in the extremities or trunk, and rarely in the head and neck or viscera. They occur with an almost equal sex distribution and a median age of 41–46 years. The sclerosing variant of perineurioma occurs at median age of 26 years {409,1528}.

On MRI, intraneural perineuriomas show enlargement of the affected nerve, with proximal and distal tapering; they are hypointense to isointense on T1-weighted images and hyperintense on T2-weighted images, with marked homogeneous contrast enhancement {1510,23,807}.

Histopathology

Most tumours are circumscribed, with storiform, whorled, and/or fascicular growth patterns. Cellularity varies, with areas that are collagenous or mixed collagenous and myxoid stroma {409,1190,1147,581}. Mitoses are typically rare, with a mean of 1 mitosis per 2 mm^2. Rare atypical perineuriomas show pleomorphism, marked hypercellularity, or infiltration into surrounding tissue. Rarely they can show reticular {504,925} or plexiform architecture {1551,925}. Sclerosing perineurioma shows thick collagen deposition, with epithelioid tumour cells arranged as cords, trabeculae, or whorls {409,1528}. Only extremely rarely do malignant peripheral nerve sheath tumours show perineurial differentiation {563}.

Key diagnostic cytopathological features

- Low cellularity but can be variable
- Collagenous to myxoid background
- Bland elongated cells with bipolar cytoplasmic processes

Reference(s): {588,804,1532}

Discussion and differential diagnosis

The cytopathological features of perineurioma are very nonspecific, and it is therefore impossible to make the diagnosis based on FNAB alone. The differential diagnoses depend partly on the subtype of perineurioma. They include low-grade fibromyxoid sarcoma, neurofibroma, cellular myxoma, and dermatofibrosarcoma protuberans, and ICC is required.

Ancillary testing

Perineuriomas express EMA, which ranges from weak and focal to strong and diffuse {581}. Claudin-1 and GLUT1 are also often positive {431,1528}. CD34 is expressed in about 60% of soft tissue perineuriomas {581}. Staining for S100, SOX10, and GFAP is negative. In addition to EMA, sclerosing perineuriomas may show limited staining for keratin {409}. Sclerosing perineurioma overlaps morphologically with sclerosing epithelioid fibrosarcoma. Low-grade fibromyxoid sarcomas may express EMA and claudin-1, mimicking perineurioma. They do, however, express MUC4, which is also seen in the related sclerosing epithelioid fibrosarcoma, and testing for *FUS*::*CREB3L2* or *FUS*::*CREB3L1* fusions can assist in diagnosing low-grade fibromyxoid sarcoma / sclerosing epithelioid fibrosarcoma.

Cellular myxomas are typically positive for CD34 and may be positive for SMA. They typically do not express claudin-1

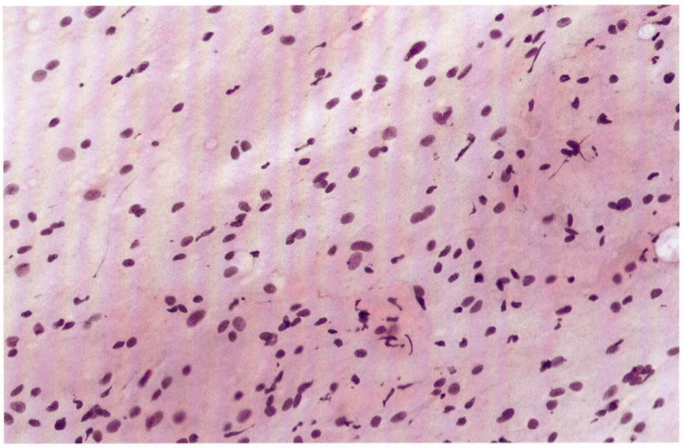

Fig. 4.115 Perineurioma. Stripped, scattered single cells with ovoid to spindle nuclei, in a thin, smoothly textured myxoid matrix (H&E).

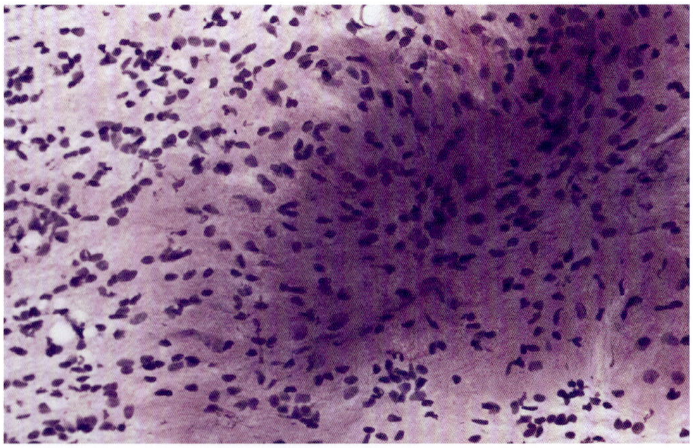

Fig. 4.116 Perineurioma. High cellularity, with small cells with predominantly ovoid to spindle nuclei with indistinct cytoplasm, embedded within focally dense myxoid matrix (Giemsa).

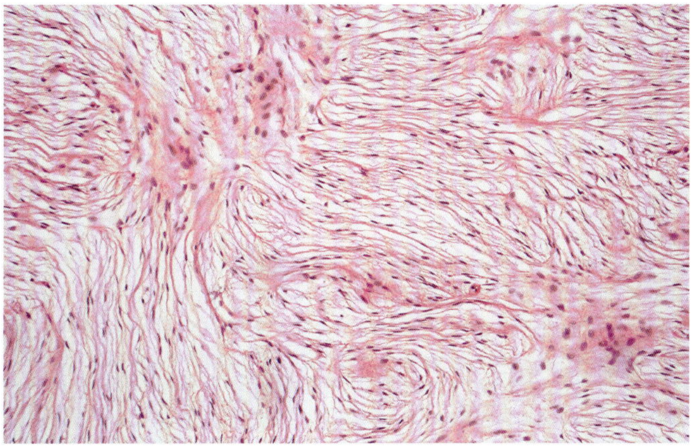

Fig. 4.117 Perineurioma. A storiform whorling architecture of thin fibres (tissue section, H&E).

or GLUT1. In difficult cases, testing for *GNAS* mutations helps classify intramuscular myxomas.

Neurofibromas may contain intermixed perineurial cells but are more diffusely positive for S100. Dermatofibrosarcoma protuberans strongly expresses CD34 but is typically more cellular at FNAB, with rare cases showing myxoid stroma. *COL1A1*::*PDGFB* fusion may be helpful in some cases.

Molecular testing for perineurioma of soft tissue is only rarely undertaken. Tumours have been associated with deletion of 22q12 and mutations in *NF2* {484,183,778}, similar to schwannomas and meningiomas.

Myofibroblastoma

Schmitt F
Silverman J
Dodd LG

Definition

Myofibroblastoma (MFB) is a benign spindle cell neoplasm occurring in the breast and extramammary sites, composed of myofibroblastic cells, bands of hyalinized collagen, and usually an adipocytic component.

Clinical features and imaging

The neoplasm is classified as mammary MFB when in the breast, as extramammary MFB when subcutaneous, as intranodal or palisaded MFB when arising in a lymph node, and as superficial MFB when involving external gynaecological sites {1488,589,909,63,1018}.

Mammary MFB was originally thought to be more frequent in the male breast, but subsequent studies demonstrated an equal sex distribution, with cases occurring especially frequently in older men and postmenopausal women {1488,589}. Intranodal or palisaded MFBs usually occur in middle-aged men in their fifth or sixth decade of life, but they have a wide age range {1018,1498,1368}. Mammary MFB generally presents as a well-circumscribed soft tissue mass, ranging from 20 mm to 130 mm, although lesions in the breast are usually 40 mm or less and extramammary sites usually 60 mm or less. Intranodal MFBs also present as a solitary circumscribed nodule up to 50 mm in diameter. The inguinal lymph nodes are most commonly involved, but a few cases have been reported in submandibular lymph nodes and rarely in other sites {1018, 1368}. Ultrasound, mammography, and MRI of the breast reveal a well-circumscribed homogeneous mass that can be confused with a fibroadenoma. Other sites, again, demonstrate a round nodule.

Histopathology

Mammary and subcutaneous MFB consists of a spindle cell proliferation arranged in irregular fascicles {1488,589,909}. The spindle cells are elongated and bland and lack any significant atypia. The spindle cells usually infiltrate bands of fibrous tissue, and focal myxoid change can be present. Admixed adipose tissue can be seen, which can cause the lesion to be confused with a spindle cell lipoma. The spindle cells have elongated nuclei and scant pale to slightly eosinophilic cytoplasm, which can resemble smooth muscle cells. Mitotic activity is low, averaging less than one mitotic figure per mm^2, and atypical mitotic figures are not seen. Mammary MFB can occasionally demonstrate a spectrum of morphological appearances, with cellular, infiltrative, epithelioid, decidua-like, collagenized/fibrous, lipomatous, and myxoid subtypes {1488}. Rarely, MFB of the breast can have bizarre mononucleated and binucleated cells that can be a potential pitfall for a malignant diagnosis, especially in CNB or FNAB specimens. The term "bizarre cell myofibroblastoma of the breast" has been proposed for this variant {63}.

Intranodal palisaded MFB consists of a cellular spindle cell proliferation that generally replaces the lymph node, although a thin peripheral rim of lymphoid tissue can be present {1018, 1498,1368}. The spindle cells are arranged in short intersecting or criss-crossing fascicles and can demonstrate subtle nuclear palisading imparting a Schwannian appearance, which can potentially lead to misdiagnosis as a schwannoma. The spindle cells are uniform, with elongated round to oval to slightly pointy-ended nuclei and surrounding pale eosinophilic cytoplasm. There is minimal cytopathological atypia, and mitotic figures are rare. The characteristic feature of intranodal palisaded MFB is the so-called amianthoid fibre, which is a stellate to globular eosinophilic extracellular band of collagen that can calcify. Admixed blood vessels, lymphocytes, red blood cells, and haemosiderin deposits can also be seen {1368}. Slit-like extracellular spaces containing erythrocytes can be present, simulating a Kaposi sarcoma–like appearance.

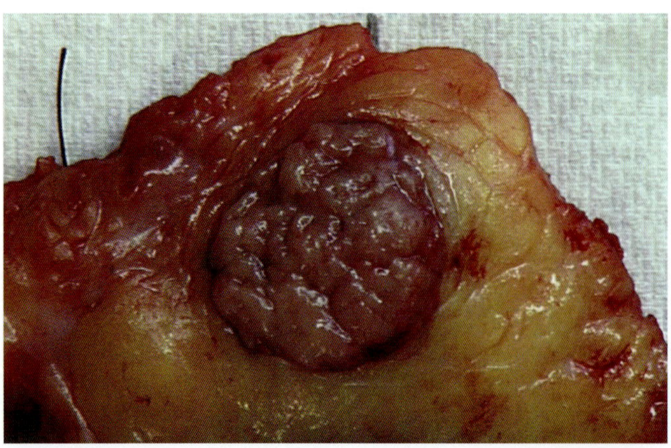

Fig. 4.118 Myofibroblastoma. A surgical specimen of well-circumscribed breast tumour.

Key diagnostic cytopathological features

Myofibroblastoma

- Moderate to high cellularity
- Cohesive tissue fragments made up of spindle cells, as well as single spindle cells in the background
- Elongated nuclei with uniformly distributed chromatin, inconspicuous nucleoli, and rare nuclear grooves; few atypical cells
- Background may contain a small amount of metachromatic stroma, which can show focal myxoid change

Reference(s): {451,56,1052,1260,1040}

Intranodal palisaded myofibroblastoma

- Usually low cellularity
- Spindle cell proliferation arranged in tissue fragments and single cells in the background
- Nuclei can align in a parallel pattern imparting a palisaded arrangement of the cells

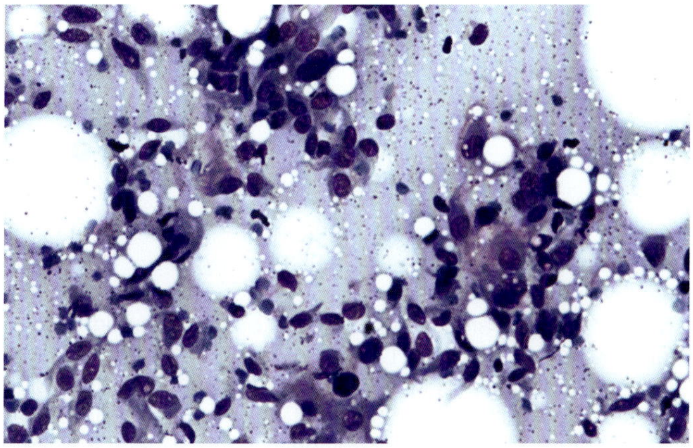

Fig. 4.119 Myofibroblastoma. Single spindle cells with fine, uniformly distributed chromatin within oval to elongated nuclei (Giemsa).

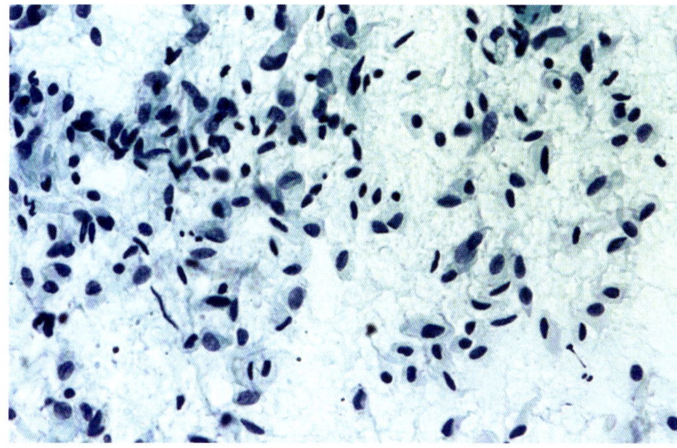

Fig. 4.120 Myofibroblastoma. A hypercellular smear consisting of single spindle cells with oval to elongated nuclei with bland, even chromatin and short spindle cytoplasm (Pap).

- Background may show haemorrhagic areas, including the presence of haemosiderin pigment and erythrocytes
- Spindle cells can surround central acellular matrix corresponding to the histopathological amianthoid fibres

Reference(s): {590,885,1523}

Discussion and differential diagnosis

The differential diagnosis of MFB is broad and encompasses a variety of reactive and neoplastic spindle cell lesions. For mammary MFB, the differential diagnosis includes solitary fibrous tumour.

Fibromatosis has long fascicles of spindle cells, in contrast to the indistinct short spindle cells of MFB, and fibromatosis is negative for desmin and positive for β-catenin, whereas MFB is positive for desmin and negative for β-catenin. Other entities to be considered in the differential diagnosis include spindle cell lipoma, which has ropy collagen in contrast to the usually diffuse collagen seen in mammary MFB, as well as spindle cell liposarcoma and low-grade malignant peripheral nerve sheath tumour, where the clinical features, cytomorphological features lacking atypia, and ICC make the diagnosis. A low-grade myofibroblastic sarcoma can also enter into the differential diagnosis, but this neoplasm has cells with hyperchromatic nuclei and moderate to severe nuclear atypia.

The differential diagnosis of intranodal palisaded MFB again includes a number of spindle cell lesions, including metastatic spindle cell carcinoma and melanoma. The metastatic malignancies demonstrate a greater degree of cellularity and nuclear atypia, and ICC assists. Benign metastasizing leiomyoma has cells with more oval and eosinophilic cytoplasm, although they do share staining for smooth muscle markers with intranodal MFB.

Ancillary testing

Mammary MFBs express CD34 and desmin, with loss of nuclear RB1 due to deletion or rearrangement of 13q14. SMA and EMA are positive in fewer than half of cases. Both solitary fibrous tumour and MFB can be CD34-positive, but mammary MFB is also desmin-positive, whereas solitary fibrous tumour is negative for desmin and positive for STAT6. In addition, MFB demonstrates loss of RB1, which is positive in solitary fibrous tumour.

Intranodal palisaded MFBs are positive for SMA and MSA. Nuclear β-catenin and cyclin D1 positivity can also be seen, but unlike in mammary MFB, desmin is infrequently positive, and CD34 is negative. Spindle cell carcinomas are cytokeratin-positive, and melanomas are positive for melan-A (MART1), SOX10, and S100. Intranodal schwannomas are S100-positive, and dendritic cell sarcomas stain for dendritic markers such as CD21 and CD35.

Myositis ossificans

Holmes BJ
Kilpatrick SE

Definition

Myositis ossificans is a benign, self-limited neoplasm of soft tissue composed of spindle cells and osteoblasts, with ossification.

Clinical features and imaging

Myositis ossificans is typically seen in athletic young adults, with an average patient age of 36 years (range: 8–84 years) and an M:F ratio of 1.5:1 {1216}. Often occurring at a site of known blunt trauma or repetitive minor trauma, myositis ossificans classically presents as a rapidly growing, painful mass in a large skeletal muscle group {7,1216}. The most frequently affected muscles include the quadriceps femoris muscle and flexor muscles of the arm, although some cases arise in the subcutis or soft tissue without muscle involvement {7,1216}. As the process matures, the pain resolves, and late-stage myositis ossificans may be painless. CT and MRI features evolve as the lesion progresses.

Histopathology

The histopathological findings evolve as myositis ossificans matures, with a variable time course but predictable pattern (Table 4.01, p. 73) {7,318}. During the initial 3–6 weeks, spindle cells proliferate in association with oedematous and vascular stroma, often with a component of organizing haemorrhage. Mitotic figures may be frequent but are not atypical. As the process matures, the spindle cell proliferation becomes surrounded by an osteoblastic proliferation that produces osteoid, mineralizing into woven bone at the periphery in a distinctive zonal pattern with a circumscribed border. Over time, the woven bone develops into lamellar bone, occasionally with a cartilaginous component that undergoes enchondral ossification. The zonal pattern is retained, with dense lamellar bone at the periphery and woven bone with or without a residual spindle cell component in the centre.

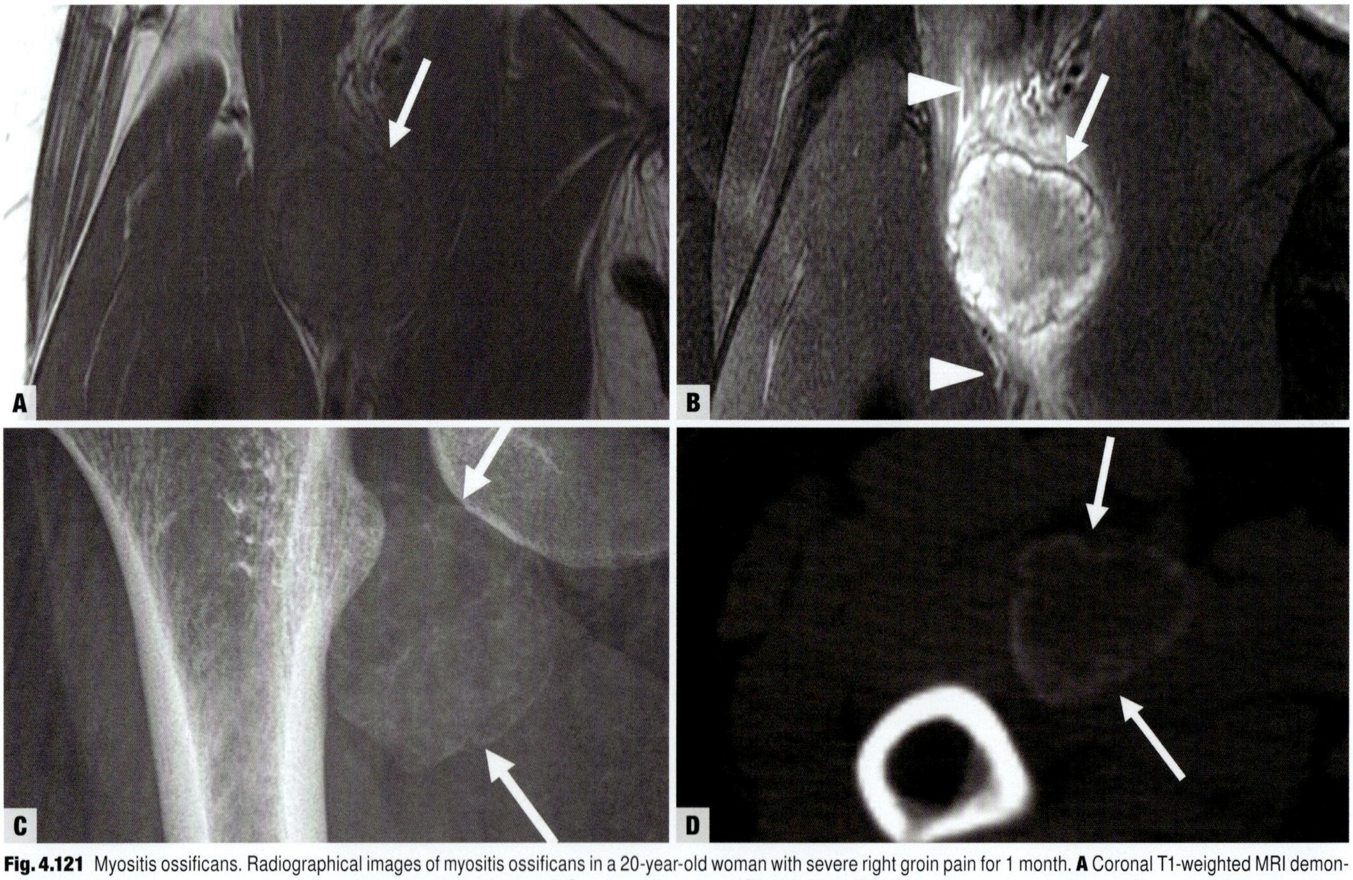

Fig. 4.121 Myositis ossificans. Radiographical images of myositis ossificans in a 20-year-old woman with severe right groin pain for 1 month. **A** Coronal T1-weighted MRI demonstrates a rounded mass anteromedial to the right proximal femur (arrow). **B** Corresponding coronal T2-weighted MRI with fat saturation shows a mass-like region of heterogeneous increased T2 signal intensity (arrow) with ill-defined surrounding soft tissue oedema (arrowheads). **C** Anterior posterior radiograph of the right medial thigh 5 weeks after onset of symptoms demonstrates a well-defined calcified lesion in the right medial thigh (arrows). **D** Axial CT shows the characteristic peripheral calcification (arrows) and lucent centre consistent with myositis ossificans. Contrast this with a soft tissue sarcoma, which typically demonstrates an ill-defined periphery and calcified, ossified centre.

Table 4.01 Clinical, radiographical, and pathological features of evolving myositis ossificans

Feature	Early	Intermediate	Mature
Approximate time course	Initial 3–6 weeks	4–8 weeks	8 weeks – 6 months
Radiographical findings	• Soft tissue mass without calcification • Oedema of surrounding tissues	• Zonal pattern: peripheral rim of calcification, initially flocculent then becoming coarse; lucent centre • Oedema of surrounding tissues • Periosteal reaction of adjacent bone may be present with retained plane between bone and lesion	• Dense peripheral calcification with lucent or lightly calcified centre
Histopathology	• Spindle cell proliferation with granulation tissue and extravasated erythrocytes • May be associated with organizing haematoma	• Zonal pattern: peripheral mature lamellar bone; intermediate osteoblastic proliferation with osteoid mineralizing to woven bone (may have cartilage with enchondral ossification); central non-ossified spindle cell proliferation with prominent vasculature	• Predominantly lamellar bone • Focal residual woven bone and spindle cell proliferation centrally
Cytopathology	• Spindle cells with wispy tapered or stellate cytoplasm, ovoid nuclei, smooth nuclear contours, fine chromatin, and increased mitotic activity • Haemorrhagic or myxoid background with granular debris • Degenerating or atrophic muscle fibres • Foamy or haemosiderin-laden histiocytes may be present	• Osteoblasts and multinucleated osteoclast-like giant cells • Spindle cells, similar to early phase • Uninucleated or binucleated chondrocytes may be present • Amorphous or fibrillary metachromatic stroma consistent with osteoid or chondroid matrix	• Paucicellular sample • Osteoblasts and osteoclast-like giant cells • Fragments of osteoid and mineralized bone • Adipocytes from marrow fat may be present

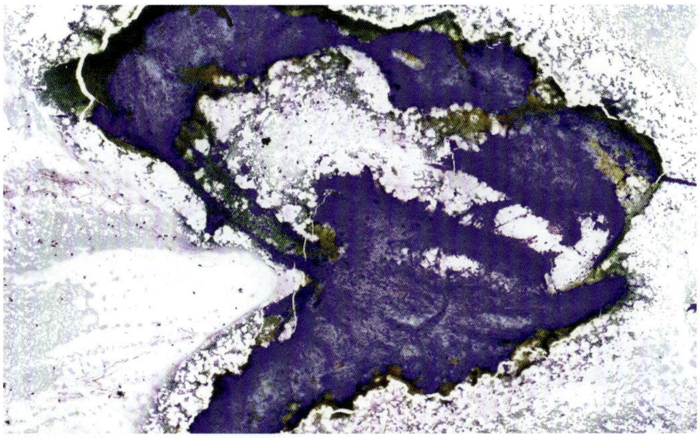

Fig. 4.122 Myositis ossificans. Tissue fragments of spindle cells, osteoblasts, and stroma, along with singly dispersed cells in a haemorrhagic background (Giemsa).

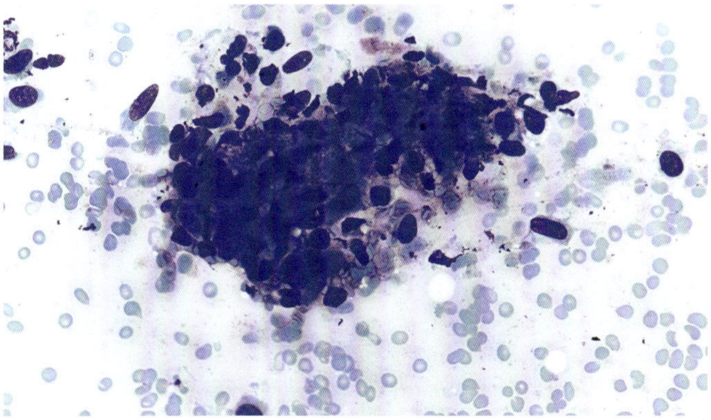

Fig. 4.124 Myositis ossificans. Spindle cells arranged in a loosely cohesive tissue fragment and singly, with delicate tapered cytoplasm and ovoid nuclei with smooth nuclear contours; there is minimal pleomorphism (Giemsa).

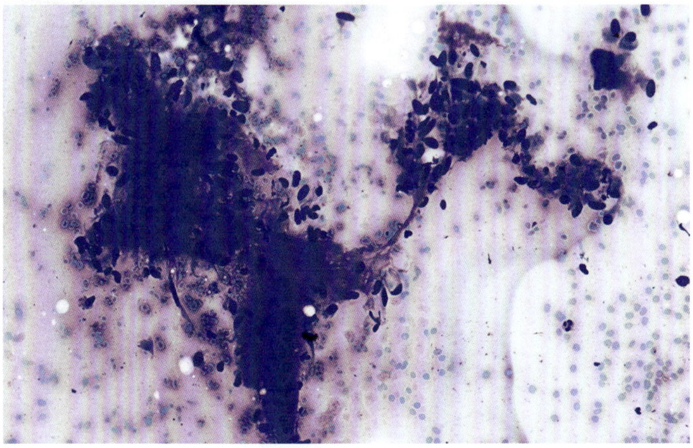

Fig. 4.123 Myositis ossificans. Variably cohesive tissue fragments of spindle cells, osteoblasts , and stroma, along with single dispersed cells in a haemorrhagic background (Giemsa).

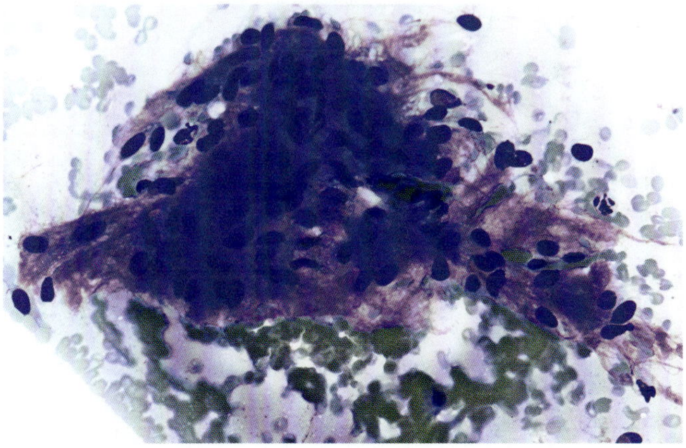

Fig. 4.125 Myositis ossificans. Spindle cells arranged in a tissue fragment, separated by magenta stroma (Giemsa).

Key diagnostic cytopathological features

- Low to moderate cellularity
- Heterogeneous at low power, depending on the phase of the progression of the lesion
- Osteoblasts cluster around osteoid in tissue fragments, and spindle cells form loose 3D tissue fragments amid single dispersed spindle cells and multinucleated giant cells
- Multiple cell types include spindle fibroblast-like cells, osteoblasts, and multinucleated osteoclast-like giant cells
- Background may be haemorrhagic or myxoid, often with granular debris and stripped nuclei
- Amorphous or fibrillary osteoid is present, associated with osteoblasts; cartilaginous matrix and degenerating muscle fibres are sometimes present

Reference(s): {721,1196,1153,968,114,333,390,295,1467,1120}

Discussion and differential diagnosis

For cases with a classic clinical history and imaging findings, biopsy is often not required. For cases with atypical imaging findings, biopsy can help to distinguish a benign process from sarcoma, although a definitive diagnosis of myositis ossificans is not always possible.

In the early phase, when spindle cells predominate, the differential diagnosis includes nodular fasciitis and proliferative myositis. Nodular fasciitis typically yields more cellular smears with a more prominent inflammatory infiltrate and delicate, branching blood vessels in myxoid stroma {333,295}. Proliferative myositis demonstrates ganglion-like cells with one or more enlarged rounded nuclei, prominent nucleoli, and basophilic cytoplasm, which are not seen in myositis ossificans {721}. Multinucleated giant cells may raise the possibility of tenosynovial giant cell tumour when abundant {1153}.

In the intermediate to mature phases, when bone is present, the differential diagnosis includes benign and malignant bone-forming tumours, particularly extraskeletal osteosarcoma and other high-grade sarcomas with heterologous osteosarcomatous differentiation {968}. In cases with prominent enchondral ossification, chondrosarcoma may also enter the differential {968}. The lack of cytopathological atypia or abnormal mitotic figures in myositis ossificans argues against sarcoma, and the finding of degenerating muscle fibres is helpful when present.

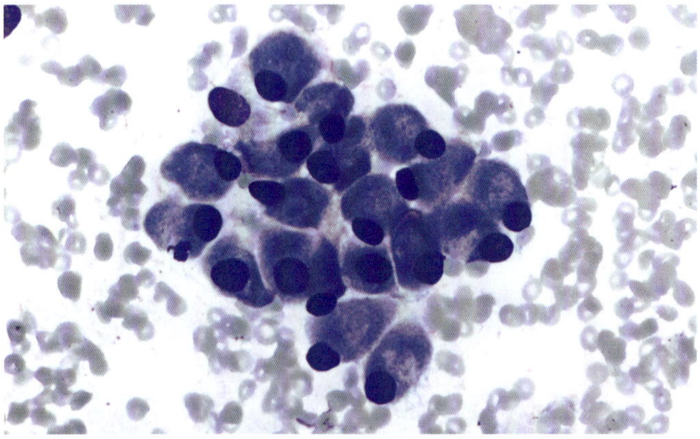

Fig. 4.126 Myositis ossificans. Osteoblasts characterized by round single nuclei and abundant eccentric basophilic cytoplasm with perinuclear clearing. Osteoblasts may be associated with osteoid, which appears as amorphous or fibrillary stroma (Giemsa).

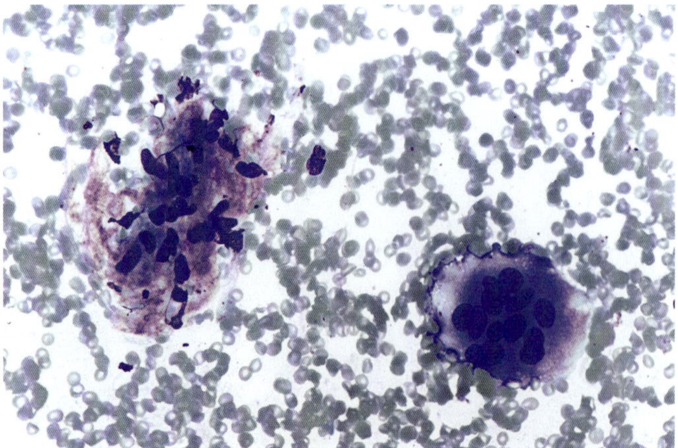

Fig. 4.127 Myositis ossificans. A multinucleated osteoclastic giant cell characterized by regular, uniform nuclei with smooth nuclear contours and small nucleoli, as well as a minute tissue fragment of spindle cells and magenta stroma (Giemsa).

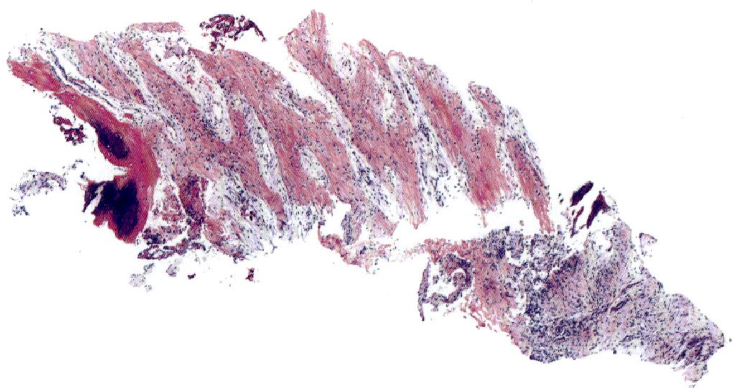

Fig. 4.128 Myositis ossificans. CNB demonstrates a zonal pattern, with woven bone located at the periphery of the lesion, surrounding an intermediate zone of collagenous stroma containing osteoblasts with variably mineralized osteoid. Cellular fragments composed of spindle cells and multinucleated giant cells are from the centre of the lesion (H&E).

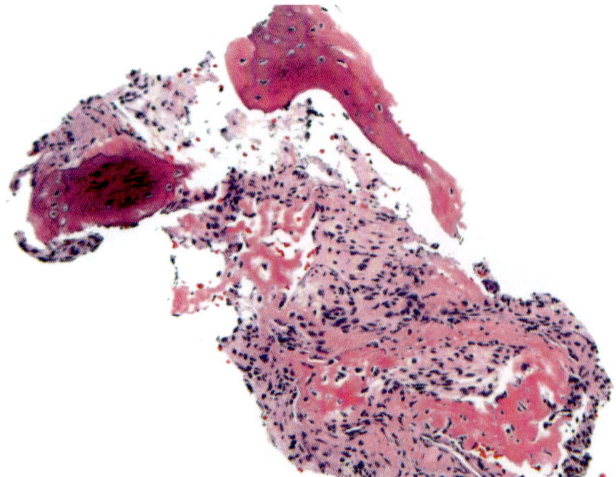

Fig. 4.129 Myositis ossificans. CNB demonstrates a zonal pattern, with woven bone (at 12 o'clock) located at the periphery of the lesion, surrounding an intermediate zone of collagenous stroma containing osteoblasts with variably mineralized osteoid (H&E).

Correlation with imaging findings showing peripheral ossification with a circumscribed border is essential.

Ancillary testing

ICC is of limited value. SMA is expressed in the spindle cells and SATB2 in the osteoblasts, but this immunoprofile is not specific for myositis ossificans {721,1467}. *USP6* rearrangements are present in the majority of myositis ossificans, as well as in nodular fasciitis and primary aneurysmal bone cyst {1358,118,1482}.

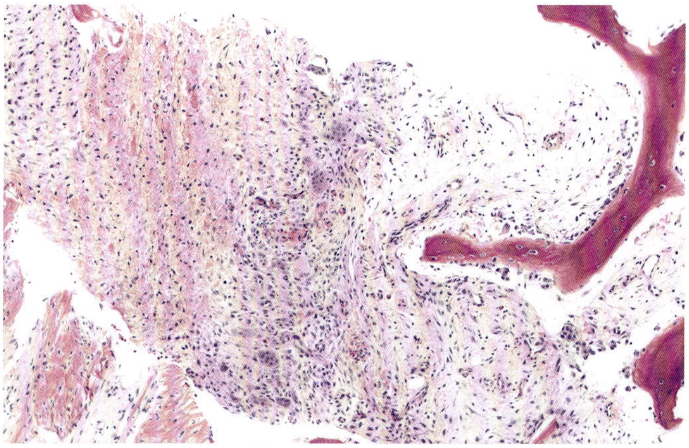

Fig. 4.130 Myositis ossificans. CNB demonstrates a zonal pattern, with osteoblasts ringing trabecular bone (3 o'clock), and then graduating cellularity with osteoblasts and osteoclastic giant cells centrally (towards 9 o'clock) (H&E).

Soft tissue chondroma

Dodd LG
Kerr DA

Definition

Soft tissue chondroma is a benign neoplasm composed of chondrocytes that produce hyaline or myxoid cartilage, arising in the extraosseous and extrasynovial soft tissues.

Clinical features and imaging

Soft tissue chondroma most commonly arises in the distal extremities, with the hands and feet being the most common sites {476, 598}. There are extremely rare examples reported in unusual sites such as the head and neck region {396}, dura {1357}, and oral cavity {716}. Chondromas of the digit are typically centred in the periarticular tissues. Affected individuals tend to be adults (middle-aged or older), and there is a slight male predominance, with an M:F ratio of 1.5:1. The tumours present clinically as slow-growing, painless masses and tend to remain small, typically < 30 mm. Depending on the extent of intralesional calcification, chondromas may or may not be visible on conventional X-ray. On MRI, they appear as circumscribed nodules that are bright on T2-weighted sequences {571}.

Histopathology

Soft tissue chondromas are typically lobulated or multilobulated, with sharp borders, and they are surrounded by a fibrous pseudocapsule. Individual chondrocytes reside in lacunae and are plump with a small, dark nucleus. Mild to moderate nuclear atypia and pleomorphism may be present, but mitotic activity is usually very limited, and atypical mitoses are absent {227,598}. There may be focal calcification of the matrix. In some instances, there may be a pattern of calcification surrounding individual chondrocytes, imparting a chondroblastoma-like appearance {185}. Degenerative changes such as myxoid or cystic degeneration are common. Individual chondrocytes may show subtle atypia and bi-nucleation, but multinucleated cells are typically not identified.

Key diagnostic cytopathological features

- Low cellularity
- Extracellular matrix material, which may appear as chondroid, myxoid, or myxofibrillary
- Chondrocytes arranged singly or in small groups, within chondroid matrix
- Nuclei are usually small, round, and dark
- Mild to moderate cytopathological atypia and pleomorphism are possible

Reference(s): {1399,699}

Discussion and differential diagnosis

Due to the frequent proximity of chondroma to bones and joints of the phalanges, the differential diagnosis includes a number of periosteal-based lesions that frequently arise in the digits, including florid reactive periostitis and bizarre parosteal osteochondromatous proliferation (Nora lesion). Both of these lesions occasionally show chondroid or chondromyxoid matrix, but this is seldom a predominant feature. Overall cytopathological and histopathological features are shared with a number of benign cartilage-forming tumours, including enchondroma, periosteal chondroma, and synovial chondromatosis. Enchondroma of the digits in particular is relatively common. Therefore, correlation with imaging studies is crucial to confirm that the lesion is located within the soft tissues and exclude tumours based in the medullary cavity, attached to the surface of the bone, or within the synovium. Chondrosarcoma of soft tissue displays more pronounced cellularity, mitotic activity, and cytopathological atypia and pleomorphism.

Ancillary testing

Soft tissue chondroma stains positively for S100. A gene fusion involving *FN1* and *FGFR1* or *FGFR2* has been identified by both FISH and RNA sequencing in a subset of soft tissue chondromas {57}. Usually the diagnosis is apparent, and ancillary studies are unnecessary.

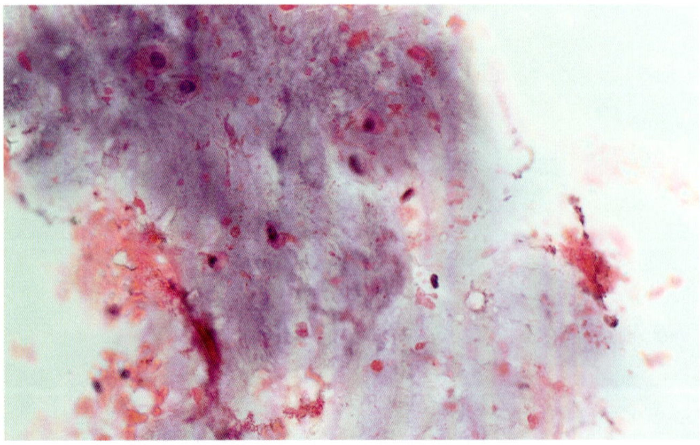

Fig. 4.131 Chondroma. Abundant cartilaginous matrix and small bland chondrocytes in lacuna (H&E).

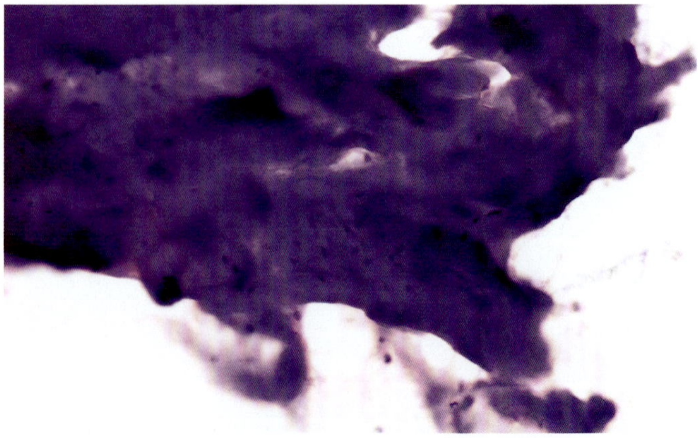

Fig. 4.132 Chondroma. Dense hyaline cartilage matrix with scattered small chondrocyte nuclei (Giemsa).

Rhabdomyoma

Monaco SE
Agaram NP

Definition

Rhabdomyomas (RMs) are benign neoplasms showing skeletal muscle differentiation.

Clinical features and imaging

RMs are divided into extracardiac RMs, which are uncommon benign tumours that occur most frequently in the oral cavity and head and neck of adults, with a male predominance, and cardiac RMs, which are the most common paediatric cardiac tumour, presenting before 2 years of age and associated with tuberous sclerosis, with mutations in *TSC1* or *TSC2* {40,659}. Genital-type RMs typically occur in women, in the vulvovaginal region. Histopathological subtypes have been described based on the differentiation of the skeletal muscle cells, such as adult-type/well-differentiated and fetal-type/immature {268}. Fetal-type RMs are associated with naevoid basal cell carcinoma in Gorlin syndrome {1534,690}. The diagnosis of cardiac tumours is typically by echocardiography, and extracardiac tumours are typically incidental findings on imaging or palpable lesions. Treatment is complete surgical excision, with recurrences reported if excision is incomplete.

Histopathology

RMs are well-circumscribed proliferations of skeletal muscle cells that appear polygonal, with eosinophilic granular cytoplasm and round nuclei. The cytoplasm can show cross-striations or intracytoplasmic rod-like inclusions. Spider cells with abundant clear glycogen vacuoles separated by strands of cytoplasm can be seen, but they are less common in the adult type {165}. Fetal types have immature thin skeletal muscle cells with variable striations and myxoid stroma with inflammatory cells, and they can infiltrate skeletal muscle.

Key diagnostic cytopathological features

- Variable cellularity
- Cohesive tissue fragments of polygonal cells with round nuclei and abundant, eccentric cytoplasm
- Cross-striations and intracytoplasmic inclusions are typically not as conspicuous on smears but can be seen on cell block

Reference(s): {349,528,905,374}

Discussion and differential diagnosis

Extracardiac RMs can be diagnosed on FNAB and small biopsies {349,528}. The differential diagnosis includes gangliocytic lesions and proliferative myositis with ganglion-like cells {161}; histiocytic proliferations, including crystal storage histiocytosis with prominent rhomboidal crystals and CD68 positivity; and glycogen storage diseases in paediatric cases. Granular cell tumours also overlap in cytomorphology, but they are strongly positive for S100 and SOX10 {638}. Paragangliomas can show similar features but are positive for neuroendocrine markers and GATA3, in addition to showing S100 staining restricted to the sustentacular cells. Oncocytoid tumours of the salivary glands or thyroid, along with alveolar soft part sarcoma and embryonal rhabdomyosarcoma, can also enter the differential diagnosis.

Ancillary testing

Diagnosis is supported by ICC positivity for desmin, MSA, myogenin, and MYOD1, with negativity for S100, neuroendocrine markers, CD68, and keratins. Positive S100 staining of variable intensity has been reported {1065}.

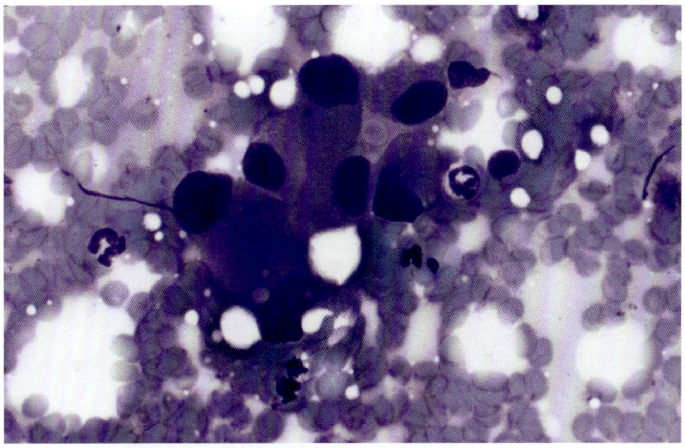

Fig. 4.133 Rhabdomyoma. Rhabdomyoma with a minute tissue fragment consisting of polygonal cells with eccentric abundant cytoplasm (Giemsa).

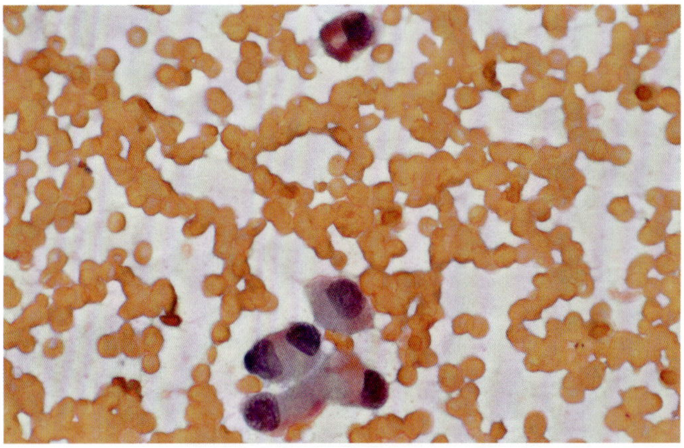

Fig. 4.134 Rhabdomyoma. Rhabdomyoma showing a minute tissue fragment of epithelioid cells with abundant eccentric cytoplasm and round nuclei (Pap).

Glomus tumour

Klijanienko J
Agaram NP

Definition

Glomus tumour (GT) is a mesenchymal neoplasm composed of cells resembling the perivascular modified smooth muscle cells of the normal glomus body.

Clinical features and imaging

GTs mainly affect young adults, with no sex predominance. The most common presentation is as a subcutaneous painful lesion in the lower or upper extremity, especially in the subungual region {435,1303,1351,535,1438}. Other presentations occur at a variety of sites, including gastrointestinal tract {946,682, 512,1454,298}, genitourinary tract {887,1220,1293,1317}, and lung {457}. Deeply located GTs present as a nonspecific mass. Some GTs may behave aggressively {678,897,854}. Multifocality is present in 10% of cases.

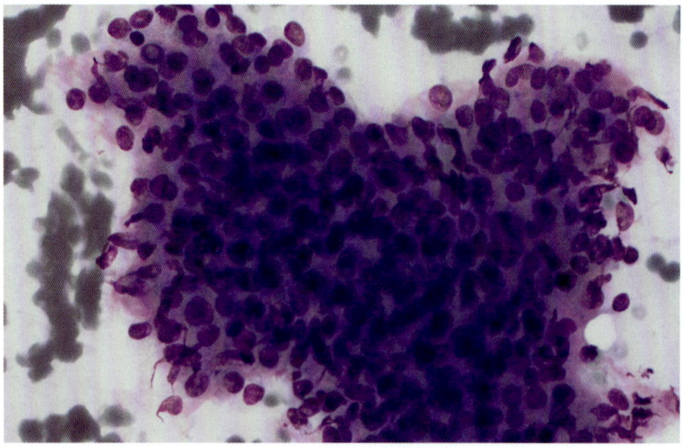

Fig. 4.135 Glomus tumour. Epithelioid to round cells with crowded nuclei (Giemsa).

Histopathology

Tumour cells are uniform and epithelioid to round with a central nucleus. The cytoplasm is lightly eosinophilic, with prominent cell borders {1133,1320}. Malignant GTs show marked nuclear atypia and/or atypical mitotic figures.

Key diagnostic cytopathological features

- Variable cellularity
- Tightly packed, well-demarcated nests and/or tissue fragments of small, round to polygonal epithelioid cells
- Distinct cytoplasmic borders and variable cytoplasm
- Round, hyperchromatic nuclei with homogeneous fine chromatin
- Magenta (Giemsa) intercellular myxoid material and a few spindle cells

Discussion and differential diagnosis

Cytopathological descriptions of GT are limited {569,964,955, 26,988,1450,1454,298,512,682,535}. The epithelioid tumour cell population may appear indistinct.

In superficial localizations, GT should be differentiated from eccrine spiradenoma {1450}, solitary fibrous tumour, and paraganglioma {988}. Eccrine spiradenoma is composed of uniform cells along with basement membrane–like magenta intercellular material {1450}. In solitary fibrous tumour, smears show tissue fragments of oval to spindle cells with ill-defined granular cytoplasm. In paragangliomas, tumour cells may show nuclear pleomorphism, with delicate intracytoplasmic reddish (Giemsa) granulations {988}.

GTs located in the gastrointestinal tract should be differentiated from gastrointestinal stromal tumours, smooth muscle tumours, and neuroendocrine tumours {1454,888}. The cells of

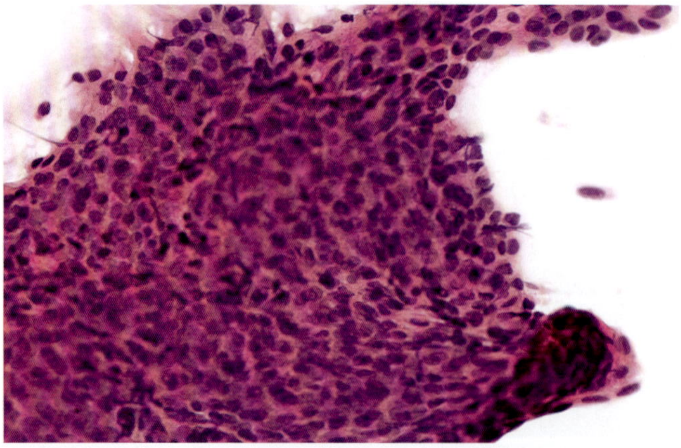

Fig. 4.136 Glomus tumour. Tightly packed, well-demarcated tissue fragments of small, round to polygonal cells (H&E).

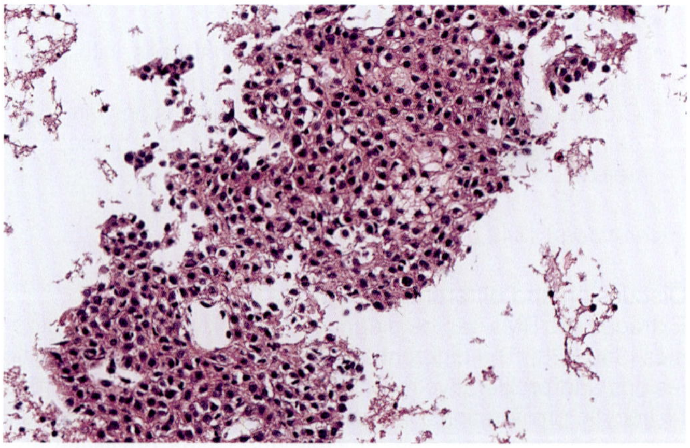

Fig. 4.137 Glomus tumour. A large tissue fragment showing polygonal to epithelioid cells with well-defined cytoplasmic borders and round, hyperchromatic nuclei (cell block, H&E).

neuroendocrine tumours are isolated or in loose small sheets with frequent pseudorosettes.

Ancillary testing

GTs are positive for SMA, MSA, collagen IV, and h-caldesmon, whereas CD34, CD56, KIT, DOG1, desmin, S100, chromogranin, and synaptophysin are usually negative {435,986}.

More than half of GT cases harbour recurrent NOTCH gene family rearrangements, with *MIR143::NOTCH1*, *MIR143::NOTCH2*, or *MIR143::NOTCH3* fusion genes {981}. Detection of NOTCH gene rearrangements and/or *BRAF* mutations may be a useful diagnostic tool, especially in malignant tumours {678,270}.

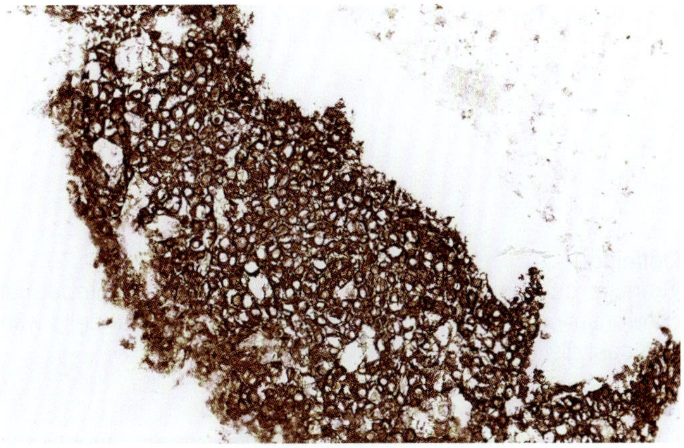

Fig. 4.138 Glomus tumour. Positive for SMA (cell block, ICC).

Granular cell tumour

Dodd LG
Klijanienko J
Silverman J

Definition
Granular cell tumour is a neoplasm showing neuroectodermal differentiation, composed of epithelioid to polygonal cells with copious, distinctively granular cytoplasm.

Clinical features and imaging
Granular cell tumour occurs in soft tissue and other body sites, including breast, tongue, gastrointestinal tract, and respiratory tract. The vast majority of granular cell tumours are benign, with very rare instances of malignant behaviour. Granular cell tumours most commonly occur in adults, with a female predominance. Soft tissue–based granular cell tumours involve the dermis and subcutis. They manifest as slow-growing, small (< 30 mm) lumps or ill-defined firm lesions that may be painful. In the gastrointestinal tract or other visceral organs, they may be incidental findings or may lead to obstructive symptoms. Approximately 10% of patients with granular cell tumours have multiple lesions. It is estimated that < 1–2% of all granular cell tumours behave in a malignant fashion. Malignant tumours tend to be larger (> 40 mm) and grow rapidly, and they can recur and metastasize {984,960, 1503}. On imaging, granular cell tumours may have irregular borders and can appear spiculated and denser than normal host tissue. On MRI, granular cell tumours have distinctive signal characteristics {141}.

Histopathology
In the dermis and other mucosal sites such as the tongue and oesophagus, granular cell tumour is often accompanied by pseudoepithelial hyperplasia, which can mimic invasive squamous carcinoma. The underlying tumour is most often infiltrative and ill-defined. Tumour cells are arranged in nests, trabeculae, or cords. Tumour cells are often very infiltrative and can occasionally cause a stromal fibrosis. Individual cells are large,

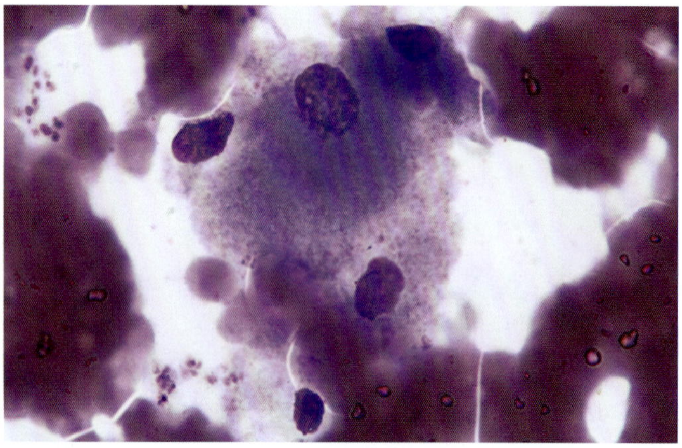

Fig. 4.139 Granular cell tumour. High-power photomicrograph showing abundant cytoplasm with a coarsely granular appearance (Giemsa).

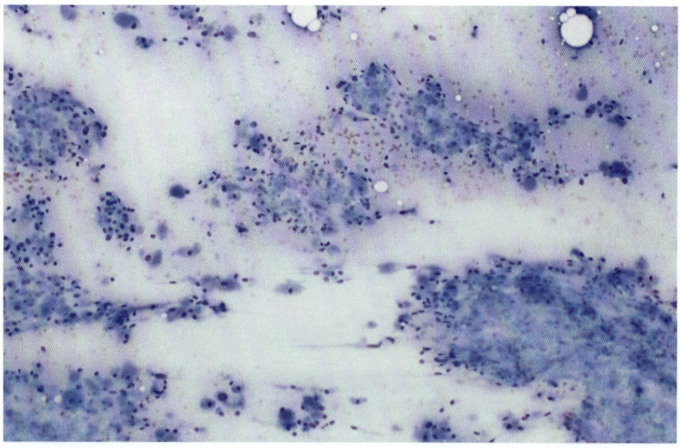

Fig. 4.140 Granular cell tumour. Moderate cellularity with loosely cohesive epithelioid cells with abundant, ill-defined cytoplasm (Giemsa).

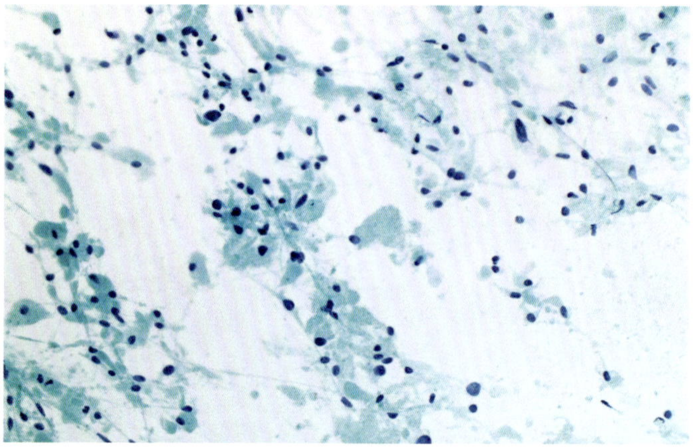

Fig. 4.141 Granular cell tumour. Loosely cohesive cells with abundant finely granular cytoplasm (Pap).

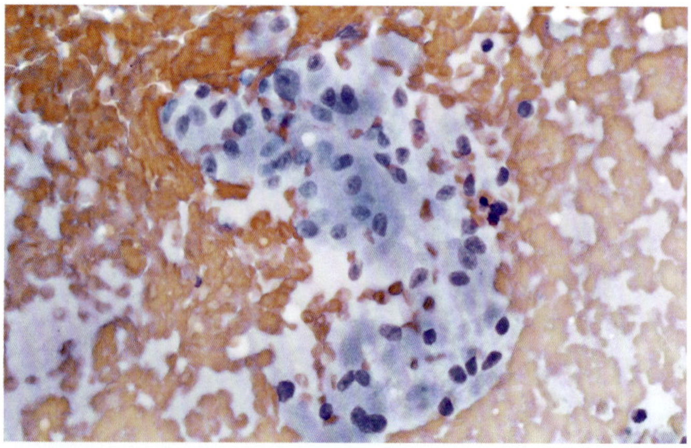

Fig. 4.142 Granular cell tumour. A loosely cohesive tissue fragment consisting of epithelioid to polygonal cells with round to oval nuclei (Giemsa).

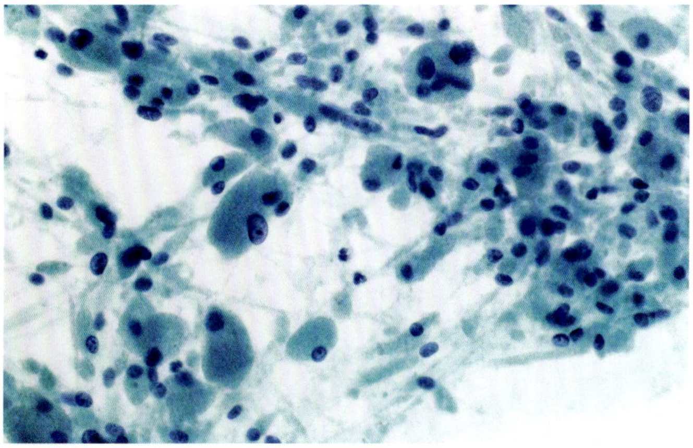

Fig. 4.143 Granular cell tumour. Epithelioid cells with abundant cytoplasm and large round nuclei with prominent nucleoli (Pap).

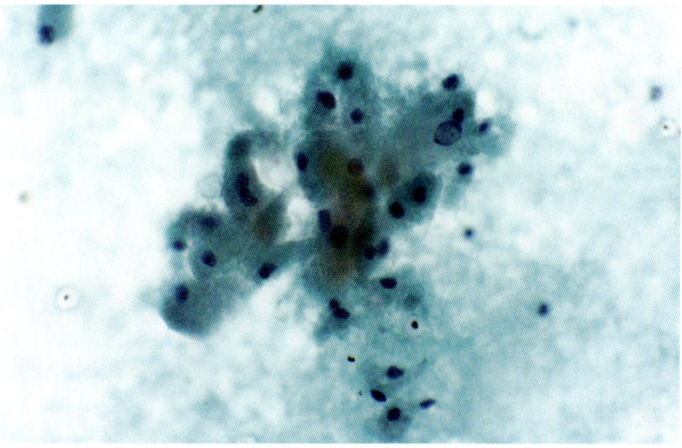

Fig. 4.144 Granular cell tumour. A loosely cohesive syncytial tissue fragment (Pap).

epithelial, or polygonal in shape, and they have abundant, faintly granular to eosinophilic cytoplasm. Cytoplasmic eosinophilia is attributable to an abundance of lysosomes and accumulation of intracytoplasmic granules.

Histopathological features associated with malignancy include necrosis, individual cell spindling, vesicular nuclei with large nucleoli, increased mitotic rate (> 2 mitoses per 2 mm^2), high N:C ratio, and pleomorphism {400}.

Key diagnostic cytopathological features

- Moderate cellularity
- Small, loosely cohesive tissue fragments or sheets and single cells
- Epithelioid cells with abundant eosinophilic cytoplasm
- Uniform, round nuclei with a single small nucleolus
- Granular debris in the background with stripped nuclei, indicating disruption of individual cells
- Features that suggest malignancy include hyperchromasia, coarse chromatin, increased N:C ratio, nuclear pleomorphism, perinucleolar clearing ("vesicular" in Pap), and enlarged nucleoli

Reference(s): {1505,287,1413,1064,835,171}

Discussion and differential diagnosis

Alveolar soft part sarcoma displays some similarities to granular cell tumour, with epithelioid cells and eosinophilic or granular cell cytoplasm, but unlike granular cell tumours, alveolar soft part sarcomas usually show nuclear pleomorphism and frequently have large and prominent nucleoli. Granular cell tumour may also be confused with epithelioid sarcoma of the classic, distal subtype, because both lesions are often located in the superficial soft tissues of the extremities. Epithelioid sarcoma has epithelioid or polygonal cells, but it usually has dense cytoplasm instead of the finely granular cytoplasm of granular cell tumour. Histiocytes also show some similarities to the cells of granular cell tumour, with abundant cytoplasm and an overall pale or eosinophilic appearance, but the nuclei of histiocytes are small, often irregular, and indented, and they lack nucleoli. Granular cells may also be confused with oncocytes, leading to difficulty in the interpretation of thyroid-based tumours {541}.

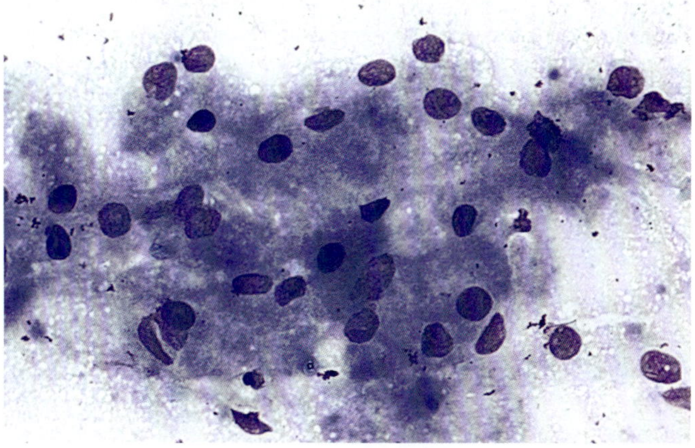

Fig. 4.145 Granular cell tumour. Epithelioid cells with granular and ill-defined abundant basophilic cytoplasm (Giemsa).

Ancillary testing

The vast majority of granular cell tumours show S100 positivity within the granular cytoplasm. They are also immunoreactive for SOX10, inhibin, calretinin, and CD68, and they display positive nuclear staining for MITF. Nuclear expression of TFE3 has been demonstrated in a subset of cases, a finding that may lead to confusion with alveolar soft part sarcoma. TFE3-positive granular cell tumour does not demonstrate a translocation of the corresponding *TFE3* gene {790,834}.

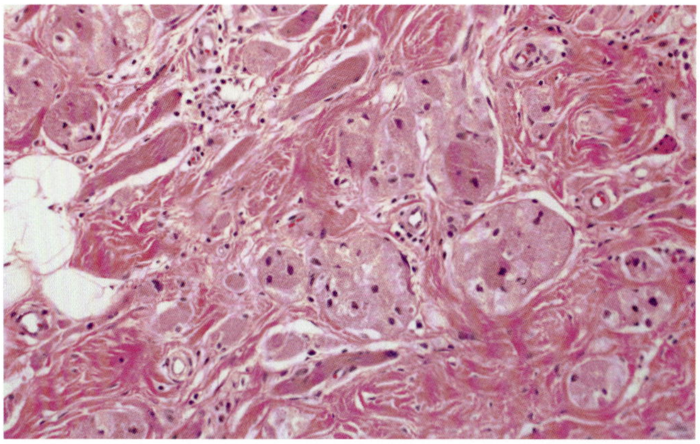

Fig. 4.146 Granular cell tumour. Granular cell tumour infiltrating stroma, eliciting a dense desmoplastic response (tissue section, H&E).

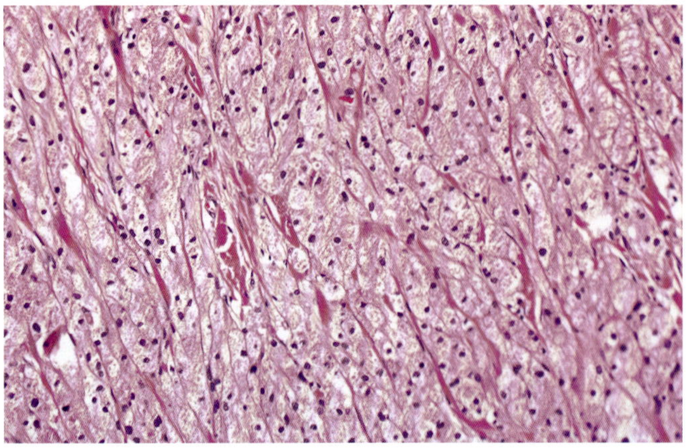

Fig. 4.147 Granular cell tumour. Rounded epithelioid cells with abundant granular eosinophilic cytoplasm and uniformly small round nuclei (tissue section, H&E).

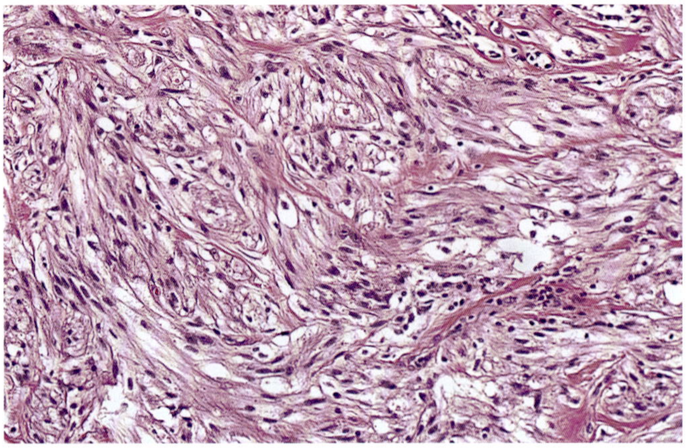

Fig. 4.148 Granular cell tumour. Spindle cells, which are a feature associated with potentially aggressive behaviour (tissue section, H&E).

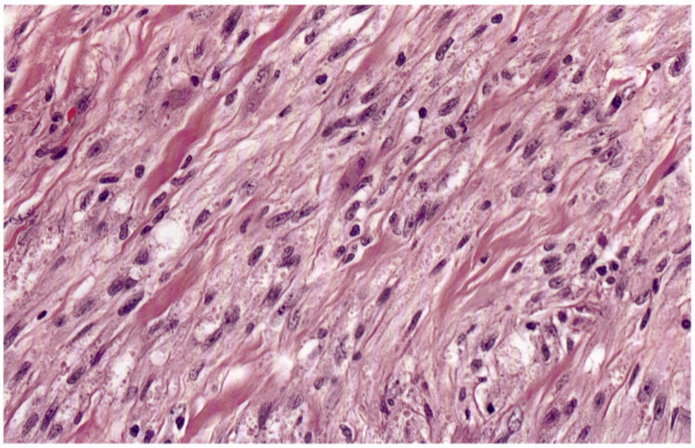

Fig. 4.149 Malignant granular cell tumour. This clinically aggressive granular cell tumour shows spindle cells, pleomorphic elongated nuclei, and enlarged nucleoli with perinuclear chromatin clearing (tissue section, H&E).

Tenosynovial giant cell tumour

Kilpatrick SE
Kerr DA
Silverman J

Definition

Tenosynovial giant cell tumour (TGCT) is a neoplasm with synovial differentiation arising from the synovium of joints, bursae, and tendon sheaths, involving the articular and/or extra-articular soft tissues.

Clinical features and imaging

TGCTs encompass a group of lesions most often arising from the synovium of joints, bursae, and tendon sheaths, and they are subdivided, based mostly on their growth characteristics, into localized TGCT, which is also known as giant cell tumour of tendon sheath and forms a discrete mass, and diffuse TGCT, which is also known as pigmented villonodular synovitis and displays an infiltrative and multinodular growth pattern. Clinical and imaging features correlate with the specific subtype. The localized form is most commonly observed in adults aged 30–50 years, arising most frequently in the hands (especially the fingers), followed in decreasing order of frequency by the toes, ankle and foot, knee, and wrist {1434}. Clinical symptoms may include a painless to painful soft tissue swelling, often present for years prior to diagnosis, and limitation of movement. On imaging, localized TGCTs form well-circumscribed masses, frequently overlying a joint and sometimes associated with underlying bone erosion.

Diffuse TGCT most commonly occurs in adults aged 20–40 years. Although virtually any joint may be affected, the larger joints, most commonly the knee, followed by the ankle and foot, hip, and shoulder, are most frequently involved. Extra-articular examples are more often seen arising in the knee or wrist {1327}. Clinical symptoms include localized pain (often of a long duration), tenderness, swelling, joint effusion, haemarthrosis, and limitation of motion. Given the tendency of TGCT to involve intra-articular spaces, MRI is the most sensitive imaging modality for detection. Imaging features include soft tissues masses, sometimes extending outside of the joint, and single to multiple cortical bone defects, rarely large and mimicking a primary bone neoplasm {855}.

Histopathology

Localized TGCTs form well-circumscribed, lobulated masses, which may be connected to the underlying synovium or tendon sheath. Collagenous septa divide the tumour into lobules, composed of variable numbers of predominantly smaller histiocyte-like cells with pale cytoplasm and round to reniform nuclei and larger polygonal to epithelioid cells with amphophilic cytoplasm and a peripheral rim of haemosiderin deposition. Aggregates of foamy histiocytes, osteoclast-type giant cells, and haemosiderin deposits are virtually always admixed at least focally. The background stroma may be significantly collagenized. Identical histological features are observed in diffuse tenosynovial giant cell tumours, but the growth pattern is infiltrative and expansile, often causing significant and grossly visible enlargement of the synovial fronds. Osteoclast-type giant cells tend to be less common and may be absent in up to 20% of cases. Tissue tears and cyst-like spaces, sometimes filled with blood, are observed in a minority of examples {1327}. Infarct-like necrosis, leaving residual "tombstones" of osteoclast-type giant cells, is not infrequently observed and may encompass virtually the entire tumour, presumably the result of torsion of the tumour nodule(s). Mitotic activity, especially among the diffuse form of tenosynovial giant cell tumour, may exceed 10 mitoses per 10 HPF, but in the absence of significant nuclear pleomorphism or frank sarcoma-like changes, this has no prognostic relevance.

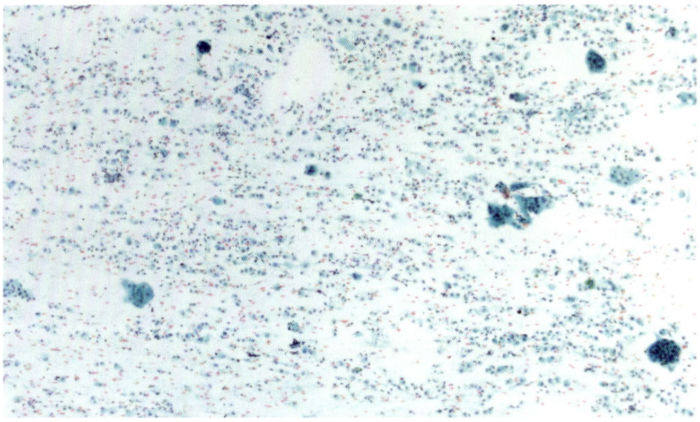

Fig. 4.150 Tenosynovial giant cell tumour. Scattered multinucleated giant cells in a background of mononuclear cells (Pap).

Key diagnostic cytopathological features

- High cellularity
- Predominantly discohesive cells and occasional 3D tissue fragments
- Polymorphous population of polygonal to histiocytoid mononuclear cells
- Round to ovoid nuclei with evenly distributed chromatin and inconspicuous nucleoli
- Variable numbers of osteoclast-type giant cells, foamy histiocytes, lymphocytes, and haemosiderin-laden macrophages
- Infarct-like necrosis may be present focally but is rarely extensive
- Mitotic figures may be abundant, but atypical forms are never observed
- Chondroid metaplasia has been described

Reference(s): {1560,623,221,525,3}

Discussion and differential diagnosis

The differential diagnosis for TGCT is largely dependent on the site and growth pattern (localized vs diffuse), encompassing both neoplastic and non-neoplastic conditions made up of a predominantly histiocytoid to epithelioid cell population, with or without abundant osteoclast-type giant cells. Correlation with imaging studies, when available, considerably narrows the differential, helping to provide a more definitive diagnosis.

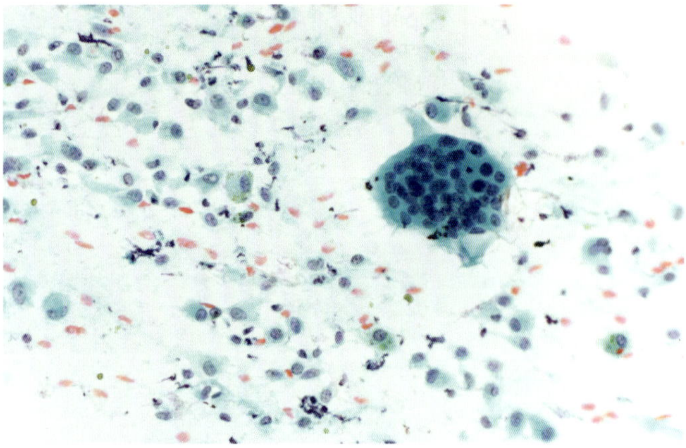

Fig. 4.151 Tenosynovial giant cell tumour. A multinucleated giant cell with relatively uniform nuclei stands out from the small mononuclear cells in the background (Pap).

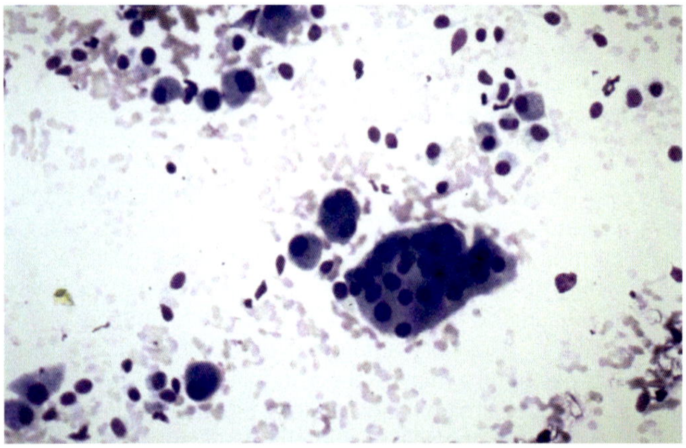

Fig. 4.152 Diffuse tenosynovial giant cell tumour (pigmented villonodular synovitis). Characteristic discohesive histiocytoid cells, admixed lymphocytes, and an osteoclast-type giant cell (Giemsa).

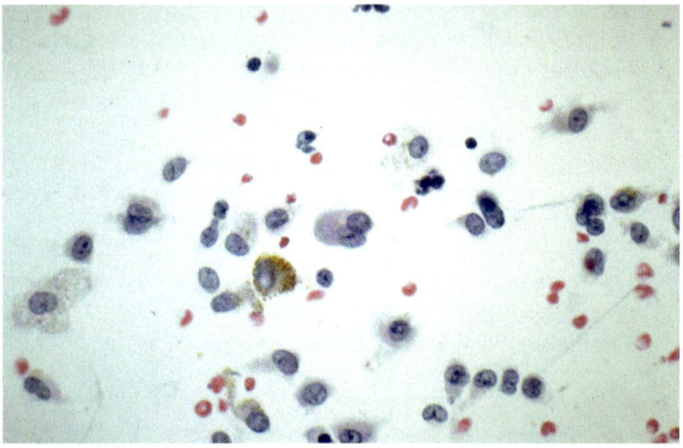

Fig. 4.153 Diffuse tenosynovial giant cell tumour (pigmented villonodular synovitis). Histiocytoid cells, one of which contains haemosiderin pigment granules (Pap).

In the extremities, especially the hand, it is important to distinguish localized TGCT from epithelioid sarcoma, which usually lacks osteoclast-type giant cells, admixed inflammatory cells, and haemosiderin pigment deposition. Giant cell tumours of soft parts are another differential diagnosis of localized TGCT, and they arise in the superficial soft tissues of the dermis or subcutis, primarily in the extremities, and are less polymorphous than TGCT, with uniform ovoid to slightly spindle mononuclear cells, a prominent fibrovascular stroma, and frequently secondary haemorrhagic and cystic changes {1037,1049}.

Revision arthroplasty rarely undergoes FNAB, but the clinical setting, with polarizable foreign material and histiocytic giant cell reaction, is diagnostic {508}.

Intra-articular haemorrhage can produce haemosiderin deposits and villous hyperplasia of the synovium.

Giant cell tumour of bone (GCTB) should only rarely be a problem for the differential diagnosis from TGCT when clinical and imaging correlation is carried out. GCTBs generally affect patients between 20 and 40 years of age, usually arising in the epiphyseal regions of long bones, with less frequent involvement of the sacrum and vertebral body, pelvis, and small tubular bones of the hands and feet. In the vast majority of cases, these tumours remain confined to the bone, and soft tissue extension is the exception {1429}. Locally recurrent GCTBs presenting in the soft tissue are a differential diagnosis of giant cell tumour of soft tissue and TGCT. GCTBs produce hypercellular smears that are more cohesive, with a dual population of uniform oval to slightly spindle mononuclear cells admixed with usually distinctly larger osteoclast-type multinucleated giant cells. Like TGCT, infarct-like necrosis may be present and sometimes extensive, and foamy histiocytes are not uncommon.

High cellularity and the presence of mitotic activity may raise the differential of malignant TGCT, but these extraordinarily rare tumours demonstrate overtly malignant cells with high nuclear grade, tumour necrosis, atypical mitotic figures, and areas of overt pleomorphic spindle cell sarcomatous differentiation {48}. Most resemble undifferentiated pleomorphic sarcomas or high-grade myxofibrosarcomas. As mentioned previously, mitotic activity, especially in the diffuse form of an otherwise typical TGCT, may be brisk, and this finding alone does not equate to "malignant" TGCT.

Ancillary testing

ICC is generally not required to establish the diagnosis of TGCT. Clusterin is frequently positive in the larger mononuclear cells, some of which may also show desmin reactivity. Histiocytic markers (CD68 and CD163) are diffusely expressed by the predominant smaller histiocyte-like cells and osteoclasts. Cytokeratins, EMA, S100, SOX10, CD21, and CD35 are uniformly negative. Cytogenetic analysis has revealed that 1p13 (*CSF1*) is most frequently involved by structural aberrations, most often fused with 2q37 (*COL6A3*), in a minority of the lesional cells {971,1270}. GCTB also demonstrates a different molecular pathogenesis with *H3-3A* (*H3F3A*) mutations, readily assessed by the diagnostic ICC surrogate H3 p.G34W {525,1254}.

Sample reports: Benign

Rekhi B
Field AS
Qian X

The sample reports provided here are based on the standardized cytopathology report in the *Diagnostic categories and report structure* section of the first chapter. See that section for a discussion on the structure and components.

These are sample reports that include the components required in one possible format; the final report format depends on local practice and local laboratory information system requirements. For brevity, demographics and ROSE are not presented here.

Each institution should select a term for the main heading of the diagnostic summary, such as "Diagnostic summary" (as used in the examples below), "Diagnosis", or "Final diagnosis", and use it consistently.

Sample report 1

Specimen type:
FNAB
Clinical and imaging information:
44-year-old female. Soft 40 mm lump in right thigh, 1-year duration. MRI shows well-defined, encapsulated, expansile, homogeneously intense 44 mm lesion with thin septa in the adductor muscle.

Diagnostic summary:
Site: Right mid-thigh adductor muscle
Category: Benign
Diagnosis: Consistent with a lipoma

Material received:
Three air-dried Giemsa slides and one alcohol-fixed slide. 3 mL pink fluid with possible fatty flecks on its surface received, but there was no pellet on spinning down for cell block.

Microscopic description:
These mildly cellular smears show tissue fragments consisting of mature adipocytes and occasional single adipocytes in a lipoproteinaceous background, consistent with a lipoma.

Sample report 2

Specimen type:
FNAB
Clinical and imaging information:
45-year-old male. Superficial soft tissue 20 mm swelling inner aspect of right thigh. Nonspecific findings on ultrasound.

Diagnostic summary:
Site: Inner aspect of lower right thigh
Category: Benign
Diagnosis: Spindle cells and fat (see comment below)

Material received:
Two air-dried slides, one alcohol-fixed slide. No fluid for cell block.

Microscopic description:
These moderately cellular smears show tissue fragments of fat and spindle cells with bland elongated nuclei seen singly and in minute tissue fragments.

Comment: The features are benign but not diagnostic of a specific lesion, and the findings may not represent the targeted lesion. Correlation with clinical and imaging findings is recommended, and repeat FNAB should be considered.

(Editor's note: The lesion has no specific clinical or ultrasound findings. Some cytopathologists may categorize the findings as "Non-diagnostic"; others, as illustrated here, categorize the findings as "Benign", report what they see on the smears, and add the caveat that "the findings may not represent the targeted lesion".)

Sample report 3

Specimen type:
FNAB
Clinical and imaging information:
35-year-old female. History of diffuse large B-cell lymphoma and bone marrow transplant. Now enlarging superficial left paraspinal mass on back in T10 region growing from 7 mm to 13 mm in 3 months.

Diagnostic summary:
Site: FNAB of superficial lesion left T10
Category: Benign
Diagnosis: Nodular fasciitis (see Supplementary reports 1 and 2 below)

Material received:
Four air-dried Giemsa-stained smears from ROSE and two alcohol-fixed smears. 2 mL of bloodstained fluid prepared for cell block (rather than for original request for flow cytometry).

Microscopic description:
These moderately cellular smears show scattered myxoid tissue fragments containing mildly pleomorphic spindle cells and occasional larger cells with a low to moderate N:C ratio and oval large nuclei with prominent single nucleoli. Similar single spindle and larger cells are present in the background, with occasional lymphocytes. The cell block shows similar material.

Comment: The features are consistent with nodular fasciitis. Confirmatory immunocytochemistry and molecular testing for *USP6* gene rearrangements have been ordered.

Supplementary report 1:
On cell block, the tumour is diffusely positive for SMA, and H3 p.K28me3 (K27me3) expression is retained. Desmin, caldesmon, S100P, SOX10, CD34, MDM2, ALK, and β-catenin are negative.

Supplementary report 2:
RNA sequencing–based fusion profiling demonstrated the *MYH9::USP6* fusion, confirming the diagnosis of nodular fasciitis.

(Editor's note: In this case, the initial categorization as "Benign" and diagnosis as "consistent with nodular fasciitis" have been issued with a note that ancillary tests are underway. The ICC findings and then the molecular results have then been issued as two supplementary reports in one integrated report, and the final diagnosis has been modified to reflect the additional ancillary test results.)

Sample report 4

Specimen type:
EUS-guided FNAB
Clinical and imaging information:
70-year-old female. History of skin cancers and chronic lymphocytic leukaemia, now found to have an 18 × 12 mm bilobed hypoechoic submucosal lesion in the gastric cardia.

Diagnostic summary:
Site: EUS-guided FNAB gastric cardia
Category: Benign
Diagnosis: Leiomyoma (see comment below)

Material received:
Six air-dried Giemsa smears from ROSE, three alcohol-fixed slides for Pap staining. 4 mL bloodstained fluid spun down for cell block.

Microscopic description:
These highly cellular smears show large tissue fragments made up of bland spindle cells with a fascicular architecture and elongated ovoid nuclei, in a bloody background. No mitoses are seen. There is no necrosis. The cell block sections show similar bland spindle cells with elongated nuclei and abundant eosinophilic cytoplasm in fascicles with small vessels. Immunocytochemistry shows the tumour cells to be diffusely positive for desmin, SMA, and h-caldesmon. S100 is negative. Both DOG1 and KIT (CD117) highlight occasional admixed interstitial cells of Cajal.

Comment: Overall, the findings best support a diagnosis of leiomyoma with an increased number of interstitial cells of Cajal. The presence of increased interstitial cells of Cajal, which are positive for KIT (CD117) and DOG1 by immunocytochemistry, in a leiomyoma may be a result of entrapment and/or hyperplasia and is a finding recognized as a mimic of gastrointestinal stromal tumour (see reference below). Clinical and imaging correlation is recommended.

Reference: Deshpande A, Nelson D, Corless CL, et al. Leiomyoma of the gastrointestinal tract with interstitial cells of Cajal: a mimic of gastrointestinal stromal tumour. Am J Surg Pathol. 2014 Jan;38(1):72–7 {316}

(Editor's note: In this case, the cytopathologist has not issued a cytopathological report but rather waited until the ICC was available to make the specific diagnosis and issue the report as a final report.)

Chapter 4

Sample report 5

Specimen type:
FNAB
Clinical and imaging information:
25-year-old male. Slow-growing superficial lump upper arm. MRI shows well-defined, lobulated lesion right forearm with hyperintensity on T2-weighted images. Note: The FNAB caused intense pain, and only one pass was performed.

Diagnostic summary:
Site: Upper right arm
Category: Benign
Diagnosis: Schwannoma

Material received:
Two air-dried slides and one alcohol-fixed slide. 2 mL of pink fluid received and processed for cell block.

Microscopic description:
Moderately cellular smears showing spindle cells in branching, anastomosing tissue fragments and scattered singly, in a relatively clean background with occasional scattered lymphocytes. The tumour cells have elongated, tapering, often angled "fishhook" nuclei and occasional intranuclear inclusions, with a moderate amount of pale spindle cytoplasm. The cell block shows similar features, and the tumour cells are diffusely positive for S100 and SOX10.

(Editor's note: In this case, the cytopathologist has not issued a cytopathology report but rather waited to include the ICC on the cell block in one integrated final report.)

Sample report 6

Specimen type:
FNAB
Clinical and imaging information:
25-year-old female patient with a well-defined lesion on the dorsum of wrist of 6 months' duration.

Diagnostic summary:
Site: Dorsum of left wrist
Category: Benign
Diagnosis: Ganglion cyst

Material received:
Four air-dried slides and one alcohol-fixed slide.

Microscopic description:
A large amount of thick proteinaceous material is present, with occasional macrophages with foamy cytoplasm.

Sample report 7

Specimen type:
FNAB
Clinical and imaging information:
36-year-old male. Left anterior axillary fold 15 mm firm fixed lesion. Ultrasound shows spiculated lesion fixed to fascia.

Diagnostic summary:
Site: Left anterior axillary fold
Category: Benign
Diagnosis: Granular cell tumour

Material received:
Three air-dried smears and two alcohol-fixed smears. 3 mL pink fluid for cell block.

Microscopic description:
Moderately cellular smears composed of cohesive sheets and scattered polygonal cells containing abundant granular cytoplasm and small round nuclei with inconspicuous nucleoli. There is no material in the cell block.

Comment: The features are those of a granular cell tumour. Correlation with clinical and imaging findings is recommended, and if clinical suspicion is high, repeat FNAB (to obtain material for immunoperoxidase studies) or CNB is recommended.

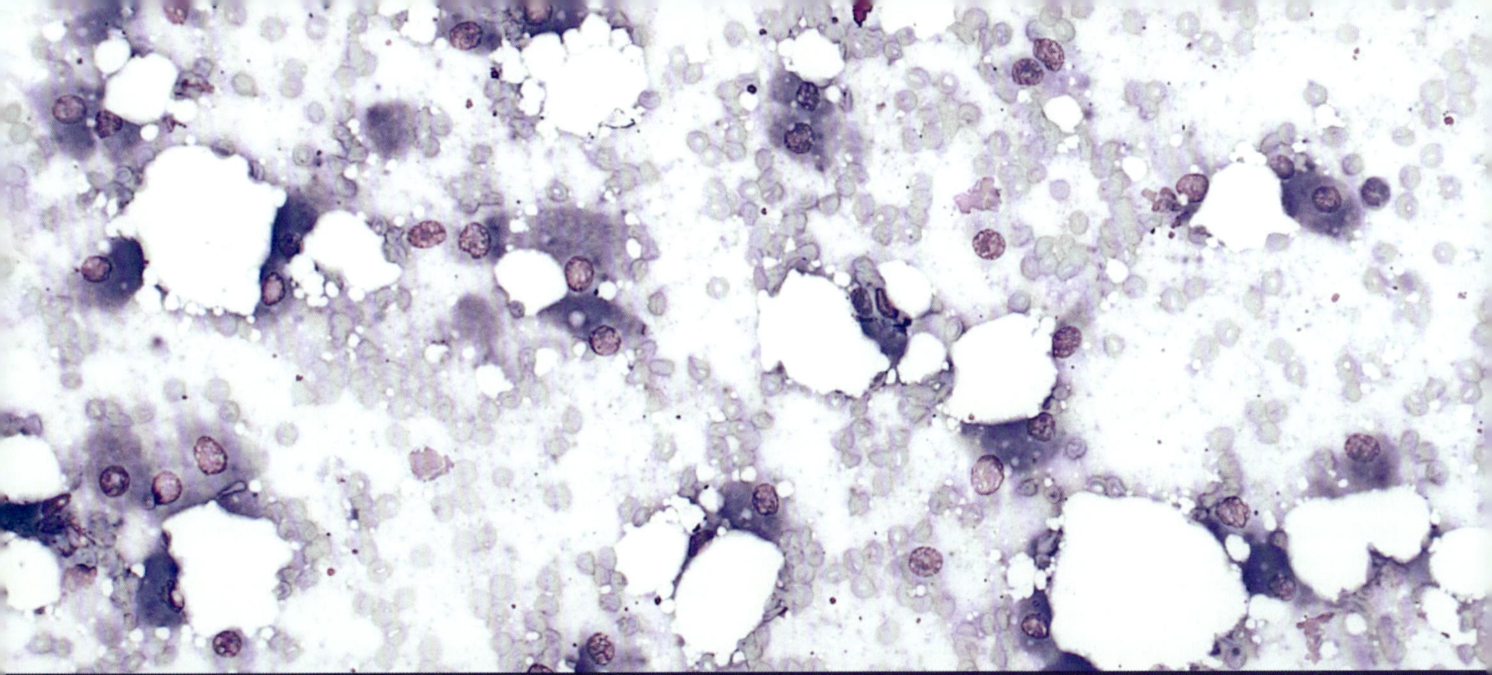

5

Diagnostic category: Atypical

Edited by: Klijanienko J, Pitman MB, Schmitt F

Introduction

Raymond WA

The "Atypical" category is used when there are cytopathological features present that are essentially benign, but with occasional features uncommon in benign lesions that raise the remote possibility of a malignancy and thus cannot be ignored. This indeterminate category is included to increase the negative predictive value of a "Benign" categorization.

Whenever atypical features are present, the FNAB is categorized as "Atypical", even if the overall material shows technical faults and would otherwise be categorized as "Insufficient", or when suboptimal preparation has resulted in a degree of artefactual or degenerative change but sufficient atypical cytomorphological features are present and a malignancy cannot be entirely excluded. Most of the specimens in this category are likely to be from reactive, inflammatory, or reparative processes, but specific features sufficient for a definitive benign diagnosis are lacking. The category must be used in conjunction with the clinical history, physical examination, and imaging findings. The report should always state that "correlation with clinical and imaging findings is required".

Definition

Raymond WA

A specimen categorized as "Atypical" demonstrates features seen predominantly in benign lesions and minimal features that may raise the possibility of a malignant lesion, but with features insufficient, either in number or in quality, to diagnose a benign or malignant process or lesion.

Discussion and background

Raymond WA

There is no consistent definition of atypia in relation to soft tissue lesions, and there are no standardized criteria for an "Atypical" categorization. The term "Indeterminate" has been used for this category in the literature, but the WHO Reporting System for Soft Tissue Cytopathology (WHO System) favours the term "Atypical" to allow consistency with other WHO Reporting Systems and to separate the more likely benign "Atypical" category from the more likely malignant category "Suspicious for malignancy", thereby maintaining a moderate to high negative predictive value for the "Atypical" category, a high positive predictive value for the "Suspicious for malignancy" category, and a hierarchical increased ROM within the WHO System categories.

Categorization of a soft tissue FNAB as "Atypical" may be based on the cellular pattern, high cellularity, nuclear features such as variable nuclear enlargement or degenerative or symplastic features as can be seen in ancient change in a schwannoma or granular cell tumour, and the stromal component. Potential problems arise due to cytomorphological overlap between different tumour types, in particular low-grade spindle cell tumours {753}. Lipomatous tumours may show atypical cells in an otherwise adipocyte-rich smear in atypical lipomatous tumours {753}.

Soft tissue inflammatory lesions may have nuclear pleomorphism and atypia, such as ganglion-like cells in nodular fasciitis, or fibroblastic proliferation after infarction or reparative changes after biopsy, traumatic haematoma, or radiotherapy, and the features may overlap with those of a neoplastic process. Other cases categorized as "Atypical" are those in which there is insufficient material present to confidently categorize the lesion subtype.

A specimen may also be rendered "Atypical" for technical reasons related to the expertise of the operator performing the FNAB, the quality of smear preparation and staining, the nature and accessibility of the site of the lesion, and the experience of the cytopathologist interpreting the specimen.

In the report, the atypical features should always be specified in the microscopic description and the differential diagnosis discussed, with a favoured diagnosis provided if possible.

This category should be used judiciously and not as a "wastebasket" for unknown diagnoses. In a large review of 1114 bone and soft tissue lesions, 3% showed atypical cells, of which 17 of the 22 with follow-up (77%) were confirmed as malignant {696}. One text {233} suggests using atypical and suspicious categories for FNAB, but most studies do not provide ROM for

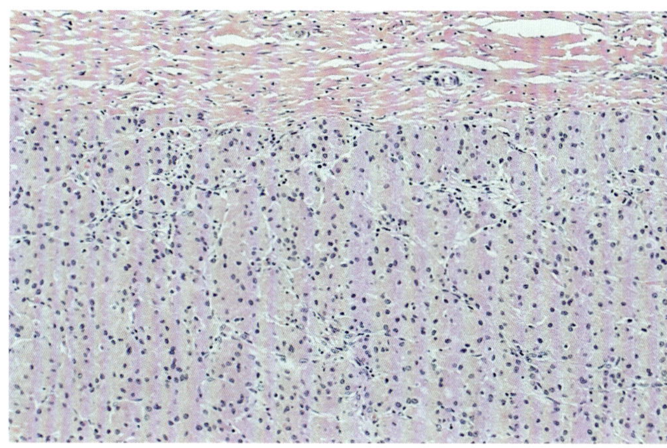

Fig. 5.02 Granular cell tumour of the subcutaneous tissue in the chest wall. Corresponding section of a benign granular cell tumour (H&E).

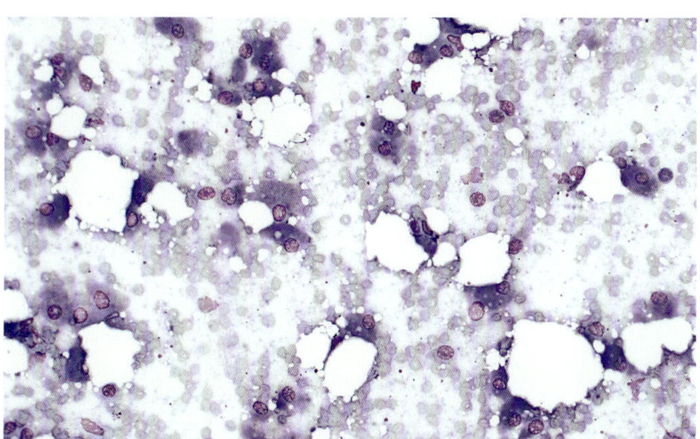

Fig. 5.01 Granular cell tumour of the subcutaneous tissue in the chest wall. Dissociated cells with rounded nuclei, showing some crush artefact, and abundant dense cytoplasm. The features are atypical, and the differential diagnosis is of granular cell tumour and an apocrine neoplasm (Giemsa).

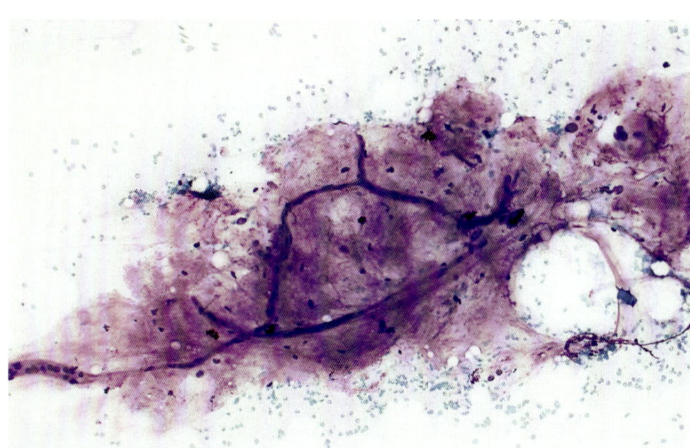

Fig. 5.03 Myxoid myofibroblastoma of the breast/subcutis. A tissue fragment of myxoid stroma with embedded spindle nuclei showing mild hyperchromatism and branching vasculature. There is a broad differential diagnosis, and the features are categorized as "Atypical" (Giemsa).

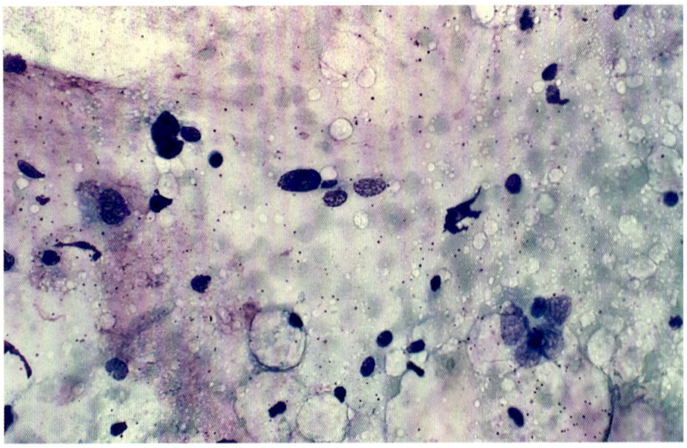

Fig. 5.04 Myxoid myofibroblastoma of the breast/subcutis. Dissociated spindle nuclei showing some size variation and hyperchromatism, and a variable amount of cytoplasm. The features raise a broad differential diagnosis and are categorized as "Atypical", suggestive of a spindle cell neoplasm (Giemsa).

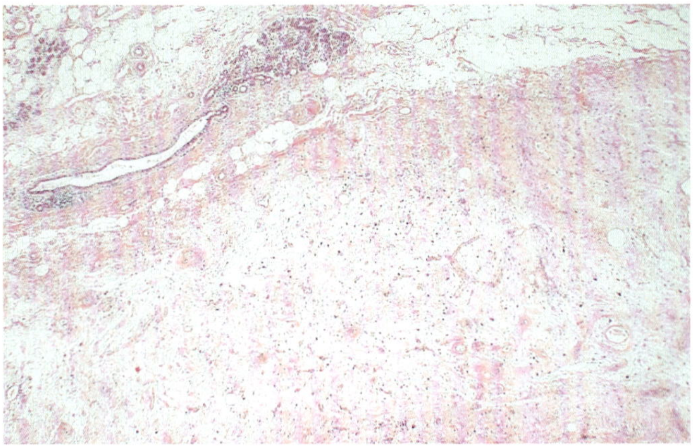

Fig. 5.05 Myxoid myofibroblastoma of the breast/subcutis. A circumscribed myxoid lesion arising in the breast, with no cytopathological features of malignancy, most consistent with a myxoid myofibroblastoma (tissue section, H&E).

atypical/suspicious FNAB and only indicate overall sensitivity and specificity in distinguishing benign from malignant. Several other studies have reported the proportion of cases in the atypical/suspicious category as 1–2%, usually representing only 1 or 2 cases {1330,1470}.

Risk of malignancy and diagnostic management recommendations

Raymond WA

This category includes reactive, inflammatory, or reparative processes that lack the specific criteria that would allow a definitive benign diagnosis, as well as cases in which the sample lacks sufficient qualitative or quantitative features to differentiate between a non-neoplastic and a neoplastic lesion. In addition, atypical specimens may represent a benign lesion or normal tissue in which there has been suboptimal preparation resulting in a degree of artefactual degenerative change, but in which there are sufficient atypical morphological features such that a malignancy cannot be entirely excluded.

The ROM has been reported as 46% in one study of soft tissue and bone lesions {753}. A recent single-institution retrospective review of more than 2200 cases categorized using the WHO System reported a ROM of 39.62%, and it was observed that the ROM varied across all categories when the pattern was taken into account; that is, ROM varied from 3% for lipomatous tumours to 62.78% for spindle cell, 78.15% for epithelioid, 84.58% for myxoid, 94.26% for pleomorphic, and 100% for round cell tumours {460}.

Correlation with clinical findings, imaging, and any available ancillary tests on FNAB material are essential once a soft tissue FNAB is categorized as "Atypical", and discussion by a multidisciplinary team is recommended. If these findings indicate that the process is highly likely to be a benign neoplasm or a reactive or inflammatory process, then observation and clinical follow-up may be considered, but in most cases, and in particular any cases where there is discrepancy in the triple approach, a repeat FNAB is recommended, ideally with ROSE and where available CNB. Incisional biopsy with frozen section or excisional biopsy may be considered if the imaging and clinical suspicion is high.

Sample reports: Atypical

Qian X
Field AS
Rekhi B

The sample reports provided here are based on the standardized cytopathology report in the *Diagnostic categories and report structure* section of the first chapter. See that section for a discussion on the structure and components.

These are sample reports that include the components required in one possible format; the final report format depends on local practice and local laboratory information system requirements. For brevity, demographics and ROSE are not presented here.

Each institution should select a term for the main heading of the diagnostic summary, such as "Diagnostic summary" (as used in the examples below), "Diagnosis", or "Final diagnosis", and use it consistently.

Sample report 1

Specimen type:
CT-guided FNAB
Clinical and imaging information:
62-year-old male. Past history of right upper arm soft tissue sarcoma, followed by radiation therapy. MRI reveals 10 mm subcutaneous lesion adjacent scar.

Diagnostic summary:
Site: Right upper anterior arm
Category: Atypical
Diagnosis: Spindle cell lesion with focal atypia (see comment below)

Material received:
Four air-dried Giemsa-stained smears from ROSE, two alcohol-fixed smears. 4 mL pink fluid.

Microscopic description:
One mildly cellular smear shows a few stromal fragments containing plump single cells along with scattered single spindle cells showing nuclear enlargement and focal atypia, against a background of inflammatory cells and red blood cells. There are no mitotic figures, markedly pleomorphic cells, or necrosis in the background. The other smears show blood only. Cell block contains limited material showing inflammatory cells and fibroblastic/myofibroblastic cells positive for SMA and negative for MDM2.

Comment: The features are considered atypical and raise a differential diagnosis of reactive changes following surgery and possibly residual sarcoma. CNB or excision biopsy is recommended.

(Editor's note: In this case, there is limited material categorized as "Atypical".)

Sample report 2

Specimen type:
FNAB
Clinical and imaging information:
28-year-old male. 30 mm soft tissue lump right forearm slow-growing over 4 years. MRI shows well-defined, lobulated 27 mm soft tissue lesion.

Diagnostic summary:
Site: FNAB right forearm
Category: Atypical
Diagnosis: Spindle cell tumour with atypia

Material received:
Two air-dried slides and one alcohol-fixed slide. 3 mL bloodstained fluid, which yielded no pellet for cell block.

Microscopic description:
Mildly cellular smears show syncytial fragments of spindle cells with occasional poorly formed nuclear palisades. Spindle cells have elongated, occasionally angulated nuclei and are embedded in a fibrillary metachromatic stroma. Occasional larger cells show nuclear enlargement, hyperchromasia, and atypia. There is no diagnostic material in the cell block.

Comment: A spindle cell neoplasm is present, showing atypia, and the differential diagnosis includes ancient schwannoma. Repeat FNAB (to obtain material for ancillary studies) or CNB is recommended.

Sample report 3

Specimen type:
FNAB
Clinical and imaging information:
25-year-old female with a slowly growing hard 60 mm mass in left flank. Ultrasound shows an irregular ill-defined mass attached to muscle and in deep subcutis.

Diagnostic summary:
Site: Left flank
Category: Atypical
Diagnosis: Spindle cell neoplasm

Material received:
Six air-dried slides. 3 mL pink fluid.

Microscopic description:
One moderately cellular smear shows spindle cells in tissue fragments with pale cytoplasm separated by magenta stroma, with elongate tapering nuclei. Occasional similar spindle cells are present in the background. There are no mitotic figures or necrosis. The other slides show only blood. The cell block has no diagnostic material.

Comment: The features are atypical and raise broad differential diagnoses, including fibromatosis. Correlation with clinical findings and further imaging is recommended. FNAB (to obtain material for immunocytochemistry) or CNB is recommended.

Sample report 4

Specimen type:
FNAB
Clinical and imaging information:
75-year-old male. Recently noticed posterior lower neck soft mass.

Diagnostic summary:
Site: Posterior left-sided neck mass
Category: Atypical
Diagnosis: Adipocytic neoplasm

Material received:
Two air-dried smears and one alcohol-fixed smear. 2 mL pink fluid. Cell block prepared.

Microscopic description:
There is scant material, consisting of tissue fragments of fat cells separated by spindle cells and occasional atypical cells with hyperchromatic large nuclei. Occasional adipocytes are in the background. Nucleoli are inconspicuous. No definite lipoblasts are seen. There is no necrosis. There is no diagnostic material in the cell block.

Comment: The features are considered atypical. The features favour an adipocytic neoplasm rather than subcutaneous fat.

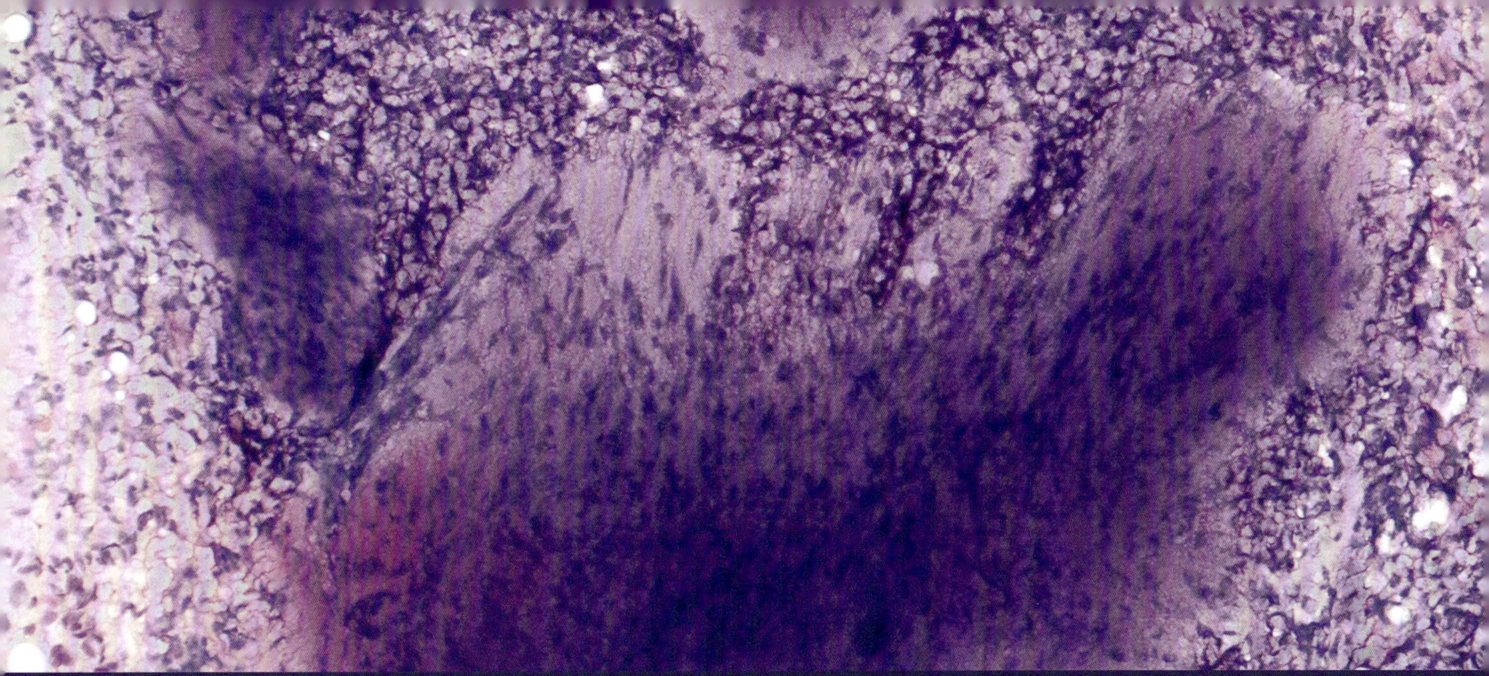

6

Diagnostic category: Soft tissue neoplasm of uncertain malignant potential (STNUMP)

Edited by: Chebib I, Dodd LG, Jo VY, Lazar AJ, Rekhi B, Schmitt F

Introduction

Layfield LJ

The category of "Soft tissue neoplasm of uncertain malignant potential" ("STNUMP") represents a diverse group of neoplasms whose biological behaviour cannot be predicted on an FNAB or CNB, or in some cases on histopathology, even if a definitive diagnosis of a specific tumour type can be made by routine cytomorphological analysis with or without ancillary testing. This section includes several neoplasms that are classified by the WHO classification of soft tissue and bone tumours as having an "intermediate (locally aggressive)" biological risk or "intermediate (rarely metastasizing)" biological risk, as well as tumour types whose criteria for risk stratification or malignancy are based on histopathological parameters that can be applied only on resection specimens.

Definition

Layfield LJ

Neoplasms in the "Soft tissue neoplasm of uncertain malignant potential" ("STNUMP") category are mesenchymal neoplasms that cannot be unequivocally diagnosed as benign or malignant on cytopathological analysis and ancillary testing, including tumours with intermediate biological potential and tumours requiring the application of histopathological criteria to determine whether they are benign or malignant.

Discussion and background

Layfield LJ

Prediction of the likelihood of a neoplasm giving rise to local recurrences or distant metastases is a principal goal in the pathological evaluation of soft tissue neoplasms. Cytopathological and histopathological evaluation can accurately separate benign from malignant neoplasms using morphological criteria and ancillary studies for the majority of tumours. However, it is well established that there are neoplasms that rarely metastasize, and the risk of metastasis is unpredictable on the basis of histopathological parameters; the fifth-edition WHO classification of soft tissue and bone tumours categorizes these as "intermediate (locally aggressive)" and "intermediate (rarely metastasizing)" tumours {1503}. Specifically, in the latter category, these are locally aggressive tumours with frequent recurrences, and they show a well-documented ability to give rise to distant metastases, albeit rarely and unpredictably.

The categories "Atypical" and "STNUMP" address two fundamentally different diagnostic issues. The category "Atypical" is used when the cytopathologist cannot recognize a specific type of soft tissue neoplasm and so cannot definitively assign the specimen to the "Benign" or "Malignant" category, or when a specific line of differentiation is identified but there are not sufficient cytopathological features to warrant assignment to the "Suspicious for malignancy" category. The category "STNUMP" is used when the cytopathologist is able to recognize a specific neoplasm or line of differentiation, but either definitive criteria cannot be applied for risk stratification or assessment of malignancy, or the tumour type has an inherent but unpredictable risk of metastasis.

This chapter includes a broad range of soft tissue neoplasms that are commonly encountered in routine practice. Three tumours of intermediate biological risk are included: dermatofibrosarcoma protuberans, a locally aggressive, frequently recurring fibroblastic neoplasm with a small risk of high-grade fibrosarcomatous transformation; inflammatory myofibroblastic tumour, a locally aggressive, rarely metastasizing neoplasm; and angiomatoid fibrous histiocytoma, another locally aggressive, rarely metastasizing neoplasm.

Myoepithelial neoplasms of soft tissue and perivascular epithelioid cell tumour (PEComa) are also included in this chapter, because the criteria for malignancy for these neoplasms are best assessed on histopathological features {579,439,358,121}.

Solitary fibrous tumour and gastrointestinal stromal tumour are also included in this diagnostic category, because risk stratification schemes predicting their risk of malignant behaviour are best applied to CNB and excision specimens rather than FNAB material {306,310}.

Risk of malignancy and diagnostic management recommendations

Layfield LJ

Currently, there is insufficient published data associated with the cytopathological category "STNUMP" to establish a ROM. However, estimates of ROM for each of the diverse tumour types have been developed based on histopathology, and accurate FNAB diagnosis with appropriate ancillary testing can establish appropriate management for the patients. A recent single-institution retrospective study of 2214 soft tissue cases showed a ROM of 51.43% {460}.

Subsequent management after FNAB biopsy requires clinical, imaging, and cytopathological correlation. If material for ancillary testing is not available, repeat FNAB with cell block and/or CNB (if available and if the lesion is accessible) is recommended. In most cases, complete resection is usually performed as the definitive treatment, and for some specific tumours, an appropriate risk stratification scheme can be applied to the histopathological specimen to determine the risk of metastasis.

Dermatofibrosarcoma protuberans

Domanski HA
Chebib I

Definition

Dermatofibrosarcoma protuberans (DFSP) is a superficial, locally aggressive fibroblastic neoplasm, with cellular storiform and spindle cell features and harbouring a *COL1A1::PDGFB* or related fusion.

Clinical features and imaging

DFSP presents most commonly as plaque-like to nodular or multinodular cutaneous masses in young to middle-aged adults (most commonly 20–30 years of age) {1387,1061}. Rarely, they present as an atrophic depressed area of skin {881} or a subcutaneous mass {90}. Related tumours include giant cell fibroblastoma and hybrid DFSP–giant cell fibroblastoma, which are seen in paediatric patients {1390,635,906,615}. DFSPs often show slow, persistent growth, unless they undergo fibrosarcomatous transformation. They occur most commonly on the trunk, proximal extremities, and head and neck region. Less commonly they occur in the perineum or genital skin {624}, breast {327}, or distal extremities {1279}.

Histopathology

Classic DFSP is characterized by a cellular spindle cell infiltration within the dermis and subcutaneous fat. Cytopathologically, tumour cells are uniform elongate spindle cells arranged in a storiform or whorled pattern. Tumour cells typically surround skin appendages and do not involve the epidermis. Characteristically, they invade into subcutaneous fat, surrounding individual adipocytes and imparting a "honeycomb" appearance to the deep edge of invasion. Subtypes include pigmented DFSP with intermixed pigmented melanocytes {369}; myxoid DFSP, which shows prominent myxoid stroma, nodular growth, and prominent vessels with mural fibrosis {1155,927}; and DFSP with myoid differentiation, which shows nests of cells with myofibroblastic differentiation and eosinophilic hyalinized stroma {168}. Importantly,

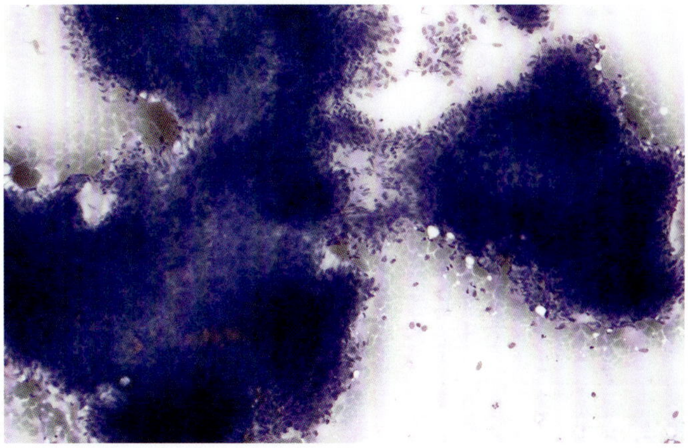

Fig. 6.02 Dermatofibrosarcoma protuberans. Cohesive, 3D tissue fragments of spindle cells and a few single cells (Giemsa).

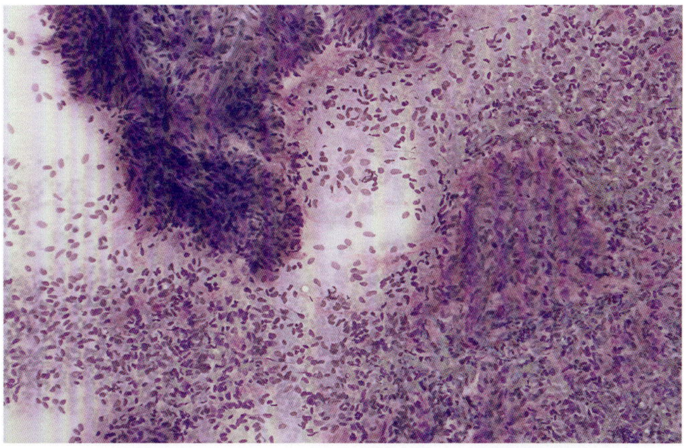

Fig. 6.03 Dermatofibrosarcoma protuberans. Cohesive tissue fragments of spindle cells within a collagenous matrix and some dispersed spindle cells and stripped nuclei (Giemsa).

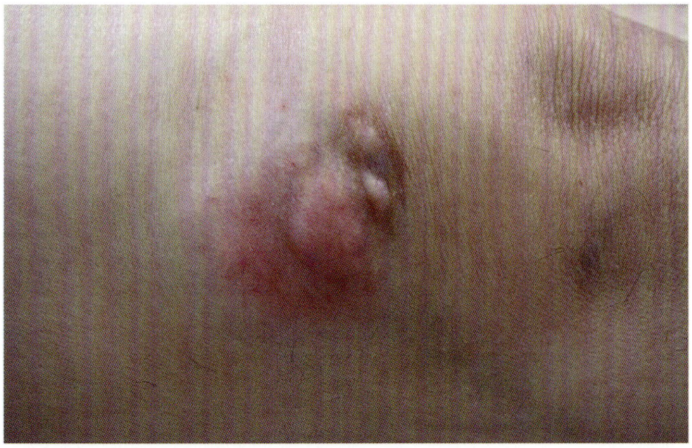

Fig. 6.01 Dermatofibrosarcoma protuberans. Dermatofibrosarcoma protuberans presenting as multinodular cutaneous masses.

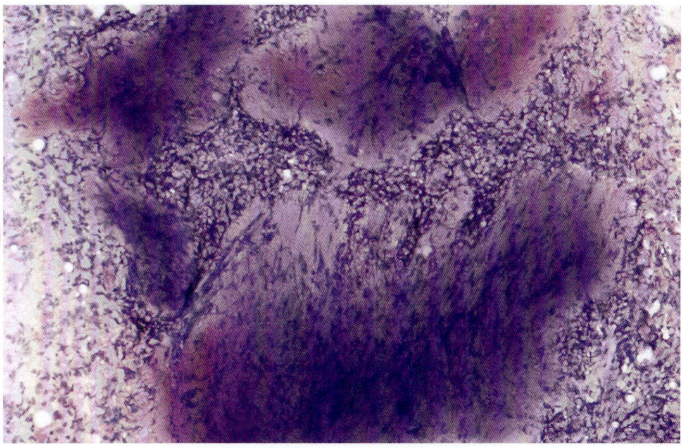

Fig. 6.04 Dermatofibrosarcoma protuberans. Large tissue fragments of spindle cells in a myxoid or metachromatic matrix and dispersed spindle cells in the background (Giemsa).

DFSP with fibrosarcomatous transformation shows a transition to a fascicular or herringbone growth pattern, increased cellularity, nuclear atypia, and mitotic activity {920,496,2}.

Key diagnostic cytopathological features

- Variable cellularity
- Tissue fragments of cohesive spindle cells showing a storiform architecture within a collagenous matrix
- Background of single cells and stripped nuclei
- Many cells with poorly defined cytoplasm
- Occasionally bipolar cytoplasmic processes in cells with better-defined cytoplasm
- Mild to moderate nuclear atypia, but uniform chromatin and typically lacking nucleoli
- May have myxoid or metachromatic matrix (Giemsa)
- Rarely tissue fragments of adipose tissue infiltrated by spindle tumour cells

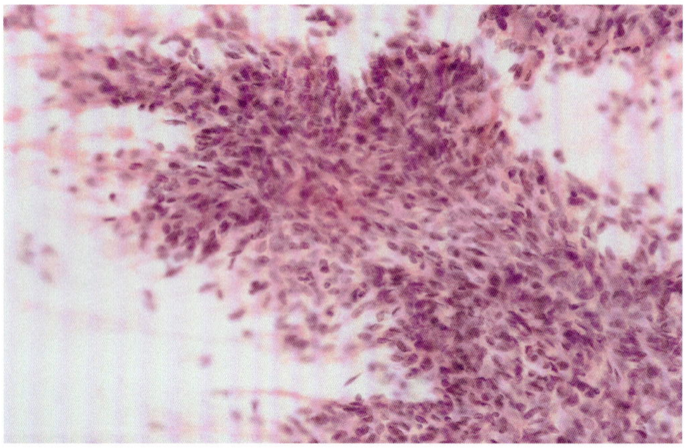

Fig. 6.05 Dermatofibrosarcoma protuberans. A cohesive tissue fragment of crowded spindle cells with a hint of a storiform pattern (H&E).

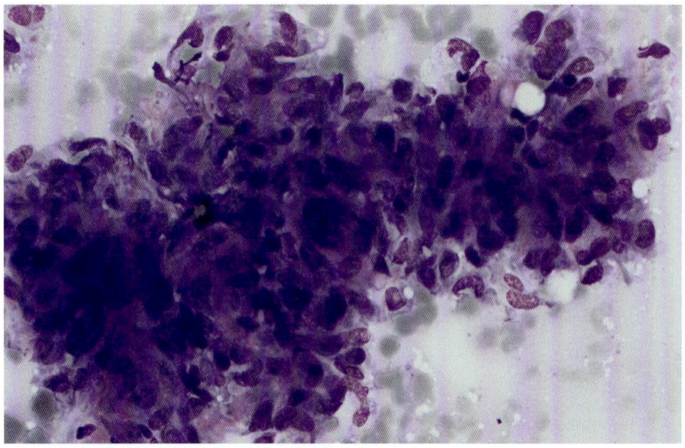

Fig. 6.06 Dermatofibrosarcoma protuberans. A cohesive tissue fragment of spindle cells with mild to moderate nuclear atypia and wispy cytoplasm in magenta matrix (Giemsa).

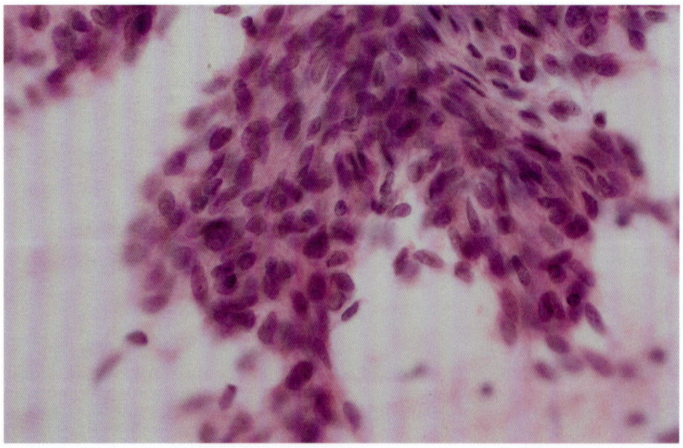

Fig. 6.07 Dermatofibrosarcoma protuberans. A cohesive tissue fragment of spindle cells with mild to moderate nuclear atypia (H&E).

Reference(s): {1125,743,1549,350,727,340,1425,715,100,1100}

Discussion and differential diagnosis

Clinical features may be helpful in distinguishing DFSP from other spindle cell neoplasms. A spectrum of benign and malignant cellular spindle cell neoplasms of soft tissue constitute the differential diagnoses for DFSP, including benign fibrous histiocytoma, peripheral nerve sheath tumours (including schwannoma, neurofibroma, and soft tissue perineurioma), nodular fasciitis, solitary fibrous tumour, "fat-poor" and "fat-free" variants of spindle cell lipoma, low-grade malignant peripheral nerve sheath tumour, low-grade fibromyxoid sarcoma, and adult fibrosarcoma {350,727,340}.

Benign fibrous histiocytoma tends to present as smaller, pigmented dermal nodules, and smears show an admixture of fibroblasts and epithelioid, xanthomatous, and multinucleated histiocytes, helping to distinguish fibrous histiocytoma from DFSP {726}. Schwannomas are characterized by tissue fragments of different sizes with irregular borders ("jigsaw puzzle pieces"), with scant dispersed cells and occasional nuclear palisading and Verocay bodies in the tissue fragments. The spindle cells of schwannoma have elongate, slender, and "boomerang" or "fishhook" nuclei {345}, with the cells within a fibrillary stroma.

Nodular fasciitis typically presents as a rapidly growing subcutaneous mass, and FNAB smears shows a haphazard distribution of single cells and small myxoid fragments of spindle cells and plump ganglion-like cells, often associated with scattered inflammatory cells {1124,1146}.

Smears of solitary fibrous tumour often have a bloody background {47}. Spindle cell lipoma presents in the posterior neck or upper back and shows bright eosinophilic fragments of collagen matrix, which helps to differentiate it from DFSP {347}.

Smears in low-grade malignant peripheral nerve sheath tumour are composed of spindle cells with wavy nuclei and comma-shaped naked nuclei, as well as polymorphous oval to rounded cells {731}. Low-grade fibromyxoid sarcoma may occasionally show cytopathological features overlapping those of DFSP {351}.

Adult fibrosarcoma is a vanishingly rare entity and was a histopathological diagnosis of exclusion {93}. It is not longer included as a specific neoplasm in the sixth-edition *Soft tissue and bone tumours* volume of the WHO Classification of Tumours series.

Ancillary testing

DFSP is characterized by diffuse strong expression of CD34 {497}, which is lost in areas of fibrosarcomatous DFSP {920}. Myoid nodules express SMA. Schwannoma and neurofibroma express S100 and SOX10, which are negative in DFSP. Soft tissue perineurioma and neurofibroma may be positive for CD34, but they also express other perineurial markers, GLUT1, claudin-1, and EMA (which is also expressed in 20% of DFSPs)

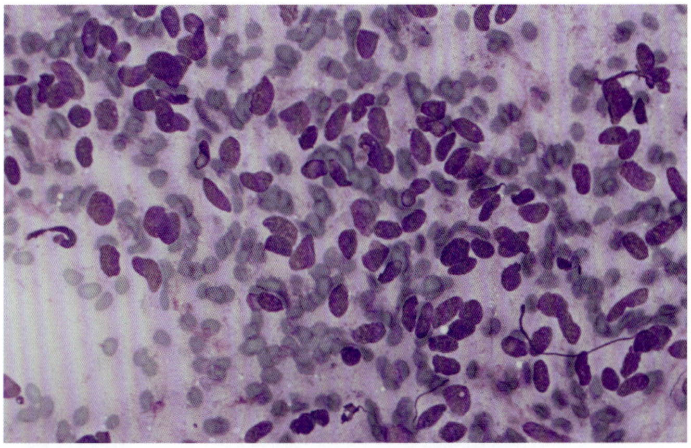

Fig. 6.08 Dermatofibrosarcoma protuberans. Dispersed stripped nuclei with mild nuclear atypia and uniform chromatin, lacking nucleoli, along with an occasional spindle cell (Giemsa).

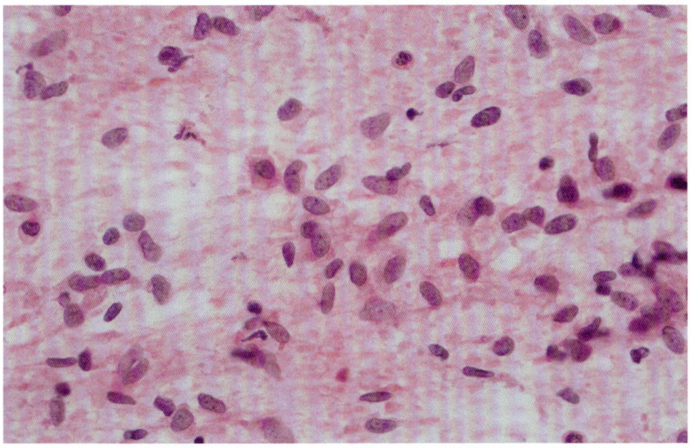

Fig. 6.09 Dermatofibrosarcoma protuberans. Dispersed single cells with poorly preserved cytoplasm, mild nuclear atypia and uniform chromatin, and stripped nuclei (H&E).

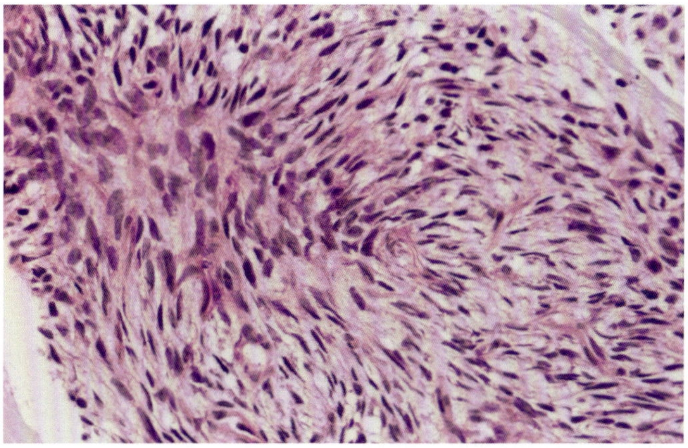

Fig. 6.10 Dermatofibrosarcoma protuberans. Distinct storiform pattern in the corresponding cell block (cell block, H&E).

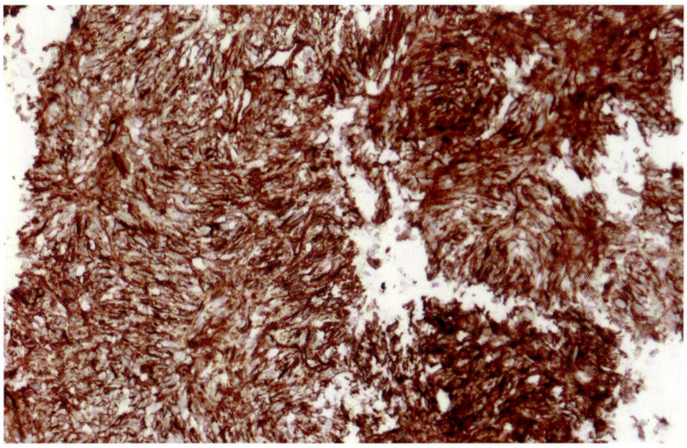

Fig. 6.11 Dermatofibrosarcoma protuberans. Strong diffuse positive CD34 staining in cell block (cell block, CD34).

{1548}. Solitary fibrous tumours also express CD34 but also express nuclear STAT6 {1380}. Both DFSP and spindle cell lipoma express CD34. Malignant peripheral nerve sheath tumours do not express CD34. A limited panel of antibodies, such as MUC4, EMA, SMA, and CD34, as well as molecular tests to confirm *FUS* rearrangements in low-grade fibromyxoid sarcoma, can be helpful for reaching the correct diagnosis.

Cytogenetic analysis has identified supernumerary ring chromosomes {997,1089,1087,1088,1090} derived from translocation t(17;22) {956} in DFSP. Rare variant translocations t(2;17) and t(9;22) have also been described {1314,1331}. The most common gene fusion, *COL1A1*::*PDGFB* {1309}, can be identified on PCR or NGS {1085}. Break-apart FISH may be used to identify *PDGFB* rearrangements. DFSPs with alternative translocations have been shown to harbour *COL6A3*::*PDGFD* or *EMILIN2*::*PDGFD* {274,327,169}. In difficult cases, the diagnosis of nodular fasciitis can be confirmed by the presence of *USP6* fusions.

Solitary fibrous tumour

Chebib I
Monaco SE
Rajwanshi A

Definition

Solitary fibrous tumour (SFT) is a spindle cell neoplasm with fibroblastic differentiation, characterized by prominent, branching, thin-walled dilated ("staghorn") vasculature and *NAB2*::*STAT6* gene rearrangement.

Clinical features and imaging

SFT presents as a painless mass arising in the superficial or deep soft tissues of the extremities, abdomen, pelvis, pleura, meninges, retroperitoneum, trunk, head and neck, and (rarely) visceral organs. SFTs have been described over a wide age range (median: 50–60 years) and with equal sex distribution. Rarely, they present with a hypoglycaemic paraneoplastic syndrome, called Doege–Potter syndrome {309,1267,1083,310, 1225,1323,481,445}.

Histopathology

SFTs tend to be well-circumscribed, lobulated masses. They show a wide histopathological spectrum, with variable cellularity and haphazard growth of fibroblast-like spindle cells with pale cytoplasm, as well as variable paucicellular fibrotic, collagenous keloidal stroma. They contain characteristic thin-walled dilated vessels showing a branching "staghorn" or haemangiopericytoma-like vasculature. Subtypes may contain mature adipocytes and are known as fat-forming or lipomatous SFT {1020, 433,516}, or they contain multinucleated giant cells {517} or myxoid stroma {315}. Rarely, they may undergo dedifferentiation to high-grade sarcoma {980,250}.

Key diagnostic cytopathological features

- Variable cellularity
- Tissue fragments, single cells, and stripped nuclei
- Uniform spindle cells with thin and wispy cytoplasmic processes

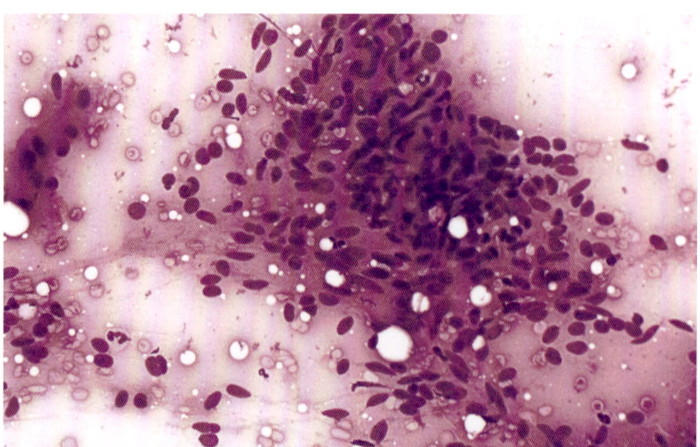

Fig. 6.12 Solitary fibrous tumour. A loosely cohesive tissue fragment and plump single cells on air-dried preparation (Giemsa).

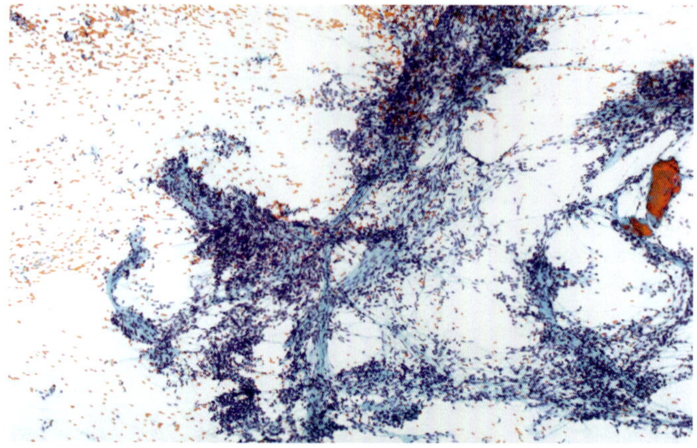

Fig. 6.13 Solitary fibrous tumour. Low power. A cellular smear showing prominent branching vasculature (Pap).

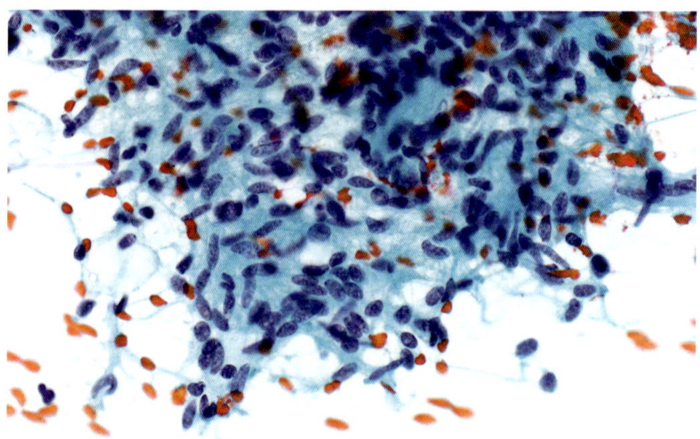

Fig. 6.14 Solitary fibrous tumour. High power. Haphazard arrangement of uniform spindle cells (Pap).

- Nuclei have finely granular chromatin and inconspicuous to absent nucleoli
- Hypocellular fragments of fibrous tissue and small fragments of ropy or wispy collagen
- Often have bloody background
- May have fat, multinucleated giant cells, myxoid stroma, or rarely mast cells
- Increased mitoses, atypia, hypercellularity, and necrosis can be associated with high-grade transformation or dedifferentiation

Reference(s): {47,236,339,527,1380,1472}

Discussion and differential diagnosis

The differential diagnosis includes desmoid-type fibromatosis, low-grade fibromyxoid sarcoma, neurogenic tumours (including peripheral nerve sheath tumours), vascular tumours, breast myofibroblastoma, dermatofibrosarcoma protuberans (DFSP),

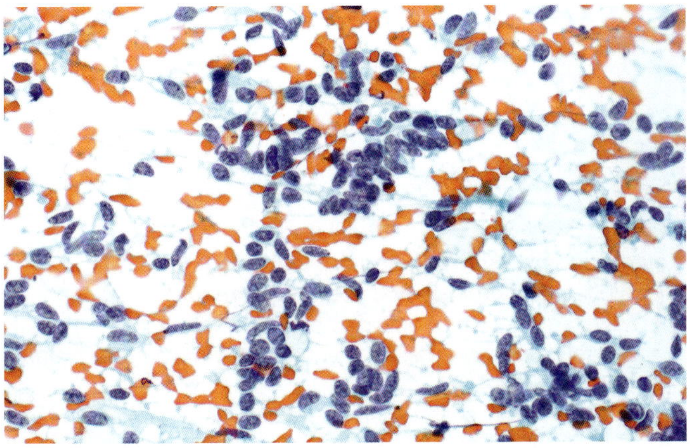

Fig. 6.15 Solitary fibrous tumour. High power. Prominent single cells and naked nuclei (Pap).

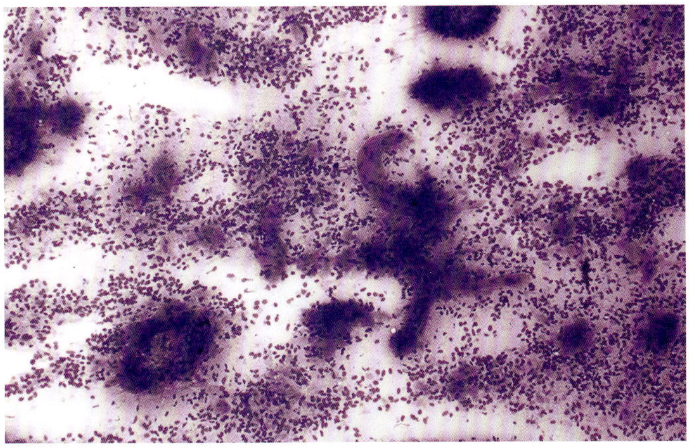

Fig. 6.16 Solitary fibrous tumour with myxoid features. Metastatic solitary fibrous tumour with myxoid features, low power (Giemsa).

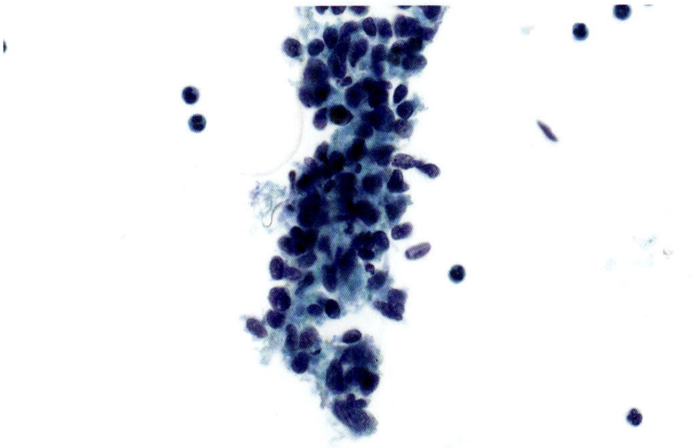

Fig. 6.17 Solitary fibrous tumour. High power. A cohesive crowded tissue fragment of haphazardly arranged spindle cells showing mild nuclear pleomorphism (LBC, Pap).

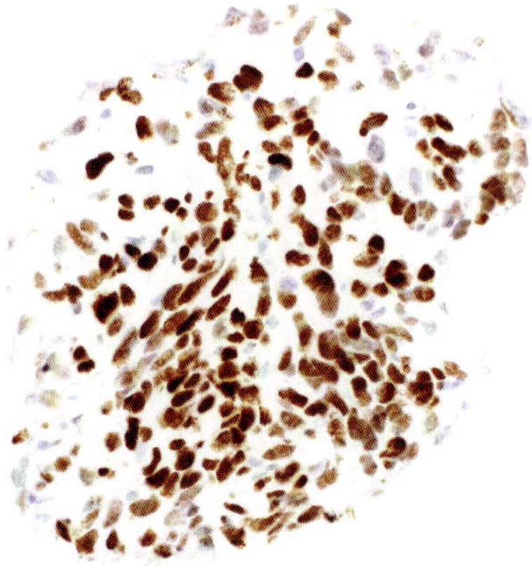

Fig. 6.18 Solitary fibrous tumour. STAT6 ICC on cell block preparation.

and synovial sarcoma. The differential for fat-forming SFT includes well-differentiated liposarcoma.

The primary diagnosis of SFT on FNAB is difficult due to the cytomorphological overlap with other entities in the differential diagnosis. Definitive diagnosis typically requires the use of ancillary testing on a cell block or concurrent core biopsy. Risk stratification for SFT cannot be performed on cytopathology material and requires evaluation of the resection specimen.

Ancillary testing

By ICC, SFT expresses CD34, BCL2, and CD99, although these markers are nonspecific, but nuclear positivity for STAT6 is a sensitive and specific surrogate for the fusion in SFT {361, 746,308,1380,1472}. Identification of *NAB2::STAT6* is difficult on conventional cytogenetics and FISH due to the proximity of the gene partners on chromosome 12q, and the gene fusion can be better characterized by PCR and NGS {1189,214,963}.

Low-grade fibromyxoid sarcoma is positive for MUC4. Peripheral nerve sheath tumours, such as schwannoma and neurofibroma, express S100 and/or SOX10. Desmoid-type fibromatosis shows nuclear expression of β-catenin. Synovial sarcomas may be positive for keratin and/or EMA, and they also express TLE1, although this may be diffusely positive in a subset of SFTs. However, synovial sarcoma is positive for *SSX1::SS18*, *SSX2::SS18*, or *SSX4::SS18* in the vast majority of cases, and ICC for SSX C-terminus or SSX::SS18 fusion–specific antibodies can be used to support the diagnosis.

CD34 expression may be seen in DFSP, vascular tumours, and a subset of breast myofibroblastomas. In difficult cases, STAT6 can differentiate SFT from DFSP, and positive *COL1A1::PDGFB* supports DFSP. Vascular tumours express other vascular markers, such as CD31, ERG, and FLI1, in addition to CD34. Myofibroblastomas are positive for desmin, and a subset show loss of RB1 expression by ICC. Finally, MDM2, which is positive in well-differentiated liposarcoma, is negative in SFT, although a subset of liposarcomas express STAT6 by ICC.

Inflammatory myofibroblastic tumour

Kerr DA
Hiroshima K
Ozawa M

Definition

Inflammatory myofibroblastic tumour (IMT) is a distinctive, rarely metastasizing neoplasm composed of myofibroblastic and fibroblastic spindle cells accompanied by an inflammatory infiltrate of plasma cells, lymphocytes, and/or eosinophils.

Clinical features and imaging

IMT typically affects children and young adults, although it may occur in older adults {239,243,225,492}. Clinical presentation varies by site of origin, and the anatomical distribution of IMT is wide, with frequent occurrence in the abdominopelvic and retroperitoneal regions, lung, and mediastinum. The head and neck, visceral organs, and somatic soft tissues are less common sites {243,492,755,694}. Systemic symptoms (e.g. fever and malaise) and laboratory abnormalities may be present {225,243,679,1352}.

Epithelioid inflammatory myofibroblastic sarcoma (EIMS) is a distinct clinicopathological subtype presenting almost exclusively as an intra-abdominal mass in male patients, and it is associated with an aggressive clinical course {879,802,818}.

IMT demonstrates variable imaging findings. Lesions are lobulated to infiltrative, and they enhance after contrast administration – frequently heterogeneously {1375,1363}. Calcifications may be present {679}.

Histopathology

Variable histopathological features characterize IMT and can be conceptualized as three main but often overlapping patterns: myxoid granulation tissue–like, hypercellular spindle cell, and hypocellular fibrous. Each pattern is characterized by different proportions of cytopathologically bland spindle fibroblastic/myofibroblastic cells, myxoid matrix, vascularity, and collagen {239,243,492,103}.

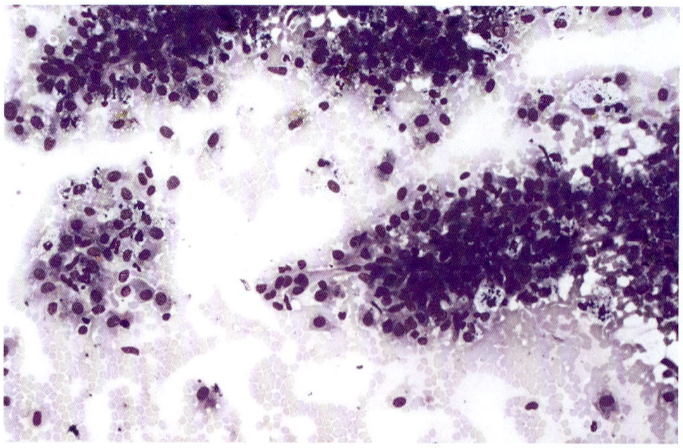

Fig. 6.19 Pulmonary inflammatory myofibroblastic tumour. Loosely cohesive tissue fragments containing small blood vessels and plentiful tingible-body macrophages are present with scattered single cells (Giemsa).

Key diagnostic cytopathological features

Classic inflammatory myofibroblastic tumour

- Low to moderate or occasionally high cellularity
- Loosely cohesive tissue fragments with scattered single cells
- Bland spindle cells of intermediate size with bipolar cytoplasmic processes
- Eccentric, slightly dense, pale tapered cytoplasm
- Nuclei are oval to round or tapered or "coffee-bean", with smooth nuclear membranes, fine to cleared (Pap) chromatin, and nucleoli ranging from inconspicuous to small and prominent
- Focal cytopathological atypia and ganglion-like polygonal cells with abundant cytoplasm, large nuclei with perinucleolar chromatin clearing (Pap, "vesicular"), and larger prominent nucleoli in a subset of cells

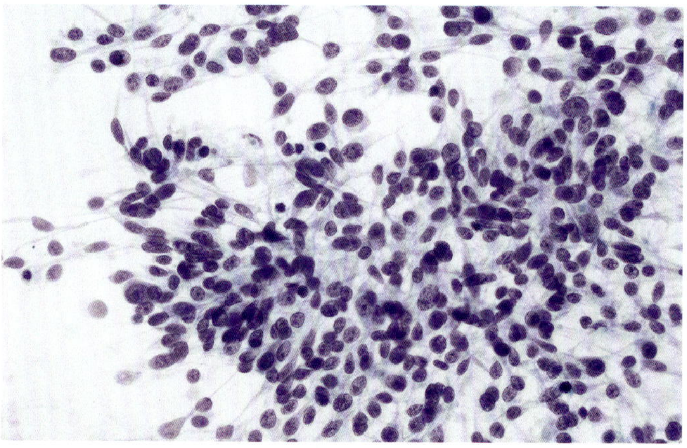

Fig. 6.20 Inflammatory myofibroblastic tumour. Loosely cohesive spindle cells with oval nuclei and small nucleoli (Pap).

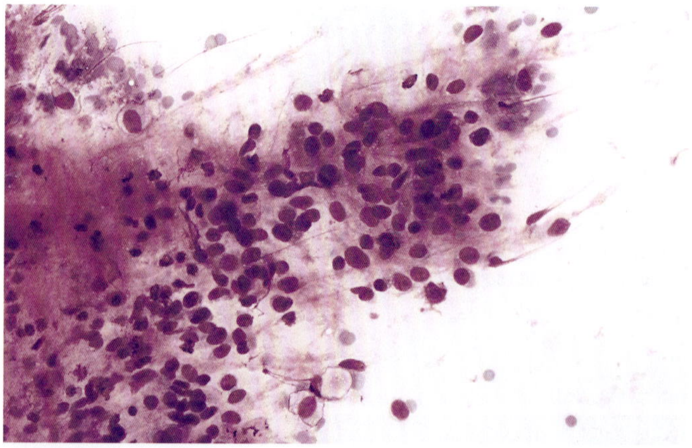

Fig. 6.21 Inflammatory myofibroblastic tumour. Spindle to polygonal cells in myxoid stroma (Giemsa).

- Possible intranuclear pseudoinclusions
- Absent to few mitoses with no atypical forms
- Background of inflammatory cells, predominantly lymphocytes, plasma cells, and histiocytes, with rare neutrophils or eosinophils
- Myxoid matrix
- Delicate vascular network; may have microvascular proliferation
- Lack of necrosis

Epithelioid inflammatory myofibroblastic sarcoma

- High cellularity
- Tissue fragments or single cells
- Tumour cells loosely attached to central, delicate, thin-walled and branching vessels
- Monotonous population of epithelioid cells with a moderate amount of pale eccentric cytoplasm
- Round nuclei with large, prominent nucleoli and perinucleolar clearing (Pap, "vesicular")
- Neutrophil-rich inflammatory infiltrate
- Myxoid stroma

Reference(s): {482,1400,1352,584,1285,28,802}

Discussion and differential diagnosis

The overall cytomorphological features of IMT are inconsistent and nonspecific, owing to its varied histopathology. EIMS demonstrates features distinct from those of classic IMT, reflecting its unique histopathological features.

The cytopathological diagnosis is challenging, and the differential spans reactive and reparative processes as well as malignancy. The differential is shaped by the predominant histopathological pattern and anatomical site of involvement. Having a high index of suspicion and applying ancillary testing judiciously improves the diagnostic accuracy {1352}.

For classic IMT, reactive fibrosis with background inflammation is a common diagnostic consideration or misdiagnosis {597, 1352,584}. IgG4-related sclerosing disease or haematopoietic malignancies may be considered in cases where the inflammatory component predominates {584}. In the hypercellular spindle cell pattern of IMT, a range of benign and malignant spindle cell tumours enters the differential, including spindle cell or embryonal rhabdomyosarcoma, smooth muscle tumours, nerve sheath tumours, and gastrointestinal stromal tumour {482,694}.

For EIMS, histiocytic sarcoma is a differential {601}, along with anaplastic large cell lymphoma, epithelioid gastrointestinal stromal tumour, dedifferentiated liposarcoma, and various

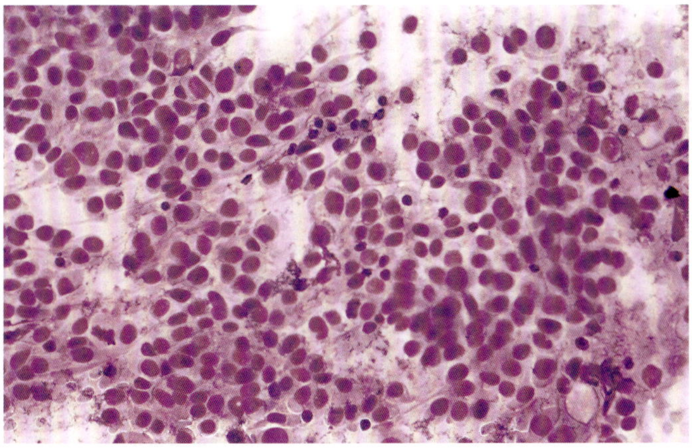

Fig. 6.22 Inflammatory myofibroblastic tumour. Spindle to mainly polygonal cells with admixed inflammatory cells, predominantly lymphocytes (Giemsa).

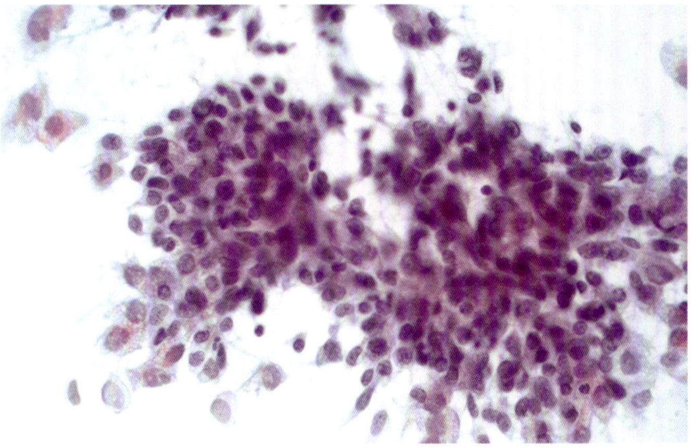

Fig. 6.23 Pulmonary inflammatory myofibroblastic tumour. Plump spindle to polygonal tumour cells with vacuolated cytoplasm, smooth nuclear contours, and fine chromatin, as well as scattered admixed inflammatory cells (Pap).

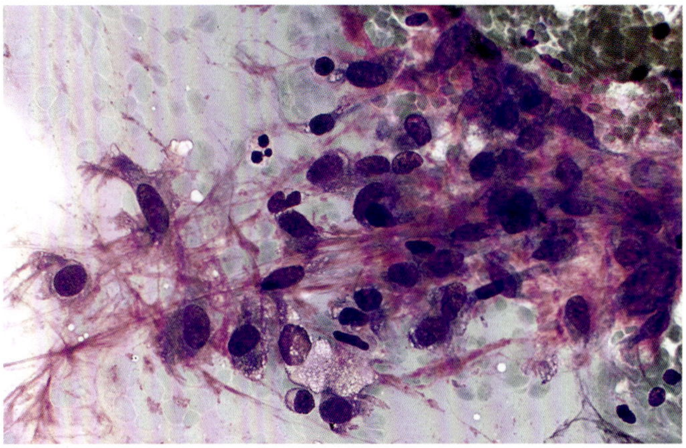

Fig. 6.24 Pulmonary inflammatory myofibroblastic tumour. Spindle to plump spindle cells with blue cytoplasm are present with admixed inflammatory cells in a magenta stromal background (Giemsa).

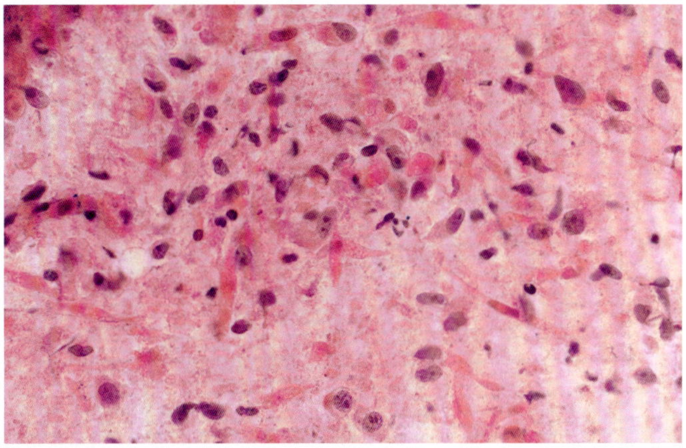

Fig. 6.25 Inflammatory myofibroblastic tumour. Spindle cells with slightly dense, tapered cytoplasm and mild nuclear atypia with small prominent nucleoli in a background of granular debris and scattered mixed inflammatory cells (rapid H&E).

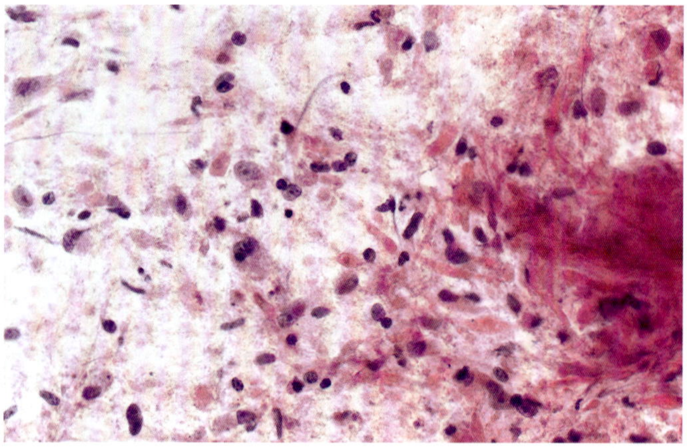

Fig. 6.26 Inflammatory myofibroblastic tumour. Very loosely cohesive plump spindle cells in a background of debris and inflammation (rapid H&E).

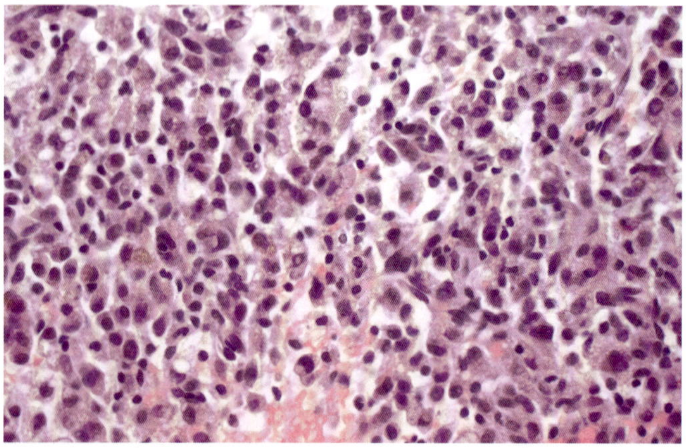

Fig. 6.27 Pulmonary inflammatory myofibroblastic tumour. Dissociated tumour cells show abundant granular to vacuolated cytoplasm with pigment, and scattered intranuclear pseudoinclusions are present (cell block, H&E).

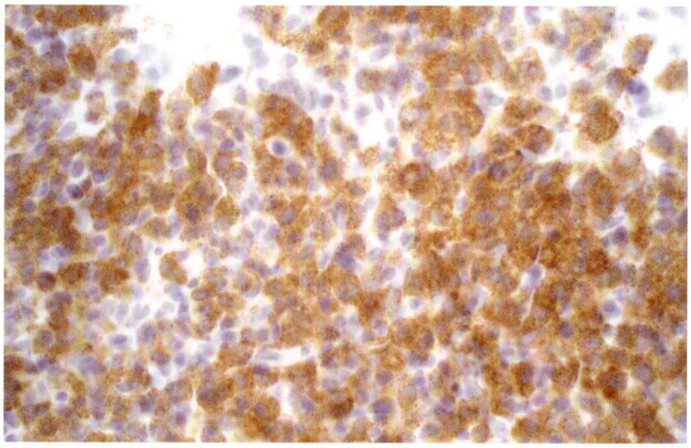

Fig. 6.28 Pulmonary inflammatory myofibroblastic tumour. A definitive diagnosis of inflammatory myofibroblastic tumour in cytopathological specimens generally requires ancillary studies. Diffuse reactivity for ALK supports the diagnosis (cell block, ALK ICC).

carcinomas. In ascites or pleural effusion samples, mesothelial proliferations (both reactive and malignant) are diagnostic considerations {802}.

Ancillary testing

A confident, specific diagnosis of IMT or EIMS is generally not possible without ancillary studies, which show ALK and ROS1 to be positive. FISH and NGS for *ALK* or other relevant kinase gene fusion can help with making the diagnosis {242,1529}.

Angiomatoid fibrous histiocytoma

Qian X
Domanski HA
Rekhi B

Definition

Angiomatoid fibrous histiocytoma (AFH) is a rare neoplasm of intermediate (rarely metastasizing) malignant potential, occurring mostly in the subcutis and characterized by varying proportions of epithelioid, ovoid, or spindle cells arranged in a nodular and often syncytial growth pattern, with haemorrhagic pseudovascular spaces and frequently a peripheral fibrous pseudocapsule with a prominent lymphoplasmacytic infiltrate.

Clinical features and imaging

AFH presents as a slow-growing, superficial, painless, 20–40 mm mass, which may simulate a haematoma or a haemangioma. It occurs most commonly in the deep dermis or subcutis of the extremities, preferentially in areas where lymph nodes are found, such as the popliteal fossa, axilla, inguinal, and neck regions {380,258,1403}. Unusual visceral, intramammary, and intracranial locations have also been increasingly reported {203,162,98,1321}. MRI shows a predominantly well-circumscribed, primarily cystic mass with a double rim and marginal infiltration {883}.

Histopathology

The classic histopathology of AFH is distinctive, with characteristic features including a well-circumscribed and lobulated margin at lower magnification; a thick fibrous pseudocapsule with variable amounts of peripheral lymphoplasmacytic infiltrate; multinodular growth in sheets, short fascicles, and sometimes whorls of uniform, bland, ovoid to spindle to histiocytoid neoplastic cells; and pseudoangiomatoid spaces filled with blood and lined by tumour cells {380,1403,67,1491}. The presence of

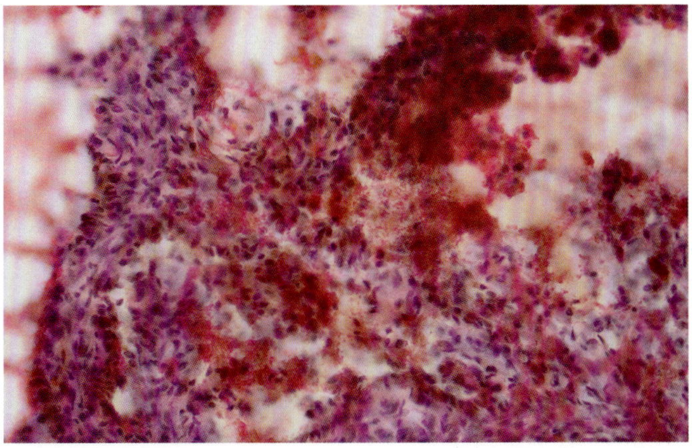

Fig. 6.29 Angiomatoid fibrous histiocytoma. Cohesive branching tissue fragments containing vessels with perivascular arrangement of tumour cells in a bloody background (H&E).

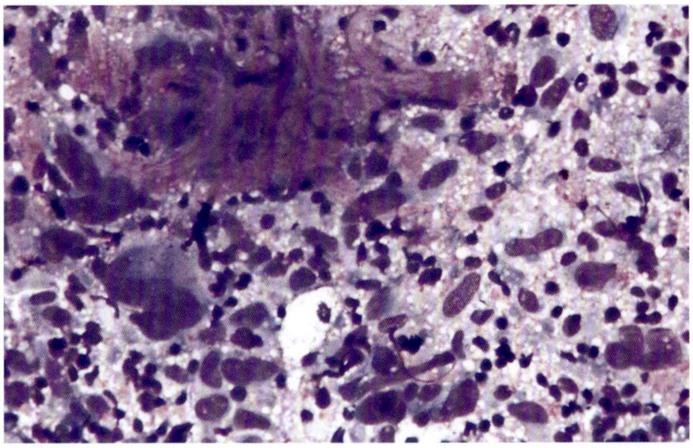

Fig. 6.30 Angiomatoid fibrous histiocytoma. A hypercellular smear composed of oval to spindle histiocytic tumour cells, including pleomorphic forms, with metachromatic stroma and interspersed lymphocytes (Giemsa).

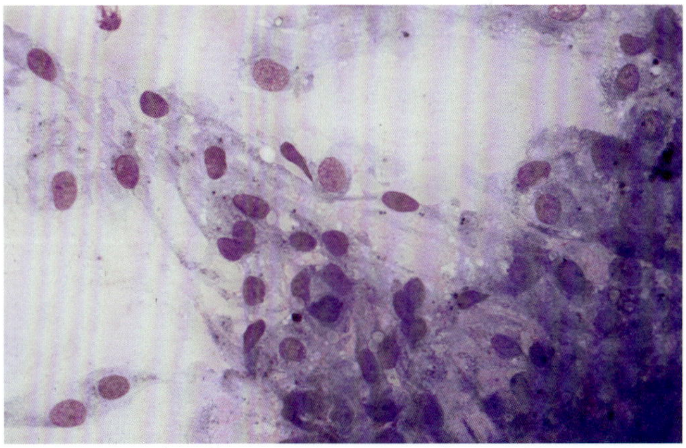

Fig. 6.31 Angiomatoid fibrous histiocytoma. A loosely cohesive tissue fragment consisting of histiocytic cells with oval to spindle nuclei with inconspicuous nucleoli and ill-defined cytoplasm (Giemsa).

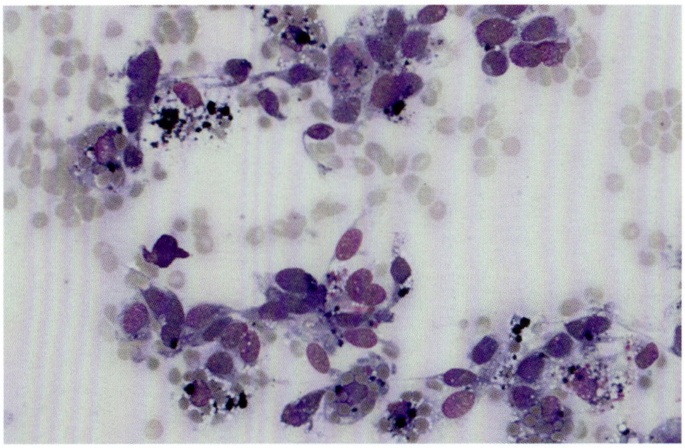

Fig. 6.32 Angiomatoid fibrous histiocytoma. Oval to spindle histiocytoid cells, most of which contain haemosiderin pigment in their cytoplasm (Giemsa).

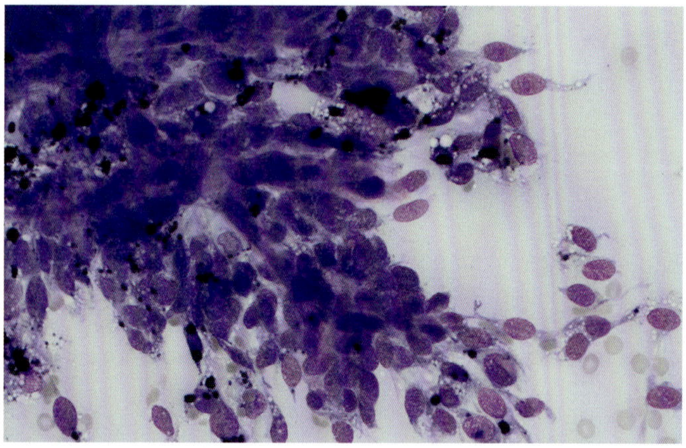

Fig. 6.33 Angiomatoid fibrous histiocytoma. A tissue fragment consisting of oval to spindle histiocytoid cells, some showing vacuolized cytoplasm and haemosiderin pigment (Giemsa).

nodules or sheets of histiocytoid cells is a consistent feature, but myxoid, reticular, small round cell, and pleomorphic subtypes have also been described {1252,1495}.

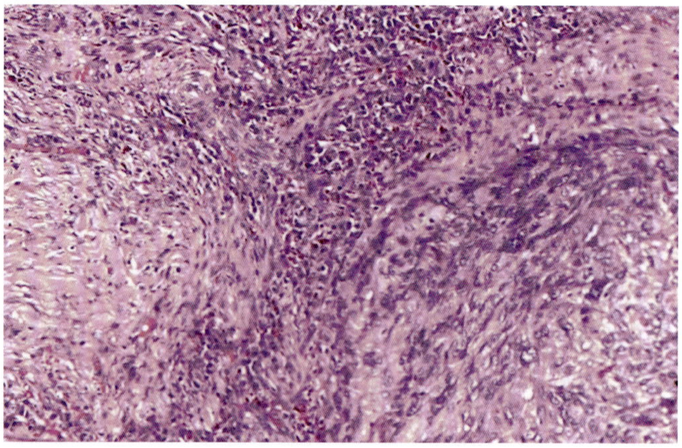

Fig. 6.34 Angiomatoid fibrous histiocytoma. Cellular tumour composed of oval to spindle histiocytic cells in a collagenous stroma along with aggregates of several pigment-laden histiocytes and lymphocytes (H&E).

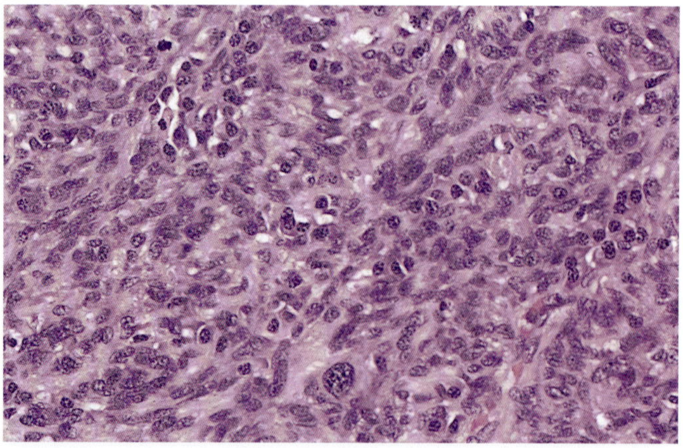

Fig. 6.35 Angiomatoid fibrous histiocytoma. Tumour cells with oval to short spindle nuclei, including a few pleomorphic forms, an occasional mitotic figure and intervening lymphocytes, and plasma cells (tissue section, H&E).

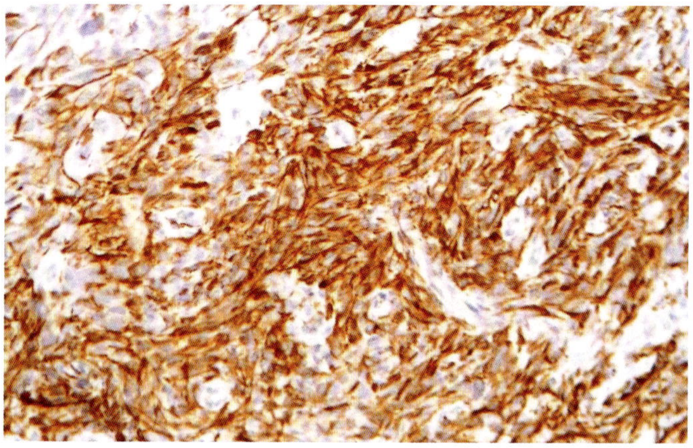

Fig. 6.36 Angiomatoid fibrous histiocytoma. Tumour cells display desmin positivity (tissue section, ICC).

Key diagnostic cytopathological features

- Moderate to high cellularity or hypocellular and bloody due to blood-filled cystic component
- Small and large cellular tissue fragments, some containing vessels
- Cohesive cellular tissue fragments, often associated with thin vessels, forming a whorl or "ball"-like structure
- Ovoid to spindle histiocytoid cells with a moderate amount of vacuolated cytoplasm and an ovoid or folded nucleus with a small inconspicuous nucleolus and perinucleolar clearing (Pap, "vesicular" nucleus)
- Occasional nuclear atypia and pleomorphism
- Variable numbers of single histiocytoid cells, haemosiderin-laden cells, lymphocytes, and plasma cells in the background

Reference(s): {1105,811,1138}

Discussion and differential diagnosis

The differential diagnosis of AFH is wide, depending on its morphology and location. For a superficial lesion, considerations include haemangioma, organizing haematoma, aneurysmal fibrous histiocytoma, and nodular fasciitis. In cases with a prominent lymphoid component resembling lymphoid tissue, considerations that enter the differential diagnosis include metastatic disease, Kaposi sarcoma, follicular dendritic cell sarcoma, and intranodal palisaded myofibroblastoma. AFH can also be confused with Ewing sarcoma, rhabdomyosarcoma, and inflammatory myofibroblastic tumour due to the frequent expression of CD99, desmin, and ALK, respectively {196,401, 1161}. In addition, pleomorphic AFH may be misdiagnosed as pleomorphic sarcoma {1495}.

Ancillary testing

The tumour cells are positive for desmin in 50–60% of cases and show variable, nonspecific staining for EMA, CD68, and CD99 {401,1161}. In ICC, ALK, especially clone D5F3, is positive in the majority of AFHs {196}. AFH is most commonly characterized by recurrent chromosomal translocations resulting in *EWSR1::CREB1* (seen in most cases), followed by *EWSR1::ATF1*, and rarely *FUS::ATF1* gene fusions, which can confirm the diagnosis of AFH {1378,1204}.

Myoepithelial neoplasms

Jo VY
Kerr DA
Kilpatrick SE

Definition

Myoepithelial neoplasms of soft tissue share morphological, immunophenotypic, and genetic features with their counterparts in salivary gland. The group includes benign myoepithelioma and mixed tumour, as well as malignant myoepithelial carcinomas.

Clinical features and imaging

Myoepithelial neoplasms of soft tissue can affect patients of all ages, with a peak incidence in early adulthood to middle age; they show an equal sex distribution {707,935,579,491}. Approximately 20% of cases occur in the paediatric population, and most of those cases are malignant {491}.

Most patients present with a palpable, often painless mass. Tumours most commonly arise in the limbs and limb girdles (particularly the lower rather than the upper) and trunk, and they are more frequently subcutaneous than deep-seated. Rarely, tumours arise in the head and neck, bone, and visceral organs {935,579,491,73,797,768}. Some present as primarily cutaneous lesions {577,427,647}.

The overall behaviour is indolent. Benign tumours show a 20% risk of recurrence and rarely metastasize, but myoepithelial carcinomas show recurrence and distant metastasis in 40–50% of cases {579,491}.

Histopathology

Myoepithelial tumours are morphologically heterogeneous; they characteristically show a wide spectrum of architectural and cytopathological features both within a given lesion and between different tumours {579,491,73}. Growth patterns vary, from reticular to trabecular, nested, or solid. Myxoid or hyalinized stroma is common. Tumour cells can be ovoid or epithelioid, usually with uniform nuclei and eosinophilic or clear cytoplasm. Some cases may show abundant cytoplasmic vacuolization, whereas others can have predominant spindle or plasmacytoid forms with hyaline cytoplasmic inclusions {408,707,579}. Osseous and/or cartilaginous differentiation is seen in as many as 15% of cases, with squamous or adipocytic metaplasia seen less frequently. Approximately 10% of benign myoepithelial tumours are mixed tumours, defined by the presence of ductal differentiation.

Myoepithelial carcinomas show appreciable moderate to severe nuclear atypia – the most reliable criterion for malignancy – often with high mitotic activity and necrosis. Malignant tumours in children often show an undifferentiated round cell component {579,491}.

Key diagnostic cytopathological features

- Moderate to high cellularity
- Small tissue fragments and/or singly dispersed cells
- Frequent extracellular fibrillary myxoid matrix, which may be abundant
- Tumour cells embedded within myxoid stromal fragments
- Spindle, epithelioid, or plasmacytoid cells
- Some tumours show a range of cell types, others show a single predominant cell type
- Occasionally purely spindle cell tumour with bipolar cytoplasmic processes and prominent rhabdoid morphology
- Myoepithelial carcinoma demonstrates nuclear atypia and pleomorphism, but definitive classification as malignant may not be possible on cytopathological material

Reference(s): {1480,857,1473}

Discussion and differential diagnosis

The differential diagnosis is broad and depends on the clinical presentation and anatomical site. In somatic soft tissue, diagnostic considerations include extraskeletal myxoid chondrosarcoma, epithelioid sarcoma, and ossifying fibromyxoid tumour.

In adult patients, myoepithelial carcinoma of soft tissue should be separated from metastatic carcinoma and melanoma, which requires clinical correlation and ICC. In paediatric patients, myoepithelial carcinomas can show predominant round cell morphology, and a wide range of round cell sarcomas may need to be excluded. Ancillary testing is useful in resolving most diagnostic considerations.

Ancillary testing

The diagnosis of myoepithelial neoplasms typically requires confirmation of myoepithelial differentiation with PLAG1 ICC positivity and *PLAG1* rearrangements – a feature of mixed tumours. *EWSR1* gene rearrangements are common in myoepitheliomas and myoepithelial carcinomas {92,75}. Occasionally, FISH to detect *EWSR1* rearrangement is required. Definitive classification is typically challenging on cytopathological material, and the diagnosis is suggested on FNAB in less than

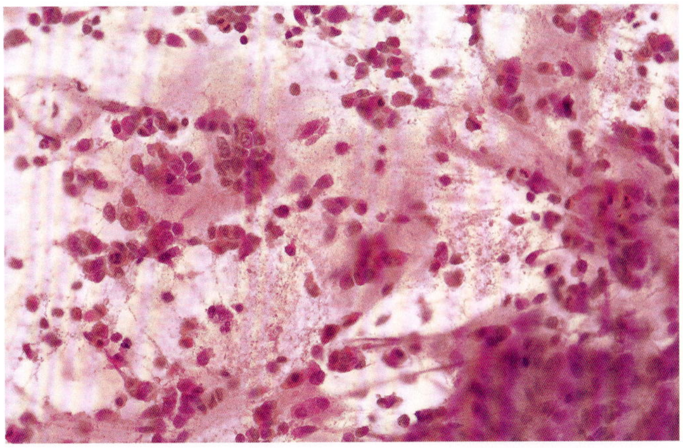

Fig. 6.37 Myoepithelial carcinoma. Small to minute tissue fragments and singly dispersed myoepithelial cells admixed with myxoid stromal fragments (H&E).

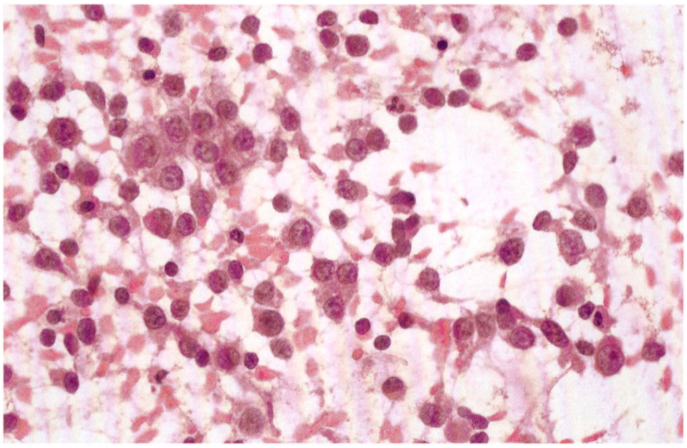

Fig. 6.38 Myoepithelial carcinoma. Low-grade myoepithelial carcinoma shows a high N:C ratio, with eccentric cytoplasm, mild to moderate nuclear atypia, and prominent nucleoli with perinucleolar clearing in some cells (H&E).

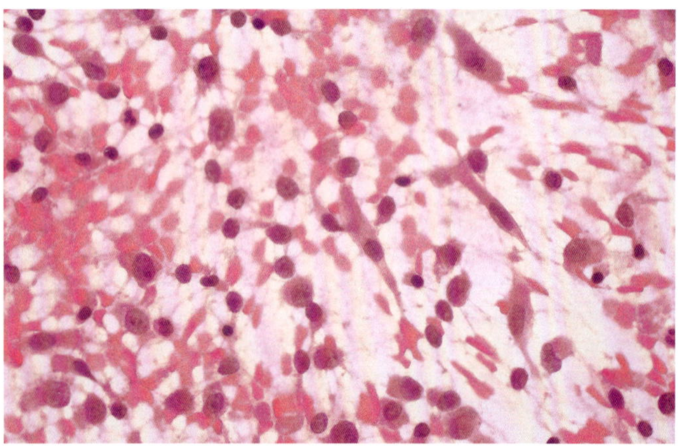

Fig. 6.39 Myoepithelial carcinoma. Most tumours show cytomorphological heterogeneity, with a mixed population of epithelioid, plasmacytoid, and spindle cells (H&E).

half of all cases {1473}. However, in rare cases FISH alone may not be sufficient, because *EWSR1* fusions are common in a wide range of mesenchymal tumours, and NGS is required to identify characteristic specific fusion genes.

Most myoepithelial tumours express keratins, EMA, and S100 {491,579,935}. SOX10 is positive in 80% of cases, although less commonly in malignant tumours, where it is positive in 30% {945}. Other commonly positive markers are GFAP (in 50%) and p63 (in 40%) {491,579,649}. Staining for myogenic markers is variable and less diagnostically useful, but calponin is commonly positive in 90% of cases, SMA in 60%, and desmin in 20% {707,579}.

In the differential diagnosis, extraskeletal myxoid chondrosarcoma can show rare staining for S100, but it is negative for keratins and EMA; FISH for *EWSR1::NR4A3* is diagnostically specific, but *EWSR1* FISH is not. Epithelioid sarcoma shows positivity for keratin and EMA, but it shows frequent staining for CD34 and is negative for S100 and SOX10, with SMARCB1 loss as a consistent feature although it is present in a small subset of myoepithelial carcinomas. Ossifying fibromyxoid tumour can also show variable staining for S100, keratin, and GFAP, but desmin is more frequently positive in ossifying fibromyxoid tumour (in as many as 50% of cases) than in myoepithelial tumours. *PHF1* rearrangements are a feature of ossifying fibromyxoid tumour.

In the paediatric age group, the most common differential diagnoses include Ewing sarcoma, which is positive for CD99 and NKX2-2 and shows the *EWSR1::FLI1* fusion; alveolar rhabdomyosarcoma, which is positive in desmin and myogenin ICC and has the *FOXO1* rearrangement; poorly differentiated synovial sarcoma showing *SS18*::SSX; high-grade myxoid liposarcoma, which is positive for DDIT3 or *DDIT3* FISH; and *CIC*-rearranged sarcoma, positive for WT1, ETV4, and the *CIC* rearrangement.

Extrarenal malignant rhabdoid tumour may also be considered; it shows variable staining for keratin, EMA, and S100 but lacks *EWSR1* rearrangement and shows SMARCB1 loss.

FISH can be used to detect *EWSR1* rearrangements, which are present in approximately half of all myoepitheliomas and myoepithelial carcinomas of soft tissue, as well as in skin and bone lesions {73,427,647,13,646}. Fusion partners are heterogeneous and include *POU5F1*, *PBX3*, *PBX1*, *ZNF444*, *KLF15*, *KLF17*, and *ATF1*, and rarely there are alternative *FUS* gene rearrangements {73,595,13,426,1370}. Some genotype–phenotype associations have been suggested; for example, the most common fusion, *EWSR1::POU5F1*, is found in as many as 28% of cases, and it tends to be associated with malignant deep-seated tumours in the limbs and nested and sheet-like growth of epithelioid cells with clear cytoplasm {73,1370}.

A small subset (< 10%) of myoepithelial carcinomas show loss of SMARCB1 expression, in most (if not all) cases occurring secondary to homozygous deletions of *SMARCB1* {491, 576,797}.

PEComa

Qian X
Layfield LJ
Yang E

Definition

Perivascular epithelioid cell tumours (PEComas) are mesenchymal neoplasms composed of perivascular epithelioid cells, which are distinctive epithelioid cells that are often closely associated with blood vessel walls and that express both melanocytic and smooth muscle markers on ICC.

Clinical features and imaging

PEComas occur most often in middle-aged individuals, with a female predominance, and they consist of a family of related tumours that include angiomyolipoma (AML) and lymphangioleiomyomatosis (LAM). Tumours may arise from any part of the body, including the kidney, lung, liver, pancreas, gastrointestinal tract, gynaecological tract, and soft tissues {580}. PEComas are commonly seen as well-circumscribed masses {1433,1228}, but imaging is nonspecific, overlapping with other more common tumours at the corresponding site. Specific imaging may be seen in some scenarios, such as pulmonary LAM demonstrating diffuse abundant cysts in bilateral lungs, or renal AML with high fat content.

Histopathology

PEComas are composed of variable proportions of epithelioid and spindle cells, which are characterized by ovoid to round nuclei with clear to eosinophilic granular cytoplasm with well-defined borders. Tumour cells are present as solid sheets, expansile nests, and cords. Perivascular distribution with radial arrangement of tumour cells surrounding a vascular lumen may be seen, but this is not a required diagnostic feature. Thin and delicate vessels in a sinusoidal pattern are common. Stromal hyalinization may be present; when it is extensive, this subtype is called sclerosing PEComa {824}. Giant cells and melanin pigment may be present. By convention, PEComas with predominantly clear, epithelioid cells may be referred to as "clear cell" tumours, and those composed predominantly of plump spindle cells that are arranged around dilated lymphatics are designated as LAM or lymphangiomyoma if present as a localized mass. AML is morphologically distinct, typically composed of smooth muscle, fat, and thick-walled vessels in varying proportions.

The criteria for malignancy are not well-defined in PEComa, although cases with aggressive clinical behaviour tend to exhibit large size (> 50 mm), an infiltrative growth pattern, lymphovascular invasion, significant cytopathological atypia, necrosis, and mitotic activity {439}. Organ system–specific modifications to these criteria have been proposed and continue to be revised as data accumulates for these rare entities {1264,121,1014}. Given these limitations, malignant potential should be reported cautiously in cytopathological specimens, unless it is a metastatic lesion in a patient with a known history.

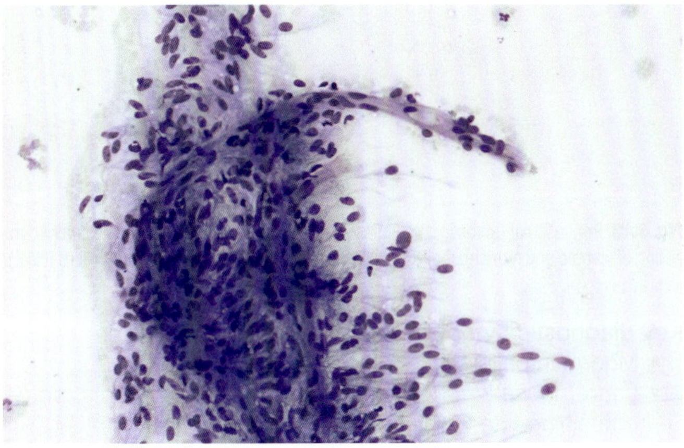

Fig. 6.40 Perivascular epithelioid cell tumour (PEComa). A syncytial tissue fragment with fine vessels and spindle to epithelioid cells (Giemsa).

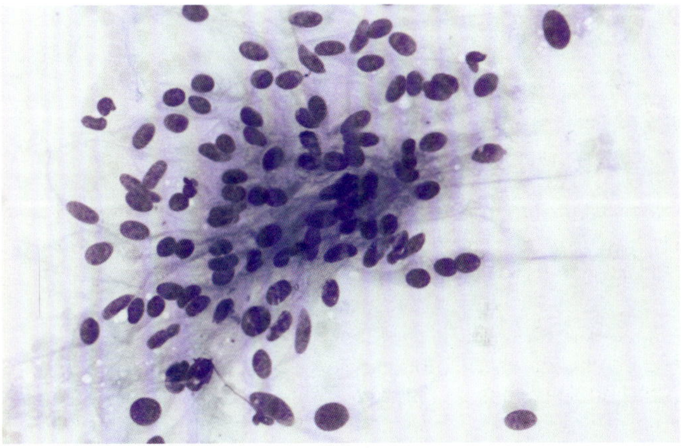

Fig. 6.41 Perivascular epithelioid cell tumour (PEComa). A loosely cohesive syncytial tissue fragment with oval to elongated nuclei in predominantly spindle cells (Giemsa).

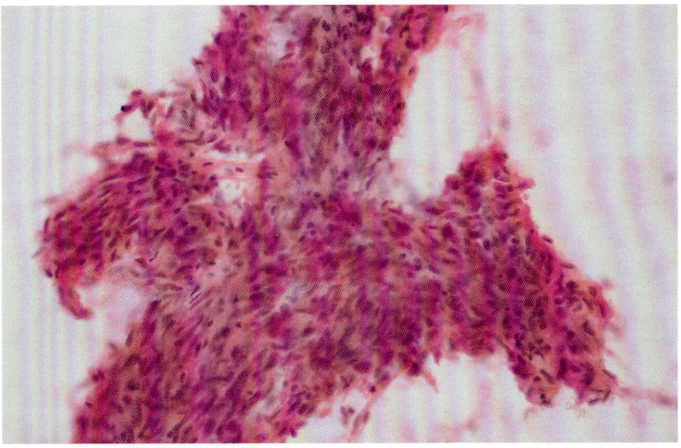

Fig. 6.42 Perivascular epithelioid cell tumour (PEComa). A cohesive dense tissue fragment of spindle cells (H&E).

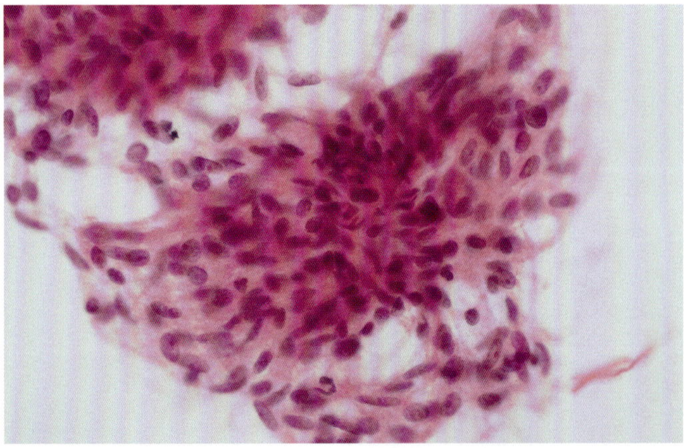

Fig. 6.43 Perivascular epithelioid cell tumour (PEComa). A cohesive tissue fragment consisting of spindle and more epithelioid cells with poorly defined cytoplasmic borders (H&E).

Key diagnostic cytopathological features

- Moderate cellularity
- Large, loosely cohesive syncytial tissue fragments, some containing fine vessels
- Epithelioid to spindle cells with moderate amounts of delicate, finely vacuolated to granular cytoplasm

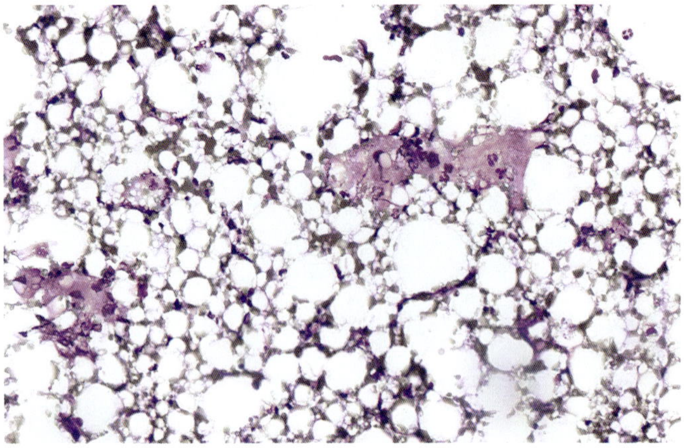

Fig. 6.44 Perivascular epithelioid cell tumour (PEComa). Scattered epithelioid cells with abundant finely vacuolated granular cytoplasm in bloody background (Giemsa).

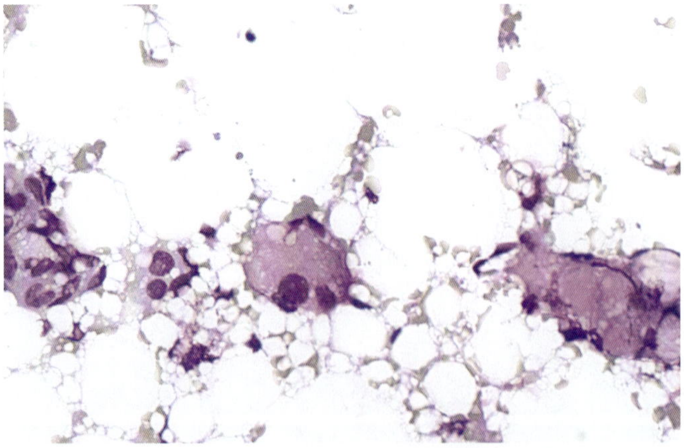

Fig. 6.45 Perivascular epithelioid cell tumour (PEComa). Minute tissue fragments and single cells showing abundant, usually eccentric finely vacuolated cytoplasm and some spindle cells with mildly pleomorphic nuclei (Giemsa).

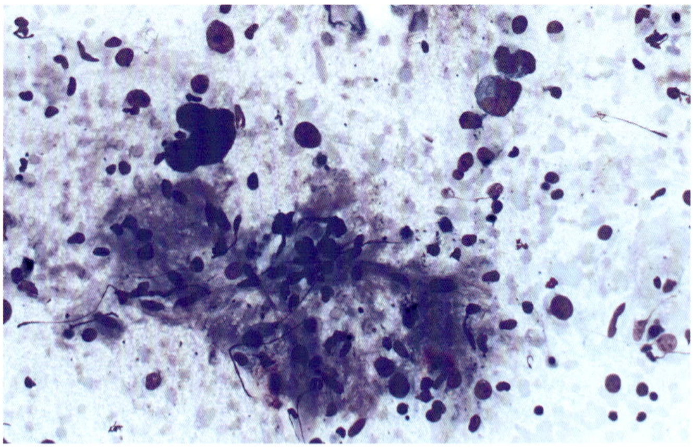

Fig. 6.46 Malignant perivascular epithelioid cell tumour (PEComa). A loosely cohesive tissue fragment containing a small vessel, with cells showing round to irregular nuclei with prominent nucleoli, granular cytoplasm, and indistinct cell borders. Scattered single cells with granular eccentric cytoplasm and prominent nucleoli, as well as large, bizarre, hyperchromatic bare tumour nuclei, are a common find in malignant PEComa (Giemsa).

- Oval to elongated nuclei with variable cytopathological atypia, ranging from smooth nuclear contours, even chromatin texture, and inconspicuous nucleoli to nuclear pleomorphism with prominent nucleoli
- Nucleoli stain bright purple (Giemsa) and light blue (Pap)
- Intranuclear pseudoinclusions may be seen
- A significant fat component may be present in AML, although lesions that require a diagnostic biopsy tend to be fat-poor AML

Reference(s): {251,1487,1228,262,1564}

Discussion and differential diagnosis

The differential diagnosis of PEComa varies depending on the spindle or epithelioid cell type and tumour location. Given PEComas' expression of melanocytic markers, the differential includes melanoma in every site, but smooth muscle ICC is positive in PEComa and negative in melanoma. PEComas with predominantly epithelioid morphology may be confused with carcinomas with clear cytoplasm, such as clear cell renal cell carcinoma, hepatocellular carcinoma, and clear cell carcinoma of Müllerian origin, but carcinomas are distinguished by diffuse cytokeratin expression and lack of smooth muscle and melanocytic marker expression.

PEComas with spindle cells may be confused with true smooth muscle neoplasms, and the cytomorphological evaluation is critical for this distinction, because smooth muscle neoplasms show cigar-shaped nuclei, eosinophilic fibrillary cytoplasm, and a predominance of thick-walled vessels without a delicate capillary network.

Ancillary testing

The hallmark of PEComa is coexpression of melanocytic markers – including HMB45, melan-A (MART1), and MITF – and smooth muscle markers – including desmin, caldesmon, and SMA – although the extent and intensity of expression may be quite variable. Cathepsin K, a protease regulated by *MITF*, may also be positive {121}. Melanocytic markers tend to be more strongly expressed in the epithelioid cells, and smooth muscle markers are more prominent in spindle cells. PEComas

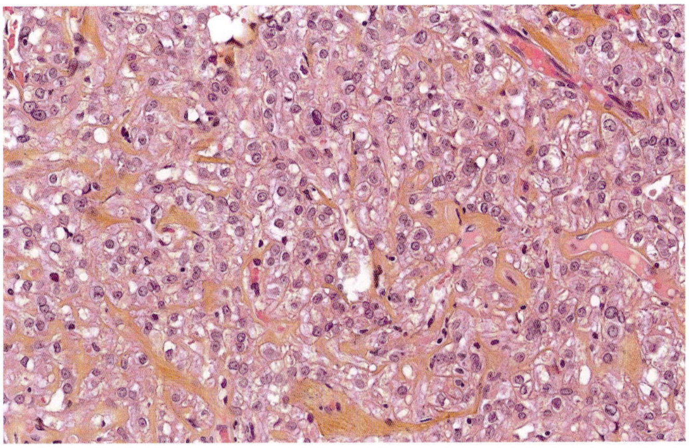

Fig. 6.47 Perivascular epithelioid cell tumour (PEComa). Cords and nests of cells separated by fine fibrovascular septa, showing abundant granular cytoplasm with well-defined borders (tissue section, H&E).

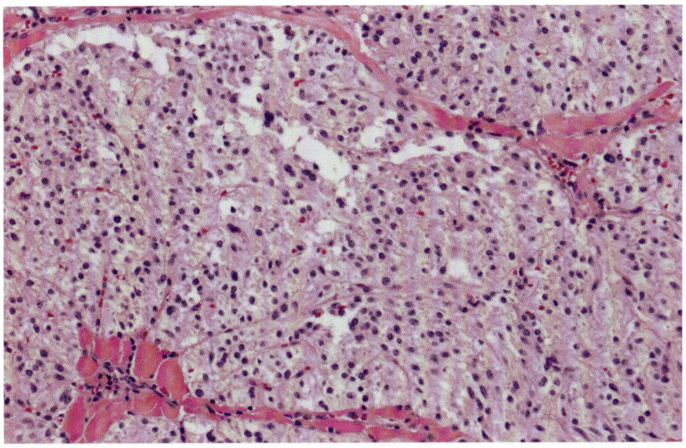

Fig. 6.48 Perivascular epithelioid cell tumour (PEComa). Large sheets of epithelioid cells with granular cytoplasm (tissue section, H&E).

are typically negative for S100, SOX10, CD10, and cytokeratin. Melanocytic markers are usually negative in smooth muscle neoplasms, but aberrant HMB45 positivity has been reported {1310}, making the interpretation of ICC less straightforward. Gastrointestinal stromal tumours may also be considered in the differential, and ICC is helpful in this scenario because gastrointestinal stromal tumours are positive for KIT (CD117) and DOG1 but negative for melanocytic markers and also usually negative for smooth muscle markers.

There are two well-defined molecular subgroups of PEComa: those with *TSC1*/*TSC2* alterations that result in activation of the mTOR pathway and those with *TFE3* fusions that result in a predominance of epithelioid and clear cell cytomorphology {15}. *TFE3*-rearranged PEComas strongly express TFE3 by ICC and tend to have little or no MITF or myogenic marker expression.

Sample reports: STNUMP

Field AS
Qian X

The sample reports provided here are based on the standardized cytopathology report in the *Diagnostic categories and report structure* section of the first chapter. See that section for a discussion on the structure and components.

These are sample reports that include the components required in one possible format; the final report format depends on local practice and local laboratory information system requirements. For brevity, demographics and ROSE are not presented here.

Each institution should select a term for the main heading of the diagnostic summary, such as "Diagnostic summary" (as used in the examples below), "Diagnosis", or "Final diagnosis", and use it consistently.

Sample report 1

Specimen type:
CT-guided FNAB and CNB
Clinical and imaging information:
54-year-old female, right retroperitoneal mass.

Diagnostic summary:
Site: Right retroperitoneum
Category: Soft tissue neoplasm of uncertain malignant potential
Diagnosis: ALK-positive spindle and epithelioid neoplasm (see comment below)

Material received:
Eight air-dried Giemsa-stained slides from ROSE, three alcohol-fixed slides. 4 mL bloodstained fluid for cell block.

Microscopic description:
These moderately cellular smears show uniform spindle cells with tapered cytoplasm and oval to coffee-bean nuclei, with scattered larger polygonal cells with large nuclei, prominent nucleoli, and abundant cytoplasm, in a background of lymphocytes and plasma cells. There is no necrosis. The cell block shows considerable similar material. Immunocytochemistry shows that the spindle cells are positive for ALK and negative for AE1/AE3 pancytokeratin, claudin-4, CD30, CD45RB, ERG, DOG1, desmin, SMA, S100, SOX10, CD34, and MDM2.

Comment: The features suggest a myofibroblastic tumour. It is noted that the CNB shows limited but similar material. FISH to assess for *ALK* gene rearrangements is underway and will be reported in a supplementary report.

Supplementary report 1:
ALK rearrangement is detected by FISH, supporting the diagnosis of inflammatory myofibroblastic tumour.

(Editor's note: In this case, the cytopathologist has waited to include the ICC on the cell block rather than issuing a cytopathology report to be later followed up with a supplementary report. FISH has confirmed the diagnosis and has been reported in a supplementary final integrated report. They have also mentioned the concurrent CNB, which provided limited material.)

Sample report 2

Specimen type:
CT-guided FNAB

Clinical and imaging information:
43-year-old male, left presacral 40 mm soft tissue mass.

Diagnostic summary:
Site: Presacral mass
Category: Soft tissue neoplasm of uncertain malignant potential
Diagnosis: Solitary fibrous tumour (see comment below)

Material received:
Nine air-dried Giemsa-stained smears from ROSE, three alcohol-fixed smears. 4 mL bloodstained fluid processed for cell block.

Microscopic description:
These moderately cellular smears show uniform spindle cells in tissue fragments and as single cells in the background. The spindle cells show fine cytoplasmic processes and nuclei with fine granular chromatin and no nucleoli. Some fat and tissue fragments that vary from minute, collagenous, and hypocellular to myxoid are also present. There is no necrosis and mitoses are not seen. There is considerable similar material in the cell block. The spindle cells are positive for CD34 and STAT6, and negative for desmin, S100, SMA, and MDM2.

Comment: The overall features support the diagnosis of solitary fibrous tumour. Cellular atypia, mitoses, and necrosis are not seen in this small sample of a large tumour, and risk stratification to assess metastatic potential based on a multivariate risk stratification model for solitary fibrous tumour (see reference below) can be performed only on resection specimens.

Reference: Demicco EG, Wagner MJ, Maki RG, et al. Risk assessment in solitary fibrous tumors: validation and refinement of a risk stratification model. Mod Pathol. 2017 Oct;30(10):1433–42 {310}

(Editor's note: In this case, the cytopathologist has issued a single integrated report with ICC and the final diagnosis.)

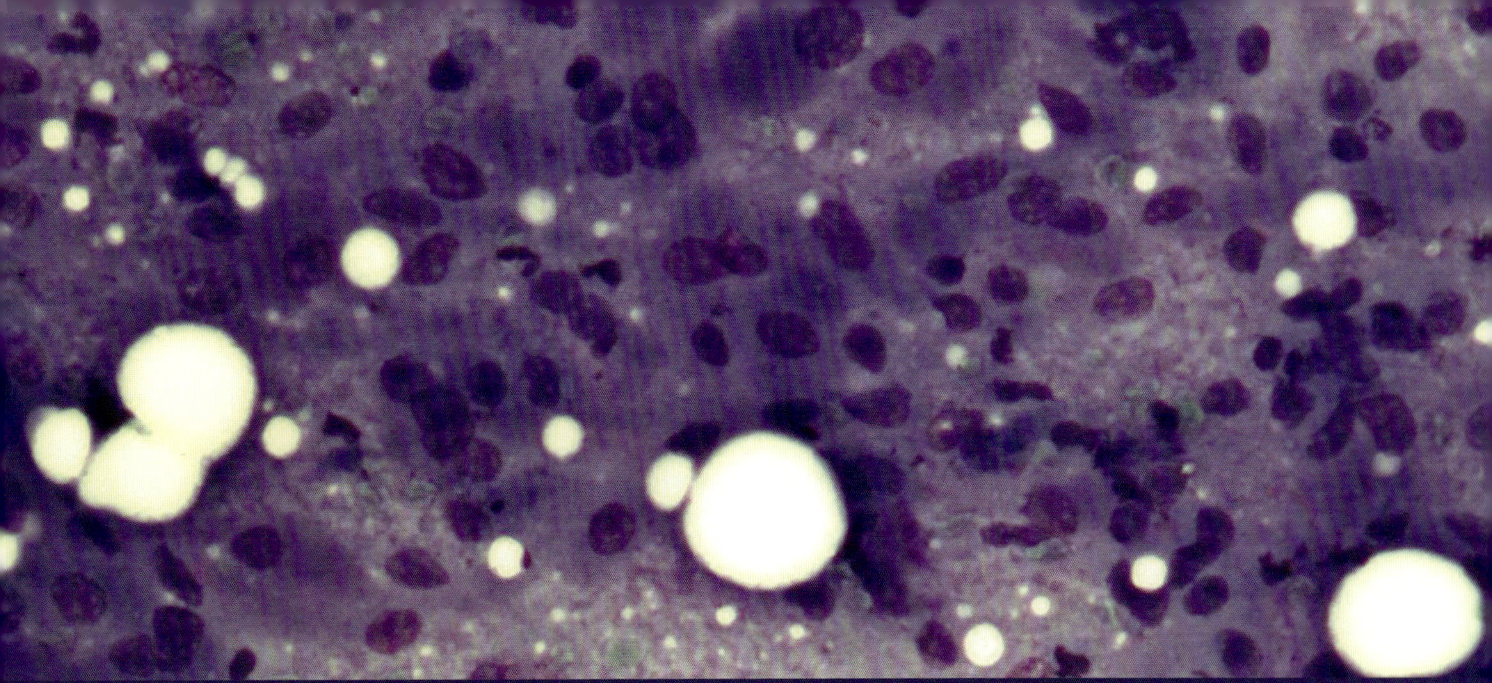

7

Diagnostic category: Suspicious for malignancy

Edited by: Pitman MB, Schmitt F

Introduction
Definition
Discussion and background
Risk of malignancy and diagnostic management recommendations
Sample reports

Introduction

Raymond WA
Klijanienko J

The "Suspicious for malignancy" category is used when cytopathological features are present that suggest a malignant diagnosis but these features are insufficient in number or specificity to permit a definitive diagnosis. Atypical cells may show features suggestive of malignancy but do not allow a confident diagnosis of malignancy due to suboptimal preparation, smearing, preservation, or staining. Such specimens cannot be regarded as "Inadequate/Insufficient/Non-diagnostic". Specimens in the "Suspicious for malignancy" category are generally from lesions that yield hypocellular smears or from neoplasms with a continuum of low-risk to high-risk features.

There is likely to be wide interobserver variability in this category. The diagnosis of malignancy is dependent in part on the cytopathologist's experience and confidence, in part on the quality of the material for assessment, and in part on the nature of the lesion. The nature of the lesion is a particular problem in soft tissue neoplasms, which may show considerable intratumoural morphological heterogeneity, as well as overlap between lesions.

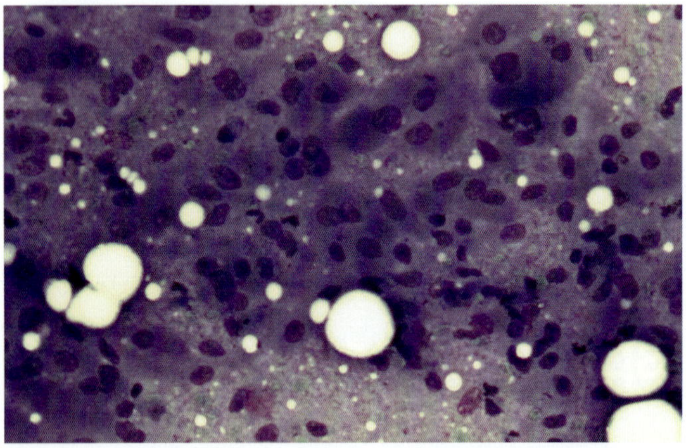

Fig. 7.01 Granular cell tumour. Numerous epithelioid cells with abundant granular cytoplasm and poorly preserved cytoplasmic borders; mild nuclear atypia (Giemsa).

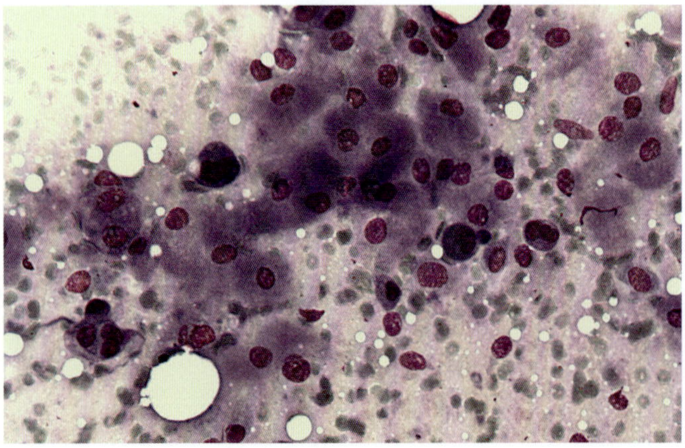

Fig. 7.02 Granular cell tumour. Pseudoepithelioid cells with irregular nuclei and poorly defined cytoplasmic borders (Giemsa).

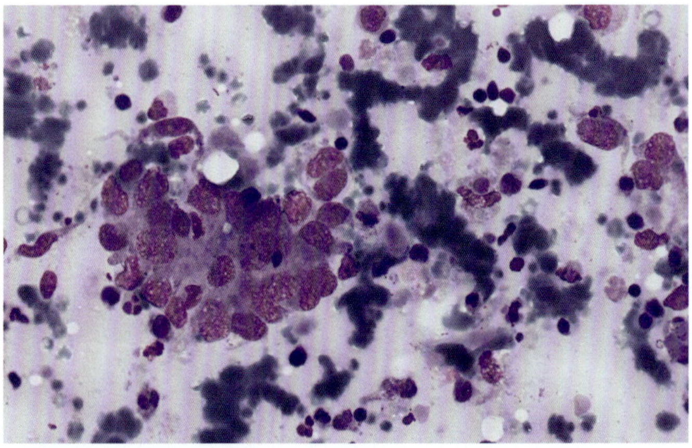

Fig. 7.03 Epithelioid angiosarcoma. Epithelioid and spindle cells showing some nuclear enlargement and atypia, categorized as "Suspicious for malignancy", because of scant cellularity and lack of diagnostic ICC.

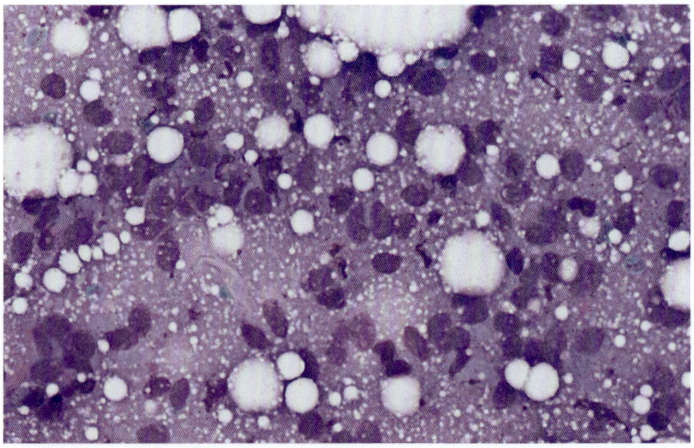

Fig. 7.04 Angiosarcoma. Dispersed round and spindle cells with moderate nuclear atypia, categorized as "Suspicious for malignancy" (Giemsa).

Definition

Raymond WA
Klijanienko J

A specimen categorized as "Suspicious for malignancy" demonstrates some cytopathological features suggestive of malignancy, but with features insufficient, in either number or quality, for an unequivocal diagnosis of malignancy.

Discussion and background

Raymond WA
Klijanienko J

The "Suspicious for malignancy" category should have a high positive predictive value for malignancy, because the WHO Reporting System for Soft Tissue Cytopathology (WHO System) includes a separate "Atypical" category for atypical FNAB samples, which are most likely benign, with a lower ROM. The category reduces the risk of false positive diagnoses and ensures a high positive predictive value in the "Malignant" category, close to 100%.

The "Suspicious for malignancy" category is expected to show a degree of interobserver variability due to the significant heterogeneity of tumours arising in the soft tissue, as well as the variation in diagnostic threshold among pathologists for the diagnosis of malignancy.

The "Suspicious for malignancy" category includes cellular smears showing nuclear enlargement, anisonucleosis, irregularity of nuclear membranes, and coarse chromatin, possibly with prominent nucleoli and mitotic figures. The background features may include necrosis, myxoid material, and inflammatory cells. Many cases are from entities that show a range of cytopathological appearances, which require specific histopathological features, such as mitotic count, infiltrative growth, or focal necrosis, for a specific diagnosis. Typical examples are smooth muscle or neural neoplasms and spindle cell lesions such as gastrointestinal stromal tumour.

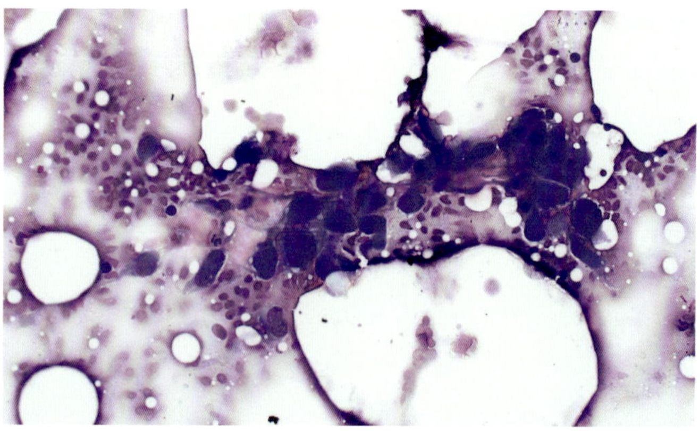

Fig. 7.05 Suspicious for malignancy – epithelioid haemangioendothelioma. FNAB of external iliac region mass showing poorly cohesive atypical epithelioid cells with occasional cytoplasmic vacuoles (Giemsa).

This category is particularly dependent on the expertise of the FNAB operator, the quality of material provided, the quality of the smear preparation, the availability of material for cell block and ancillary testing, and the inherent nature of the lesion. Many soft tissue neoplasms are of low cellularity, such as lipomatous tumours, and it may be difficult to obtain sufficient atypical cells in a cytopathology preparation to allow a diagnosis of malignancy. Other tumours show considerable intratumoural variation in cellularity, which may be reflected in hypocellular smears.

The rate of "Suspicious for malignancy" cases varies in published studies. In a review of 1114 bone and soft tissue lesions, 1% showed cells suspicious for malignancy, of which 5 of the 7 with follow-up (71%) were confirmed as malignant on histopathology {696}. One text {233} suggests using atypical and suspicious categories for FNAB, but most studies do not provide ROM for atypical/suspicious FNAB and only indicate overall sensitivity and specificity in distinguishing benign from malignant. Several other studies have reported the proportion of cases in the atypical/suspicious category as 1–2%, usually representing only 1 or 2 cases {1330,1470}.

Ancillary techniques, such as ICC on cell block material, can assist in confirming a specific tumour type, but in many soft tissue tumours the cellularity is insufficient for definitive assessment, or the ICC may suggest a cell lineage but not define the malignant nature of the neoplasm. Molecular studies in a few specific tumours, such as *MDM2* FISH analysis for liposarcoma, may allow a definitive diagnosis; if one of these tumours is suspected on the FNAB, such ancillary tests can be requested. In all cases, the tumour type suspected, or a differential diagnosis, should be stated in the cytopathology report.

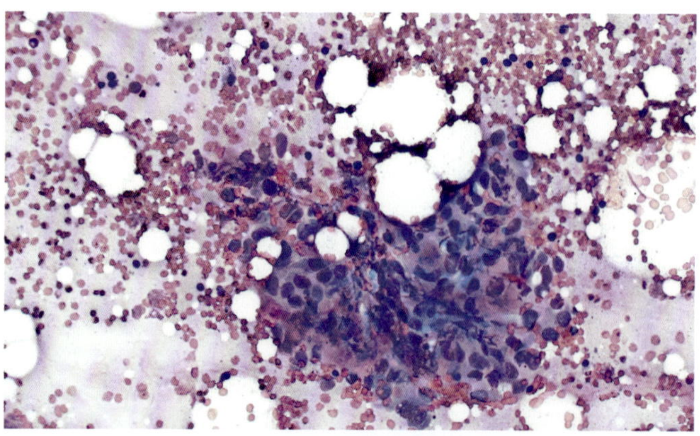

Fig. 7.06 Epithelioid haemangioendothelioma. A cohesive tissue fragment consisting of atypical cells with no specific differentiation and a moderate amount of cytoplasm, categorized as "Suspicious for malignancy" (Giemsa).

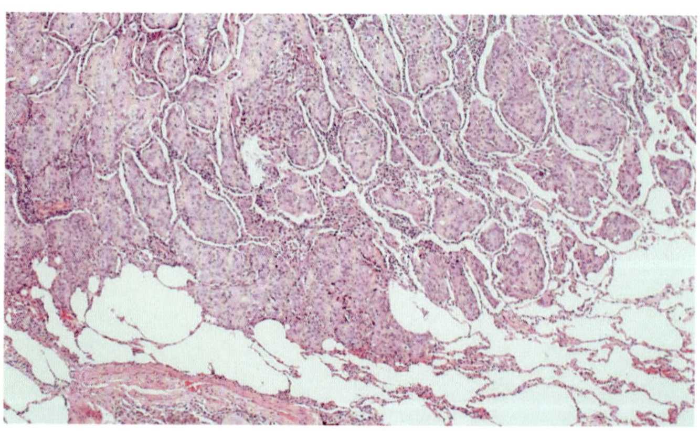

Fig. 7.07 Epithelioid haemangioendothelioma. Wedge resection of lung deposit demonstrates intra-alveolar spread, and the features are consistent with metastasis from the hepatic region mass (H&E). CD34, ERG, and CD31 confirmed positive by ICC; cytokeratins negative.

Risk of malignancy and diagnostic management recommendations

Raymond WA
Klijanienko J

The category has a high positive predictive value for malignancy, with a reported ROM of 71–80% {696,753}, and in one recent retrospective single-institution study of more than 2200 cases, the ROM was 68.42% based on using the six categories of the WHO System {460}. The authors of the study made the interesting observation that the ROM varies not only with categorization into the six categories but also with the FNAB pattern seen, from 3% for lipomatous tumours, which include one of the most common FNAB targets (superficial lipoma), to 62.78% for spindle cell, 78.15% for epithelioid, 84.58% for myxoid, 94.26% for pleomorphic, and 100% for round cell tumours. Further research around this finding will be worthwhile to guide cytopathologists and clinicians.

Clinical and imaging findings should always be correlated with the cytopathological report and the results of any ancillary testing available, ideally in a multidisciplinary meeting. If there are discrepancies, repeat FNAB should be recommended to confirm the malignancy, preferably with ROSE to effectively triage material for cell block, ICC, FISH, or NGS, along with CNB whenever available. In some situations, incisional biopsy with or without frozen section or a surgical excision biopsy may be required.

Sample reports: Suspicious for malignancy

Rekhi B
Field AS
Qian X

The sample reports provided here are based on the standardized cytopathology report in the *Diagnostic categories and report structure* section of the first chapter. See that section for a discussion on the structure and components.

These are sample reports that include the components required in one possible format; the final report format depends on local practice and local laboratory information system requirements. For brevity, demographics and ROSE are not presented here.

Each institution should select a term for the main heading of the diagnostic summary, such as "Diagnostic summary" (as used in the examples below), "Diagnosis", or "Final diagnosis", and use it consistently.

Sample report 1

Specimen type:
FNAB
Clinical and imaging information:
74-year-old male, with rapidly increasing, firm, painful 40 mm lump in left frontoparietal scalp region of 3 months' duration. Ultrasound shows lesion involving dermis and possibly bone.

Diagnostic summary:
Site: Left frontoparietal scalp
Category: Suspicious for malignancy
Diagnosis: Suspicious for sarcoma

Material received:
Three air-dried smears and one alcohol-fixed smear.

Microscopic description:
Predominantly haemorrhagic smears show scant material consisting of occasional minute tissue fragments of markedly pleomorphic spindle cells, along with a few scattered large polygonal cells with atypical nuclei. One tissue fragment shows a possible vasoformative architecture. Occasional haemosiderin-laden macrophages are also seen.

Comment: The features are suspicious for a sarcoma such as angiosarcoma. Correlation with clinical and imaging findings is required. Repeat FNAB (to obtain material for ancillary studies) or CNB is recommended.

Sample report 2

Specimen type:
FNAB
Clinical and imaging information:
55-year-old female with a rapidly growing 70 mm soft tissue mass fixed to skin in left thigh, 4 months' duration. MRI reveals a well-defined 75 mm heterogeneous soft tissue mass involving the deep fascia and the surrounding muscles.

Diagnostic summary:
Site: Left mid-thigh vastus medialis muscle
Category: Suspicious for malignancy
Diagnosis: Suspicious for sarcoma with necrosis (see supplementary report below)

Material received:
Six air-dried slides, three alcohol-fixed slides. 3 mL pink fluid processed for cell block.

Microscopic description:
These paucicellular smears show several minute tissue fragments consisting of spindle and pleomorphic cells, as well as several similar single intact cells, in a background of limited necrosis. Several minute tissue fragments of fat are also present.

Comment: The features are suspicious for sarcoma with necrosis, suggesting a high-grade neoplasm. Immunocytochemistry will be performed on the limited material in the cell block.

Supplementary report 1:
There are a very limited number of tumours cells in the cell block, positive for MDM2 and CDK4 and negative for pankeratin AE1/AE3. The features are "Suspicious for malignancy" and raise the possibility of a dedifferentiated liposarcoma. Correlation with the clinical and imaging findings is recommended along with CNB or incisional biopsy.

(Editor's note: There is limited material, and the cytopathologist has issued a "Suspicious for malignancy" categorization report and alerted the clinical team that ICC will be attempted on the cell block. The cell block ICC, again on limited material, supports the diagnosis of sarcoma and raises the possibility of a dedifferentiated liposarcoma.)

Sample report 3

Specimen type:
FNAB
Clinical and imaging information:
70-year-old male with a 45 mm firm mass over his left deltoid. MRI shows a T2-hyperintense, septate multilobulated mass involving the subcutaneous region.

Diagnostic summary:
Site: Left deltoid
Category: Suspicious for malignancy
Diagnosis: Suspicious for sarcoma, including possibility of myxofibrosarcoma

Material received:
Five air-dried Giemsa-stained smears from ROSE and two alcohol-fixed smears. 3 mL bloodstained fluid.

Microscopic description:
There is scant material, consisting of small tissue fragments of predominantly myxoid material containing scattered spindle and stellate cells (including occasional cells showing nuclear atypia), foamy macrophages (which may represent pseudolipoblasts), and lymphocytes. There are thin blood vessels within these myxoid fragments. There is no diagnostic material in the cell block.

Comment: The features are "Suspicious for malignancy" and raise the possibility of low-grade myxofibrosarcoma, although cellular myxoma cannot be completely excluded. Correlation with clinical and imaging findings and CNB or incisional biopsy is recommended.

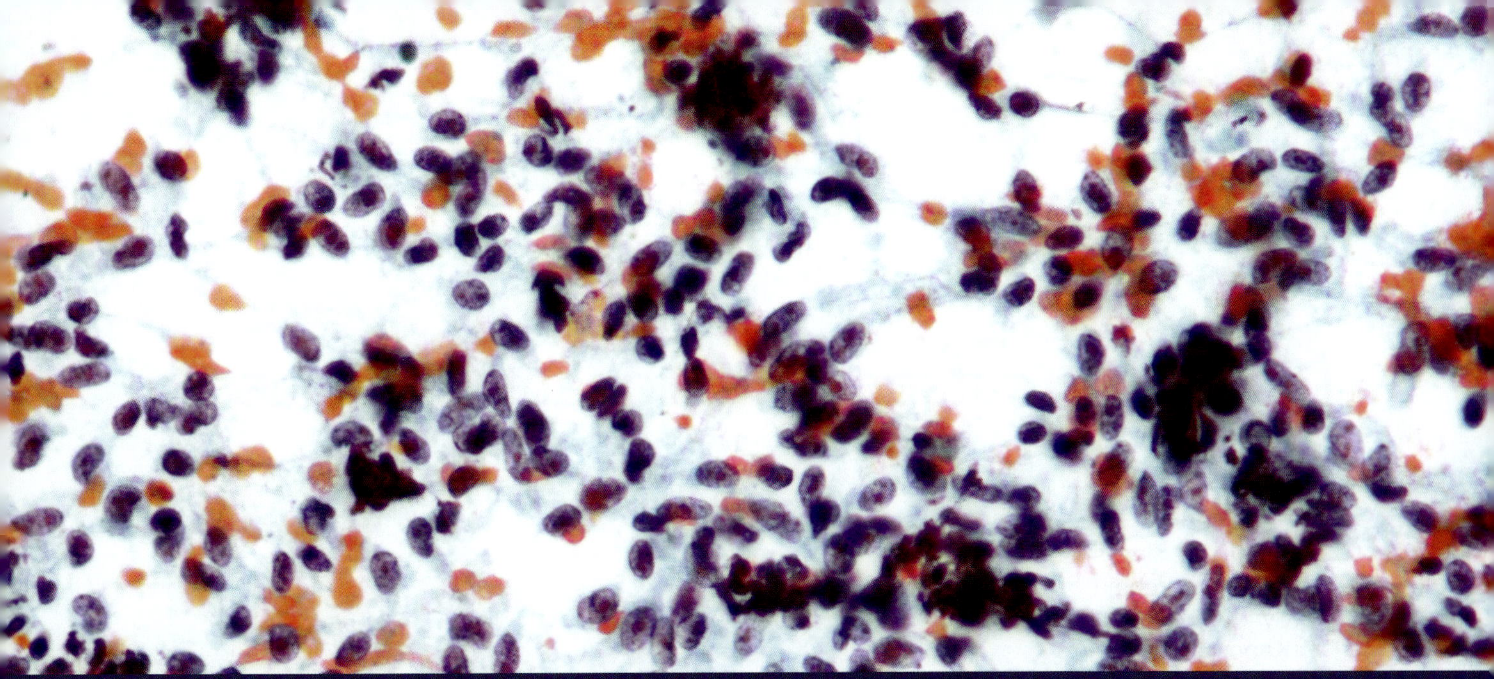

8

Diagnostic category: Malignant

Edited by: Bode-Lesniewska B, Carrilho C, Chebib I, Dodd LG, Field AS, Jo VY, Lazar AJ, Mehrotra R, Qian X, Rekhi B, Schmitt F

(Continued on next page)

8

Diagnostic category: Malignant (continued)

Introduction

Klijanienko J
Domanski HA
Layfield LJ

The diagnosis of malignancy is dependent in part on the quality of the material provided for assessment, in part on the nature and location of the lesion, and in part on the cytopathologist's experience and confidence. ICC, FISH, and molecular analysis for specific mutations are also important for the diagnosis of malignancy in some soft tissue tumours.

The "Malignant" category is used when unequivocal cytomorphological features of malignancy are present. No single cytopathological feature is diagnostic of malignancy, but the presence of round cells, prominent nuclear atypia, marked abnormalities of N:C ratio, atypical mitotic figures, marked variability in cell size and shape, necrosis, and hypercellularity are highly suggestive of malignancy.

Non-lymphoid proliferations composed of round or oval cells from soft tissue neoplasms are almost always malignant, whereas tumours composed of pleomorphic cells are frequently malignant. Tumours composed of bland uniform spindle cells lacking nuclear atypia and mitotic figures are often benign but require careful analysis and correlation with imaging and clinical features to avoid false negative and false positive diagnoses. Correlation with histopathological features in CNB is also helpful in avoiding a false positive diagnosis. Hypercellular specimens may be malignant, whereas a hypocellular specimen favours a benign diagnosis. Some soft tissue malignancies have characteristic molecular features; for example, *MDM2* amplification is particularly helpful in establishing malignancy in fat tumours. Other sarcomas are associated with specific translocations, including *ASPSCR1*::*TFE3* in clear cell sarcoma, *FUS*::*CREB3L2* in low-grade fibromyxoid sarcoma, and *FUS*::*DD1T3* in myxoid liposarcoma {404,111}.

After confirmation of malignancy, cytopathological examination should establish the type of malignancy by differentiating between sarcomas, metastatic carcinomas, melanoma, and lymphomas. When possible, further subtyping into a

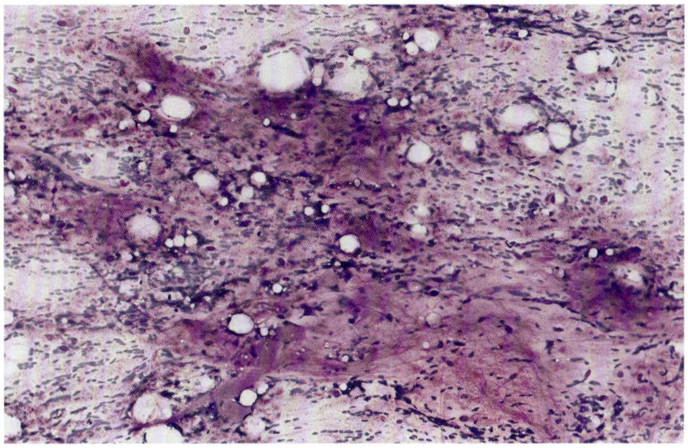

Fig. 8.02 Myxofibrosarcoma. Low cellularity; slightly atypical spindle and polygonal cells with abundant myxoid matrix, a pattern that can be seen in both benign and malignant tumours (Giemsa).

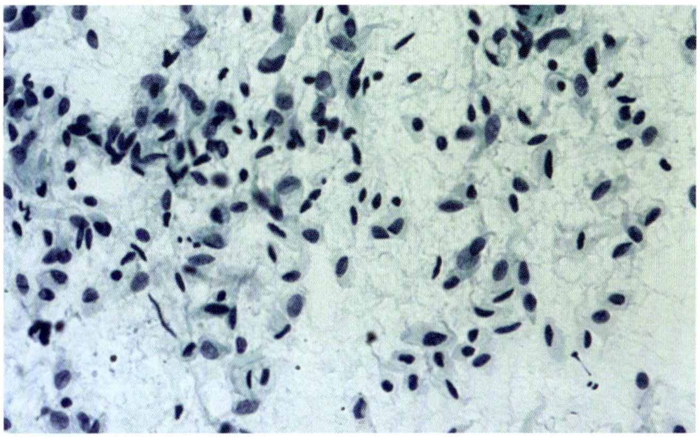

Fig. 8.03 Myofibroblastoma. Numerous dispersed spindle cells, which can be seen in both benign and malignant spindle cell tumours (Pap).

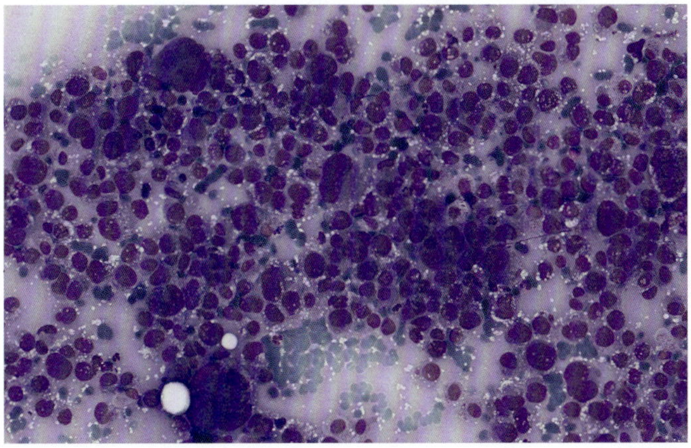

Fig. 8.01 Dedifferentiated liposarcoma. Polymorphous, spindle, and oval cells with high-grade nuclei (Giemsa).

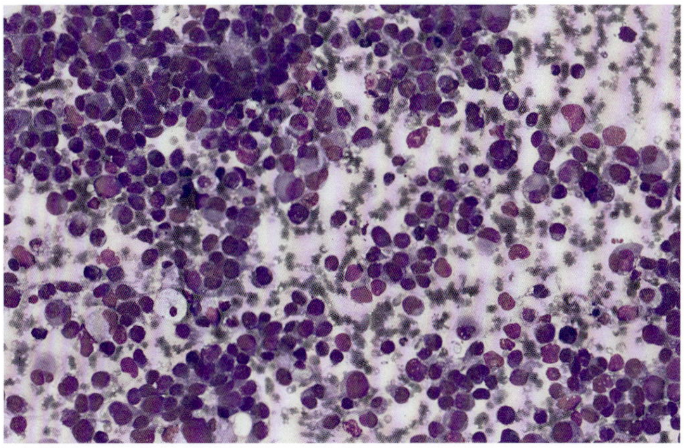

Fig. 8.04 Alveolar rhabdomyosarcoma. A cell-rich smear showing round and more pleomorphic polygonal atypical cells (Giemsa).

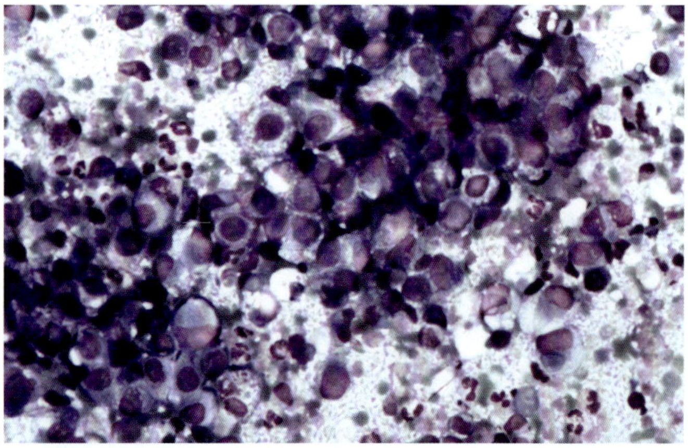

Fig. 8.05 Epithelioid sarcoma. Dispersed epithelioid cells with high-grade pleomorphic nuclei (Giemsa).

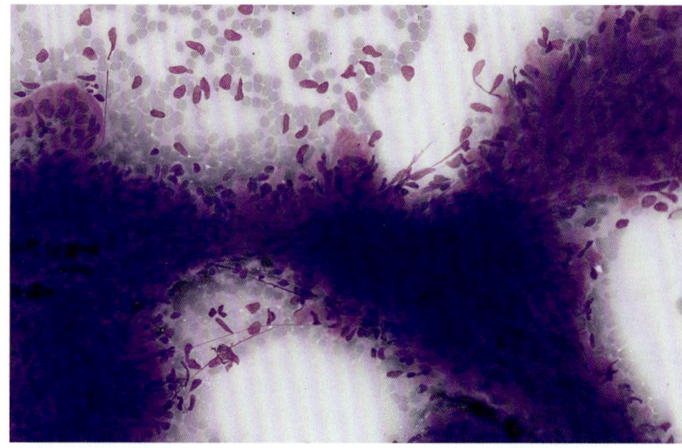

Fig. 8.06 Dermatofibrosarcoma protuberans. Tissue fragments of spindle cells within magenta stroma, with single spindle cells and stripped nuclei in the background (Giemsa).

specific sarcoma type or at least designation of the sarcoma as low-grade or high-grade should be performed, and ICC and molecular analysis can aid in the specific identification of some sarcoma types.

Definition

Klijanienko J
Domanski HA
Layfield LJ

Specimens categorized as "Malignant" demonstrate unequivocal cytopathological features of malignancy.

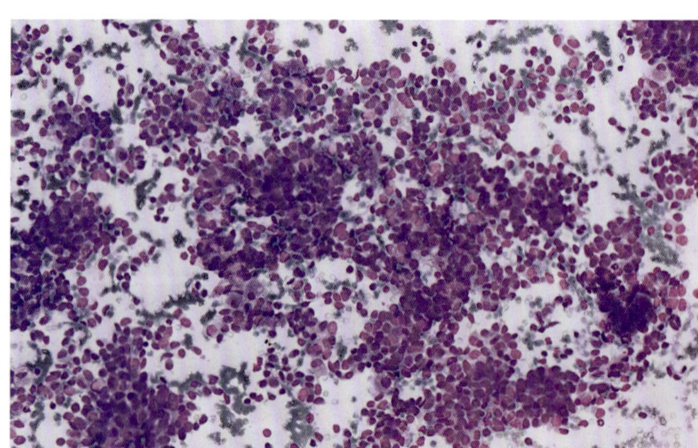

Fig. 8.07 Round cell sarcoma (sarcoma with *CIC* alteration). Round cell sarcoma showing high cellularity and discohesive sheets and single intact cells (Giemsa).

Discussion and background

Domanski HA
Field AS

The "Malignant" category encompasses all cases in which the material is unequivocally malignant, characterized either by cellular smears with distinctly malignant cytomorphological features or by smears showing key cytopathological features diagnostic of a specific malignant tumour or tumour group. The "Malignant" category must be used in conjunction with clinical history, physical examination, and imaging findings. The report should almost always state that "correlation with clinical and imaging findings is required".

This category includes both primary low- or high-grade sarcomas and secondary tumours occurring in the soft tissues. In addition to the "Malignant" diagnosis, distinguishing primary sarcoma from metastatic lesions of non-mesenchymal origin in the initial diagnostic process has significant impact on further clinical management. Clinical data and information about previous malignancies, together with the cytopathological features of the FNAB smears, are usually sufficient to render a correct diagnosis in many cases of secondary malignancies {342,1423, 1017}. However, when a mass in soft tissue is the first manifestation of a carcinoma, melanoma, or lymphoma, ancillary tests are often necessary to determine the site of the primary malignant lesion and to assist with potential treatment targets.

Regarding primary soft tissue sarcomas, if a specific tumour diagnosis cannot be rendered, the case should at least be categorized as "Malignant", and a differential diagnosis is required. In some cases, diagnosis of high-grade or low-grade sarcoma can provide a diagnostic level sufficient to plan surgical treatment and further management. However, for some types of sarcomas, optimal treatment includes neoadjuvant or adjuvant therapy, which typically requires a specific histopathological type and grade of sarcoma. In such cases ancillary testing of FNAB material and CNB may be essential for the accurate determination of the precise histopathological diagnosis {783,1062,342,198}. Small round cell neoplasms are a typical example of this necessity; the categorization of small round cell neoplasms as "Malignant" based on the FNAB smears is usually straightforward, but these entities share many cytopathological features and can be difficult to specifically diagnose on the basis of cytomorphology alone {343,463}. Because most small round cell sarcomas are characterized by specific patterns of protein expression or genetic changes, ancillary tests are essential to reach a specific histopathological diagnosis {22,463,343}. Similarly, myxoid soft tissue neoplasms often pose diagnostic challenges in FNAB examination due to the overlapping cytopathological features of many entities {1231,1463}. Although the sensitivity and specificity for detecting malignancy in this group of neoplasms is high {1231}, additional ICC or molecular tests can assist in establishing a definitive diagnosis for certain specific entities {785,1241}.

Risk of malignancy and diagnostic management recommendations

Domanski HA
Field AS

The ROM for the "Malignant" category ranges from 91% to 100% based on several retrospective studies {753,1001,176,1017,705, 1231}. A more recent large retrospective study reported a ROM of 97.69%, noting that the ROM varies depending on both the cytomorphological pattern and the WHO Reporting System for Soft Tissue Cytopathology (WHO System) categorization {460}.

Clinical and imaging correlation is always necessary in evaluating neoplasms within the "Malignant" category {289,158}, and management decisions as to any further diagnostic workup and definitive management should be made by a multidisciplinary team. If FNAB does not provide enough material for diagnosis, or if the cytopathological findings are inconsistent with clinical and imaging assessments, the imaging findings should be carefully reviewed and correlated. If suspicion remains high, repeat FNAB – preferably with ROSE and triaging of material for appropriate ancillary tests – or CNB or simple excision biopsy should be conducted before proceeding with any major surgical or oncological interventions.

Atypical lipomatous tumour / well-differentiated liposarcoma

Bode-Lesniewska B
Jo VY

Definition

Atypical lipomatous tumour / well-differentiated liposarcoma (ALT/WDLPS) is a locally aggressive, non-metastasizing mesenchymal neoplasm composed either entirely or partly of a proliferation of adipocytes showing at least focal nuclear atypia in both adipocytes and stromal cells, and characterized by an amplification of *MDM2* and *CDK4*.

Clinical features and imaging

ALT/WDLPS occurs in middle-aged and elderly patients of both sexes. The ALT designation is applicable to resectable tumours of the extremities occurring as large, deeply located, slowly growing masses most commonly occurring in the thigh and buttock or trunk, shoulder, or back {1512}, whereas the WDLPS designation is used for prognostically less favourable retroperitoneal or mediastinal tumours in the retroperitoneum and paratesticular region and less commonly in the mediastinum or head and neck. ALT/WDLPS in deep locations and especially in the retroperitoneum is often asymptomatic until it exceeds 200 mm. On CT or MRI, a homogeneous fatty mass is seen, sometimes with pronounced septation but without solid areas {742,86}. Curative complete resection is possible in extremity or trunk locations, but the retroperitoneal tumours tend to spread diffusely and recur (often repeatedly) due to the inherent difficulties of a complete resection. ALT/WDLPS carries a risk of dedifferentiation in the recurrent tumours, most commonly in the retroperitoneum – in as many as 20% of cases; in the extremities this risk is 2%.

Histopathology

ALT/WDLPS consists of solid sheets of adipocytes showing variability of cell size and fibrotic septation, with variable nuclear atypia of both the adipocytes and stromal cells. The nuclei of the adipocytes are variably enlarged, showing hyperchromasia and pleomorphism, with occasional multinucleation. Multinucleated cells showing a wreath-like arrangement of hyperchromatic nuclei around an eosinophilic cytoplasm resembling flowers and known as "floret" cells may be encountered. The presence

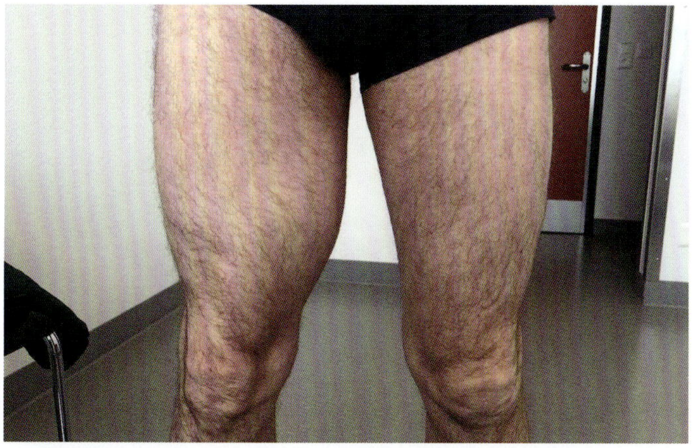

Fig. 8.08 Atypical lipomatous tumour / well-differentiated liposarcoma. A patient presenting with a large, slowly growing mass on the lower anterior aspect of the right thigh.

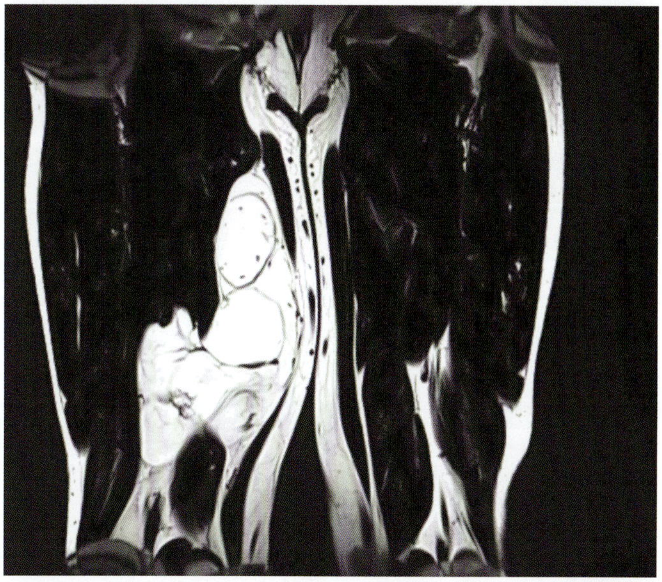

Fig. 8.09 Atypical lipomatous tumour of the thigh. Coronal MRI showing a large, deeply located lipomatous mass in the right thigh.

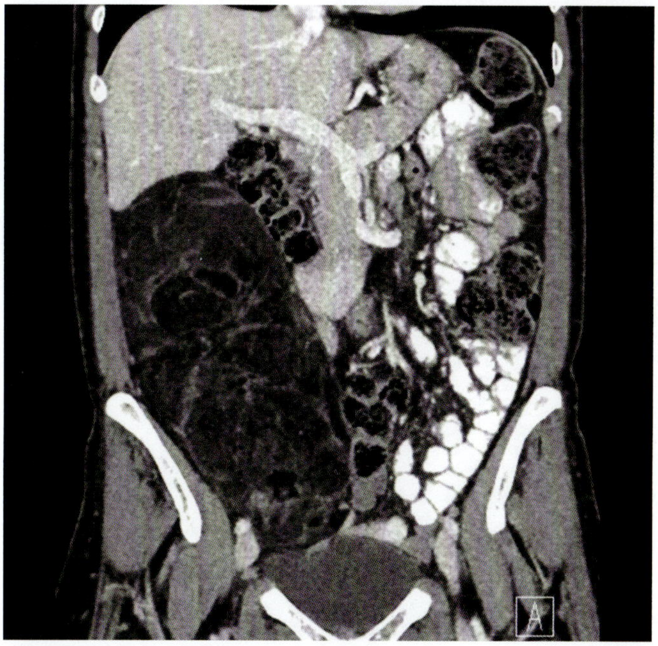

Fig. 8.10 Right-sided retroperitoneal atypical lipomatous tumour / well-differentiated liposarcoma. Coronal CT.

of lipoblasts neither makes nor is required for a diagnosis of ALT/WDLPS {1503}. Occasionally, areas with abundant myxoid matrix may be present. In the inflammatory variant, numerous lymphocytes and plasma cells, as well as neutrophils and eosinophils, may be observed, whereas collagenous regions with atypical stromal cells and sometimes rare atypical adipocytes dominate in the sclerosing subtype. Lipoma-like, inflammatory, and sclerosing areas may all be a part of the same tumour. There are no solid, nodular, or spindle cell regions or pleomorphic areas lacking a lipomatous component in adequately sampled ALT/WDLPS. If these non-lipogenic nodular components are present, mostly with an abrupt transition, the progression to dedifferentiated liposarcoma has occurred.

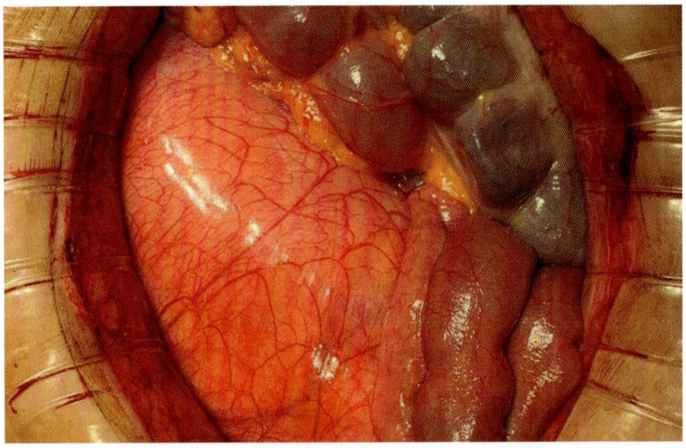

Fig. 8.11 Retroperitoneal atypical lipomatous tumour / well-differentiated liposarcoma. Intraoperative finding of the retroperitoneal mass.

Key diagnostic cytopathological features

- Variable cellularity
- Cohesive tissue fragments of adipocytes showing variability of size and nuclear atypia
- Nuclear atypia of the adipocytes varies from slight hyperchromasia to pronounced pleomorphism and multinucleation
- "Floret" cells and lipoblasts may be present
- Lipoblasts have one or more clear vacuoles in cells varying in size, with the vacuoles indenting the nucleus, which often appears scalloped by the vacuoles; there may be more than one nucleus
- "Floret" cells have a wreath or circumferential arrangement of nuclei around central eosinophilic cytoplasm (Pap)
- No solid or spindle cell non-adipocytic component

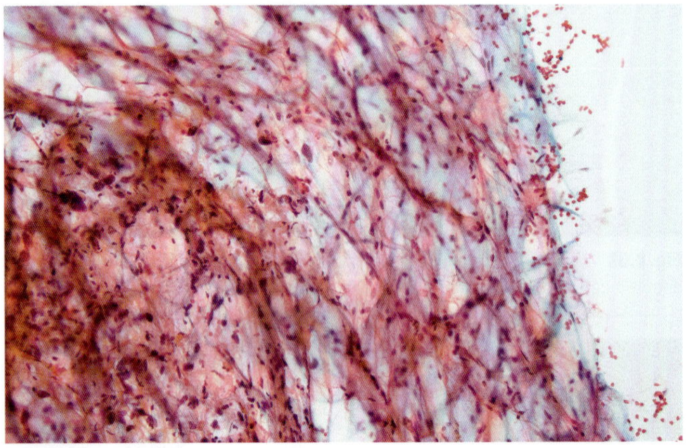

Fig. 8.12 Atypical lipomatous tumour / well-differentiated liposarcoma. A large tissue fragment consisting of adipocytes showing size variation and increased cellularity, with scattered, atypical, enlarged nuclei (Pap).

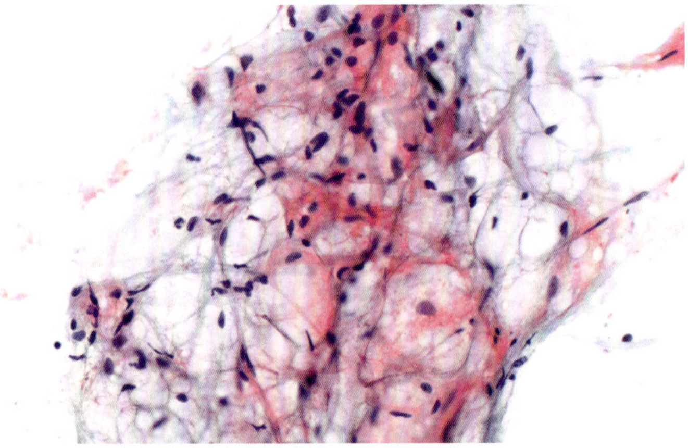

Fig. 8.14 Atypical lipomatous tumour / well-differentiated liposarcoma. Recurring tumour deeply located in the thigh. A direct smear showing mild hypercellularity and mild nuclear hyperchromasia, enlargement, and atypia. *MDM2* gene amplification on FISH (Pap).

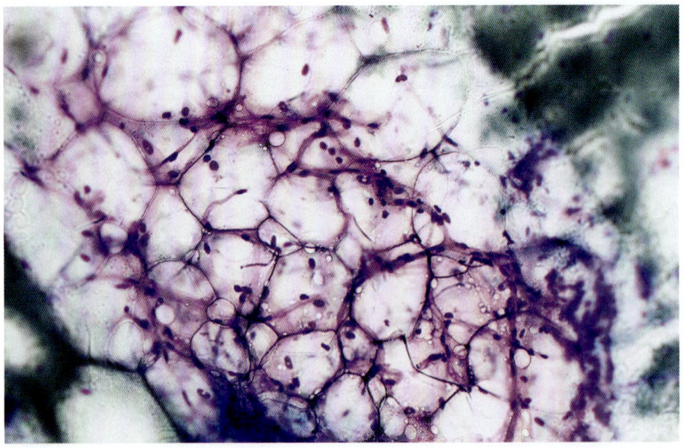

Fig. 8.13 Atypical lipomatous tumour / well-differentiated liposarcoma. A tissue fragment consisting of lipocytes indistinguishable from normal fat (Giemsa).

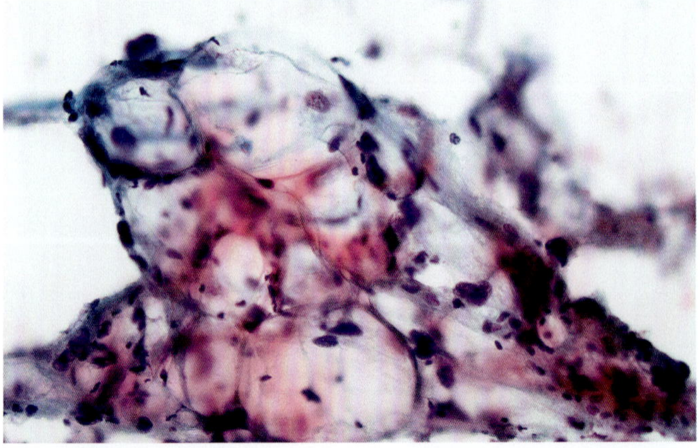

Fig. 8.15 Atypical lipomatous tumour / well-differentiated liposarcoma. Enlarged hyperchromatic atypical nuclei (Pap).

Discussion and differential diagnosis

Typical lipoma is the main differential diagnosis of ALT/WDLPS, and it may show similar clinical and imaging findings. Deeply located large intramuscular lipomas are rare in the extremities and are extremely rare in the retroperitoneum. Spindle cell and pleomorphic lipomas occur mostly in the subcutaneous tissue of the neck and shoulder and usually measure < 50 mm.

Ancillary testing

ICC demonstrates the overexpression of MDM2 or CDK4 in the atypical nuclei of ALT/WDLPS, but this may be difficult to detect in the lipoma-like variant. Lipomas do not carry the 12q13-q15 amplicon and do not usually contain MDM2-positive nuclei on ICC. FISH of the *MDM2* gene reliably discriminates between lipoma and lipoma-like ALT/WDLPS {421,234, 1555,1410}, whereas ICC has a low sensitivity of 45% in this setting {235}.

Overexpression of MDM2 in the nuclei of macrophages found in fat necrosis poses a diagnostic pitfall, but FISH, which may be performed on direct smears and cell blocks, is a reliable method for the detection of the diagnostic amplification of the *MDM2* gene {1566,573}.

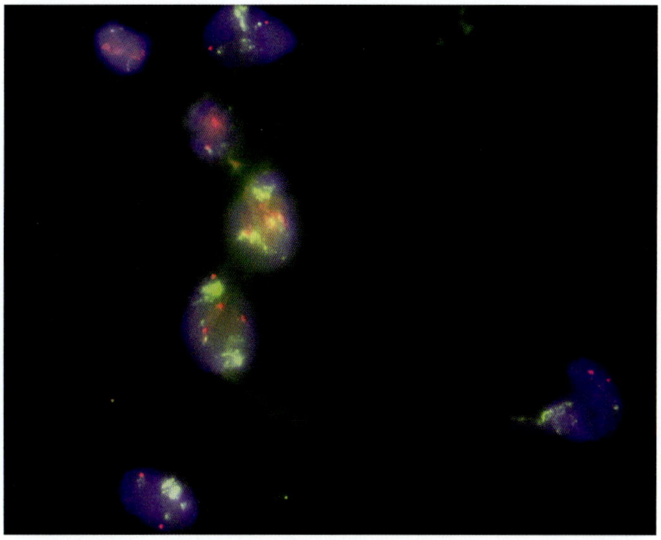

Fig. 8.16 *MDM2* amplification in FISH of recurring thigh tumour. FISH on direct smear showing adipocyte nuclei containing 2–4 centromere signals (red) of the chromosome 12 (CEP12) and clusters of *MDM2* gene signals (green), corresponding to the amplification of the *MDM2* gene (FISH, *MDM2*).

Chapter 8

Dedifferentiated liposarcoma

Qian X
Dodd LG

Definition

Dedifferentiated liposarcoma (DDLPS) is an atypical lipomatous tumour / well-differentiated liposarcoma (ALT/WDLPS) showing progression, either in the primary or in a recurrence, to a usually non-lipogenic sarcoma of variable histopathological grade, in most cases characterized by amplification of *MDM2* and *CDK4*.

Clinical features and imaging

DDLPS occurs most commonly in middle-aged to elderly adults, without sex predilection. Patients frequently present with a large painless mass, most commonly in the retroperitoneum and abdominal cavity. Other sites include the spermatic cord, deep soft tissue of proximal extremities, trunk, and head and neck region. MRI shows coexisting lipogenic and non-lipogenic components, and the latter should be targeted by FNAB {1027,1187}.

Histopathology

The classic histopathological feature is transition, abrupt or gradual, from ALT/WDLPS to non-lipogenic sarcoma with a wide range of morphological patterns, but the well-differentiated lipogenic component may be absent {555,307}. Common patterns include cellular pleomorphic, myxofibrosarcoma-like, fascicular spindle cell, fibromatosis-like, and a storiform meningothelial-like pattern. Other less common patterns include inflammatory cell–rich or inflammatory myofibroblastic tumour–like, a predominantly epithelioid morphology, and even a nested pattern resembling paraganglioma. Many tumours display mixed patterns {224,1401,402,1409,830}. Heterologous elements showing skeletal muscle, bone, cartilage, and vascular or smooth muscle differentiation can occur {138,1296,1162}. Some cases exhibit homologous lipoblastic differentiation, resembling pleomorphic liposarcoma {876}.

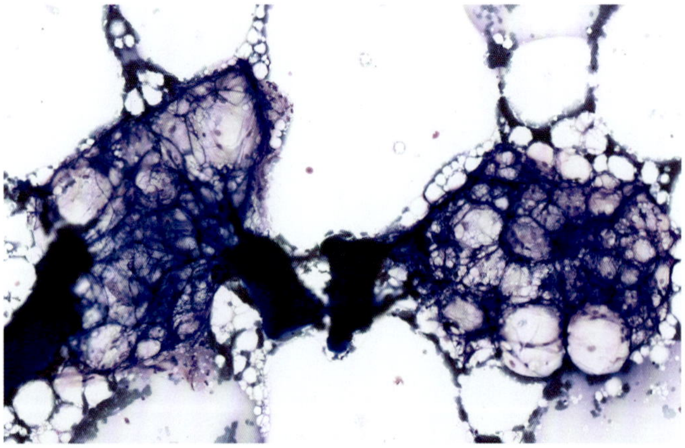

Fig. 8.17 Dedifferentiated liposarcoma. A well-differentiated region showing lipocytes and lipoblasts (Giemsa).

Key diagnostic cytopathological features

- Variable cellularity
- Variable smear patterns
- Dispersed single cells and loosely cohesive tissue fragments sometimes arrayed around vessels in an often myxoid background
- Spindle to stellate to pleomorphic tumour cells with variable degrees of atypia
- Occasional "floret" cells, with a wreath-like circumferential arrangement of nuclei around a central eosinophilic cytoplasm (Pap) can be a clue
- A coexisting lipogenic component may or may not be present
- Heterologous elements such as osteosarcoma or homologous elements of liposarcoma with lipoblasts may be present

Reference(s): {877,725,329}

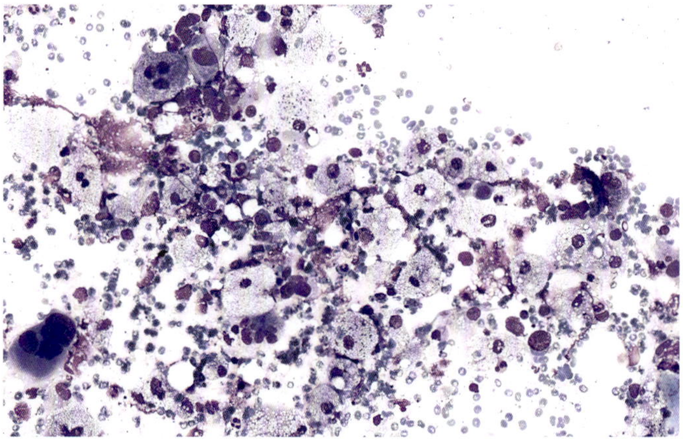

Fig. 8.18 Dedifferentiated liposarcoma. Microvacuolated lipocytes and a small number of large polymorphous cells with large hyperchromatic atypical nuclei (Giemsa).

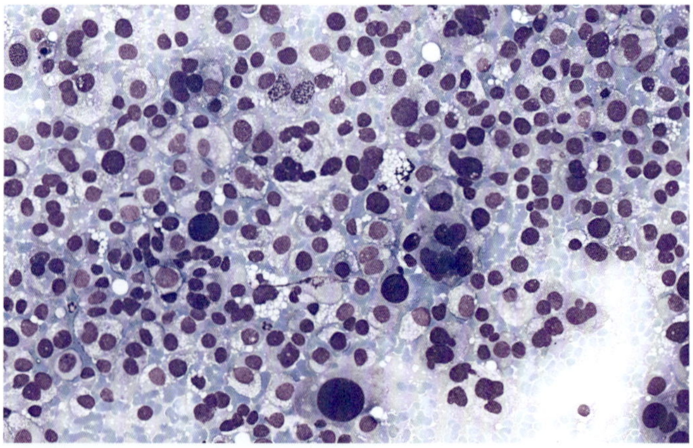

Fig. 8.19 Dedifferentiated liposarcoma. A less-differentiated region showing lipocytes with eccentric cytoplasm containing fine vacuoles and large lipoblasts with large atypical nuclei. Several atypical mitoses are present (Giemsa).

Discussion and differential diagnosis

Various spindle and pleomorphic sarcomas constitute a very broad range of differential diagnoses, depending on the cytomorphological pattern and location. The most common mimics are undifferentiated pleomorphic sarcoma, myxofibrosarcoma, and pleomorphic liposarcoma {232,877,791}, and ICC is usually required, with or without FISH and NGS.

Ancillary testing

MDM2 amplification, along with co-amplification of *CDK4*, is considered pathognomonic for ALT/WDLPS. Nuclear expression of MDM2 by ICC and/or *MDM2* gene amplification detected by FISH or NGS is desirable in establishing the diagnosis of DDLPS {139,1406,307,877}. Undifferentiated pleomorphic sarcoma, myxofibrosarcoma, and pleomorphic liposarcoma lack *MDM2* amplification in most cases. Given that *MDM2* gene amplification is also a hallmark of intimal sarcoma (an aggressive sarcoma arising in the wall of large vessels), tumour location and the presence of a lipogenic component warrant significant consideration of DDLPS {744,143}.

DDLPS with loss of H3 p.K28me3 (K27me3) expression is difficult to differentiate from a malignant peripheral nerve sheath tumour, especially because a small subset of these tumours exhibit MDM2 expression and/or *MDM2* amplification {863}. DDLPS with heterologous differentiation may lead to erroneous diagnoses, such as extraskeletal osteosarcoma and spindle cell rhabdomyosarcoma, and homologous differentiation can lead to misdiagnosis as pleomorphic liposarcoma {138,1296,1162}.

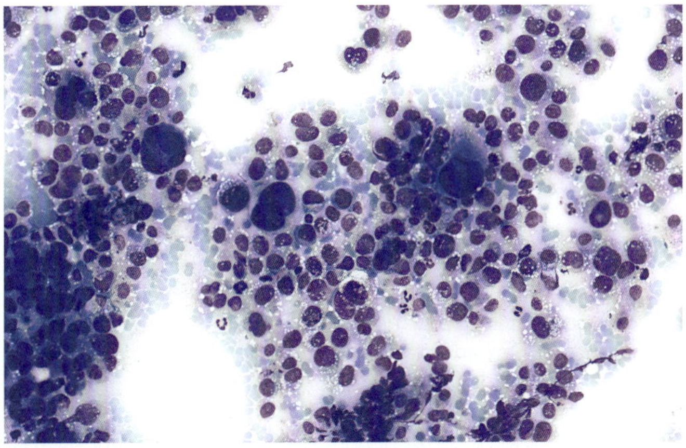

Fig. 8.20 Dedifferentiated liposarcoma. Tissue fragments and single cells, which are lipocytes with finely vacuolated cytoplasm and larger cells, some of which are binucleated or multinucleated with large pleomorphic nuclei (Giemsa).

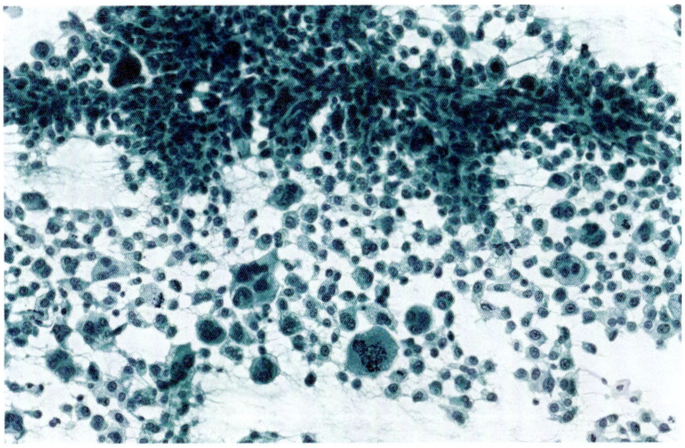

Fig. 8.21 Dedifferentiated liposarcoma. A tissue fragment with a thin vessel and plentiful lipocytes, along with singly dispersed lipocytes and scattered large lipoblasts with highly pleomorphic atypical nuclei. Several atypical mitoses are present (Pap).

Pleomorphic liposarcoma

Rekhi B
Qian X

Definition

Pleomorphic liposarcoma (PLPS) is a pleomorphic high-grade sarcoma containing a variable number of pleomorphic lipoblasts and lacking any other specific differentiation.

Clinical features and imaging

Pleomorphic liposarcoma occurs over a wide age range, from 18 to 93 years. Patients frequently present with a rapidly growing painless mass, most commonly in the lower extremity (including the thigh), followed by the upper extremity and trunk. Other sites are the retroperitoneum, head and neck, abdomen, pelvis, and spermatic cord {474,575}.

On CT and MRI, a well-circumscribed tumour with a negligible amount of fat is noted. The MRI features resemble those of other high-grade sarcomas, including areas of necrosis and haemorrhage {1053}.

Histopathology

Tumours display varying admixtures of lipogenic and non-lipogenic areas, including pleomorphic sarcomatous, round cell, epithelioid, and spindle cell components, along with tumour necrosis, vascular invasion, and frequent mitotic figures. Rarely, myxofibrosarcoma-like and pericytic growth patterns are noted {474,575}. ICC shows S100 expression in areas of lipogenic differentiation in as many as 48% cases {474,575}.

Key diagnostic cytopathological features

- Moderate to high cellularity

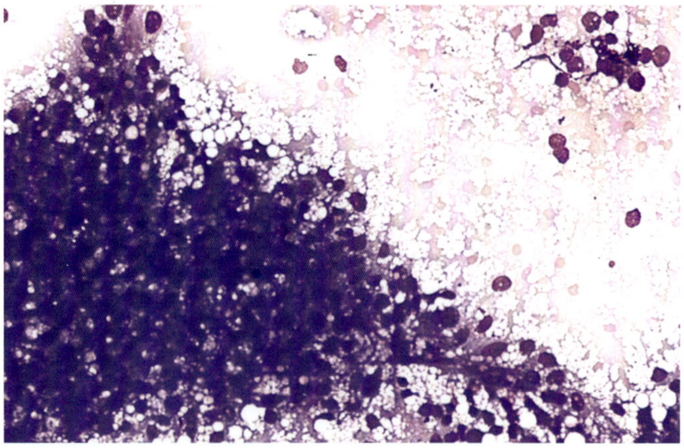

Fig. 8.22 Pleomorphic liposarcoma. A hypercellular smear showing a cohesive tissue fragment and few scattered pleomorphic cells, which are pleomorphic lipoblasts with moderate to abundant vacuolated cytoplasm (Giemsa).

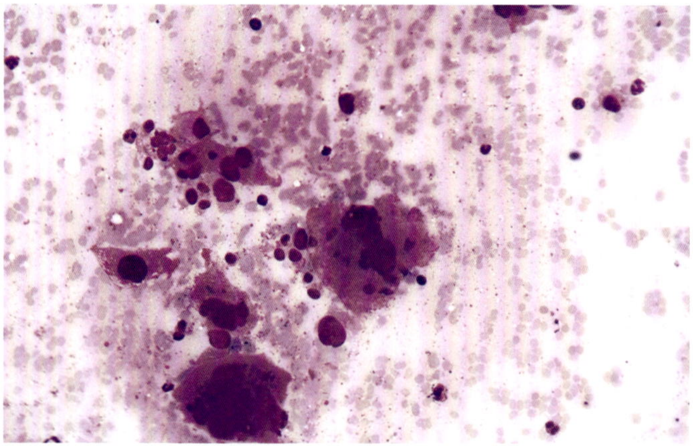

Fig. 8.24 Pleomorphic liposarcoma. Markedly pleomorphic and large cells, including multinucleate forms, but no vacuolated cells (Giemsa).

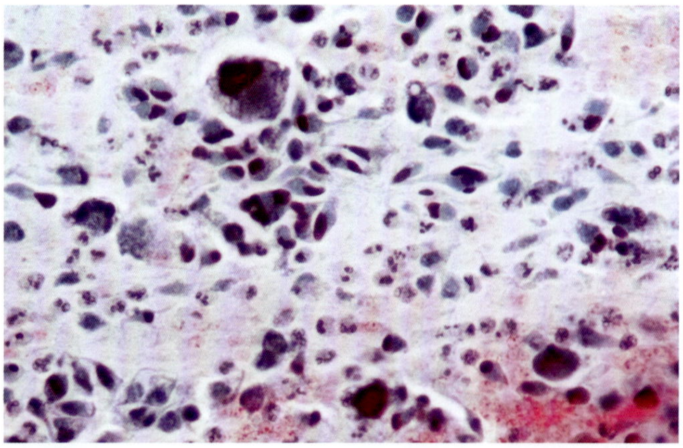

Fig. 8.23 Pleomorphic liposarcoma. A hypercellular smear with many polygonal, spindle, and pleomorphic cells, including large pleomorphic giant cells with abundant granular to vacuolated cytoplasm and highly pleomorphic nuclei (Pap).

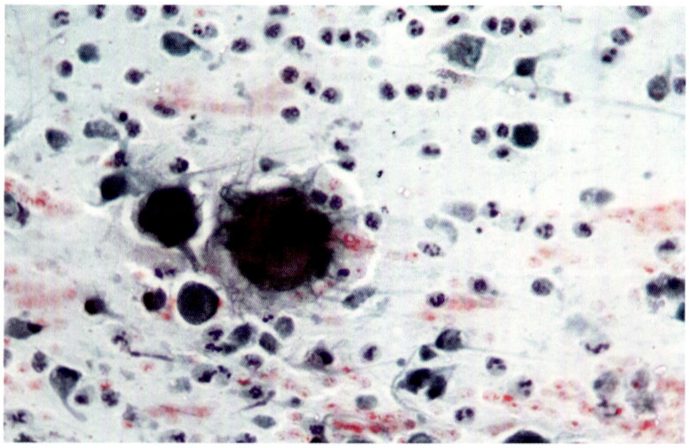

Fig. 8.25 Pleomorphic liposarcoma. A hypercellular smear displaying large multivacuolated pleomorphic lipoblasts (Pap).

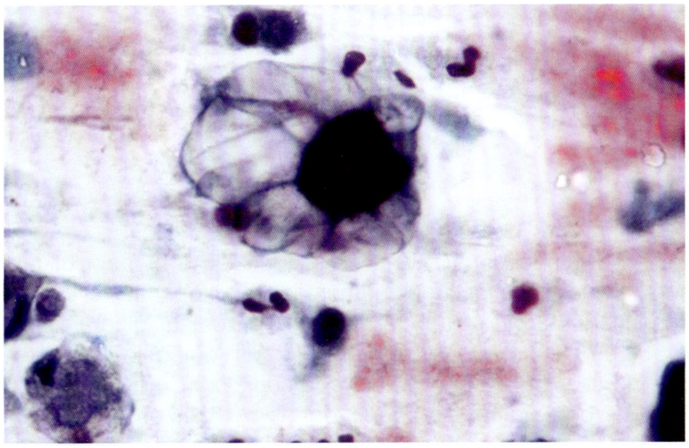

Fig. 8.26 Pleomorphic liposarcoma. A multivacuolated pleomorphic lipoblast (Pap).

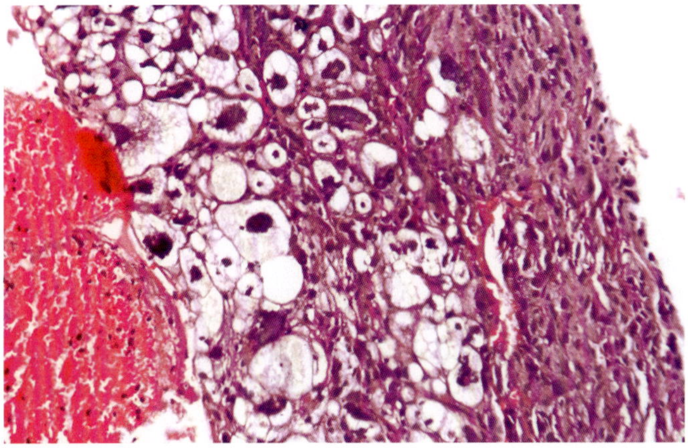

Fig. 8.28 Pleomorphic liposarcoma. A tissue section displaying pleomorphic sarcomatous cells, including multivacuolated forms (pleomorphic lipoblasts) (H&E).

- Loosely cohesive tissue fragments and scattered single cells displaying marked pleomorphism, as well as stripped nuclei
- Variable numbers of lipoblasts and cells with fibrillary cytoplasm and microvesicles
- Epithelioid and spindle cells are seen
- Inflammatory cells and mitotic figures
- Lipoproteinaceous background and necrosis
- Rarely, myxoid background and branching blood vessels have been reported

Reference(s): {334,877,1169,1193,725,1164}

Discussion and differential diagnosis

PLPS can be misdiagnosed as a pleomorphic sarcoma, a dedifferentiated liposarcoma, or a well-differentiated liposarcoma. Well-differentiated liposarcoma lacks pleomorphic sarcomatous cells {334}. Dedifferentiated liposarcoma with homologous differentiation is difficult to differentiate from pleomorphic liposarcoma {876}. Myxoinflammatory fibroblastic sarcoma and myxofibrosarcoma constitute other differential diagnoses because they display "pseudolipoblasts" {776,1059,1463}. The epithelioid variant of PLPS can mimic carcinoma {939,304}. The newly characterized myxoid pleomorphic liposarcoma enters the diagnostic consideration in young adults {265,568}.

Ancillary testing

There is no pathognomonic genetic alteration, but mutations of *TP53* and *NF1*, as well as copy loss of *RB1* (50%), have been reported in PLPS {479,1263,110}.

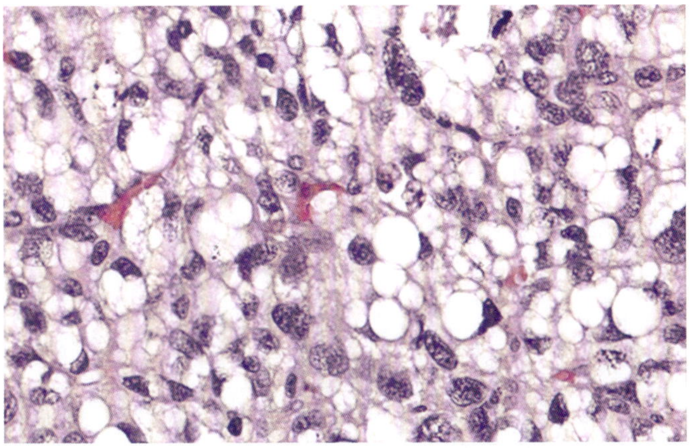

Fig. 8.27 Pleomorphic liposarcoma. A tissue section displaying pleomorphic lipoblasts arranged in a diffuse pattern with intervening thin-walled blood vessels and an occasional mitotic figure (H&E).

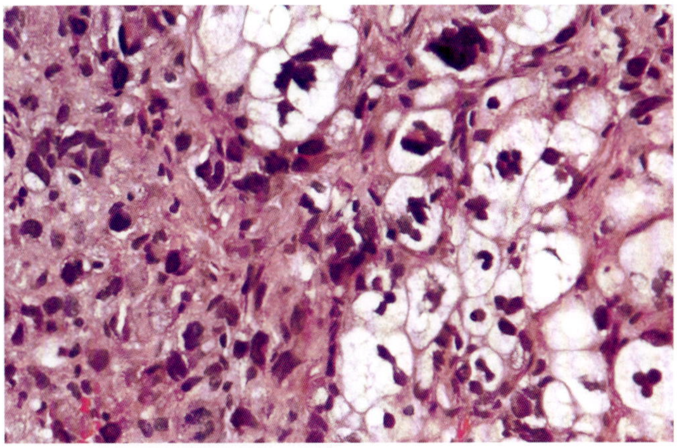

Fig. 8.29 Pleomorphic liposarcoma. A tissue section displaying pleomorphic sarcomatous cells, including several pleomorphic lipoblasts with vacuolated cytoplasm (H&E).

Chapter 8

Myxoid liposarcoma

Dodd LG
Bui M

Definition

Myxoid liposarcoma (MLPS) is a malignant tumour composed of uniform round to ovoid cells with a variable number of small lipoblasts set in a myxoid stroma with a branching capillary vasculature, with a pathognomonic translocation of *FUS*::*DDIT3* or *EWSR1*::*DDIT3* fusion.

Clinical features and imaging

MLPS occurs in a wide age range of patients, but young to middle-aged adults are most commonly affected {1503}. Rare cases of MLPS have been documented in children and adolescents {42}. MLPS is typically located in the extremities and rarely in the trunk or chest wall, and the deep soft tissue compartment of the thigh is the single most common site {706}. Affected individuals often present with a history of a painless lump or mass of variable duration.

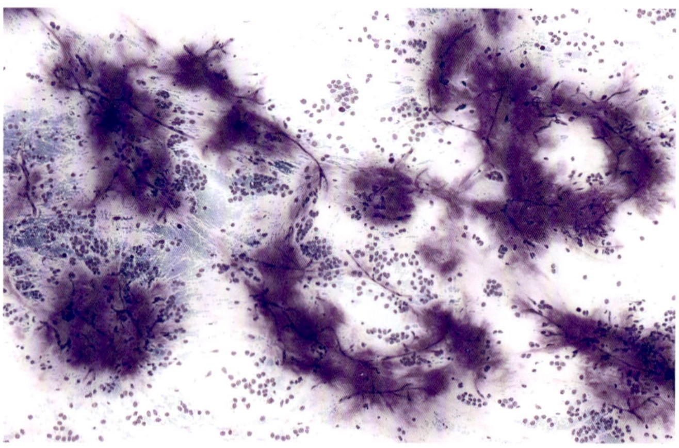

Fig. 8.30 Myxoid liposarcoma. Myxoid tissue fragments with branching thin vessels and round cells in the background (Giemsa).

The prognosis of MLPS is dependent on a number of factors, including patient age, tumour location, adequacy of tumour resection, margin status, and degree of tumour differentiation {1563,993,810}. MLPS differentiation is determined by the "round cell" component within a tumour, with > 5% round cell regions portending a poorer prognosis {1324,706,72,417,976}. Local recurrence or metastases occurs in as many as 60% of cases {417,536}. MLPS has a tendency to metastasize to unusual sites, including other soft tissue locations, which may account for its occasional presentation as multifocal disease {69}.

MLPS has a variable appearance on imaging. It is usually lobulated with discrete borders, and necrosis within the tumour results in a heterogeneous appearance. Like other tumours with myxoid stroma, MLPS tends to show high signal intensity on T2-weighted MRI.

Histopathology

MLPS displays a spectrum, from a low-grade tumour with abundant myxoid material and low cellularity to a high-grade densely cellular tumour made up of small primitive round cells (previously known as "round cell liposarcoma"). MLPS is usually a multinodular lesion with central hypocellular regions and increased concentration of tumour cells near the periphery of individual lobules. The tumour is composed of abundant extracellular myxoid matrix material containing a variable number of branching capillary vessels arranged in a plexiform pattern. Individual tumour cells vary in shape, from spindle primitive cells to lipoblasts in various states of maturity. Nuclear atypia is usually minimal, and mitoses are seldom seen. Variations on classic morphology include chondroid metaplasia, stromal hyalinization, and foci of mature lipomatous areas {446}.

In some MLPSs, myxoid areas transition to a higher-grade component, with distinctive round cells with increased N:C ratio

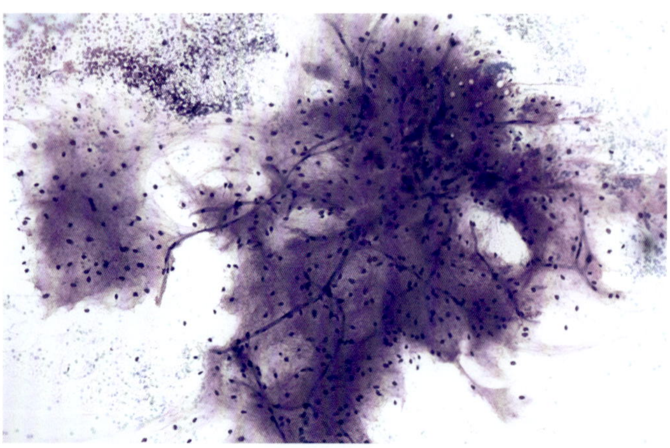

Fig. 8.31 Myxoid liposarcoma. Plexiform vascular arcade embedded in a myxoid stroma (Giemsa).

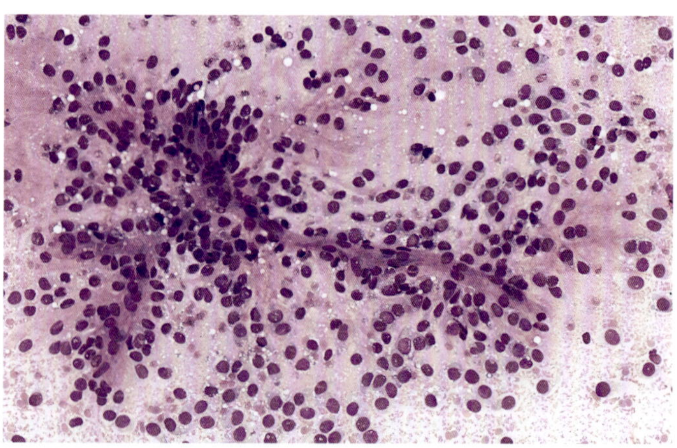

Fig. 8.32 Myxoid liposarcoma. Round cells arranged along a branching thin vessel in a myxoid background (Giemsa).

producing dense cellularity and less myxoid background, fewer vascular arcades, and fewer individual lipoblasts. If present, these higher-grade foci tend to concentrate at the periphery of the tumour lobules, but some MLPSs with a higher percentage of round cells may show dispersion throughout the entire tumour.

Key diagnostic cytopathological features

Low-grade myxoid liposarcoma

- Variable cellularity
- Abundant extracellular myxoid stroma in tissue fragments
- Myxoid tissue fragments contain small anastomosing capillary vessels in a plexiform or arcade pattern
- Small, uniform spindle to ovoid cells with slightly irregular nuclear membranes and small prominent nucleoli
- Small and large lipoblasts with one or more eccentric clear cytoplasmic vacuoles and a displaced nucleus

High-grade (round cell) liposarcoma

- High cellularity
- Dispersed population of small round cells with very high N:C ratio
- Inconspicuous matrix material and vascular tissue fragments
- Mild cellular and nuclear pleomorphism
- Irregular nuclear membranes, multiple prominent small nucleoli, and occasional intranuclear pseudoinclusions
- Rare lipoblasts

Discussion and differential diagnosis

The differential diagnosis of MLPS includes other entities with myxoid stroma, including myxoma, myxofibrosarcoma, extraskeletal myxoid chondrosarcoma, myxoinflammatory fibroblastic sarcoma, and lipoblastoma {785,711}.

Intramuscular and juxta-articular myxomas are hypocellular, have very rare small uniform spindle cells, and lack the vascular plexiform fragments that are the diagnostic feature of MLPS. Myxofibrosarcoma tends to be more cellular than MLPS and has obvious cellular pleomorphism, a feature not associated with MLPS. Myxofibrosarcoma can often have small vascular fragments identifiable, but the plexiform type is not seen. Extraskeletal myxoid chondrosarcoma shows substantial overlap with MLPS on cytopathology, with both having myxoid material and vascular fragments with associated tumour cells, but lipoblasts are not seen in extraskeletal myxoid chondrosarcoma. Myxoinflammatory fibroblastic sarcoma has a myxoid background, but it can be eliminated from the differential diagnosis because it is

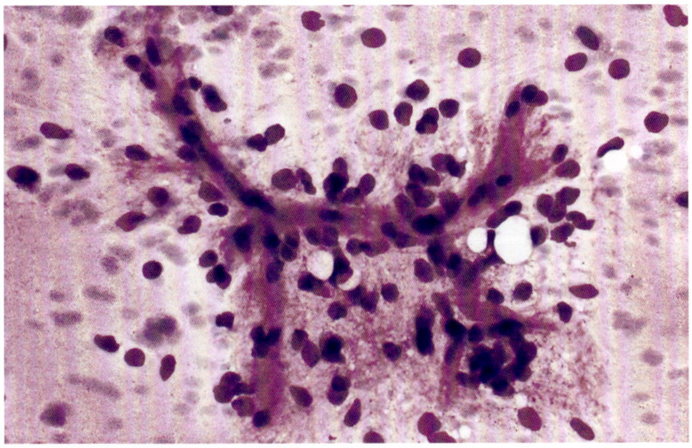

Fig. 8.33 Myxoid liposarcoma. Small branching vascular arcade in a background of thick myxoid material. The tumour cells are small, spindle to ovoid cells with indistinct cytoplasm. Vacuolated lipoblasts are also present (Giemsa).

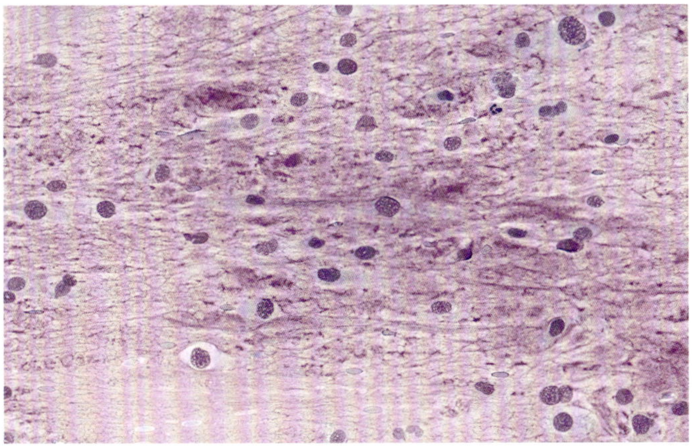

Fig. 8.34 Myxoid liposarcoma. Spindle cells with mild to moderately pleomorphic nuclei in a myxoid background (Giemsa).

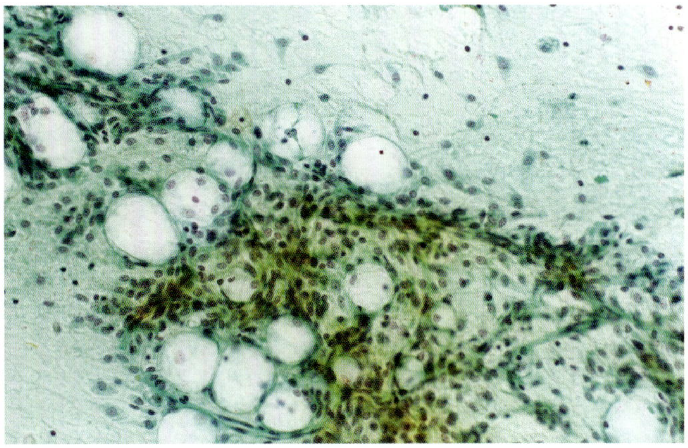

Fig. 8.35 Myxoid liposarcoma. A tissue fragment shows spindle cells, a branching vascular arcade, and numerous lipoblasts (H&E).

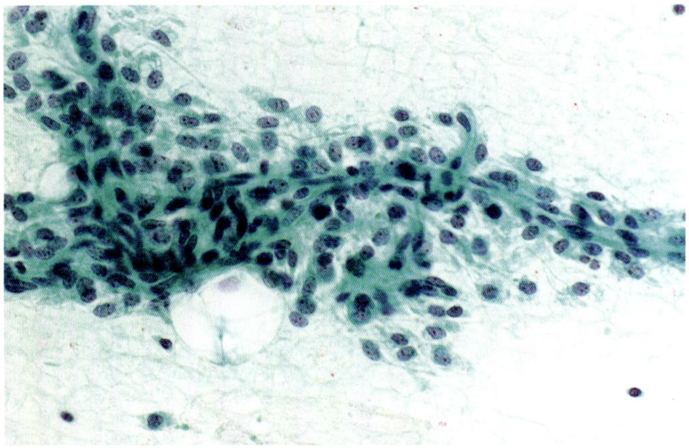

Fig. 8.36 Myxoid liposarcoma. Small, spindle to ovoid cells surrounding a capillary are individual cells that are uniform and have slightly irregular nuclear membranes and small nucleoli (Pap).

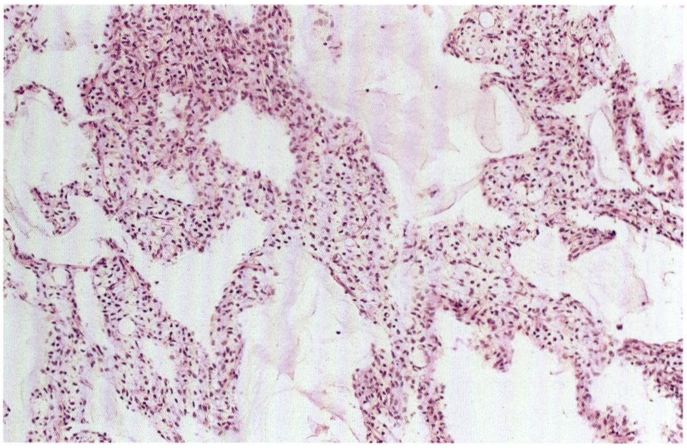

Fig. 8.37 Myxoid liposarcoma. Large pools of extracellular matrix material separated by moderately cellular tumour containing occasional small capillaries (H&E).

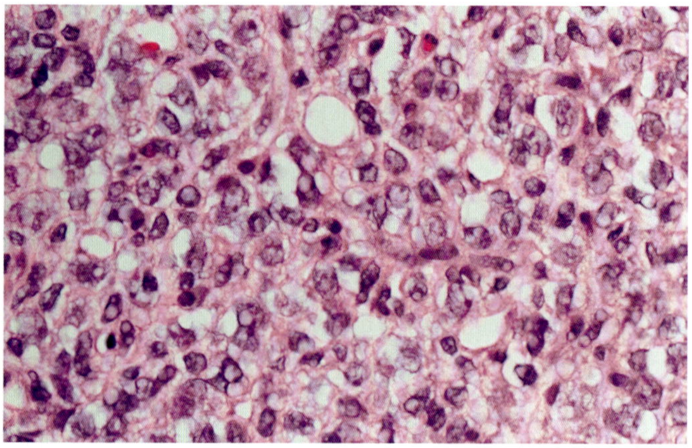

Fig. 8.38 Round cell liposarcoma. An area of tumour that has transitioned into a higher-grade round cell solid tumour with occasional lipoblasts (H&E).

a neoplasm restricted to the distal extremities, a site that is very unlikely for MLPS. Finally, lipoblastoma is a lesion that occurs almost exclusively in very young children.

Ancillary testing

MLPS is characterized by a balanced translocation involving the *DDIT3* gene on chromosome 12, with either *FUS* on chromosome 16 or less frequently *EWSR1* on chromosome 22. Detection of a fusion transcript involving the *DDIT3* gene locus is by FISH break-apart probe, which is a sensitive and specific test for MLPS {1007}.

ICC is useful in distinguishing the round cell type of high-grade MLPS from other small round blue cell tumours, with positive DDIT3 in the nuclei serving as a sensitive and specific marker for both the low-grade and high-grade forms of MLPS {102,1249}.

Myxofibrosarcoma

Klijanienko J
Bui M

Definition

Myxofibrosarcoma (MFS) is a spectrum of malignant fibroblastic neoplasms with variably myxoid stroma, a characteristic curvilinear vascular pattern, and cellular spindle cells with variable nuclear pleomorphism.

Clinical features and imaging

MFS is a relatively common sarcoma in adults, arising mainly in the limbs and less frequently in the head and neck, trunk, hands, and feet. Usually tumours present as a superficial and subcutaneous mass {921,594,799}. Deeper soft tissue locations are also seen, but the tumour is extremely uncommon in the abdomen and retroperitoneum {593,1316}.

Histopathology

MFS is an infiltrative tumour with a multinodular architecture, variably prominent pleomorphic cells, distinctive curvilinear vessels, hypercellular foci in higher-grade variations, and myxoid stroma. Low-grade MFS demonstrates large amounts of myxoid matrix, scant spindle regular cells and areas rich in curvilinear vessels. In high-grade MFS, myxoid matrix is less prominent, but spindle cells are numerous and pleomorphic. Mitotic activity, multinucleated giant cells, and necrosis may also be present {594,921, 1227}. Epithelioid variants exhibit epithelioid cells {1009}.

Key diagnostic cytopathological features

Low-grade myxofibrosarcoma

- Moderate to high cellularity
- Abundant myxoid matrix in tissue fragments showing a curvilinear vascular architecture
- Small number of isolated single, regular spindle and stellate cells with elongated nuclei
- Pseudolipoblasts
- Mild nuclear atypia

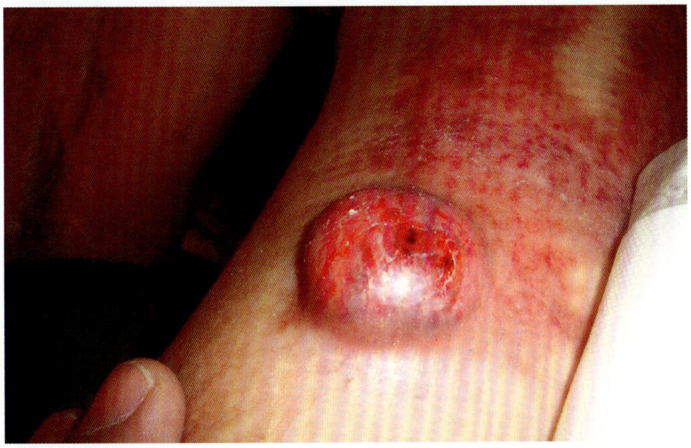

Fig. 8.39 Myxofibrosarcoma. Myxofibrosarcomas are usually superficially located.

High-grade myxofibrosarcoma

- High cellularity
- Numerous spindle or pleomorphic cells with marked cytopathological atypia
- Scant or no myxoid matrix
- Multinucleated giant cells and atypical mitotic figures may be present
- Curvilinear vessels may be present

Epithelioid myxofibrosarcoma

- High cellularity
- Numerous monotonous epithelioid cells exhibiting cytoplasmic and nuclear pleomorphism varying from mild to severe
- Macronucleoli and abundant lacy cytoplasm

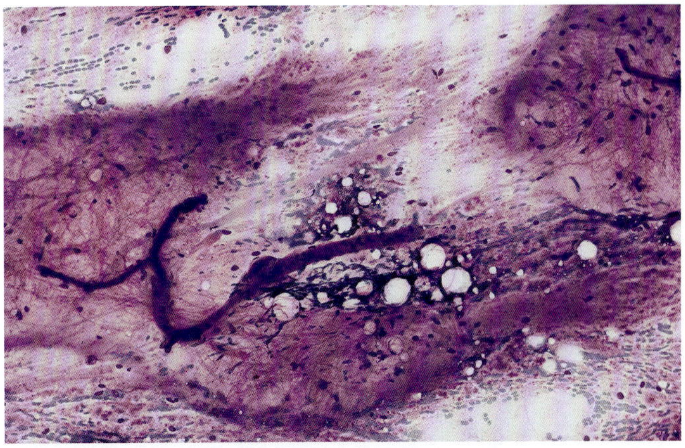

Fig. 8.40 Low-grade myxofibrosarcoma. Tissue fragments showing abundant myxoid matrix containing a small number of small and regular spindle cells and curvilinear vessels. Very occasional fat cells (Giemsa).

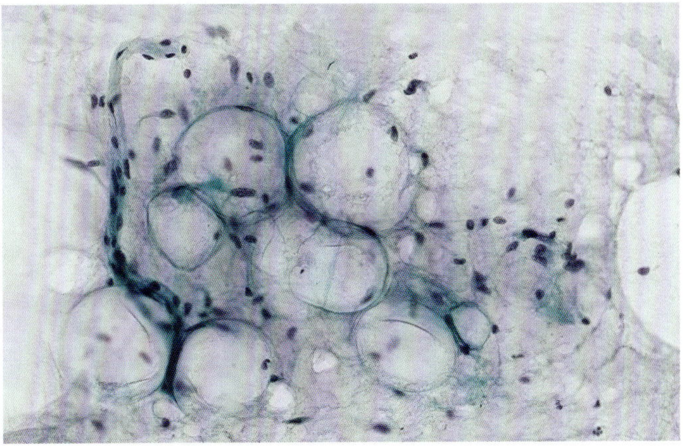

Fig. 8.41 Low-grade myxofibrosarcoma. A tissue fragment of abundant myxoid matrix, curvilinear vessels, and fat cells or pseudolipoblasts (Pap).

- Abundant myxoid matrix with curvilinear vessels in tissue fragments

Reference(s): {1493,1050,249,710,1463,928}

Discussion and differential diagnosis

Low-grade MFS should be differentiated from myxoid liposarcoma, low-grade fibromyxoid sarcoma, extraskeletal myxoid chondrosarcoma, dermatofibrosarcoma protuberans with myxoid change, and myxoma. High-grade MFS should be differentiated from dedifferentiated liposarcoma, pleomorphic liposarcoma, and undifferentiated pleomorphic sarcoma {785,725}.

Ancillary testing

MFS has no specific immunoprofile or genetic alteration. Ancillary techniques such as ICC, FISH, and NGS may be used to differentiate MFS from myxoid tumours, especially from myxoid liposarcoma. Occasional cases may show reactivity for SMA or CD34, whereas desmin and S100 are usually negative.

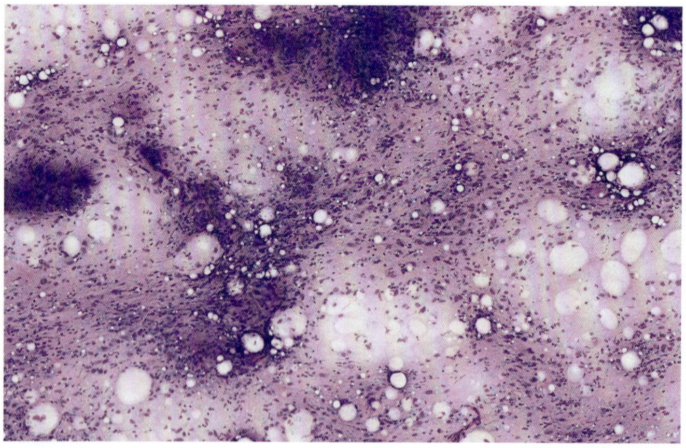

Fig. 8.42 High-grade myxofibrosarcoma. A highly cellular smear showing myxoid tissue fragments and myxoid background, with plentiful pleomorphic cells (Giemsa).

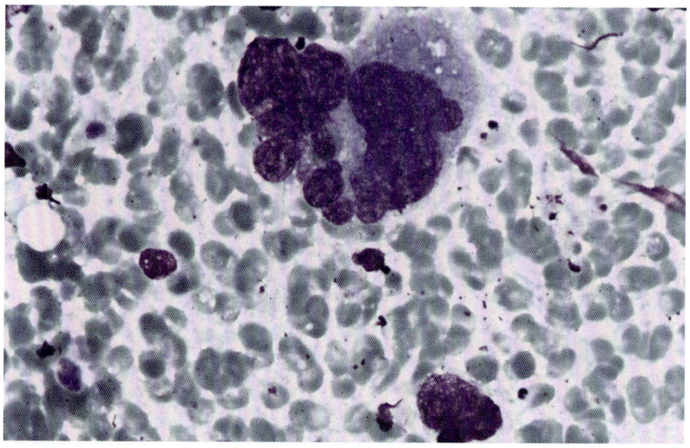

Fig. 8.44 High-grade myxofibrosarcoma. A large, multinucleated giant cell with bizarre nuclear enlargement and pleomorphism and adjacent large, stripped nucleus mimicking undifferentiated pleomorphic sarcoma (Giemsa).

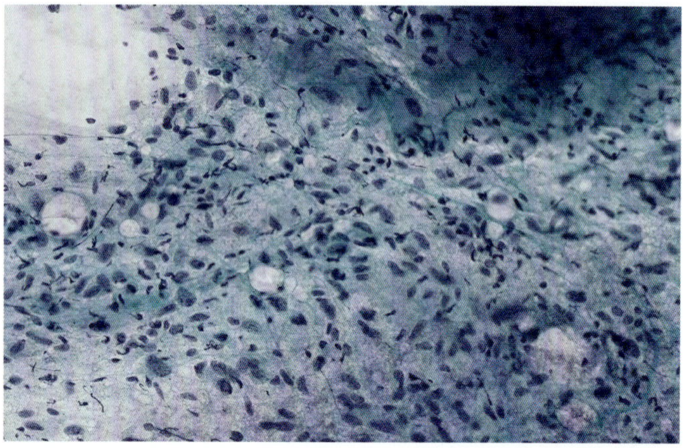

Fig. 8.43 High-grade myxofibrosarcoma. A poorly defined tissue fragment showing myxoid matrix containing numerous spindle cells with moderate to occasionally highly pleomorphic nuclei (Pap).

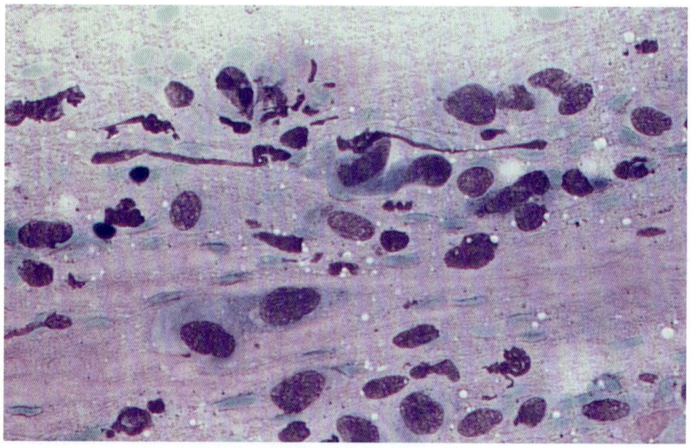

Fig. 8.45 Epithelioid myxofibrosarcoma. Epithelioid and plump spindle cells showing nuclear pleomorphism in a myxoid background (Giemsa).

Myxoinflammatory fibroblastic sarcoma

Qian X
Klijanienko J

Definition

Myxoinflammatory fibroblastic sarcoma (MIFS) is an infiltrative, locally aggressive fibroblastic neoplasm that typically arises in the distal extremities, characterized by pleomorphic fibroblastic cells with macronucleoli in a myxohyaline background with a variably prominent inflammatory cell infiltrate.

Clinical features and imaging

Young to middle-aged adults (mean age: 40 years; range: 4–91 years) frequently present with a slowly growing, painless mass. MIFS occurs commonly in the subcutaneous tissue of the fingers, hands, wrists, ankles, and feet {973,914,933,848}. MIFS recurs locally but rarely metastasizes. Unusual locations include the upper arms, thighs, shoulders, and inguinal area {661,776}. Imaging findings are nonspecific, showing an infiltrative mass located along the tendon sheath. Like other myxoid tumours, MIFS is T1-hypointense and T2-hyperintense, with homogeneous or heterogeneous enhancement on MRI {1008, 458}.

Histopathology

MIFS is characterized by a lobular architecture; an infiltrative border; and a combination of bland spindle cells, scattered large Reed–Sternberg–like or lipoblast-like cells, and abundant inflammatory cell-rich myxoid stroma {776,1366}. MIFS overlaps morphologically and genetically with two closely related entities: haemosiderotic fibrolipomatous tumour and pleomorphic hyalinizing angiectatic tumour {377,534,831}.

Key diagnostic cytopathological features

- Variable cellularity
- Prominent myxoid matrix in tissue fragments
- Mixed population of bland spindle cells and mononuclear epithelioid cells
- Scattered large, atypical Reed–Sternberg–like cells with macronucleoli
- Mixed inflammatory cells with haemosiderin and macrophages
- Pseudolipoblasts

Reference(s): {500,1504,1118,1059,1414,1486}

Discussion and differential diagnosis

The differential diagnosis of MIFS is extremely broad and depends on the tumour location and the relative amounts of each component present on the FNAB smears. The differential diagnosis ranges from benign lesions such as ganglion cyst or tenosynovial giant cell tumour to malignant neoplasms such as myxofibrosarcoma, epithelioid sarcoma, and Hodgkin lymphoma.

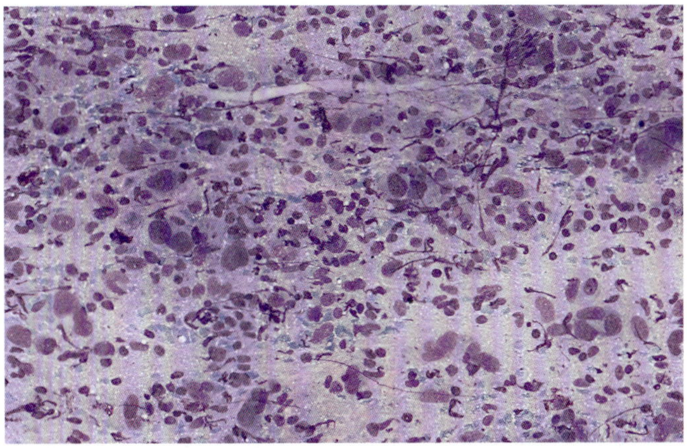

Fig. 8.46 Myxoinflammatory fibroblastic sarcoma. Highly pleomorphic cells with often large bizarre nuclei are present with stripped nuclei and some lymphocytes in a myxoid background (Giemsa).

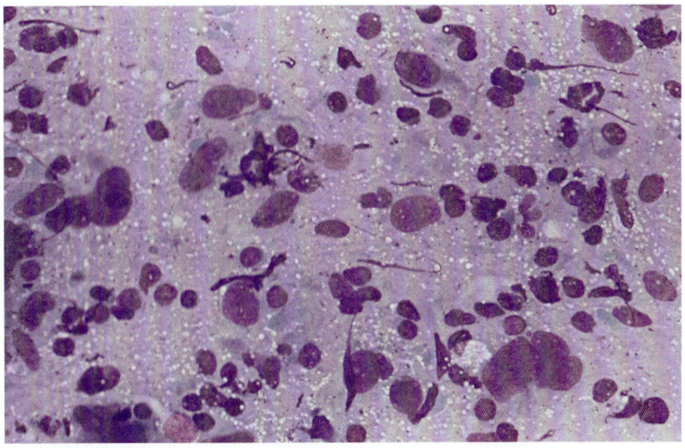

Fig. 8.47 Myxoinflammatory fibroblastic sarcoma. Pleomorphic tumour cells, often with large, multilobated bizarre nuclei, and stripped nuclei and some lymphocytes in a myxoid background (Giemsa).

Ancillary testing

The translocation t(1;10) resulting in *TGFBR3::OGA* (formerly known as *MGEA5*) and *BRAF* rearrangement have been identified in MIFS {74,428,1567}. The detection of these gene alterations is neither sensitive nor cost-effective, and there are no distinctive ICC or molecular markers that can be used in diagnosis {1366}.

Chapter 8

Extraskeletal myxoid chondrosarcoma

Qian X
Agaram NP
Rekhi B

Definition

Extraskeletal myxoid chondrosarcoma (EMC) is a malignant mesenchymal neoplasm of uncertain differentiation characterized by abundant myxoid matrix, multilobular architecture, and uniform cells arranged in cords, clusters, and reticular networks, and by an *NR4A3* rearrangement, with no evidence of cartilaginous differentiation.

Clinical features and imaging

EMC presents in middle-aged adults (mean age: 50 years; range: 4–92 years), as a slowly enlarging, deep-seated soft tissue mass. Despite high recurrence and metastatic rates, cases usually have a prolonged clinical course. EMC occurs most commonly in the lower extremities, with the thigh as the most common location, followed by the popliteal fossa, buttock, trunk, head and neck, paraspinal soft tissue, abdomen, pelvis, and foot {384,913}. Unusual locations include finger, pleura, and bone {1044,495,708,416}. MRI shows a well-circumscribed lobulated mass, which is isointense to muscles on T1-weighted images and hyperintense on T2-weighted and short-tau inversion recovery (STIR) images with peripheral/septal enhancement {676}.

Histopathology

EMC is characterized by a lobular architecture and a reticular arrangement of uniform tumour cells with oval to spindle nuclei and eosinophilic cytoplasm in a chondromyxoid stroma. A subset of high-grade tumours shows hypercellularity and prominent epithelioid to rhabdoid cytomorphology {384,849,913}.

Key diagnostic cytopathological features

- Moderate to high cellularity
- Bright magenta chondromyxoid stroma (Giemsa)

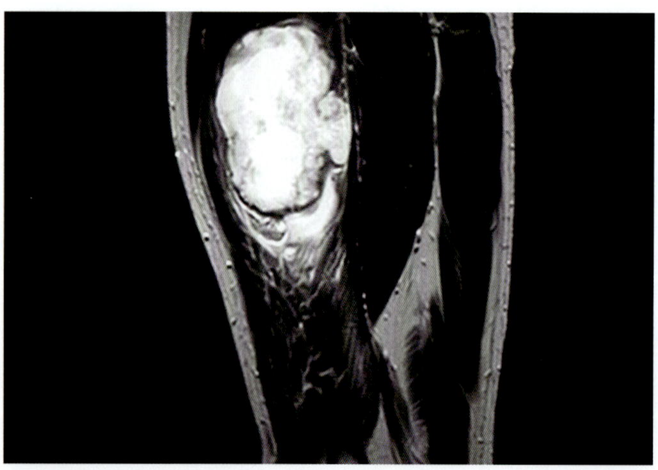

Fig. 8.48 Extraskeletal myxoid chondrosarcoma. MRI showing a well-defined, T2-hyperintense, lobulated soft tissue mass in the thigh.

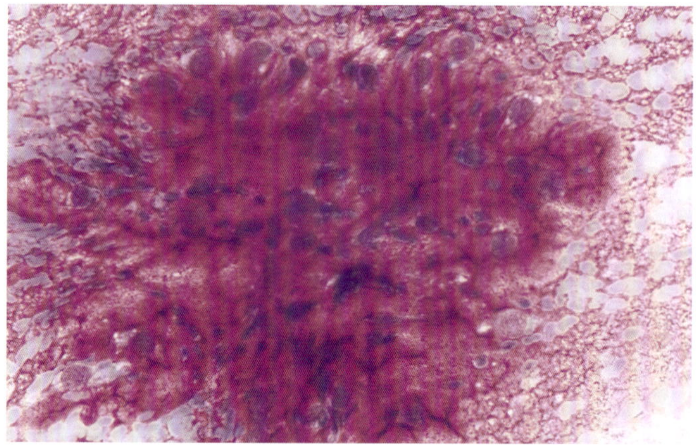

Fig. 8.49 Extraskeletal myxoid chondrosarcoma. A tissue fragment showing polygonal cells embedded in a bright magenta stroma (Giemsa).

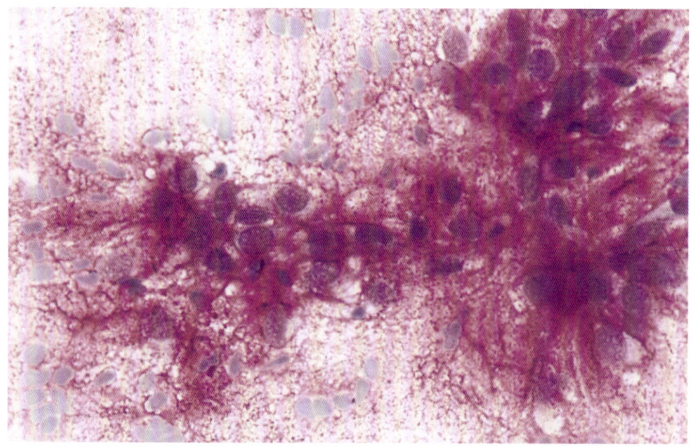

Fig. 8.50 Extraskeletal myxoid chondrosarcoma. Polygonal to epithelioid cells in a fibrillar magenta stroma (Giemsa).

- Dispersed, corded, lace-like, and occasional perivascular arrangement of uniform cells
- Variable polygonal and epithelioid to rhabdoid to spindle cells
- Oval to spindle nuclei with small nucleoli, frequent intranuclear pseudoinclusions, and grooves
- Vacuolated cytoplasm and unipolar or bipolar cytoplasmic processes of variable length

Reference(s): {762,1230,628,1464}

Discussion and differential diagnosis

The differential diagnosis of EMC includes other myxoid tumours with a monotonous appearance, including low-grade fibromyxoid sarcoma, high-grade myxoid liposarcoma, myoepithelial tumour of soft tissue, and ossifying fibromyxoid tumour. Myxoid liposarcoma displays complex and plexiform vascular networks and a variable number of univacuolated lipoblasts. NGS assists in the diagnosis. Low-grade fibromyxoid sarcoma has a more fibrillary matrix and expresses MUC4 on ICC. Myoepithelial tumour and EMC have significant morphological overlap, and NGS is required for differentiation. Despite the name "extraskeletal myxoid chondrosarcoma", there is no cartilaginous differentiated material present in EMC.

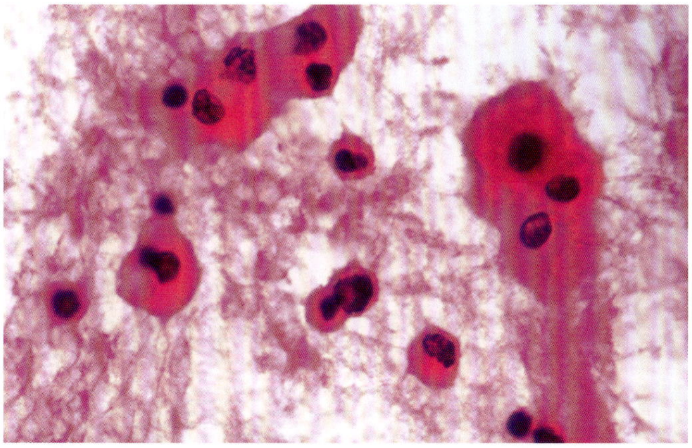

Fig. 8.51 Extraskeletal myxoid chondrosarcoma. Tumour cells of polygonal shape, containing moderate to abundant well-defined cytoplasm, arranged as single cells and in minute tissue fragments and cords against a semitransparent myxoid stroma (H&E).

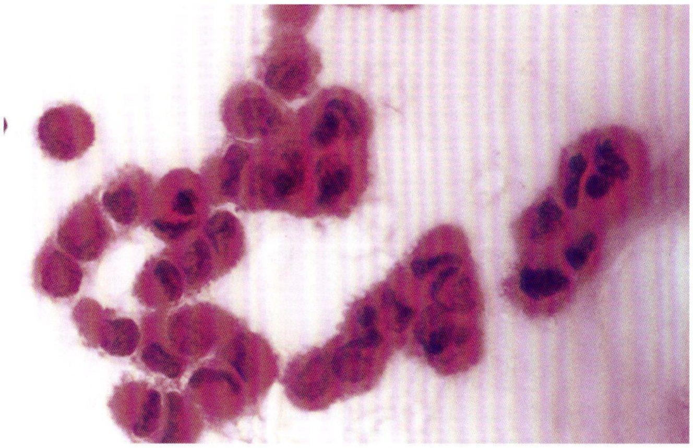

Fig. 8.52 Extraskeletal myxoid chondrosarcoma. Cord-like arrangement of tumour cells with epithelioid to rhabdoid morphology (moderate to abundant well-defined eccentric cytoplasm, including intracytoplasmic inclusions) (H&E).

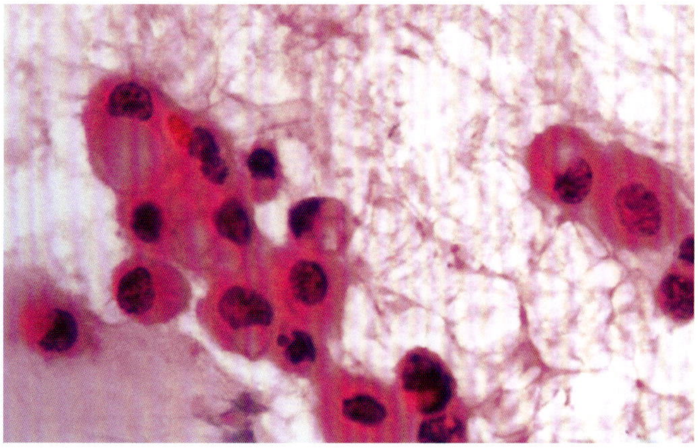

Fig. 8.53 Extraskeletal myxoid chondrosarcoma. Minute tissue fragments of non-overlapping, loosely cohesive tumour cells with well-defined, eosinophilic cytoplasm and intracytoplasmic vacuoles against a fibrillar, translucent background (H&E).

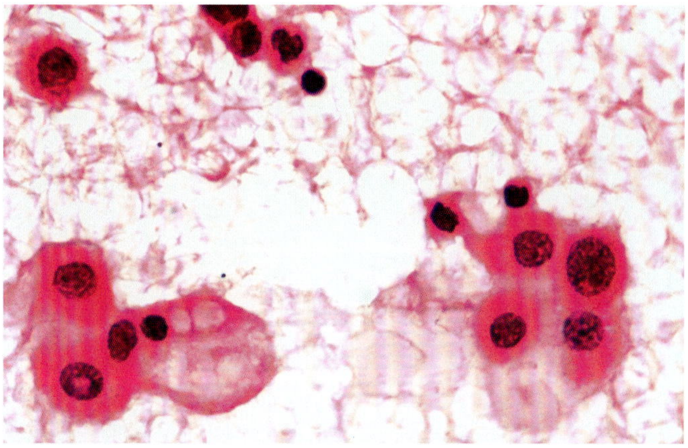

Fig. 8.54 Extraskeletal myxoid chondrosarcoma. A cohesive tissue fragment of tumour cells containing moderate to abundant well-defined eosinophilic to vacuolated cytoplasm (H&E).

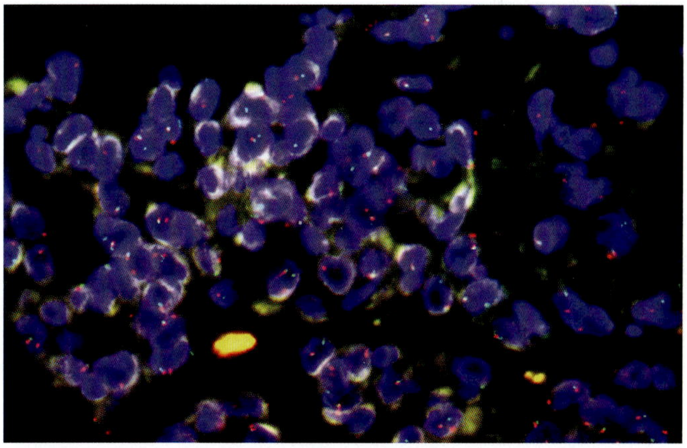

Fig. 8.55 Extraskeletal myxoid chondrosarcoma. FISH showing *EWSR1* gene rearrangement, with cells displaying red–green split signals (FISH).

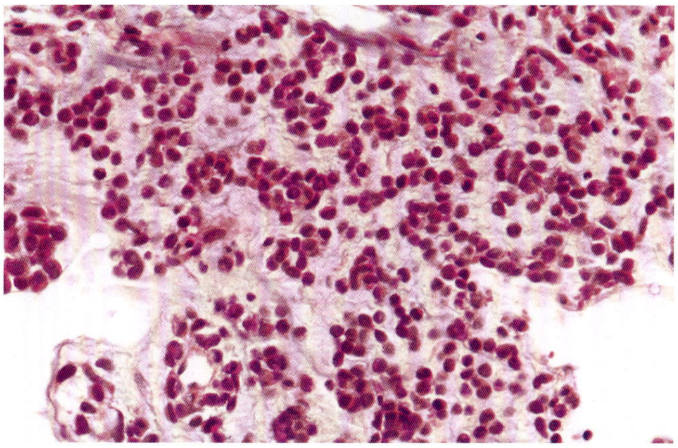

Fig. 8.56 Extraskeletal myxoid chondrosarcoma. A tissue section displaying loose strands and cords of tumour cells with epithelioid to rhabdoid-like morphology, embedded in a myxoid stroma (H&E).

Ancillary testing

EMC variably expresses nonspecific ICC markers such as S100, NSE, and KIT (CD117). SMARCB1 (INI1) loss has been reported in a subset of tumours with rhabdoid morphology. Detection of *NR4A3* arrangement by FISH or *EWSR1::NR4A3* fusion by RT-PCR or NGS can help in confirming a diagnosis of EMC {1255,428}. Myxoid liposarcoma harbours *DDIT3* rearrangement, which is negative in EMC {1013,1469}. Both EMC and myoepithelial tumours harbour *EWSR1* rearrangement, but *NR4A3* rearrangement is specific for EMC. Ossifying fibromyxoid tumour often expresses S100 and desmin and demonstrates *PHF1* and/or *TFE3* rearrangement {351,1469,428,96}.

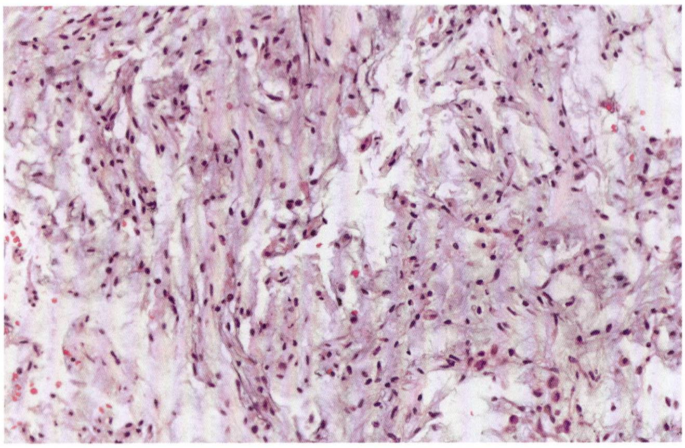

Fig. 8.57 Extraskeletal myxoid chondrosarcoma. Tumour composed of relatively uniform cells with oval to spindle nuclei and eosinophilic cytoplasm in a chondromyxoid stroma (H&E).

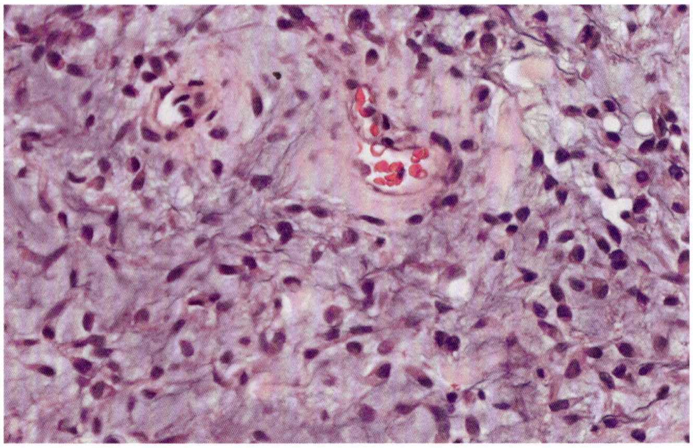

Fig. 8.58 Extraskeletal myxoid chondrosarcoma. Cells with oval to spindle nuclei and eosinophilic cytoplasm arranged in a reticular growth pattern in a chondromyxoid stroma (H&E).

Chordoma

Jo VY
Klijanienko J
Rekhi B

Definition

Chordoma is a malignant tumour that shows notochordal differentiation, usually arises in the axial skeleton, and is characterized by brachyury immunoexpression and loss of SMARCB1 expression secondary to *SMARCB1* deletion in poorly differentiated chordoma.

Clinical features and imaging

The majority of chordomas arise in bones of the axial skeleton, with relatively equal distribution to the base of skull (in 32%), mobile spine (in 32.8%), and sacrum/coccyx (in 29.2%) {907, 987}. The presentation is with pain and site-related symptoms. Most poorly differentiated chordomas arise in paediatric patients, most commonly in the base of skull {1292}. Poorly differentiated chordoma and dedifferentiated chordoma that shows transition to a high-grade sarcoma are associated with more aggressive behaviour and poor prognosis {1292}.

Imaging typically demonstrates a destructive, large mass that expands the bone, often with extension into soft tissue. Tumours appear lytic on CT, while MRI often shows a lobulated, septate, and heterogeneous mass, usually T1-hypointense and T2-hyperintense. Dedifferentiated chordomas may present with rapid growth and rapid worsening of symptoms, as well as more T2-hypointense areas on MRI {537}.

Histopathology

Chordoma shows a lobulated architecture separated by fibrous septa. Large epithelioid cells with variably clear to eosinophilic cytoplasm are arranged in nests, cords, or sheets, embedded in the abundant myxoid extracellular matrix. Tumour cells have round nuclei with small or inconspicuous nuclei. Some tumour cells show abundant bubbly cytoplasm, the so-called physaliphorous cells. Occasionally the matrix may appear chondromyxoid and mimic hyaline cartilage. Poorly differentiated chordoma is a poorly differentiated neoplasm with notochordal differentiation showing more solid growth, often with rhabdoid or signet-ring cells and a scarcity of physaliphorous cells, with minimal myxoid stroma and extensive necrosis.

Dedifferentiated chordoma is a biphasic neoplasm characterized by a high-grade sarcoma with spindle and/or pleomorphic cells, either admixed with or abruptly transitioning from conventional chordoma. The dedifferentiated component may show osteosarcomatous and rhabdomyosarcomatous differentiation.

Key diagnostic cytopathological features

- Variable cellularity
- Round, cuboidal, and epithelioid cells arranged in cords within an abundant myxoid matrix forming discohesive tissue fragments
- Extracellular matrix is granular, fibrillary, and metachromatic (Giemsa)
- Round nuclei and occasional binucleation

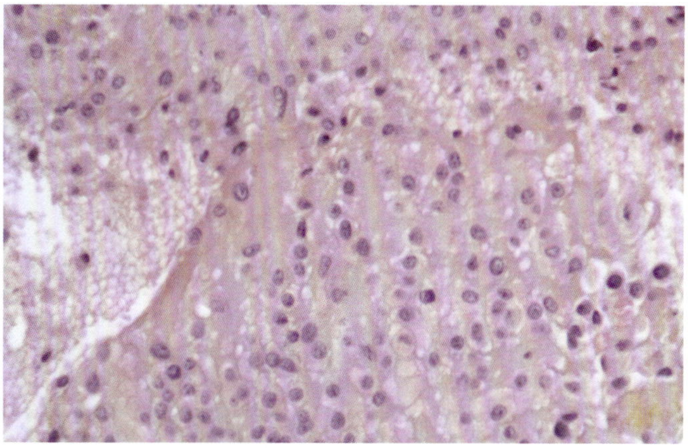

Fig. 8.59 Cell block from chordoma. Mononucleated cells and chondroid matrix are well identified on histopathological sections (HES).

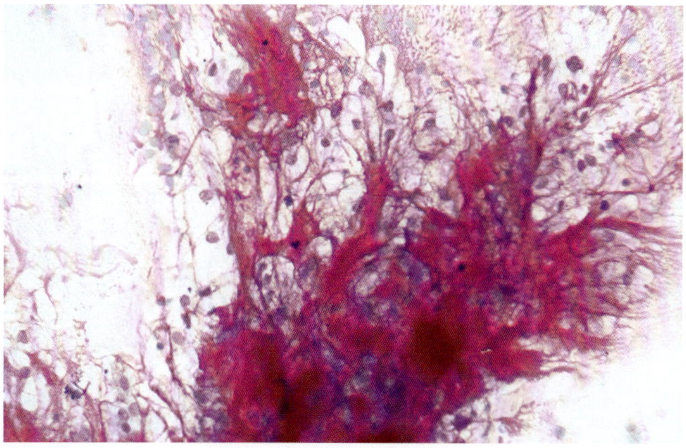

Fig. 8.60 Conventional chordoma. A cellular smear showing cells with cytoplasmic vacuoles (physaliphorous cells) in abundant fibrillary metachromatic stroma (Giemsa).

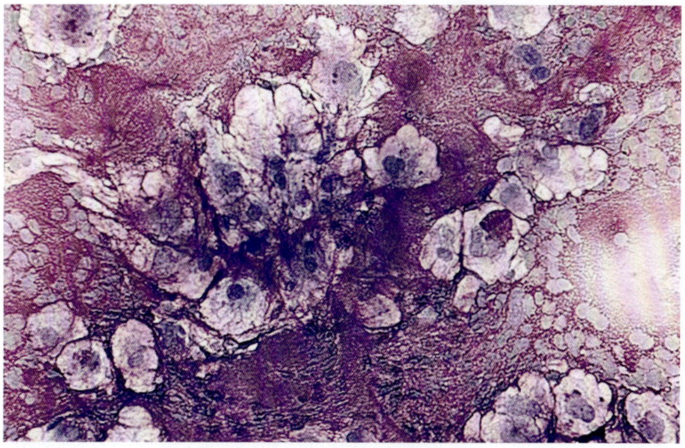

Fig. 8.61 Chordoma. A matrix-rich smear with typical physaliphorous cells (Giemsa).

Chapter 8

- Varying amounts of cytoplasm, which is granular or variably vacuolated, ranging from "signet ring" (single large eccentric vacuole impinging the nucleus) to abundant and multivacuolated physaliphorous cells
- Cytopathological atypia and pleomorphism can be more pronounced in some cases
- Poorly differentiated chordoma shows scarce matrix and rhabdoid and/or more uniform epithelioid cells with central large round nuclei and large nucleoli, with some cells showing eccentric cytoplasm
- Dedifferentiated chordoma shows a dedifferentiated component of nonspecific high-grade spindle cell or pleomorphic malignant neoplasm, with frequent necrosis, with chordoma usually present focally

Reference(s): {415,1114,685,1475,1173,1250}

Discussion and differential diagnosis

Clinical correlation is necessary to exclude benign notochordal cell tumour, which is usually found incidentally and, when presenting as a large tumour, may be challenging to distinguish from chordoma. Both entities express brachyury, but even with larger size, benign notochordal cell tumour does not show destructive growth or invasion into soft tissue, and it is composed of solid sheets of vacuolated tumour cells that resemble adipocytes, often admixed with physaliphorous cells {59}. Microcyst formation with colloid-like extracellular material may be seen, but myxoid stroma is absent in most cases of benign notochordal cell tumour. Some notochordal tumours have indeterminate features and show permeative growth, soft tissue extension, and myxoid change, and have been designated "atypical notochordal cell tumour" {182}, but standardized criteria have not been established for this provisional entity.

The differential diagnosis for conventional chordoma also includes chondrosarcoma with myxoid stroma, myxopapillary ependymoma, soft tissue myoepithelioma and myoepithelial carcinoma, pleomorphic adenoma, mucinous adenocarcinoma, and renal cell carcinoma. Correlation with clinical history and imaging is helpful. Brachyury reliably distinguishes chordoma from these mimics, which are all negative.

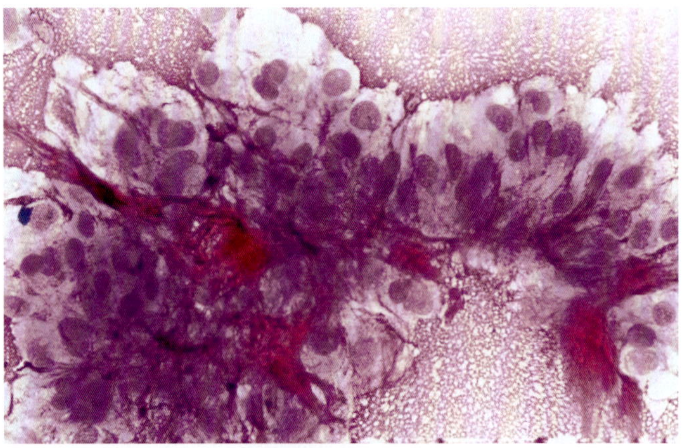

Fig. 8.62 Conventional chordoma. Polygonal cells with well-defined cell borders and abundant vacuolated cytoplasm (Giemsa).

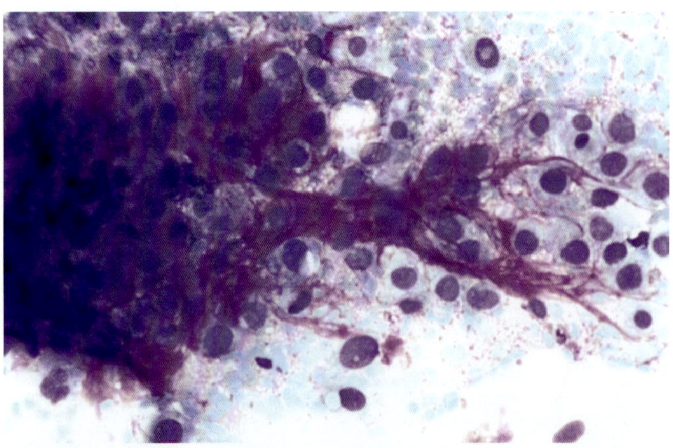

Fig. 8.63 Chordoma. Mononucleated cells from chordoma that had metastasized, showing nuclear atypia, in magenta matrix (Giemsa).

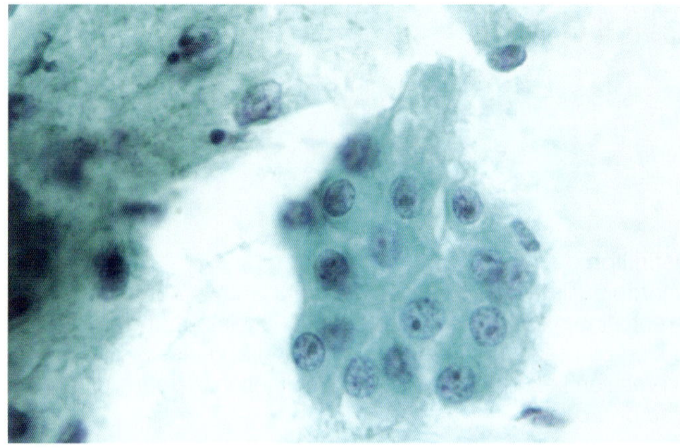

Fig. 8.64 Conventional chordoma. A cohesive tissue fragment of polygonal cells containing moderate to abundant cytoplasm with distinct nucleoli (Pap).

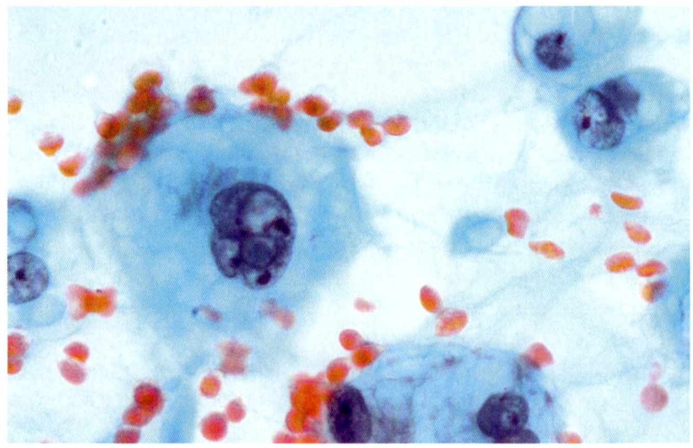

Fig. 8.65 Conventional chordoma. Tumour cells showing well-defined cell borders, abundant cytoplasm with multiple vacuoles (physaliphorous cells), large often pleomorphic nuclei, distinct nucleoli, intranuclear inclusions, and an occasional binucleated cell (Pap).

Ancillary testing

Chordoma is positive for epithelial markers, including cytokeratin and EMA, and variably positive for S100. All cases show expression of brachyury (encoded by *TBXT*), a transcription factor required for notochordal development {1126,1459}. Nuclear staining for brachyury is highly sensitive and specific for chordoma and reliably distinguishes it from cytomorphological mimics

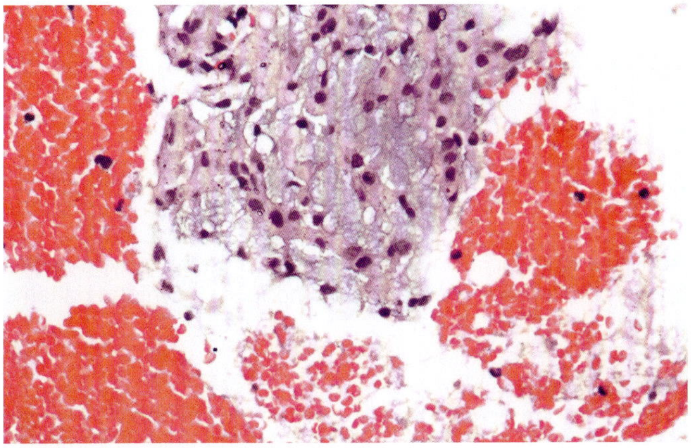

Fig. 8.66 Conventional chordoma. A cohesive tissue fragment of tumour cells containing moderate to abundant, eosinophilic to vacuolated cytoplasm in a myxoid stroma (cell block, H&E).

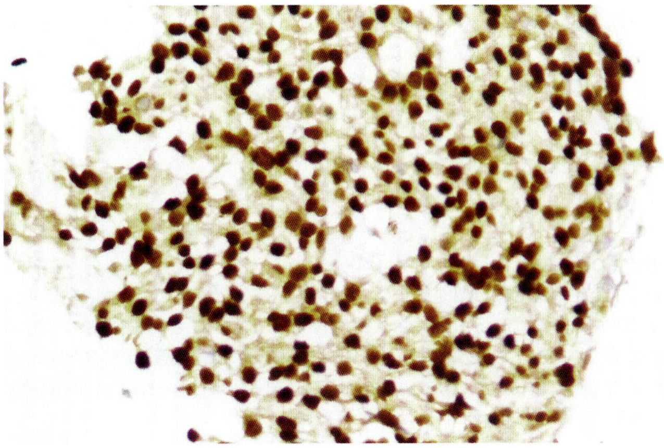

Fig. 8.67 Conventional chordoma. Tumour cells in cell block displaying diffuse nuclear brachyury positivity (ICC, brachyury).

{651}. Brachyury is positive in poorly differentiated chordoma, but expression is absent in the dedifferentiated component in dedifferentiated chordomas, and these regions may show focal keratin expression {1459,949}, necessitating correlation with clinical and imaging and a broad ICC panel if conventional chordoma is not sampled. Poorly differentiated chordoma shows SMARCB1 loss secondary to *SMARCB1* deletions {961,1291}.

Myoepithelial tumours also show positivity for S100 and keratins, but they additionally show frequent staining for GFAP, SOX10, and p63/p40, which are negative in chordoma. Most cases of metastatic renal cell carcinoma do not show the fibrillary metachromatic stroma of chordomas and are positive for PAX8. Metastatic adenocarcinomas may show 3D overlapping tumour cell tissue fragments and gland formation. Myxopapillary ependymoma shows GFAP immunopositivity {651,1411,215}.

Low-grade fibromyxoid sarcoma

Chebib I
Qian X

Definition

Low-grade fibromyxoid sarcoma (LGFMS) is a malignant fibroblastic neoplasm characterized by alternating collagenous and myxoid areas, deceptively bland spindle cells with a whorling growth pattern, and arcades of small blood vessels, and by *FUS::CREB3L2* or *FUS::CREB3L1* fusions.

Clinical features and imaging

Presentation is with a painless mass, over a wide age range (median: 30–45 years) and with a slight male predilection {502, 775,437,392}. LGFMS most often arises in the deep soft tissues of the extremities {502,775,437,515,1165}, head and neck {775, 437}, mediastinum {515}, and retroperitoneum {502,437,515, 392,1431}. Tumours rarely arise in the superficial soft tissues {137,1165} or within visceral organs {782}. On imaging, LGFMS typically appears as well-circumscribed masses, hypodense to isodense to muscle on CT and showing variably hypointense and hyperintense foci distributed in nodular or gyriform patterns on MRI {605,1236}.

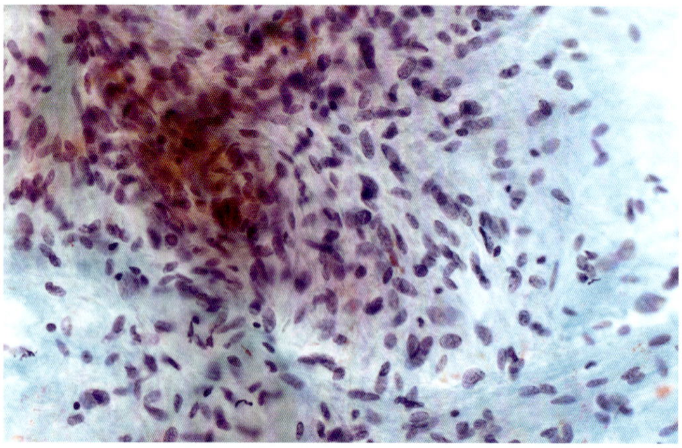

Fig. 8.68 Low-grade fibromyxoid sarcoma. Bland, uniform spindle cells lacking nuclear hyperchromasia or anisonucleosis, in a myxoid matrix (Pap).

Histopathology

LGFMS is composed of fibrous, collagenous hypocellular areas that abruptly transition into cellular myxoid areas. This mosaic pattern, with abrupt transition between the collagenous and myxoid areas, can be recognized on CNB. In addition, tumour areas may show larger collagenous rosettes. The tumour cells are spindle, bland, and uniform, arranged in short fascicles or a storiform pattern. Mitotic activity is low, and there is no necrosis. Peripheral arcades of arteriole-sized blood vessels may be present {502,775,437,137,515,1165,392}. In some tumours, areas of sclerosing epithelioid fibrosarcoma may be present, composed of monomorphic epithelioid cells arranged in cords, nests, and sheets, surrounded by hyalinized sclerotic stromal collagen {515,362,77,1129}.

Key diagnostic cytopathological features

Low-grade fibromyxoid sarcoma

- Variable cellularity
- Mix of irregular fibrotic, collagenous fragments and loosely cohesive tissue fragments showing fascicles and single cells in a myxoid background
- Uniform bland to mildly atypical, elongate spindle cells
- Nuclei show finely granular to vesicular (Pap) chromatin, without nucleoli, hyperchromasia, or significant anisonucleosis
- Naked nuclei and intranuclear cytoplasmic pseudoinclusions may be seen
- Fibrotic to myxoid matrix
- Rare arteriole-sized curvilinear vessels
- May contain an admixture of fat

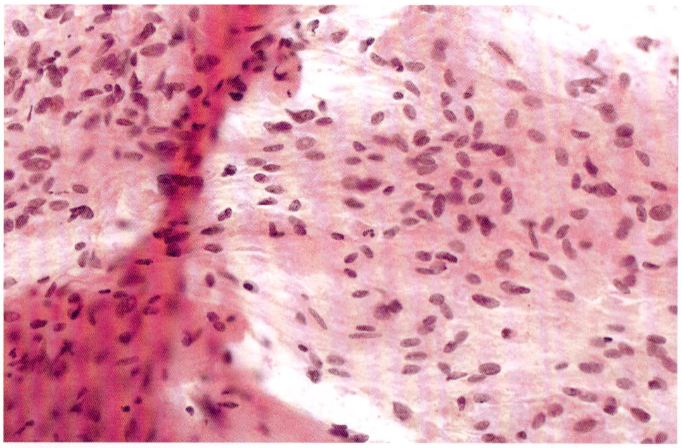

Fig. 8.69 Low-grade fibromyxoid sarcoma. Relatively uniform spindle cells in a myxofibrotic stroma, with a thin-walled blood vessel (H&E).

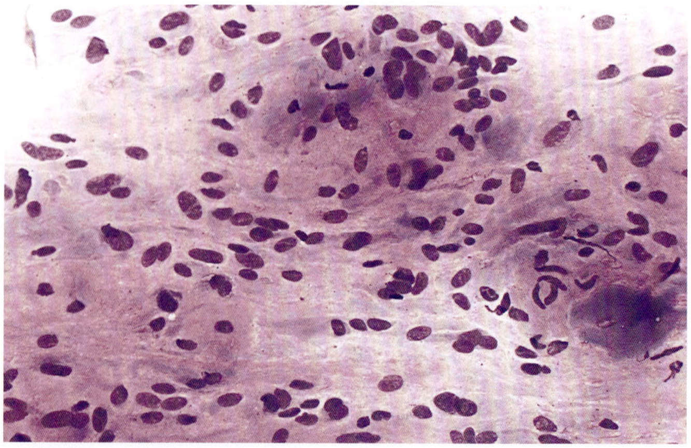

Fig. 8.70 Low-grade fibromyxoid sarcoma. Bland, uniform spindle cells, some with pale cytoplasm, within a myxoid matrix (Giemsa).

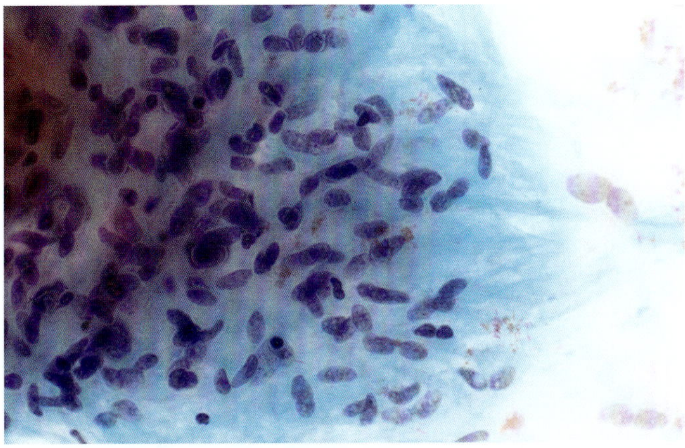

Fig. 8.71 Low-grade fibromyxoid sarcoma. High-power image showing spindle cells with elongated, mildly pleomorphic nuclei with fine, even chromatin, within a fibrillary collagenous matrix (Pap).

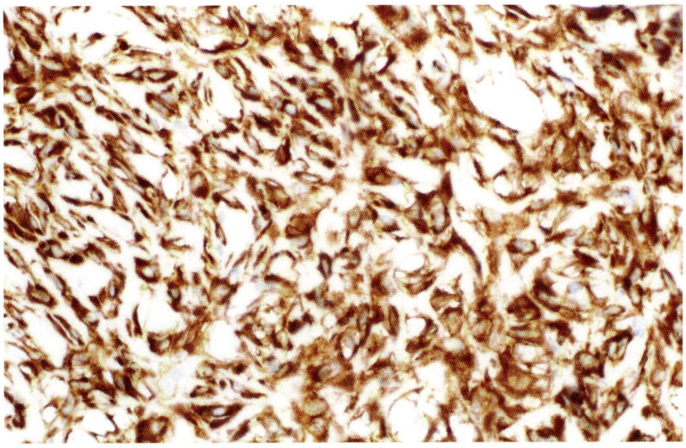

Fig. 8.72 Low-grade fibromyxoid sarcoma. MUC4 expression in low-grade fibromyxoid sarcoma (cell block, ICC, MUC4).

Sclerosing epithelioid fibrosarcoma

Low cellularity

- Cells vary from small round blue cells to ovoid spindle cells, epithelioid cells, and plasmacytoid cells
- Nuclei may be ovoid to pleomorphic
- Sclerotic, fibrotic, or myxoid stroma

Reference(s): {826,351,1121}

Discussion and differential diagnosis

A primary diagnosis of LGFMS cannot be made solely on cytopathological features {826,351}, and these tumours are likely to be placed into the "Atypical" category. The differential diagnosis is wide and includes spindle cell neoplasms such as peripheral nerve sheath tumours, schwannoma, neurofibroma, and perineurioma, as well as desmoid-type fibromatosis, dermatofibrosarcoma protuberans with myxoid differentiation, solitary fibrous tumour, and low-grade myxofibrosarcoma, as well as intramuscular myxoma.

Other differential diagnoses include myxoid liposarcoma and extraskeletal myxoid chondrosarcoma. Myxoid liposarcoma may be differentiated by the presence of lipoblasts, and round cell and spindle cell variants of myxoid liposarcoma show higher cellularity and atypia than LGFMS, although NGS can be of great assistance. Dermatofibrosarcoma protuberans with myxoid changes is a superficial tumour; the distinction from LGFMS may be difficult, requiring ICC. Cellular myxoma is an intermediate lesion between intramuscular myxoma and LGFMS, showing minimally atypical cells with some elongated nuclei in a myxoid background.

Sclerosing epithelioid fibromyxoid sarcoma should be differentiated from malignant melanoma and mucinous carcinoma {785,725,249}.

The differential diagnosis of hybrid tumours or predominantly sclerosing epithelioid fibrosarcoma include metastatic carcinoma, epithelioid vascular tumours, ossifying fibromyxoid tumour, biphasic synovial sarcoma, and extraskeletal osteosarcoma. A definitive diagnosis requires MUC4 ICC {359}.

Ancillary testing

LGFMS and subsets of sclerosing epithelioid fibrosarcoma share cytomorphological features, and they are diffusely and strongly positive in the cytoplasm for MUC4 ICC and share molecular characteristics {515,362,77,1129,359}. They may be positive for EMA and SMA {515,359}. Cytogenetic testing reveals t(7;16) or t(11;16) translocations and supernumerary ring chromosomes. *FUS* rearrangements can be detected by FISH, or *FUS*::*CREB3L1* or *FUS*::*CREB3L2* fusion by PCR/NGS-based techniques {515}.

Gastrointestinal stromal tumour

Schaefer IM
Hiroshima K
Pitman MB
Stelow EB

Definition

Gastrointestinal stromal tumour (GIST) is a mesenchymal neoplasm with variable behaviour, characterized by differentiation towards the interstitial cells of Cajal.

Clinical features and imaging

GISTs arise in the stomach (60%), small bowel (30%), rectum (4%), colon (1–2%), and oesophagus (<1%) {944,1202,947,948}, and rarely in the mesentery, omentum, and retroperitoneum {1158}. Most GISTs are sporadic, but 5–10% of cases occur in association with cancer predisposition syndromes. Most syndromic GISTs are succinate dehydrogenase (SDH)-deficient, including those associated with the non-hereditary Carney triad, which includes GIST, pulmonary chondroma, and paraganglioma {178}, as well as those associated with the autosomal dominant Carney–Stratakis syndrome, which includes GIST and paraganglioma in the context of SDH germline mutations {1081,

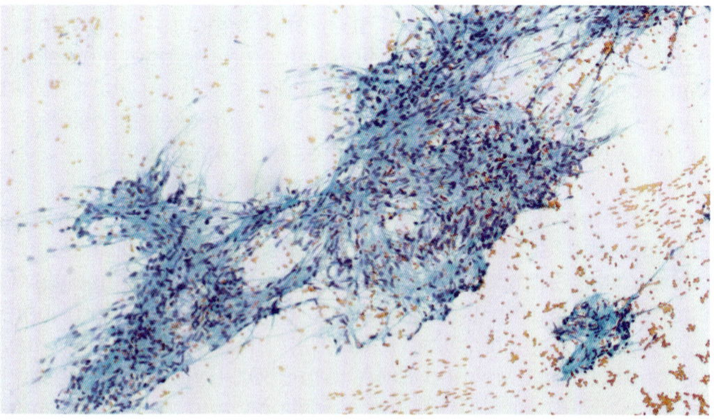

Fig. 8.73 Gastrointestinal stromal tumour, spindle cell type. Cohesive tissue fragments of spindle cells with oval nuclei with even chromatin; inconspicuous nucleoli; and long, tapered, wispy cytoplasmic processes (Pap).

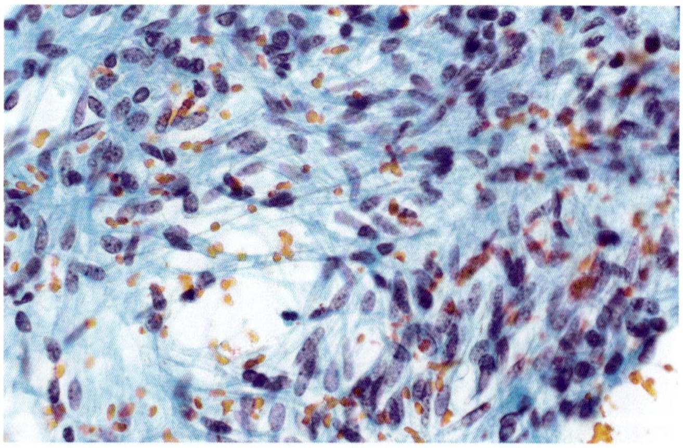

Fig. 8.74 Gastrointestinal stromal tumour, spindle cell type. A tissue fragment consisting of irregularly arranged spindle cells with long cytoplasmic processes and elongated, oval nuclei with even chromatin and inconspicuous nucleoli (Pap).

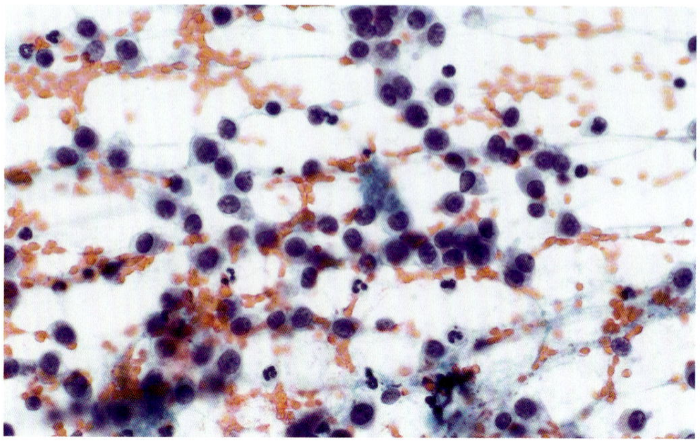

Fig. 8.75 Gastrointestinal stromal tumour, epithelioid type, succinate dehydrogenase–deficient. Relatively monomorphic polygonal cells with eccentric plasmacytoid cytoplasm seen singly and in minute tissue fragments (Pap).

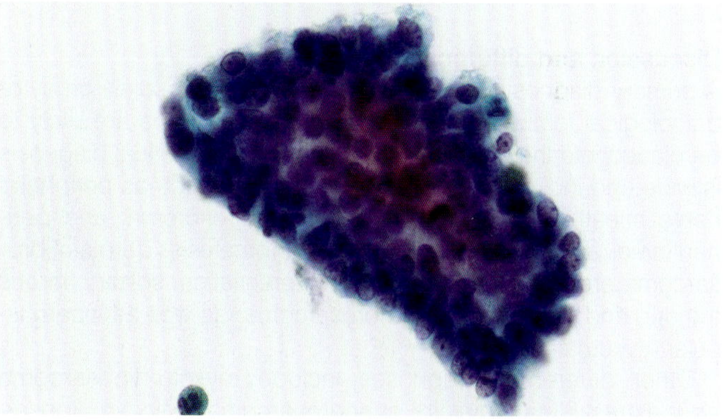

Fig. 8.76 Gastrointestinal stromal tumour, epithelioid type. A cohesive dense tissue fragment in an LBC preparation, consisting of rounds cells with relatively hyperchromatic nuclei, mimicking epithelial cells and carcinoma (Pap).

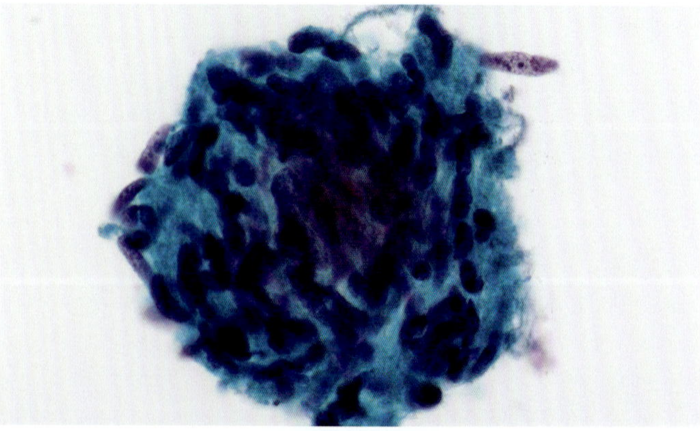

Fig. 8.77 Gastrointestinal stromal tumour, spindle cell type. A cohesive tissue fragment of spindle cells rounded up in an LBC preparation, making the long cytoplasmic processes less conspicuous than on direct smears. The elongated, oval nuclei are apparent (Pap).

1354,1503}. GISTs that are < 20 mm are usually asymptomatic and incidental findings {1442,1024}. The most common presentations are vague abdominal symptoms, acute and chronic bleeding, an abdominal mass, and pain {1442,1257,1484,255}. Advanced GISTs spread into the peritoneal cavity and often metastasize to the liver {305,1202,918}. CT and MRI, as well as FDG PET, are useful in the detection and functional characterization of GIST {480,653,306}. EUS-guided FNAB is often used to obtain diagnostic tissue material of submucosal GIST {187, 1277}.

Histopathology

GISTs display spindle (70%), epithelioid (20%), or mixed (10%) cytomorphology {257}. SDH-deficient GISTs are characterized by striking multilobular or plexiform architecture and epithelioid or mixed morphology {954,1503}. Most gastric GISTs are spindle cell tumours, with epithelioid morphology seen in approximately 20–25% of cases. Small intestinal and colonic GISTs are usually spindle cell tumours with diffuse sheets or vague storiform architecture. Risk stratification in GIST is performed on resection specimens.

Key diagnostic cytopathological features

- High cellularity
- Tissue fragments of variable size composed of uniform, bland spindle cells with delicate cytoplasm best seen in the Giemsa-stained smears, often containing thin-walled vessels
- Oval tapered to blunt-ended nuclei with fine chromatin
- Epithelioid tumour cells are rounder, with round to oval nuclei
- Mitotic figures and necrosis are uncommon in low-risk tumours
- Higher-risk tumours are composed of either spindle or epithelioid cells showing nuclear and cellular pleomorphism, mitotic figures, and rare necrosis
- Uncommon features include tissue fragments of cells in a more nested configuration, the presence of nuclear pseudoinclusions, and metachromatic (Giemsa) collagenous stromal tissue

Reference(s): {1345,1346,354,789}

Discussion and differential diagnosis

Because the cytopathological features of GIST vary according to the histopathological subtype, the differential diagnosis of GIST includes a range of mesenchymal, neural, and neuroendocrine neoplasms, such as leiomyoma of the gastrointestinal tract, which usually involves the oesophagus and colorectum, as well as leiomyosarcoma, schwannoma, malignant peripheral nerve sheath tumour, desmoid fibromatosis, inflammatory fibroid polyp, neuroendocrine tumour, and sarcomatoid carcinoma. Leiomyoma and schwannoma are among the most common differential diagnoses and consist of relatively uniform spindle cells similar to those found in GIST. The anatomical site and cytopathological features, such as the presence of thin-walled blood vessels, can support a diagnosis of GIST, but ICC is usually required.

Ancillary testing

GISTs are positive in ICC for KIT (CD117) in 95% of cases, DOG1 in 98%, PDGFRA in 80%, and CD34 in 70–80%, and they usually retain expression of SDHB and SDHA {257}. SDH-deficient GISTs are characterized by loss of SDHB expression {954,360}. Additional loss of SDHA expression is observed in *SDHA*-mutant GIST {360}. In the differential diagnosis from schwannomas and

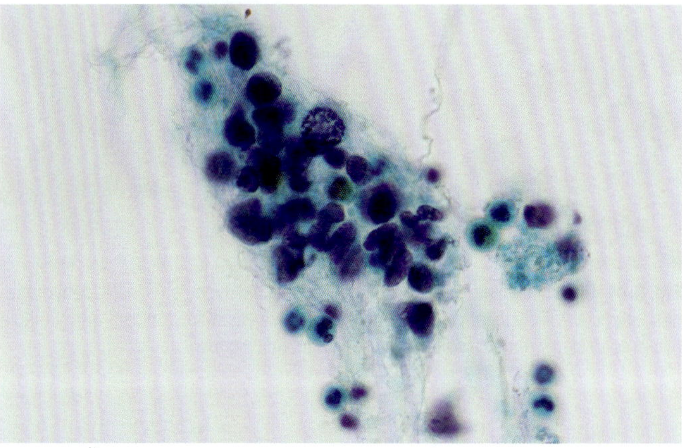

Fig. 8.78 Gastrointestinal stromal tumour, epithelioid type. Direct smears show polygonal epithelioid cells with round nuclei, which introduces carcinoma into the differential diagnosis (Pap).

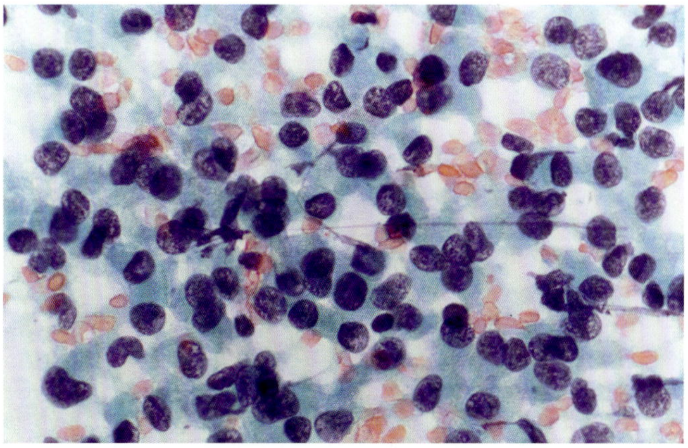

Fig. 8.79 Gastrointestinal stromal tumour, epithelioid type. A direct smear shows a monotonous population of cells with eccentric plasmacytoid cytoplasm and mildly atypical nuclei, mimicking a neuroendocrine tumour (Pap).

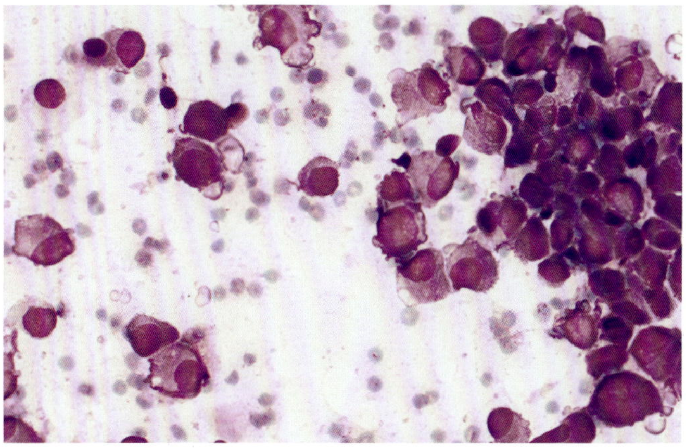

Fig. 8.80 Gastrointestinal stromal tumour, epithelioid type, succinate dehydrogenase–deficient. Large, polygonal cells with eccentric cytoplasm imparting a plasmacytoid feature, present singly and in loosely cohesive tissue fragments (Giemsa).

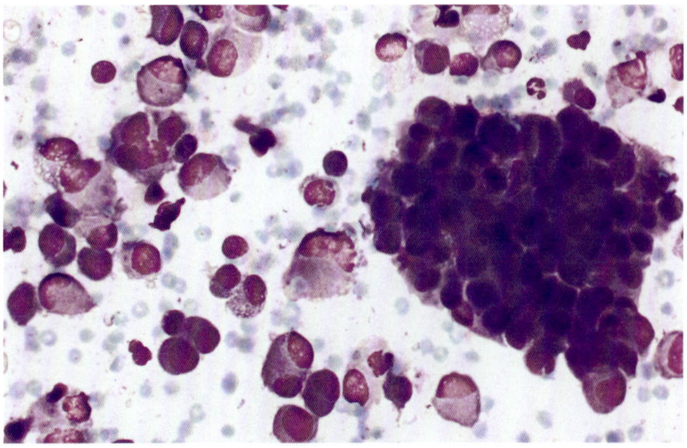

Fig. 8.81 Gastrointestinal stromal tumour, epithelioid type, succinate dehydrogenase–deficient. Polygonal cells with eccentric plasmacytoid cytoplasm and variable nuclei seen singly and in a cohesive tissue fragment (Giemsa).

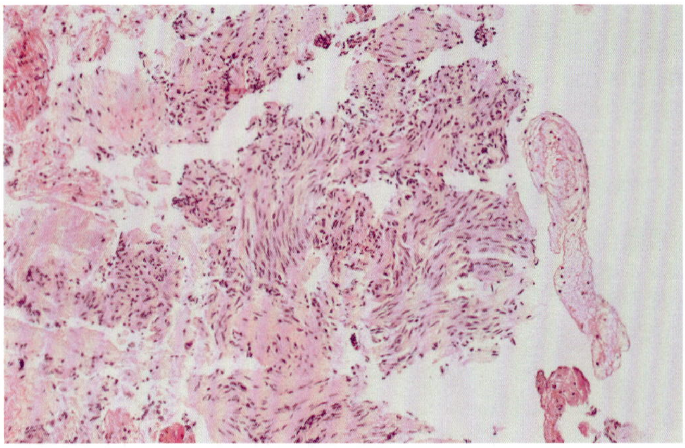

Fig. 8.82 Gastrointestinal stromal tumour, spindle cell type. Spindle cells with elongated wavy nuclei and indistinct spindle cytoplasm (cell block, H&E).

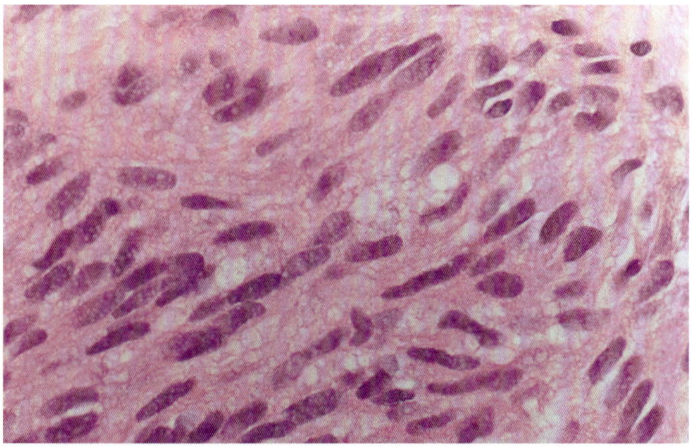

Fig. 8.83 Gastrointestinal stromal tumour, spindle cell type. Spindle cells, often with indistinct spindle cytoplasm, show elongated, mildly pleomorphic spindle nuclei, some with a perinuclear vacuole, which offer a clue to the diagnosis (cell block, H&E).

leiomyomas, positivity for KIT (CD117) and DOG1 and negativity for desmin and S100 are required {1345,604}.

Molecular testing is rarely needed for establishing the diagnosis of GIST, but it can inform therapeutic decisions. Approximately 85% of GISTs are initiated by gain-of-function mutations in the *KIT* {564} or *PDGFRA* {553} receptor tyrosine kinase gene, whereas genomic inactivation or epigenetic silencing of *NF1* {472} and SDH subunits, including *SDHA*, *SDHB*, *SDHC*, and *SDHD* {144}, can be observed in many *KIT/PDGFRA*-wildtype GISTs. The most common GIST chromosomal aberrations are deletions of 14q inactivating *MAX* {1256}, deletions of 22q inactivating *DEPDC5* {1070}, and deletions of 1p and 15q, followed by cell-cycle regulator mutations {379,1520,521} and dystrophin inactivation {1485}. SDH-deficient GISTs have occasional 1q deletion, presumably targeting *SDHC* {895,1354}.

Leiomyosarcoma

Domanski HA
Klijanienko J

Definition

Leiomyosarcoma (LMS) is a malignant neoplasm composed of cells showing smooth muscle differentiation.

Clinical features and imaging

LMS accounts for approximately 10% of all primary soft tissue sarcomas and for 10–15% of limb sarcomas; it typically occurs in adults, with a peak incidence in the sixth decade of life, although it may develop in younger individuals as well {757,1506,669,314}. LMS occurs most often in the extremities and retroperitoneum, but also in other locations such as visceral organs and bones {490,1506,1371}. Many subcutaneous and deep soft tissue LMSs originate from a small to medium-sized vein, and a subgroup of these neoplasms originate from large blood vessels such as the vena cava and other large veins {403,126}. The imaging features of LMS

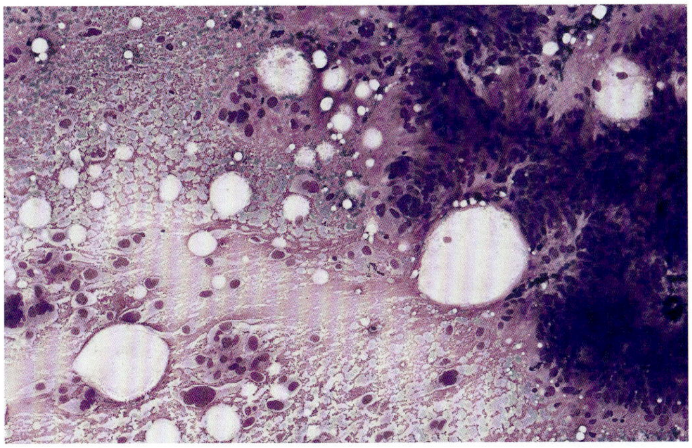

Fig. 8.84 Leiomyosarcoma. Crowded tissue fragments and single cells, showing pleomorphic cells with large pleomorphic nuclei and spindle cells in a granular background (Giemsa).

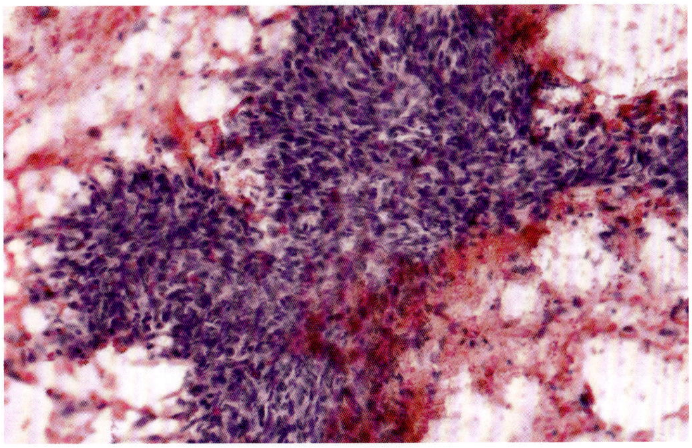

Fig. 8.85 Leiomyosarcoma. A cohesive, crowded, 3D tissue fragment of atypical spindle cells and pleomorphic cells (H&E).

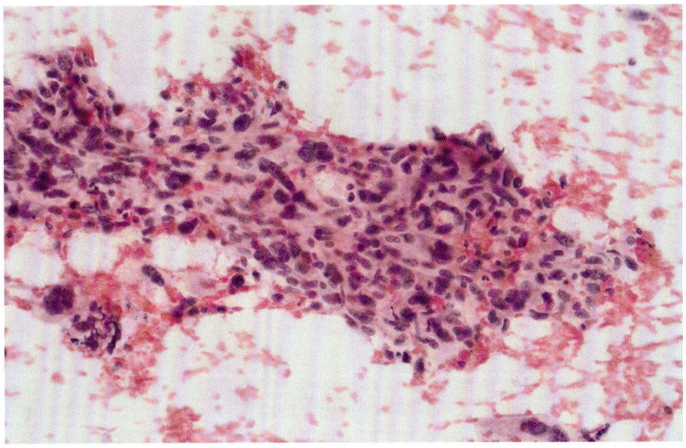

Fig. 8.86 Leiomyosarcoma. Mixed fascicular, spindle, and pleomorphic cells, some with eosinophilic spindle cytoplasm, in a tissue fragment (H&E).

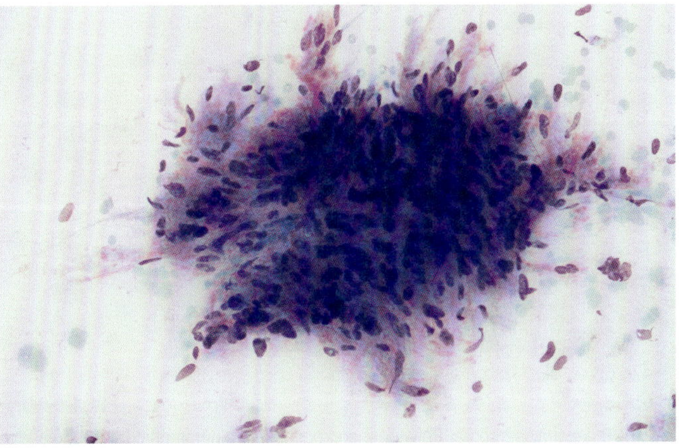

Fig. 8.87 Leiomyosarcoma. A tissue fragment of moderately pleomorphic spindle cells embedded in magenta collagenous matrix (Giemsa).

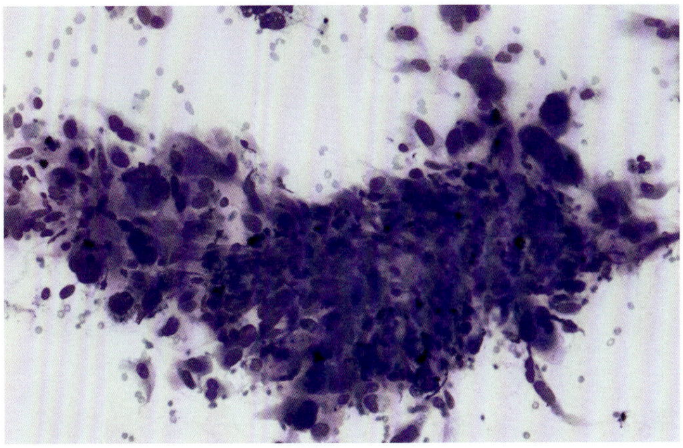

Fig. 8.88 Leiomyosarcoma. A cohesive tissue fragment of pleomorphic cells with bizarre large nuclei and some spindle cells and occasional multinucleated cells (Giemsa).

are nonspecific. The signal on T1-weighted MRI is isointense to muscle, and there is an intermediate or high signal on T2-weighted images. CT generally shows heterogeneous soft tissue masses {1055}.

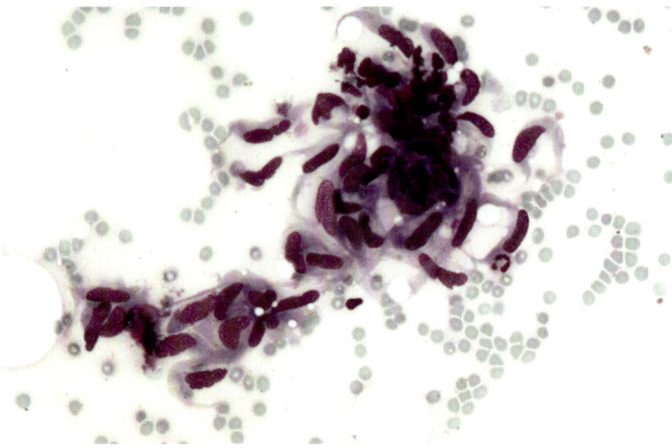

Fig. 8.89 Leiomyosarcoma. Spindle cells with elongated, cigar-shaped nuclei and well-defined elongated spindle cytoplasm (Giemsa).

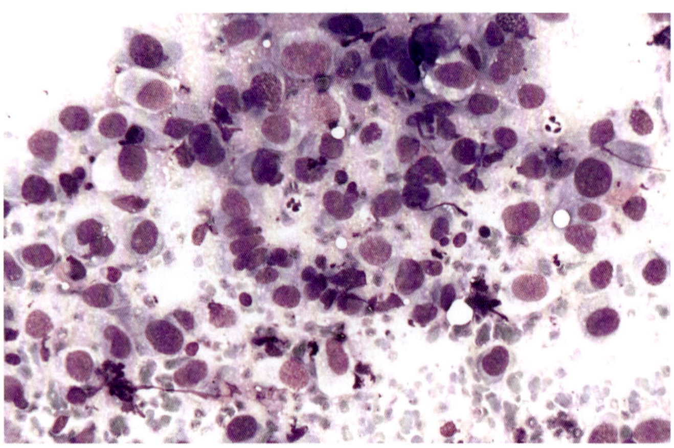

Fig. 8.90 Leiomyosarcoma. Polygonal and epithelioid pleomorphic cells, some with highly pleomorphic nuclei and prominent nucleoli, some with eccentric cytoplasm. Several mitoses are present (Giemsa).

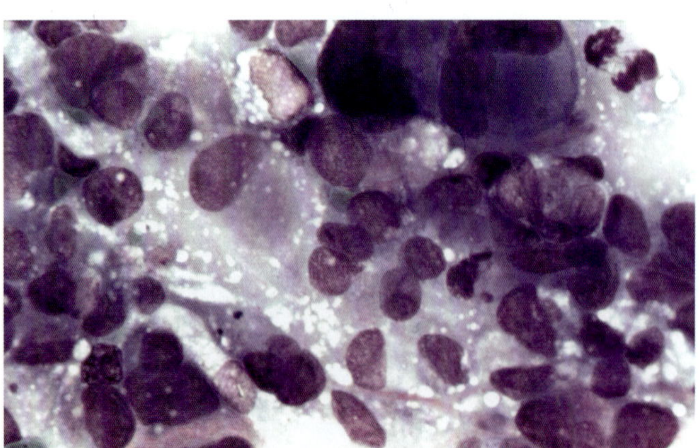

Fig. 8.91 Leiomyosarcoma. Highly pleomorphic epithelioid, spindle, and giant cells, some with large pleomorphic nuclei (Giemsa).

Histopathology

LMS shows diffuse cellularity and a predominantly fascicular pattern of growth, with the tumour bundles intersecting each other at wide angles. Storiform, palisaded, and aimless patterns may be present in some tumours or in different areas of the same tumour {1506}. Most LMSs show moderate cellular and nuclear pleomorphism and consist of spindle cells with plump, blunt-ended nuclei and moderate to abundant, pale to brightly eosinophilic fibrillary cytoplasm. The degree of cellular and nuclear atypia varies in different cases and in different areas of the same case {938}. The majority of LMSs are of high grade and show high mitotic counts, including atypical mitoses, and necrosis is often present in larger tumours {403,1506}. Pleomorphic variants of LMS are predominantly composed of pleomorphic spindle and polygonal cells admixed with varying large, bizarre, atypical cells and multinuclear giant cells, with or without abundant eosinophilic or fibrillary cytoplasm {1038}. Other findings occasionally seen include focal fibrosis, myxoid change, and hyalinized hypocellular areas {403}, while epithelioid morphology, multinucleated osteoclast-like giant cells, and areas with osseous or chondro-osseous metaplasia are rare findings.

Key diagnostic cytopathological features

- High cellularity, except in tumours with hyalinized matrix
- Tissue fragments show mixed fascicular, spindle cell, pleomorphic, predominantly fascicular and spindle cell, or predominantly pleomorphic architecture and cell type
- Fascicles and sheets of spindle cells arranged in parallel alignments
- Large, spindle or round, binucleated giant cells with intracytoplasmic granulations
- Nuclei are cigar-shaped, blunt-ended, and occasionally indented or segmented
- Stripped, atypical, poorly preserved nuclei in the background
- Blue or magenta matrix in tissue fragments (Giemsa)
- Minor component of dispersed, well-preserved spindle and round to polygonal cells with dense cytoplasm and occasional cytoplasmic projections
- Pleomorphic, bizarre, multinucleated cells
- Epithelioid tumour cells in epithelioid variant
- Occasional intranuclear pseudoinclusions
- Necrosis and inflammatory cells
- Rare osteoclast-like giant cells
- Variable mitoses

Reference(s): {277,1383,1509,732,346,499,33,705,1066}

Discussion and differential diagnosis

LMS smears are usually moderate to highly cellular and show distinctive cytoarchitectural patterns at low-power microscopy, which in most cases is a characteristic fascicular/spindle cell/pleomorphic pattern. LMS shares many cytopathological features with other spindle cell lesions, as well as with high-grade pleomorphic sarcomas of other lineage and epithelioid malignancies. In two large series of LMS cytopathology, only 24% and 34.8% of cases, respectively, were specifically diagnosed as LMS in FNAB {732,346}.

The cytopathological differential diagnosis of LMS includes benign spindle cell lesions, such as leiomyoma, nodular

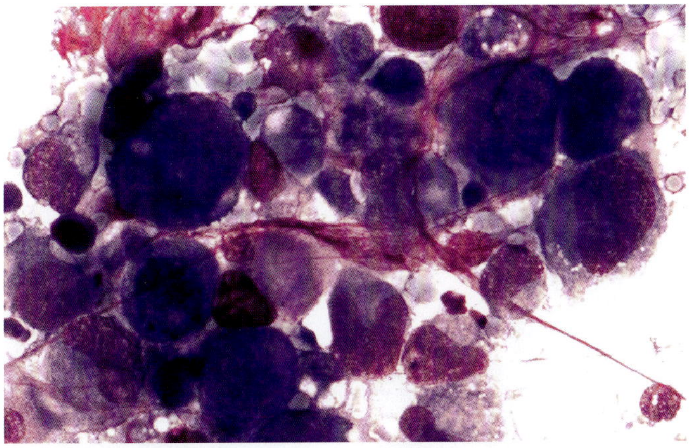

Fig. 8.92 Leiomyosarcoma. Highly pleomorphic cells with often large and bizarre nuclei, with a few strands of magenta stromal background (Giemsa).

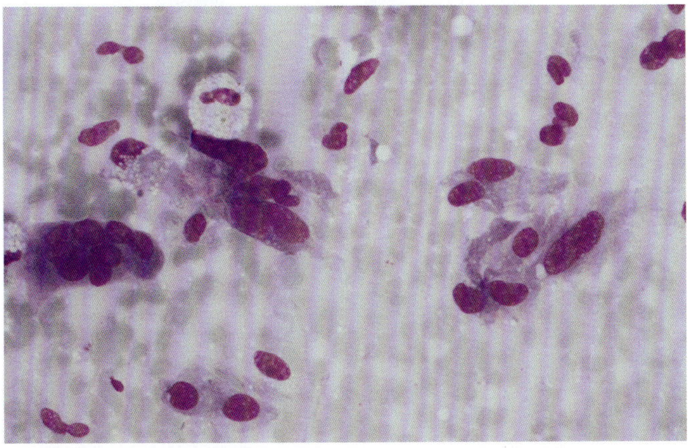

Fig. 8.93 Leiomyosarcoma. An osteoclast-like giant cell and tumour cells with oval or elongated, occasionally indented nuclei and cytoplasmic extensions (Giemsa).

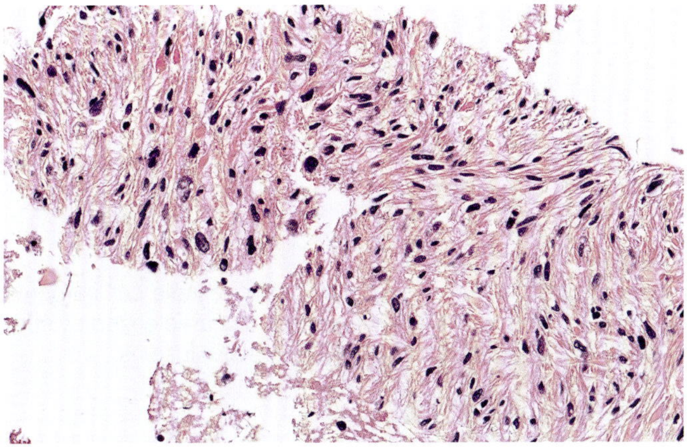

Fig. 8.94 Leiomyosarcoma. Atypical spindle cells with eosinophilic cytoplasm and pleomorphic nuclei, arranged in a fascicular architecture (cell block, H&E).

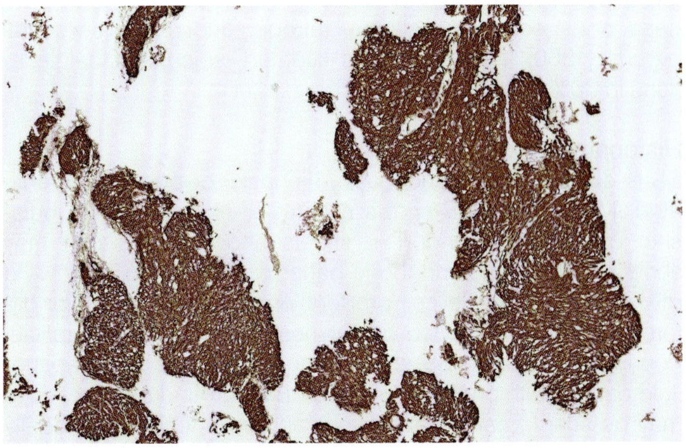

Fig. 8.95 Leiomyosarcoma. Strong desmin positivity supports diagnosis (cell block, ICC, desmin).

fasciitis, desmoid fibromatosis, and schwannoma. Both leiomyoma and LMS are positive for SMA and desmin. Increased cellularity, pleomorphic nuclei, and mitoses help to distinguish leiomyoma and LMS. The clinical presentation of nodular fasciitis differs from that of LMS in that nodular fasciitis commonly presents as a rapidly growing and occasionally painful or tender superficial nodule that regresses spontaneously in most cases {276,1343}. Smears from fibromatoses are usually of lower cellularity, showing less pronounced pleomorphism and nuclear atypia, compared with LMS {1058}. Smears from schwannoma show cohesive fascicles and sheets of variable size in a fibrillary background matrix and few dispersed cells, and the tumour cells have elongated, wavy, occasionally comma- or boomerang-shaped nuclei that are often pointed {345,724,197}. Schwannoma shows diffuse S100 positivity and stains negatively for smooth muscle markers.

Malignant entities such as monophasic synovial sarcoma, malignant peripheral nerve sheath tumour, and high-grade pleomorphic sarcomas should be considered in the differential diagnosis of LMS. A distinctive pattern of cohesive tissue fragments of bland spindle cells alternating with dispersed cells and a pericapillary arrangement of tumour cells suggests monophasic synovial sarcoma {32,729,393,1452,1341}. Malignant peripheral nerve sheath tumour occurs commonly in the setting of neurofibromatosis. Differentiation of LMS from myofibroblastic sarcoma and high-grade pleomorphic sarcomas can be difficult in individual cases, apart from blunt-ended nuclei favouring LMS, and the diagnosis relies on ICC.

Ancillary testing

LMS stains for SMA, desmin, and caldesmon, although sometimes only focally. Focal cytokeratin and EMA positivity has been reported. Synovial sarcomas show TLE1 positivity in most cases, and molecular testing with the presence of *SS18* fusion confirms the diagnosis. Malignant peripheral nerve sheath tumours express S100 and SOX10 focally, with a subset of cases showing loss of H3 p.K28me3 (K27me3); they do not express smooth muscle markers.

Synovial sarcoma

Chebib I
Domanski HA
Klijanienko J
Rekhi B

Definition

Synovial sarcoma (SS) is a monomorphic spindle cell sarcoma showing variable epithelial differentiation, characterized by specific *SS18::SSX1*, *SS18::SSX2*, or *SS18::SSX4* fusions.

Clinical features and imaging

SS presents as a painful or painless mass over a wide age range (median: 30–40 years) and shows an equal sex distribution {772,1360}. SSs most often occur in the deep soft tissue of the extremities, but they also arise in the trunk and abdomen, head and neck, mediastinum, retroperitoneum, and visceral organs {1360}. Imaging shows stippled, spiculated calcifications in 30% of cases {140,1507}.

Histopathology

SS is classified as monophasic, biphasic, or poorly differentiated. Monophasic SS shows uniform spindle cells with indistinct cytoplasm arranged in sheets and fascicles that may show whorling or herringbone patterns. Biphasic SS shows a mix of similar spindle cell proliferation and focal epithelial differentiation that includes cords, nests, glands, and papillae. Poorly differentiated SS shows round cells or a large epithelioid pattern with prominent nucleoli. Background stromal tissue may be scant to abundant, dense and collagenized, or focally myxoid. SS often shows irregular, dilated, thin-walled, so-called "staghorn" vessels, imparting the previously known "haemangiopericytoma" pattern, and calcifications are variably present. Mitotic figures are readily identified and are increased in poorly differentiated SS.

Key diagnostic cytopathological features

- High cellularity
- Branching tissue fragments and single cells
- Monophasic SS shows uniform oval to fusiform cells with scant cytoplasm, hyperchromatic nuclei, small to absent nucleoli, and stripped nuclei
- Biphasic SS shows tissue fragments of mixed uniform oval to fusiform spindle cells and epithelioid cells showing glandular, alveolar, or acinar formation better seen in the Pap stain
- Poorly differentiated SS shows small round cells and rarely rhabdoid cells
- Capillaries can be seen in some tissue fragments, with surrounding loosely cohesive tumour cells
- Mitotic figures can often be identified
- Mast cells may also be present

Reference(s): {709,1452,729,32,393,30,1341,754,1177}

Discussion and differential diagnosis

The specific diagnosis of monophasic SS on cytopathology alone may be challenging, but cellular FNAB smears from

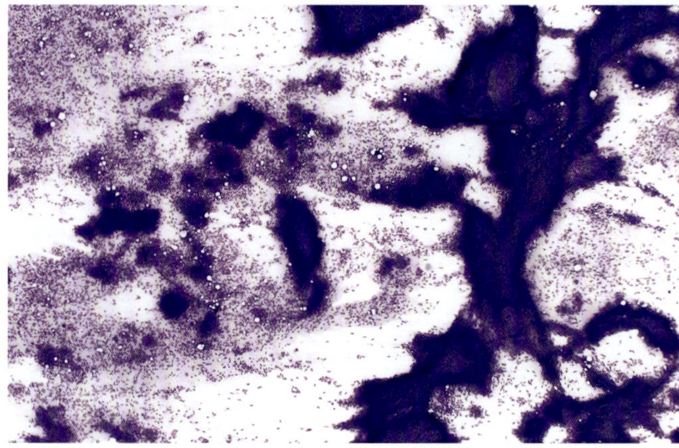

Fig. 8.96 Synovial sarcoma. Highly cellular smears composed of cohesive tissue fragments and single cells (Giemsa).

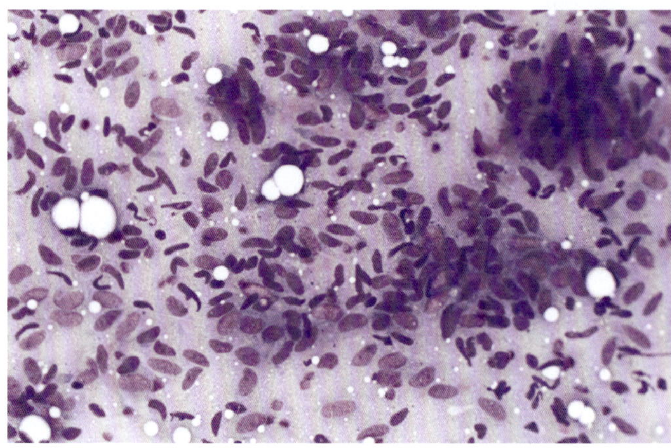

Fig. 8.97 Monophasic synovial sarcoma. A loosely cohesive and predominantly single-cell population of spindle cells with scant cytoplasm and stripped nuclei (Giemsa).

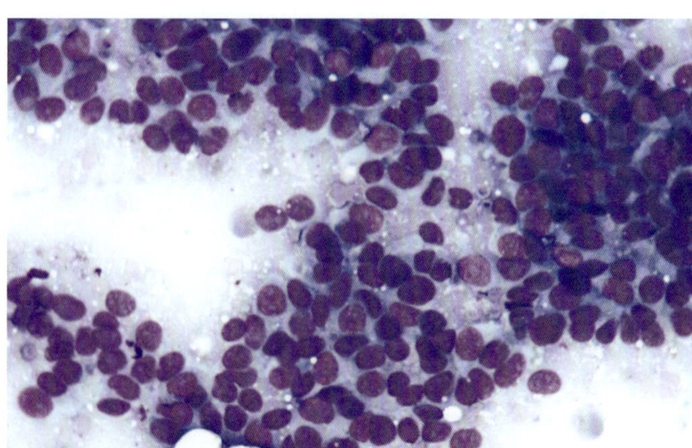

Fig. 8.98 Biphasic synovial sarcoma. Plump epithelioid cells in biphasic synovial sarcoma with round nuclei and single nucleoli (Giemsa).

SS can be categorized as "Malignant" {729}. A soft tissue sarcoma with biphasic morphology, in a patient without neurofibromatosis, is consistent with biphasic SS. The primary diagnosis of poorly differentiated SS is especially challenging {30,1177}, and definitive classification typically requires the use of ancillary studies to differentiate from cytopathological mimics.

The differential diagnosis for monophasic SS includes malignant peripheral nerve sheath tumour (MPNST), solitary fibrous tumour (SFT), dermatofibrosarcoma protuberans, gastrointestinal stromal tumour, and thymoma. MPNST occurs in the setting of neurofibromatosis, in a background of neurofibroma, or arising from a peripheral nerve. Dermatofibrosarcoma protuberans arises superficially.

The differential diagnosis for biphasic SS includes MPNST with epithelial differentiation, myoepithelial tumours of soft tissue, epithelioid sarcoma, and metastatic carcinoma, and ICC is often required. Poorly differentiated SS must be distinguished from small round cell sarcomas including Ewing sarcoma, *CIC*-rearranged sarcoma, sarcoma with *BCOR* genetic alterations, rhabdomyosarcoma, and lymphoma, and this requires ICC.

Ancillary testing

By ICC, SS typically expresses EMA and/or keratins, including pankeratins, CK7, and CK19. They may also express S100, BCL2, and CD99, but these markers are nonspecific. In the differential diagnosis, MPNSTs focally express S100 or SOX10, but a subset of cases show complete loss of H3 p.K28me3 (K27me3). SS often shows weak to patchy positivity for H3 p.K28me3 (K27me3) and rarely complete loss of expression. SFT may also express CD99 and BCL2, but STAT6 can be used as a surrogate for the *NAB2::STAT6* fusion characteristic of SFT. TLE1 is diffusely and strongly positive in SS nuclei in most cases, but TLE1 may also be expressed in MPNST and SFT {1391,751,441}. Dermatofibrosarcoma protuberans typically expresses CD34, which is negative in SS, whereas gastrointestinal stromal tumour expresses KIT (CD117), DOG1, and CD34. Myoepithelial tumours of soft tissue often show expression of epithelial markers; neurogenic markers, such as S100 and SOX10; and myogenic markers, including SMA, calponin, desmin, and p63. A subset show loss of SMARCB1 (INI1) expression. Myoepithelial tumours may harbour *EWSR1* rearrangements with various partners. Epithelioid sarcoma can also show epithelial differentiation by ICC, loss of SMARCB1 (INI1), and positivity for CD34.

Many of the differential diagnoses of poorly differentiated SS express CD99. Ewing sarcomas show diffuse strong membranous staining with CD99 and nuclear NKX2-2. They

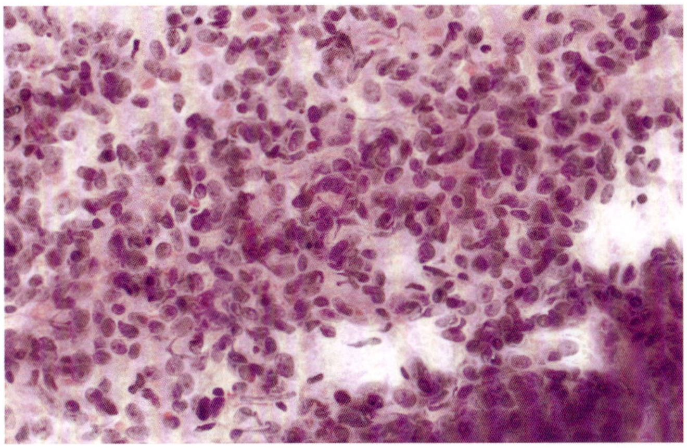

Fig. 8.100 Poorly differentiated synovial sarcoma. Small round blue cells in loosely cohesive tissue fragments are characteristic of poorly differentiated synovial sarcoma (H&E).

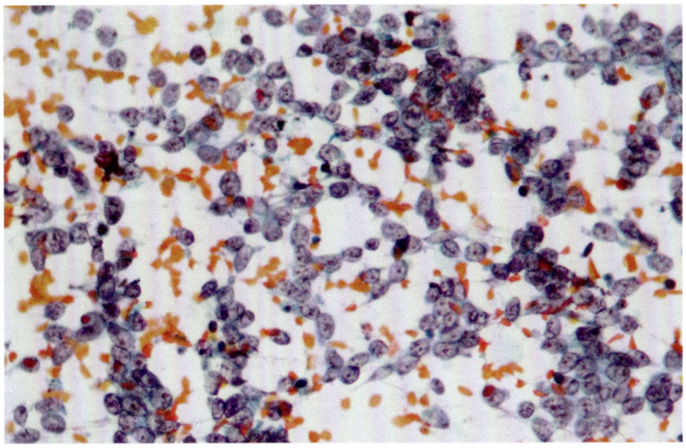

Fig. 8.101 Poorly differentiated synovial sarcoma. Synovial sarcoma with predominantly small round blue cells in minute tissue fragments and singly (Pap).

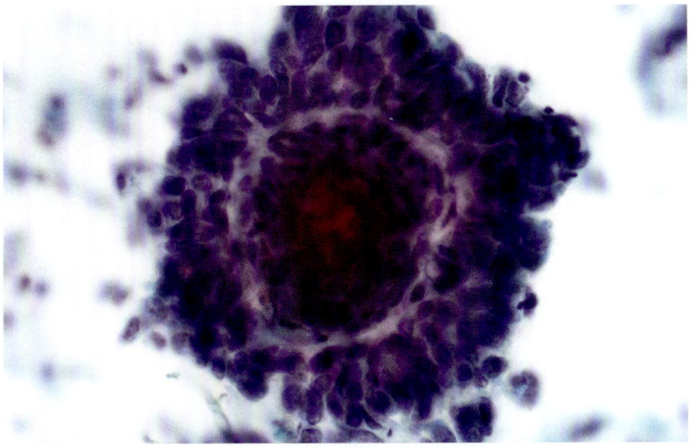

Fig. 8.99 Biphasic synovial sarcoma. A large gland-like tissue fragment consistent with biphasic synovial sarcoma (Pap).

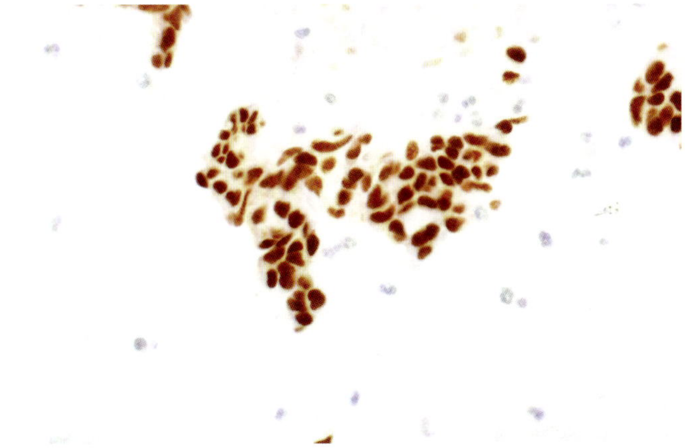

Fig. 8.102 Synovial sarcoma. Cell block preparation showing synovial sarcoma positive for SS18::SSX fusion protein (cell block, ICC).

Chapter 8

harbour *EWSR1* or *FUS* rearrangements. In *CIC*-rearranged sarcomas, CD99 expression is often multifocal, and they may also express WT1 and ETV4. Sarcoma with *BCOR* genetic alterations also expresses multifocal CD99 positivity, but it additionally expresses SATB2, BCOR, and cyclin B3 (CCNB3) in tumours that harbour *BCOR::CCNB3* fusions. SS also shows expression of BCOR, so molecular testing is typically required to confirm the presence of *SS18* fusion. Rhabdomyosarcoma expresses desmin, myogenin, and MYOD1, and the alveolar subtype harbours *PAX3::FOXO1* or *PAX7::FOXO1* fusion.

The SS18::SSX fusion–specific antibody is a surrogate for fusions of *SS18* with *SSX1*, *SSX2*, or *SSX4*; both it and the SSX C-terminus antibody are nuclear stains, sensitive and specific for SS {104}. By cytogenetics, SS harbours a t(X;18) translocation {280}. The fusion can also be demonstrated by FISH for *SS18* {1000,1364,58} or PCR and NGS to identify *SS18::SSX1*, *SSX2*, or *SSX4* fusion partners {514,772,58}.

Kaposi sarcoma

Carrilho C
Grayson W
Jo VY
Pantanowitz L
Schmitt F

Definition

Kaposi sarcoma (KS) is a locally aggressive endothelial proliferation that usually presents with cutaneous lesions in the form of multiple patches, plaques, or nodules, and can involve mucosal sites, lymph nodes, and visceral organs. It is associated with KS-associated herpesvirus / human herpesvirus 8 (KSHV/HHV8) infection.

Clinical features and imaging

KS lesions predominantly affect skin and mucosal sites as patches or macules in the "patch stage", plaques in the "plaque stage", or nodules in the "nodular stage". Nodules can coalesce and ulcerate. KS has also been described in the lymph nodes, eye, musculoskeletal system, heart, spleen, nervous system, gastrointestinal tract, and other unusual locations {466,1071,1109,1489}.

The aggressiveness and extension are related to host immune status and to four clinical-epidemiological forms: classic KS, endemic or African KS, epidemic AIDS-associated KS, and iatrogenic transplant-associated KS. Classic KS is indolent and affects skin of the lower extremities, mainly in older men. The lesions, which can be solitary or multiple, are violaceous/brownish macules, plaques, or nodules. Endemic KS affects skin as multiple lesions in the lower extremities and regional lymph nodes. When KS involves lymph nodes in children and other young people, it is more aggressive than when it occurs in adults. AIDS-associated KS is more aggressive and manifests with disseminated mucocutaneous and visceral involvement. The palate, lymph nodes (including the epitrochlear node), gastrointestinal tract, and lungs are frequently involved. Although KS presents at any stage of HIV infection, it usually occurs in patients with HIV with a low CD4+ T-cell count. Cases in patients receiving HAART exhibit a less aggressive course, and lesions may initially flare but eventually regress. Iatrogenic transplant-associated KS occurs after solid organ transplantation or drug immunosuppression; the presentation can be localized in skin and mucosal membranes or disseminated with visceral lesions {1142,1489,405,610}. The clinical course is variable, but it is usually aggressive in patients with visceral involvement.

Histopathology

The histopathology is similar in all clinical and epidemiological forms. The patch stage is characterized by a subtle proliferation of abnormal vessels lined by flattened endothelial cells, dissecting the upper dermis. Pre-existent vessels can protrude into the lumina of new proliferating vessels, a feature called the "promontory sign". Vessels are surrounded by chronic inflammatory cells (mainly lymphocytes and plasma cells), extravasated erythrocytes, and haemosiderin pigment. The plaque stage involves most of the dermis and is characterized by a proliferation of vessels and spindle cells, both of which dissect dermal collagen, along with features observed in the patch stage. The nodular stage is characterized by a nodular proliferation of spindle cells arranged in fascicles, with slit-like vascular spaces containing erythrocytes, as well as an admixed variable lymphoplasmacytic inflammatory infiltrate, hyaline globules, and haemosiderin-laden macrophages. Except in anaplastic KS lesions seen in AIDS, atypia is minimal, the mitotic index is low, and necrosis is absent {1142,603,1544}.

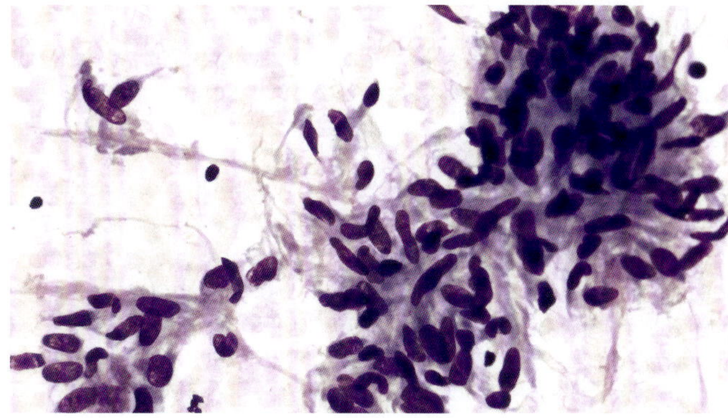

Fig. 8.103 Kaposi sarcoma. FNAB of a nodule on the leg of a man with HIV infection shows a loosely cohesive tissue fragment of bland spindle cells with elongated, sometimes comma or angled nuclei with uniform granular chromatin (Giemsa).

Key diagnostic cytopathological features

- Variable cellularity
- Bloody background
- Loosely cohesive to cohesive tissue fragments of spindle cells with radial arrangement and nuclear crush artefact centrally
- Spindle cells have a moderate amount of cytoplasm, with indistinct borders in the tissue fragments
- Nuclear pleomorphism is uncommon, chromatin is finely granular, and nucleoli are inconspicuous
- Very rarely, eosinophilic globular structures can be identified in the spindle cells or extracellularly
- Macrophages with haemosiderin can sometimes be found

Reference(s): {466,996,405,1142,1489}

Discussion and differential diagnosis

The differential diagnosis includes reactive spindle cell lesions such as granulation tissue and nodular fasciitis, as well as other mesenchymal spindle cell neoplasms, including leiomyoma, fibrohistiocytic neoplasms, and angiosarcoma {466}. In the setting of HIV infection, granulomatous lesions can also be present concomitantly, making the diagnosis difficult {405}. The anaplastic variant of KS must be distinguished from other high-grade sarcomas. Sarcomatoid carcinoma and spindle cell melanoma should be excluded.

Ancillary testing

ICC is useful to distinguish KS from other spindle cell lesions {342}. KS spindle cells express endothelial markers such as CD31, CD34, and ERG, as well as lymphatic-specific markers such as D2-40 or PROX1. Nuclear expression of KSHV/HHV8 (LANA1) is present in almost all cases {342,1071,191}.

Chapter 8

Angiosarcoma

Jo VY
Carrilho C
Schmitt F
VandenBussche CJ

Definition

Angiosarcoma is a malignant vascular neoplasm that variably recapitulates the morphological and immunocytochemical features of endothelial cells.

Clinical features and imaging

Approximately half of all angiosarcomas are cutaneous, and soft tissue angiosarcoma can occur in the lower extremities, trunk, head and neck, breast, bone, retroperitoneum, and viscera {915}. A large age range is observed, but these tumours are very rare in children, and peak incidence is during the seventh decade of life {321,1275}. There is a male predominance.

Patients typically present with a rapidly growing and often painful mass. Some tumours are associated with acute haemorrhage, and a subset of patients present with symptoms such as anaemia, coagulopathy, and haematoma {915}.

Imaging features are usually nonspecific, and tumours are often large and show infiltrative growth and frequent necrosis. Tumours show intermediate signal on T1-weighted MRI, with high signal intensity occurring with haemorrhage, and they appear bright on T2-weighted imaging {456,1182}.

A subset of angiosarcomas arise after radiation exposure or chronic lymphoedema; these cases are associated with high-level *MYC* amplification {523,870}, although *MYC* amplification also occurs in a small subset of primary angiosarcomas. Rarely, angiosarcoma may arise in association with implanted foreign material, arteriovenous fistulas, pre-existing haemangioma or vascular malformation, or prior trauma or surgery, as well as in certain syndromes, such as neurofibromatosis and Maffucci syndrome {586,634,1494,923,1201}.

Angiosarcomas are highly aggressive, with high rates of local recurrence (~20%) and distant metastases (~50%); more than half of all patients die of disease within 1 year {915}.

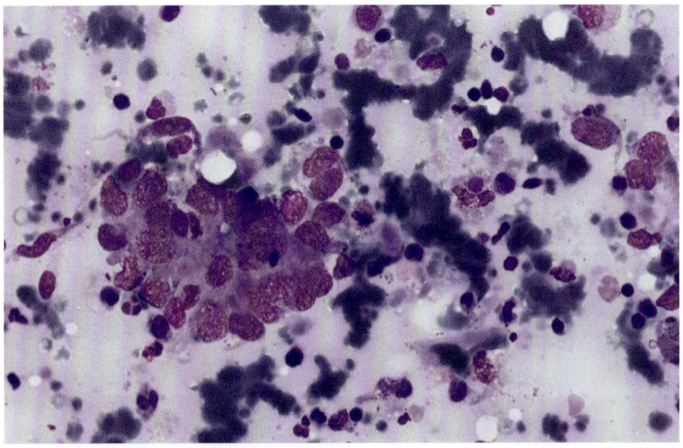

Fig. 8.104 Epithelioid angiosarcoma of breast. Numerous spindle and epithelioid cells, mimicking adenocarcinoma (Giemsa).

Histopathology

Angiosarcomas are characteristically infiltrative tumours. Their appearance can range widely in the degree of differentiation and the degree of atypia, but histopathological grade does not appear to predict prognosis. Some angiosarcomas are composed of well-formed, anastomosing vessels lined by enlarged nuclei. The presence of endothelial multilayering, "hobnailing" (where individual angiosarcoma cells bulge into the lumen), and complex dissecting growth aids in recognition, especially for subtle low-grade cases. Many tumours frequently show high-grade features with a sheet-like or solid growth of epithelioid or spindle cells, and there are often areas of anastomosing or ramifying vascular channels. Tumour cell nuclei show atypia, although marked pleomorphism is rare. Nuclei are typically large, and the chromatin is cleared or "vesicular", with prominent nucleoli and often abundant cytoplasm that is eosinophilic

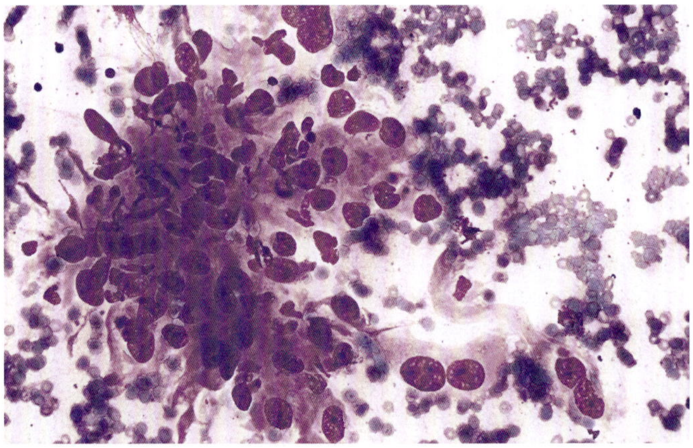

Fig. 8.105 Angiosarcoma. A large tissue fragment of spindle, epithelioid, and polygonal tumour cells, with markedly pleomorphic nuclei with nucleoli, with occasional spindle cytoplasm (Giemsa).

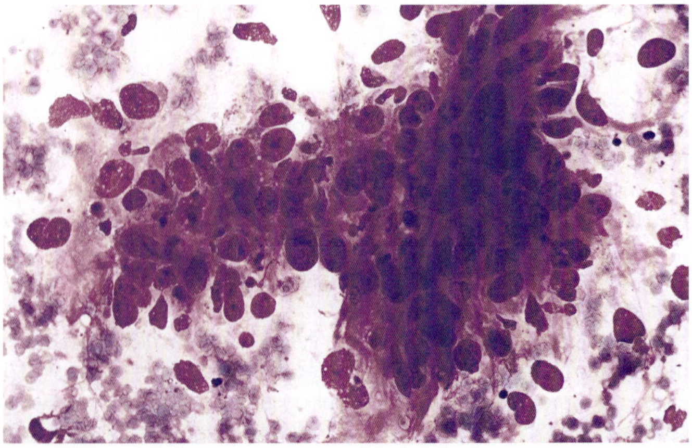

Fig. 8.106 Angiosarcoma. A crowded tissue fragment consisting of spindle and epithelioid cells, with occasional tadpole-like forms (Giemsa).

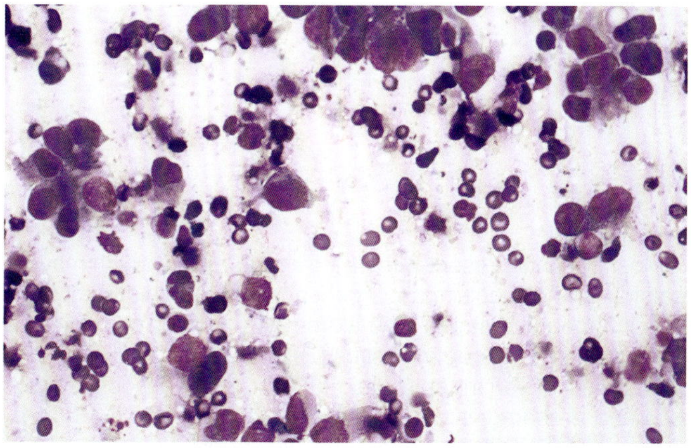

Fig. 8.107 Epithelioid angiosarcoma. Epithelioid tumour cells with large round nuclei with prominent nucleoli, often a high N:C ratio, and often eccentric cytoplasm (Giemsa).

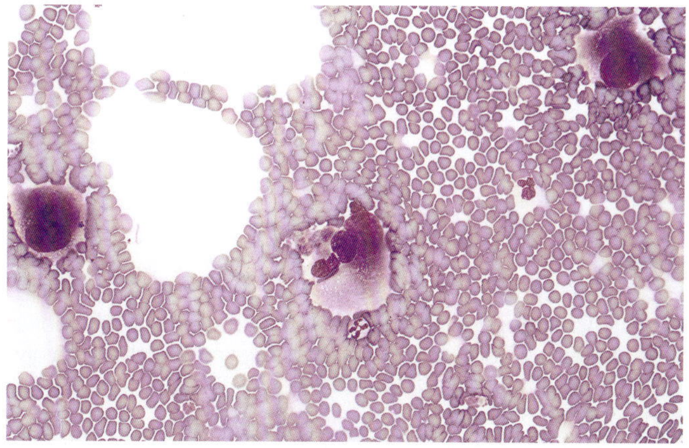

Fig. 8.108 Angiosarcoma. Smears may be paucicellular with an abundantly bloody background.

or pale. Mitotic activity and necrosis are common, especially in high-grade tumours. Some cases show extensive haemorrhage, organizing haematoma, or blood lakes. Epithelioid angiosarcoma is composed of diffuse sheets of epithelioid or polygonal cells, usually with only rare foci of vasoformation {422}.

Key diagnostic cytopathological features

- Low cellularity
- Bloody background
- Tissue fragments showing rudimentary vascular architecture or more solid spindle regions
- Single dispersed spindle, epithelioid, or polygonal cells
- Large nuclei with prominent or bar-shaped nucleoli, with eccentric cytoplasm
- Abundant cytoplasm with frequent cytoplasmic projections with spider-like or tadpole-like forms
- Cytoplasmic haemosiderin may be seen
- Vasoformative cytoplasmic features are infrequent but very helpful when present, including pseudoacini and intracytoplasmic vacuoles with associated erythrocytes
- Mitoses, including atypical forms, and necrosis may be seen, especially in high-grade and epithelioid tumours

Reference(s): {1441,475,698,148,730}

Discussion and differential diagnosis

The differential diagnosis is broad and depends on the features. Tumours with spindle and epithelioid cytomorphology may resemble malignant melanoma, and haemosiderin pigment may be mistaken for melanin. Angiosarcoma may also resemble carcinoma, especially epithelioid angiosarcoma, in which keratin staining is frequent. Clinical correlation and careful examination for any vascular architecture and vasoformative features are helpful.

It may be challenging to distinguish angiosarcoma from epithelioid haemangioendothelioma (EHE), because these tumour types share many cytomorphological features, including spindle and epithelioid morphology, round nuclei, eccentric cytoplasm, and intracytoplasmic vacuoles. EHE is more likely to show myxohyaline stroma and a more uniform cell population, with mild to moderate nuclear atypia.

Ancillary testing

Angiosarcomas are positive for the endothelial markers CD31, CD34, and ERG {953}; however, these markers do not distinguish angiosarcoma from other vascular neoplasms. Angiosarcoma may stain for keratin, and this is most frequent in epithelioid angiosarcoma (50%) {941}. Radiation-associated angiosarcomas and lymphoedema-associated angiosarcomas show nuclear MYC staining secondary to *MYC* amplification {523,870}. The differential diagnosis includes melanomas, which are positive for S100, SOX10, HMB45, and melan-A (MART1), and epithelioid sarcoma, which like angiosarcoma shows positivity for CD34, ERG, and keratin, but is characterized by loss of SMARCB1 (INI1). EHE also expresses endothelial markers, but it is defined by the *CAMTA1*::*WWTR1* fusion, resulting in ICC nuclear staining for CAMTA1, which is highly sensitive and specific for EHE {357}.

Malignant peripheral nerve sheath tumour

Jo VY
Monaco SE
VandenBussche CJ

Definition
Malignant peripheral nerve sheath tumour (MPNST) is a malignant spindle cell neoplasm with limited Schwann cell differentiation, characterized by concurrent inactivating mutations involving three pathways: *NF1*, *CDKN2A/CDKN2B*, and PRC2 core components (*SUZ12* or *EED*).

Clinical features and imaging
MPNSTs arise most commonly in patients aged 20–50 years, although they may arise in younger patients, including children, in the context of neurofibromatosis type 1 (NF1). MPNST can arise from a peripheral nerve, from a pre-existing benign nerve sheath tumour, or in a patient with NF1; approximately 50% of cases are associated with NF1 {406}, and about 10% arise after radiation therapy {430}.

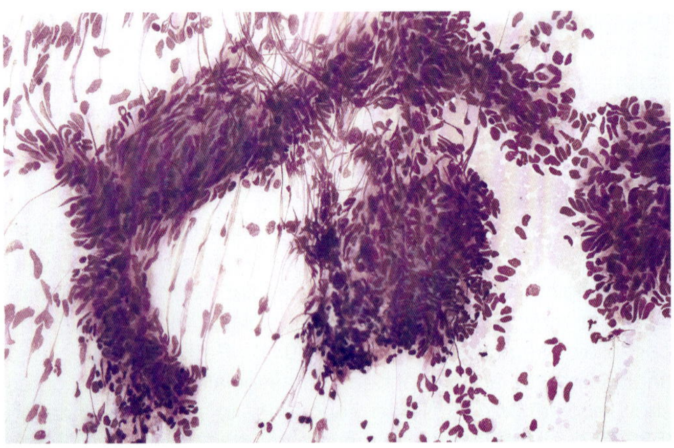

Fig. 8.109 Malignant peripheral nerve sheath tumour. Hypercellular, large cohesive tissue fragments of atypical spindle cells, with single dissociated tumour cells and stripped nuclei in the background (Giemsa).

Most patients present with an enlarging mass, which may be painful, and patients may experience neuropathic symptoms with intraneural tumours. The extremities, trunk, and head and neck are the most common sites {792,367}.

The distinct variant epithelioid MPNST is not associated with NF1 and is characterized by *SMARCB1* inactivation {648,1251}.

Overall, MPNSTs are aggressive, with poor prognosis.

Histopathology
MPNST is composed of fascicles of spindle cells, often interlacing and with alternating areas of hypercellularity and hypocellularity, imparting a marbled appearance. Tumours have characteristic thin-walled and irregular "staghorn" or haemangiopericytoma-like vessels, and many cases show dense perivascular growth of tumour cells. Geographical necrosis and high mitotic activity are common, particularly in high-grade tumours. Tumour cells have spindle, wavy, or serpentine hyperchromatic nuclei and pale eosinophilic cytoplasm. There is nuclear enlargement and mild atypia, but MPNSTs typically show an overall uniformity, with prominent pleomorphism seen in occasional cases. Heterologous differentiation occurs in about 15% of MPNSTs and can be rhabdomyoblastic in the so-called "triton tumour", osseous, cartilaginous, vascular, or epithelial, which can be glandular or squamous.

There may be infiltration into pre-existing peripheral neve sheath tissue or a precursor neurofibroma, and a spectrum of different degrees of malignant progression within a given tumour may be observed in NF1-associated cases.

Epithelioid MPNST shows predominant epithelioid morphology, with lobulated growth, frequently fibromyxoid stroma, and round nuclei with prominent nucleoli in cells with abundant eosinophilic cytoplasm.

Key diagnostic cytopathological features
- High cellularity

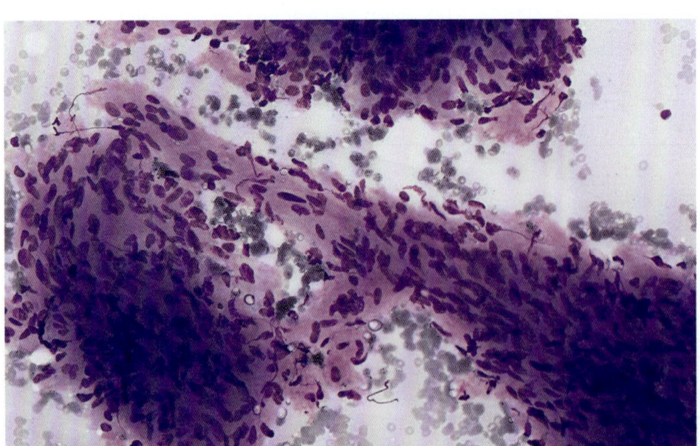

Fig. 8.110 Malignant peripheral nerve sheath tumour. Cohesive tissue fragments showing spindle cells arranged in vague fascicles (Giemsa).

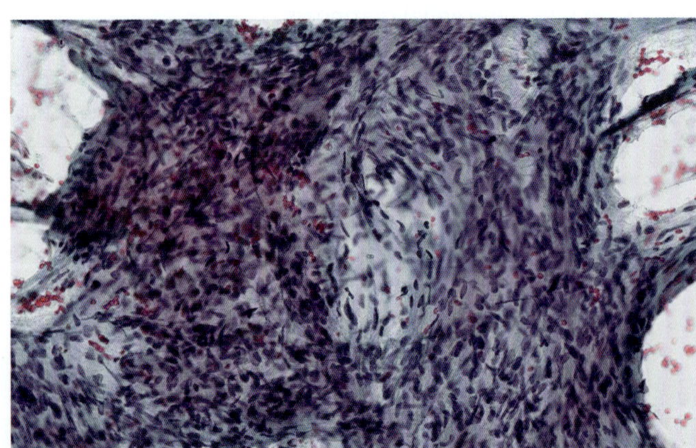

Fig. 8.111 Malignant peripheral nerve sheath tumour. A large tissue fragment consisting of spindle cells in a poorly formed fascicular growth pattern (Pap).

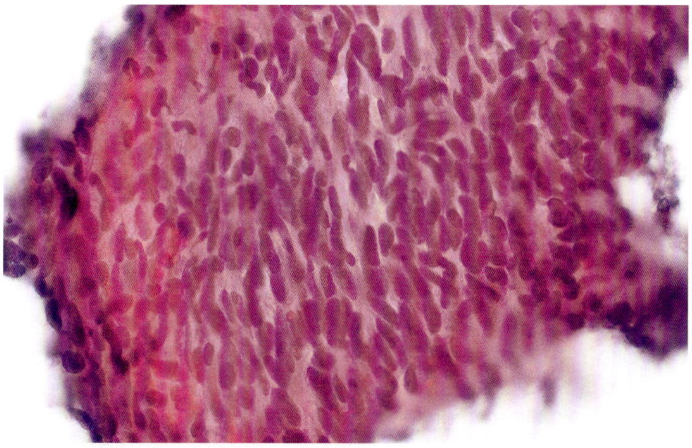

Fig. 8.112 Malignant peripheral nerve sheath tumour. Fascicular growth architecture may be seen in tissue fragments (Pap).

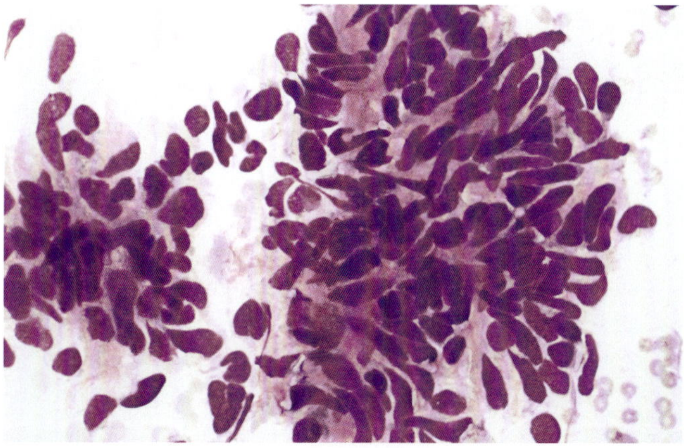

Fig. 8.113 Malignant peripheral nerve sheath tumour. Enlarged, hyperchromatic, ovoid or buckled nuclei, often with tapering ends (Giemsa).

- Large syncytial tissue fragments with vague fascicular growth, as well as single intact cells
- Overall uniform size and shape of cells, with ovoid or buckled, hyperchromatic nuclei with evenly dispersed chromatin and small or inconspicuous nucleoli and sparse to more abundant elongated cytoplasm with tapering ends
- Necrosis and stripped nuclei frequently seen in the background
- Less commonly tumours may show a fibrillary myxoid stroma
- Marked pleomorphism may be seen in high-grade tumours
- Heterologous rhabdomyoblastic differentiation with scattered large rhabdomyoblasts with abundant eccentric cytoplasm can be seen
- Epithelioid MPNSTs show large epithelioid cells, often in tissue fragments with myxoid or fibrillary extracellular matrix

Reference(s): {731,526,1466,642,1250}

Discussion and differential diagnosis

Distinguishing MPNST from other spindle cell sarcomas often requires ancillary testing. In the context of association with a peripheral nerve or schwannoma or neurofibroma, or the setting of NF1 or prior radiation therapy, MPNST should be a chief consideration. MPNSTs arising de novo are more challenging to recognize.

Mimics of MPNST include cellular schwannoma, leiomyosarcoma, synovial sarcoma, solitary fibrous tumour, and dedifferentiated liposarcoma. Cellular schwannoma lacks cytopathological atypia. Leiomyosarcomas arising in soft tissue sites are often associated with a large vessel. ICC is required for other tumours.

Epithelioid MPNST may closely mimic amelanotic malignant melanoma, and ICC is helpful.

Ancillary testing

The majority of MPNSTs are negative for the Schwann cell markers S100, SOX10, and GFAP, but positive patchy and focal staining for any of these markers occurs in 30% of cases {668}. Tumours with heterologous differentiation show expression of corresponding markers, such as desmin and myogenin in rhabdomyoblasts and keratin in epithelium. In the differential diagnosis, schwannomas show strong and diffuse staining for S100 and SOX10, which are either negative or focal in MPNST.

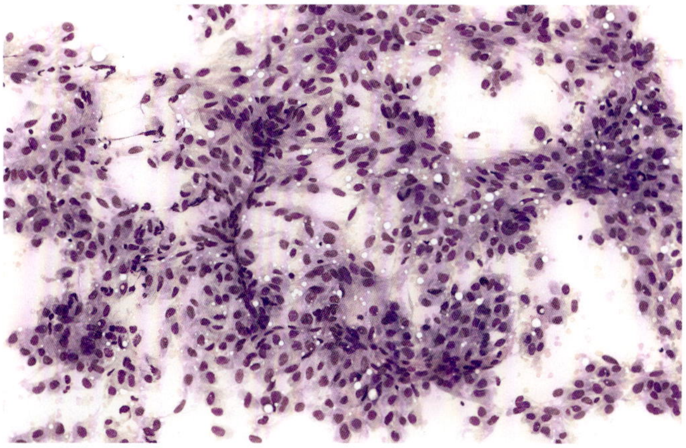

Fig. 8.114 Malignant peripheral nerve sheath tumour. A mix of spindle and epithelioid cells (Giemsa).

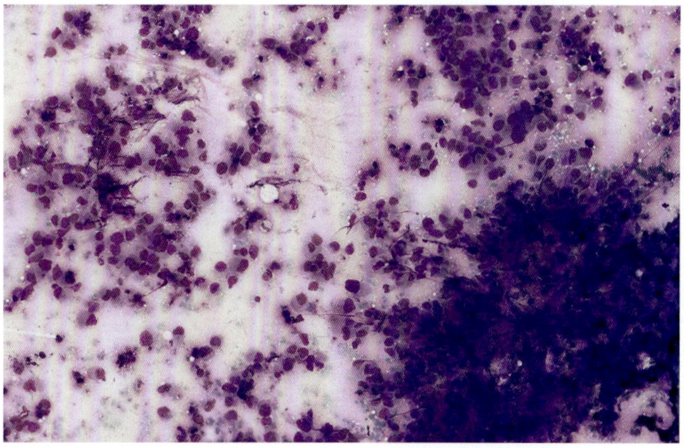

Fig. 8.115 Malignant peripheral nerve sheath tumour. Epithelioid cells in a cohesive tissue fragment and singly in background, with some stripped nuclei. The cells have a high N:C ratio and a small amount of spindle or eccentric cytoplasm (Giemsa).

Leiomyosarcomas express the smooth muscle markers SMA, desmin, and caldesmon. Molecular alterations for which sensitive and specific diagnostic ICC markers are available can differentiate synovial sarcoma with SS18-SSX and SSX, solitary fibrous tumour with STAT6, and dedifferentiated liposarcoma with MDM2 and CDK4.

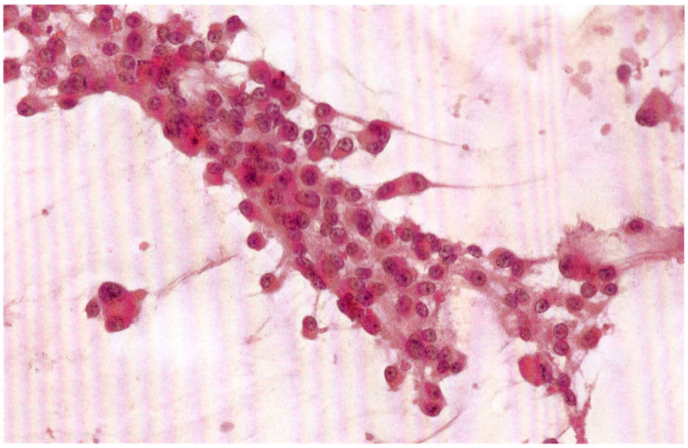

Fig. 8.116 Epithelioid malignant peripheral nerve sheath tumour. Large epithelioid cells with round to pleomorphic nuclei with prominent nucleoli; there is perinucleolar clearing ("vesicular" chromatin) in some nuclei and occasional binucleation (H&E).

Epithelioid MPNSTs show strong and diffuse staining for S100 and SOX10, with retained H3 p.K28me3 (K27me3), and they are consistently negative for the melanocytic markers HMB45 and melan-A (MART1), distinguishing them from amelanotic melanoma. Unlike in conventional MPNST, SMARCB1 loss is characteristic in epithelioid MPNST {648,1251}, but it can also be seen in other epithelioid tumours, including the mimic proximal-type epithelioid sarcoma. Epithelioid sarcoma is negative for S100 and SOX10, positive for keratins and EMA, and frequently positive for CD34.

Loss of H3 p.K28me3 (K27me3) secondary to PRC2 inactivation can be detected by ICC in MPNST, and complete loss of staining for H3 p.K28me3 (K27me3) is seen in 50–80% of all cases, typically in high-grade and radiation-induced tumours {1091,1130,1253,1056,957}. However, nonspecific partial loss may be seen in a subset of MPNSTs. ATRX loss and an alternative-lengthening-of-telomeres phenotype has been described in a small subset of NF-1 associated MPNSTs {1191,846}.

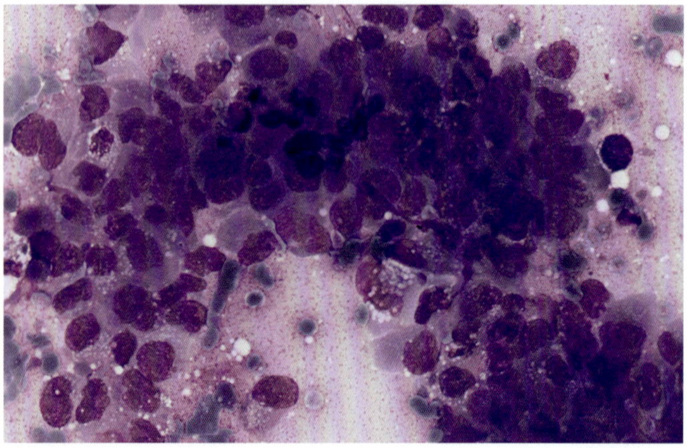

Fig. 8.117 Malignant peripheral nerve sheath tumour. Rhabdomyoblastic differentiation, with larger cells with abundant eccentric cytoplasm and highly pleomorphic nuclei among epithelioid tumour cells ("triton tumour") (Giemsa).

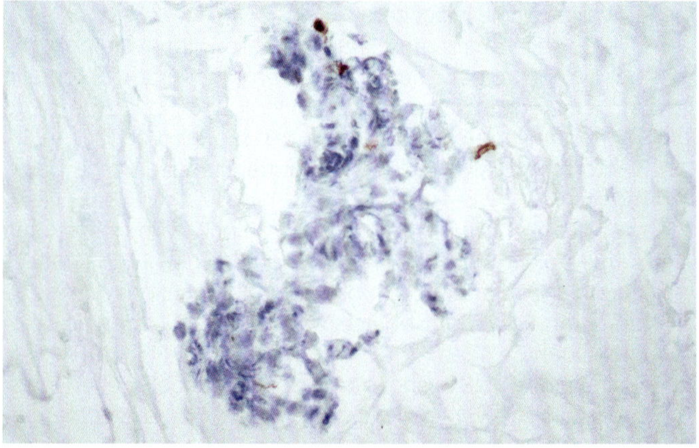

Fig. 8.118 Malignant peripheral nerve sheath tumour. Loss of expression of H3 p.K28me3 (K27me3) in malignant peripheral sheath tumour is most commonly seen in higher-grade tumours. Note the positive lymphocytes, a useful positive internal control (cell block, ICC).

Malignant melanotic nerve sheath tumour

Jo VY
Agaram NP

Definition

Malignant melanotic nerve sheath tumour (MMNST) is a rare peripheral nerve sheath tumour composed uniformly of Schwann cells showing melanocytic differentiation, usually arising in association with spinal or autonomic nerves; it is variably associated with Carney complex and frequently shows aggressive clinical behaviour. *PRKAR1A* mutations and loss of PRKAR1A protein expression are seen in the overwhelming majority of cases.

Clinical features and imaging

MMNST primarily affects adults and is rare in children. Patients with Carney complex who develop MMNST are typically younger (mean: 22.5 years) than patients with sporadic cases (mean: 33.2 years), and they tend to develop multiple tumours {179,1417}. Most cases arise in association with spinal or autonomic nerves. Although most cases have been reported in midline sites, MMNST rarely arises elsewhere in the gastrointestinal tract, soft tissues, bone, heart, bronchus, liver, and skin {208, 210}. Presenting symptoms include pain, sensory abnormalities, and tumour-related mass effects.

MMNST frequently shows aggressive behaviour, with as many as half of all affected patients developing local recurrence or metastasis {1436,1417,1483,703}.

Histopathology

MMNST is composed of short fascicles and sheets of polygonal to spindle cells, which may have heavy cytoplasmic melanin pigment deposition, varying from coarsely clumped to finely granular and often obscuring the nucleus. Tumour cells have round or spindle nuclei with characteristic nuclear grooves and pseudoinclusions, as well as small nucleoli. The cytoplasm is amphophilic or eosinophilic and may appear syncytial. Areas of vague palisading and whorled architecture may be seen. Some examples may show marked nuclear atypia and large macronucleoli, as well as high mitotic activity and necrosis. Psammoma bodies are present in at least half of all cases.

Key diagnostic cytopathological features

- High cellularity
- Tissue fragments, some of which are discohesive, composed of spindle and polygonal cells with plump or spindle nuclei having small nucleoli, nuclear grooves, and occasional pseudoinclusions
- Enlarged nuclei show mild atypia
- Thin, tapering cytoplasmic processes with variable melanin pigmentation
- Psammoma bodies may be present but are not always sampled

Reference(s): {983,1131,1326,874,269,596}

Discussion and differential diagnosis

There are only rare reports of the cytopathological features of MMNST, with just two cases in the setting of Carney complex {983} and most cases being sporadic {1131,1326,874,269, 596}. MMNST is indistinguishable from malignant melanoma in many instances, especially since psammoma bodies may not be present, and clinical correlation is required to exclude metastatic malignant melanoma. Clinical findings suggesting features of Carney complex, including myxoma, endocrine neoplasms, and pigmented skin lesions, support MMNST.

Ancillary testing

By ICC, MMNST shows strong staining for S100 and SOX10, as well as the melanocytic markers HMB45, melan-A, and tyrosinase. Loss of PRKAR1A expression is seen in most cases {1417,1483}; it is diagnostic of MMNST and is not a feature of melanoma.

Molecular testing may resolve challenging cases, because malignant melanoma arising in cutaneous sites has characteristic driver mutations, including *BRAF*, *KRAS*, *NRAS*, *NF1*, *KIT*, and *TERT* mutations, as well as ultraviolet (UV)-associated mutation signatures {769}. Notably, CNS melanocytomas, uveal melanomas, and melanomas arising in blue naevi have a distinctive molecular profile of activating *GNAQ* or *GNA11* mutations, as well as additional *BAP1* and *SF3B1* mutations {769,259}, and they may show a more uniform appearance that closely mimics that of MMNST.

Infantile fibrosarcoma

Teot LA
Jo VY

Definition

Infantile fibrosarcoma (IFS) is a malignant fibroblastic tumour most commonly occurring in infancy, frequently characterized by an *ETV6::NTRK3* fusion.

Clinical features and imaging

IFS is a locally aggressive and rapidly growing tumour that only rarely metastasizes. The superficial or deep soft tissues of the extremities are the most common sites of involvement, followed by the trunk and the head and neck {240,229}. The typical presentation is rapid growth of a painless mass or exophytic nodule {229}, and superficial tumours may ulcerate and appear vascular {1531}. Rarely, tumours may present in intra-abdominal, retroperitoneal, or visceral sites {240,229,1051,1079}. One third of cases occur congenitally {229}. Analogous tumours that arise in the kidney are termed "cellular congenital mesoblastic nephroma".

Imaging features are nonspecific, and IFS typically appears as a heterogeneously enhancing mass on ultrasound, CT, or MRI, sometimes with a prominent vascular component {671, 1012}. Extensive haemorrhage may be seen, particularly in larger tumours {1531,692,24}.

Histopathology

IFS most commonly appears as a uniform fascicular or sheet-like proliferation of monomorphic spindle to ovoid cells, but it may show a broad histopathological spectrum {293}. Some IFSs may show a haphazard architecture, a more primitive round cell population, or stellate morphology. Most tumours show a characteristic vascular component composed of ectatic, irregularly branching (haemangiopericytoma-like) vessels, which can be numerous. The stroma ranges from myxoid to collagenous, and some examples with less cellularity may resemble fibromatosis or myofibroma {238,293}. A prominent chronic inflammatory

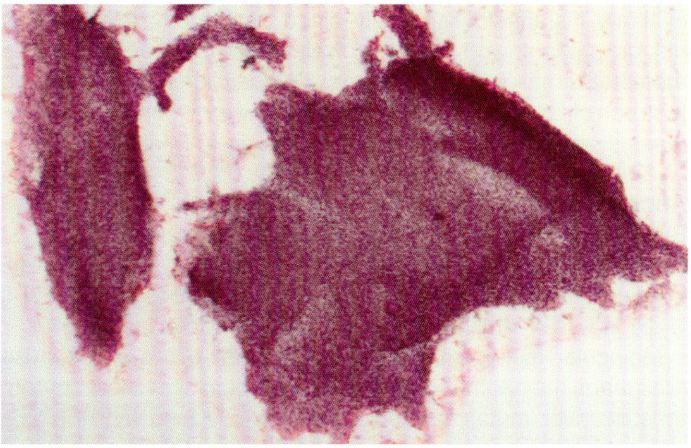

Fig. 8.119 Infantile fibrosarcoma. Cohesive large tissue fragments consisting of relatively monomorphic spindle cells (H&E).

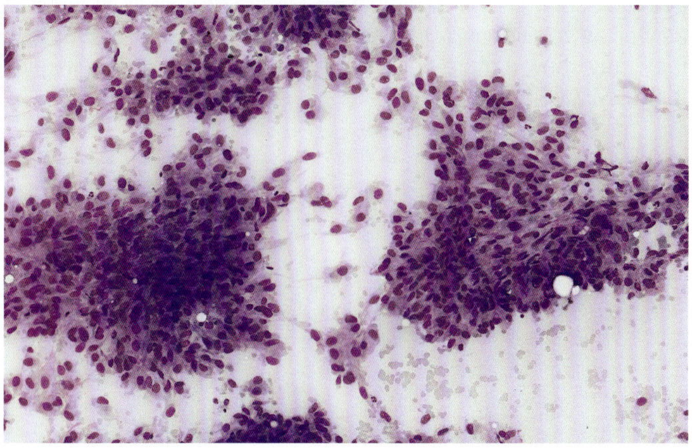

Fig. 8.120 Infantile fibrosarcoma. Tissue fragments of ovoid to spindle cells with mildly pleomorphic elongated nuclei with fine chromatin and few mitoses (Giemsa).

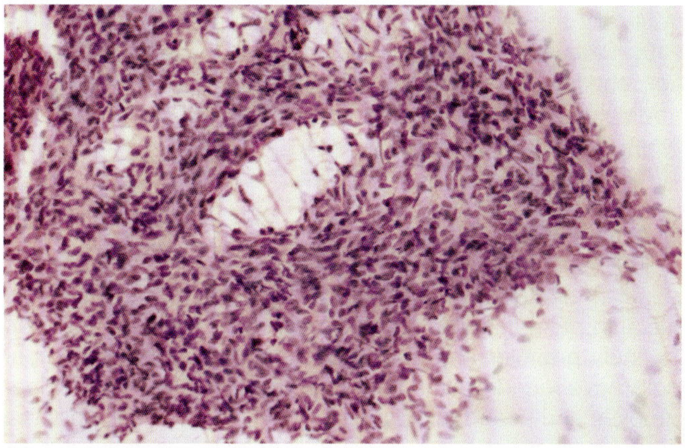

Fig. 8.121 Infantile fibrosarcoma. A cohesive dense tissue fragment of spindle cells with mildly pleomorphic elongated nuclei showing fine chromatin, arranged haphazardly (H&E).

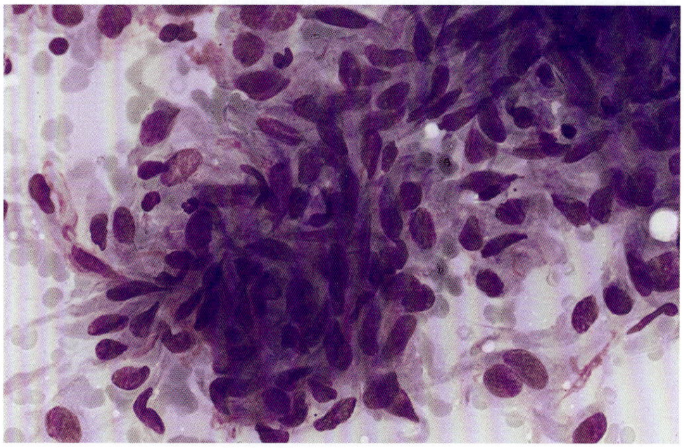

Fig. 8.122 Infantile fibrosarcoma. Plump spindle cells with elongated nuclei with fine chromatin and inconspicuous nucleoli in tissue fragments and singly (Giemsa).

infiltrate may be seen. IFS frequently shows infiltrative growth into adjacent normal tissue. Mitotic figures can range from rare to numerous, but atypical forms are rare. Necrosis may be present.

Key diagnostic cytopathological features

- Variable cellularity
- Cohesive sheets, tissue fragments, and singly dispersed cells, with scattered bare, stripped nuclei
- Haphazard to vague fascicular arrangement of cells in tissue fragments
- Monomorphic, spindle to ovoid cells with homogeneous cytoplasm
- Oval to elongate, mildly pleomorphic nuclei with smooth contours, fine chromatin, and indistinct nucleoli, with variable mitoses
- Necrosis may be present

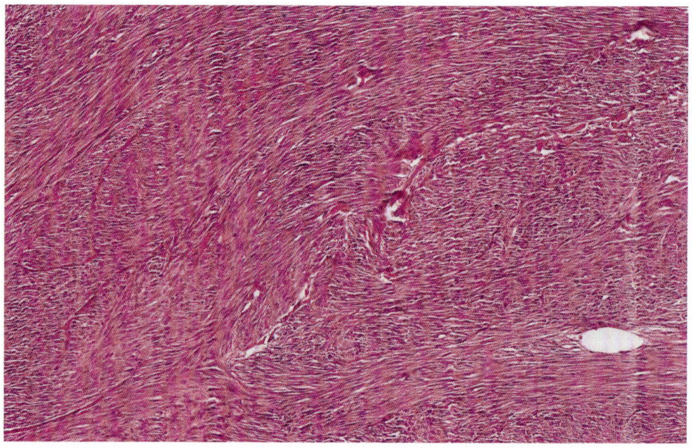

Fig. 8.123 Infantile fibrosarcoma. Densely arrayed uniform spindle cells in fascicles. Blood vessels are not prominent in this tumour (tissue section, H&E).

Discussion and differential diagnosis

Cytopathological findings have not been clearly defined in the rare reports of FNAB of IFS {712,520}. However, the cytopathological features of cellular congenital mesoblastic nephroma, a renal tumour morphologically and molecularly identical to IFS, are presumed to be similar {1122,529,760,122}.

Significant morphological overlap exists between IFS and various benign, intermediate, and malignant paediatric mesenchymal neoplasms {238}. Distinction between these entities requires ICC and often molecular studies, as well as correlation with the clinical presentation.

Ancillary testing

The immunoprofile is nonspecific. Tumours variably express SMA, CD34, S100, and desmin. IFS with NTRK rearrangements usually shows diffuse positivity for pan-TRK {238,293}. Detection of *ETV6::NTRK3* or variant rearrangements by FISH, RT-PCR, or targeted NGS is helpful for confirming the diagnosis.

Chapter 8

Spindle cell / sclerosing rhabdomyosarcoma

Agaram NP
Jo VY
Rekhi B

Definition

Spindle cell / sclerosing rhabdomyosarcoma (RMS) is a type of RMS that has fascicular spindle cell and/or sclerosing morphology.

Clinical features and imaging

"Fusion-associated spindle and sclerosing rhabdomyosarcomas", including infantile cases characterized by a recurrent *VGLL2*-related fusion {44}, and "*MYOD1*-mutant spindle cell / sclerosing rhabdomyosarcoma" {1166}, have replaced the single group "spindle cell / sclerosing rhabdomyosarcoma", based on morphology, genetic changes, and importantly clinical outcomes {1180,795} in the forthcoming sixth-edition WHO classification of soft tissue and bone tumours. The varying FNAB findings of these two new entities are yet to be fully elucidated, and the following sections are based on the fifth edition at this stage.

Spindle cell / sclerosing RMS accounts for 3–10% of all RMS cases. It affects infants, children, and adults. The tumours usually present as a rapidly growing, painless soft tissue mass, with symptoms related to local compression at the tumour site. The head and neck region is the most common site of involvement, followed by the extremities. Rarely, other locations are affected, such as viscera (uterus, prostate), retroperitoneum, or bone {1010,186,513,713,901,16,438,1492,85,779,288,972,924,1562}.

Histopathology

Spindle cell RMS is characterized by cellular fascicles of spindle cells with an intersecting or herringbone growth pattern, resembling leiomyosarcoma or fibrosarcoma. The spindle neoplastic cells have pale eosinophilic cytoplasm and blunt, ovoid, or fusiform, centrally located nuclei with small inconspicuous nucleoli. Mitotic figures, nuclear atypia, and hyperchromatic nuclei are often present. Primitive undifferentiated areas with round cells and hyperchromatic nuclei may also be present focally. Sclerosing RMSs show prominent hyalinizing sclerosis, with tumour cells arranged in cords, nests, microalveoli, or trabeculae in a pseudovascular growth pattern, with prominent intervening sclerosis noted {14,1010,186,815,924}. The recently described intraosseous spindle cell RMSs show, apart from the typical spindle cell morphology, areas of distinctly epithelioid cells arranges in sheets and fascicles {1492,288,16,795}.

Key diagnostic cytopathological features

Sclerosing rhabdomyosarcoma

- Low cellularity
- Tissue fragments of varying size consisting of round to polygonal cells with round to oval nuclei and variable amount of ill-defined cytoplasm
- Wisps of intervening metachromatic stroma between the cells may be seen in Giemsa-stained smears

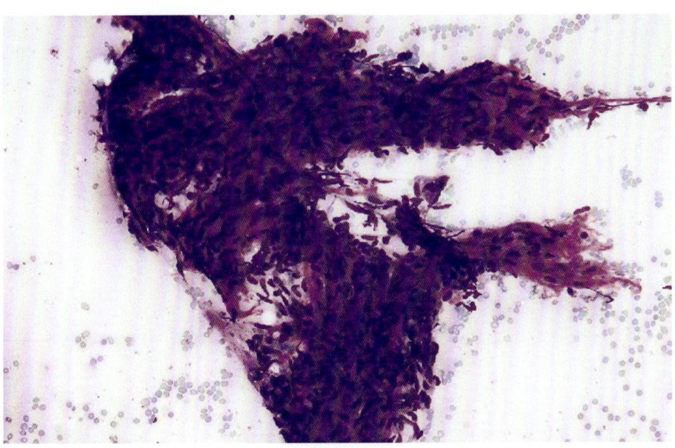

Fig. 8.124 Spindle cell rhabdomyosarcoma. A tissue fragment with fascicles of spindle cells with minimal cytoplasm (Giemsa).

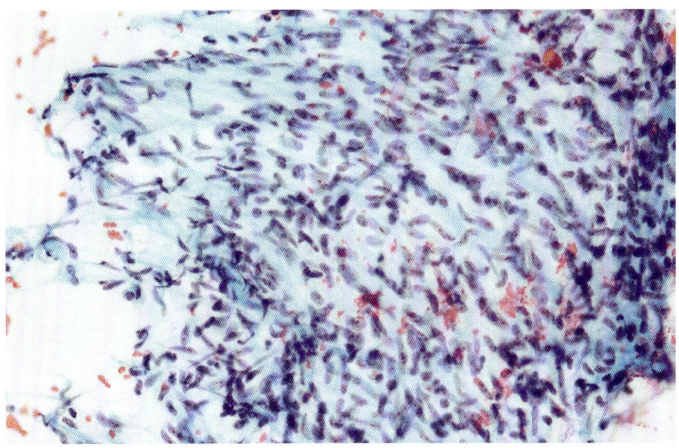

Fig. 8.125 Spindle cell rhabdomyosarcoma. A tissue fragment of poorly formed fascicles of spindle cells with moderately pleomorphic elongated nuclei with tapered ends and nucleoli (Pap).

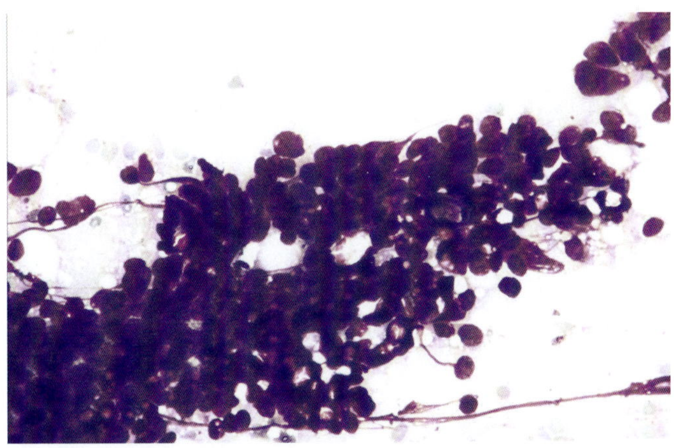

Fig. 8.126 Sclerosing rhabdomyosarcoma. A crowded, loosely cohesive tissue fragment composed of cells with round to oval nuclei and minimal to scant cytoplasm (Giemsa).

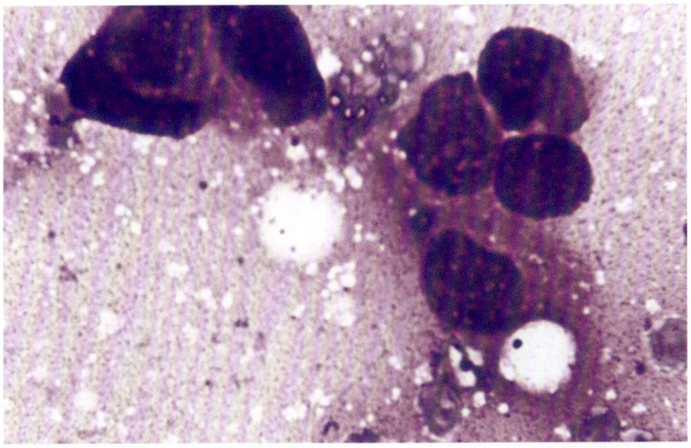

Fig. 8.127 Sclerosing rhabdomyosarcoma. A minute tissue fragment consisting of tumour cells displaying round to oval nuclei and moderate to abundant, ill-defined cytoplasm (Giemsa).

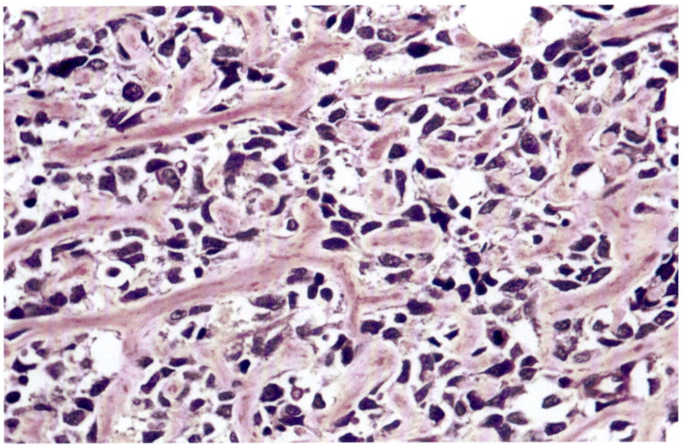

Fig. 8.128 Sclerosing rhabdomyosarcoma. Cells with round to oval, hyperchromatic nuclei and a variable amount of eosinophilic cytoplasm, embedded in a densely hyalinized sclerotic stroma (tissue section, H&E).

Spindle cell rhabdomyosarcoma

- Moderate cellularity
- Loose and tightly cohesive tissue fragments showing fascicles of spindle cells with oval to spindle hyperchromatic nuclei and a minimal to moderate amount of ill-defined bluish to vacuolated cytoplasm (Giemsa)
- Cellular stromal fragments and a variable number of macrophages

Reference(s): {1166}

Discussion and differential diagnosis

The differential diagnosis includes synovial sarcoma, malignant peripheral nerve sheath tumour, and various malignant spindle and round cell tumours {1166}. The lack of arborizing vascular structures is useful in ruling out a synovial sarcoma despite the presence of relatively monomorphic round to oval cells {1452}. Leiomyosarcomas display a variable number of spindle cells with blunt-ended nuclei and/or epithelioid cells. Malignant peripheral nerve sheath tumour is a spindle cell sarcoma that may show heterologous rhabdomyoblastic differentiation, often closely mimicking spindle cell RMS and distinguished by ICC {1101,1466}. The presence of spindle nuclei is helpful in largely ruling out Ewing sarcoma and other round cell malignancies, and ICC can be diagnostic.

Ancillary testing

Spindle cell / sclerosing RMS is characterized in ICC by variable but often diffuse expression of desmin and only focal expression of myogenin (MYF4) in most cases. MYOD1 staining can be focal or diffuse in spindle cell RMS, but the new entity in the forthcoming sixth-edition WHO classification of soft tissue and bone tumours, "*MYOD1*-mutant spindle cell / sclerosing rhabdomyosarcoma", usually shows diffuse MYOD1 positivity. A subset of cases of the recently described intraosseous spindle cell RMS can also show positivity for keratin and ALK {237}. Synovial sarcoma harbours *SS18*::SSX fusions, which can be detected by FISH for *SS18* or ICC for SS18::SSX and SSX. Leiomyosarcoma is positive for desmin, but it is also positive for SMA and caldesmon and negative for myogenin {346}. Spindle cell RMS can be differentiated from malignant peripheral nerve sheath tumour by its staining for skeletal muscle markers and negativity for Schwannian markers, as well as the expression of S100, SOX10, GFAP, and H3 p.K28me3 (K27me3) {582}.

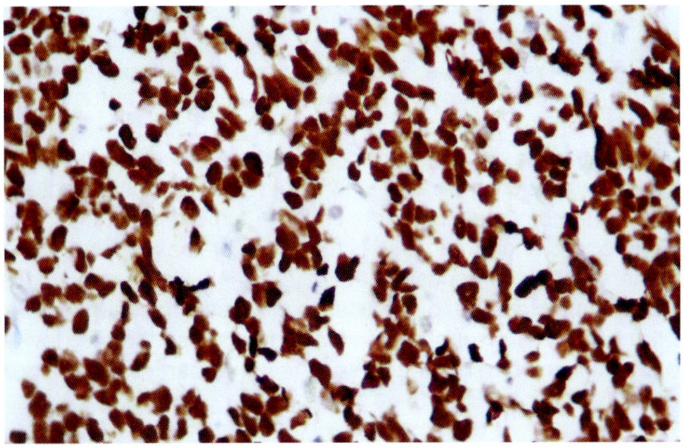

Fig. 8.129 Sclerosing rhabdomyosarcoma. Tumour cells displaying diffusely positive MYOD1 (tissue section, ICC).

Extrarenal rhabdoid tumour

Dodd LG
Monaco SE

Definition

Extrarenal rhabdoid tumour (ERT) is a highly malignant soft tissue tumour, mainly affecting infants and children, that consists of characteristic round or polygonal neoplastic cells with eccentric glassy eosinophilic cytoplasm containing hyaline-like inclusion bodies, as well as macronucleoli. Morphologically and genetically identical tumours also arise in the kidney and brain. The majority of tumours are characterized by biallelic alterations of *SMARCB1*, leading to loss of expression of SMARCB1 (INI1).

Clinical features and imaging

ERT affects very young infants and neonates. Rare congenital cases have been documented with dissemination of tumour to the placenta {150,194}. ERT arises in the deep soft tissues of the extremities; abdominal, pelvic, and retroperitoneal areas; and head and neck region. ERT can also occur in visceral organs. ERT most commonly presents as large tumorous nodules, but it can occasionally manifest as multiple metastases, commonly in the skin. The prognosis for ERT is dismal, with a majority of patients succumbing to metastases or dissemination of tumour {209,1282}. A subset of patients are predisposed to the development of one or more rhabdoid tumours as part of a predisposition syndrome {1339,10}.

Histopathology

ERT shows sheets of undifferentiated cells with a rhabdoid appearance. Individual cells have abundant eccentric dense eosinophilic cytoplasm, clear chromatin, and a large nucleolus. There is often a paranuclear dense eosinophilic inclusion or globule that corresponds to intermediate filaments. Necrosis is frequently present, and mitoses are easily identifiable.

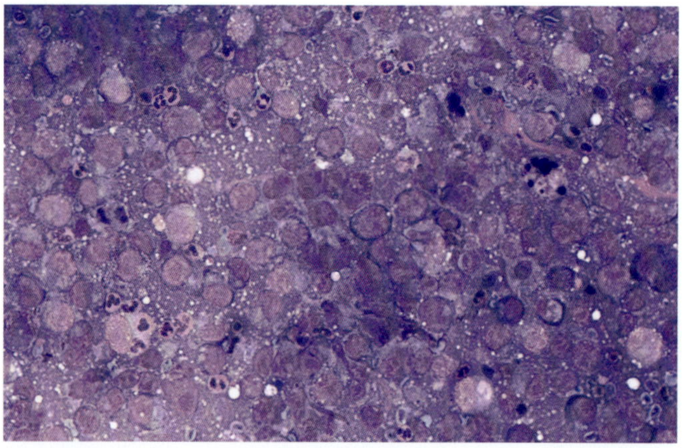

Fig. 8.130 Extrarenal rhabdoid tumour. A highly cellular smear showing large cells with a high N:C ratio, round to more pleomorphic nuclei, and macronucleoli (Giemsa).

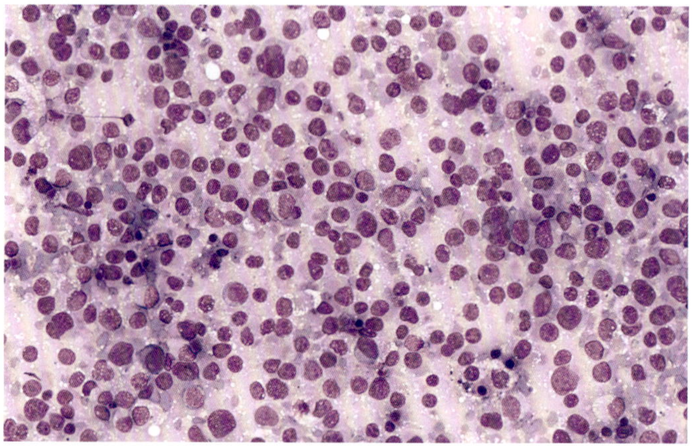

Fig. 8.131 Extrarenal rhabdoid tumour. Single large cells with round to pleomorphic nuclei, some cells with eccentric cytoplasm (Giemsa).

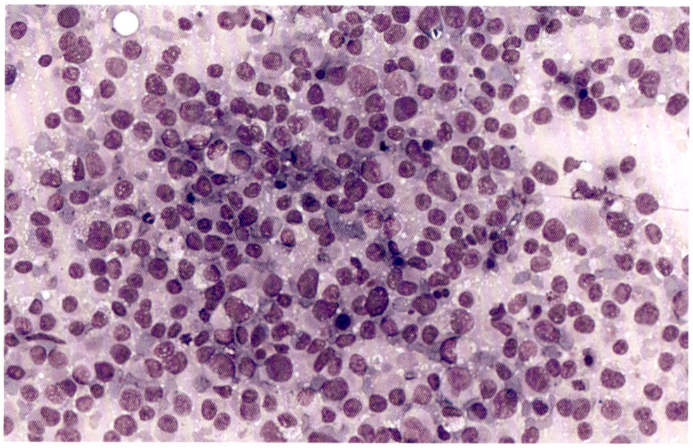

Fig. 8.132 Extrarenal rhabdoid tumour. Predominantly single cells with round to pleomorphic large nuclei, nucleoli, and eccentric cytoplasm, occasionally containing fine vacuoles (Giemsa).

Key diagnostic cytopathological features

- Variable cellularity
- Large cells seen singly and in loosely cohesive tissue fragments
- High N:C ratio
- Eccentric pale blue to basophilic (Giemsa) cytoplasm
- Large nuclei with macronucleoli
- Nuclear chromatin is fine and clear

Reference(s): {1468,366,1325}

Discussion and differential diagnosis

The differential diagnosis of malignant rhabdoid tumour includes a number of paediatric neoplasms in the "small round blue cell tumour" category, such as rhabdomyosarcoma, desmoplastic

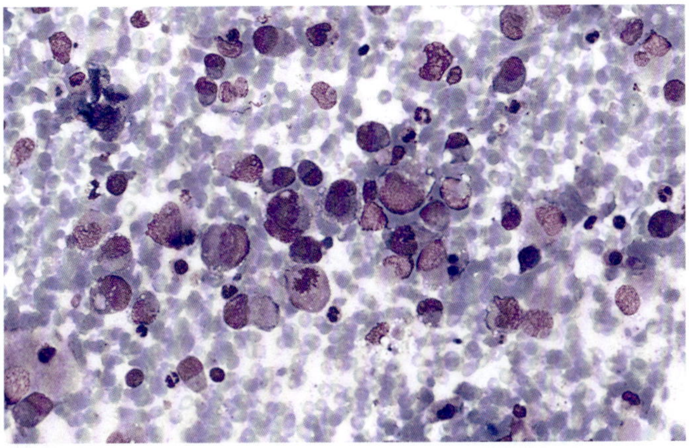

Fig. 8.133 Extrarenal rhabdoid tumour. Large cells with round to often markedly pleomorphic nuclei and abundant eccentric cytoplasm. An atypical mitosis is noted, with some apoptotic debris (Giemsa).

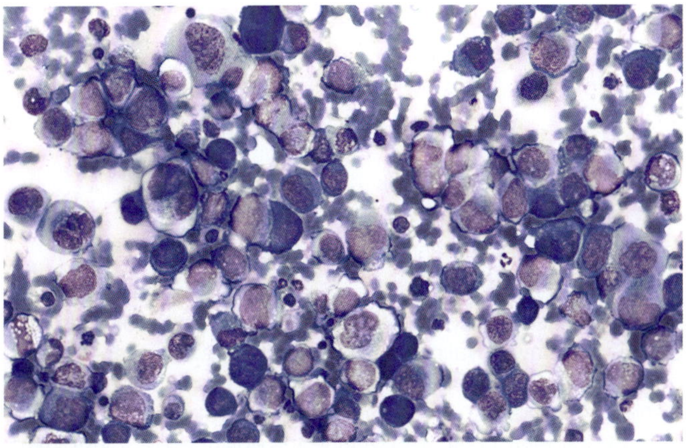

Fig. 8.134 Extrarenal rhabdoid tumour. Minute tissue fragments and single large cells with variably sized nuclei varying from round to highly pleomorphic with macronucleoli and often with abundant eccentric cytoplasm (Giemsa).

round cell sarcoma, Wilms tumour, and Ewing sarcoma, requiring ICC to make a diagnosis.

Ancillary testing

ERT is variably positive for CD99 and markers of neuroendocrine differentiation {1076,398}. ERT shows loss of SMARCB1 (INI1) expression {572}. Affected individuals have germline mutations or deletions affecting the *SMARCB1* locus on chromosome 22 {151}. Rhabdoid tumours coexpress vimentin and markers of epithelial differentiation such as EMA or keratin (which frequently presents in a paranuclear pattern).

Epithelioid haemangioendothelioma

VandenBussche CJ
Domanski HA

Definition

Epithelioid haemangioendothelioma (EHE) is a malignant vascular neoplasm composed of epithelioid endothelial cells with a distinctive myxohyaline stroma. Most cases are characterized by a *WWTR1::CAMTA1* gene fusion, but a small subset show distinct morphology, with well-formed vessels lined by epithelioid endothelial cells with abundant eosinophilic cytoplasm, and are characterized by a *YAP1::TFE3* fusion.

Clinical features and imaging

In the forthcoming sixth-edition WHO classification of soft tissue and bone tumours, *YAP1::TFE3* haemangioendotheliomas have been separated from EHE {152}, but at this stage, this entity is presented here to compare with EHE.

EHE can arise at any site but most commonly involves deep soft tissues, lung, and liver. Skin and soft tissue lesions are usually solitary {1497,1140,919}, whereas visceral and bone lesions are often multifocal and may be metastatic at presentation {618, 862,130,1428,722}.

EHE usually arises in adults and is rare in children {322}. Cases have a wide age distribution among adults, but patients with *YAP1::TFE3* fusion tumours tend to be younger than those with a *WWTR1::CAMTA1* fusion {70}. Visceral lesions have a slight female predominance {322,919,1499}.

In soft tissues, EHEs usually present as a painful mass. Those arising from large vessels can result in other symptoms of vascular occlusion, such as oedema and thrombophlebitis. EHE of the liver is usually an incidental finding, but it may cause abdominal pain, weight loss, ascites, hemoperitoneum, or portal hypertension {862,1372}. Thoracic tumours are more likely to be symptomatic, causing pain, cough, dyspnoea, or haemoptysis {780}. Approximately 20% of patients with thoracic EHE are asymptomatic, with incidentally detected disease.

EHE of soft tissues can be indolent, but approximately 21% of cases metastasize and pursue an aggressive clinical course, leading to death in approximately 17% of patients {1497,919, 322,386,429}. EHE arising in lung or bone has a worse prognosis than soft tissue tumours, and patients often present with metastatic disease {1287,62,862,780}. In contrast, cutaneous EHE has an excellent prognosis {919,1140}.

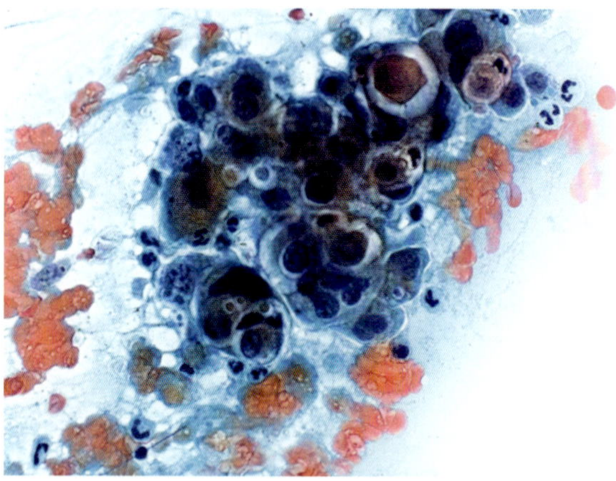

Fig. 8.135 Epithelioid haemangioendothelioma. A small tissue fragment demonstrates the complexity of vacuolization that can be seen in epithelioid haemangioendothelioma, with red cells and neutrophils in some vacuoles, and a striking "cell-within-a-cell" morphology, with cells apparently wrapped in larger cells. The nuclei vary in size, degree of pleomorphism and coarse chromatin, and prominence of nucleoli (Pap).

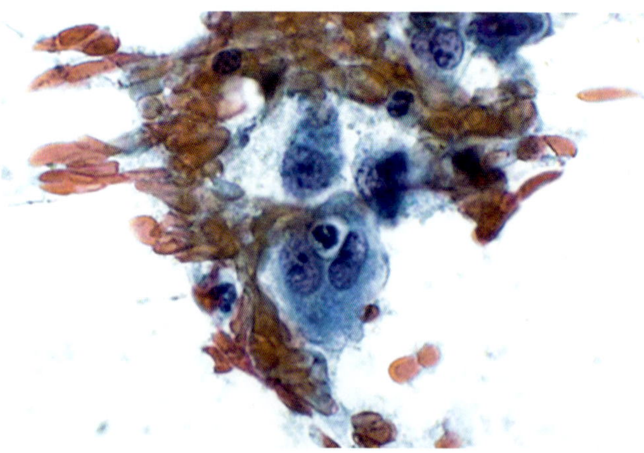

Fig. 8.136 Epithelioid haemangioendothelioma. A binucleated cell with a neutrophil in an intracytoplasmic lumen between the two nuclei (centre) and several other large neoplastic cells containing variable amounts of cytoplasm and showing large pleomorphic nuclei (Pap).

Histopathology

EHEs form cords and nests of cells in a myxohyaline stroma. The cells are epithelioid, with a moderate amount of eosinophilic cytoplasm. The cytoplasm sometimes contains intracytoplasmic vacuoles, which may be empty or contain red blood cells. The cells have round nuclei and inconspicuous nucleoli {919,1367}. EHEs with *YAP1::TFE3* fusion are more likely to have a solid growth pattern, show brightly eosinophilic cytoplasm, and form vascular spaces {70}. A small subset (< 10%) of EHEs have atypical features, such as nuclear pleomorphism, increased mitotic activity, solid sheet-like growth, and necrosis, and these cases may resemble epithelioid angiosarcomas {322,919}.

Key diagnostic cytopathological features

- Variable cellularity
- Predominantly single cells and less commonly small tissue fragments, which may be pseudopapillary or pseudoglandular
- Bloody background with haemosiderin-laden macrophages
- Cells may be associated with a scant amount of dense stromal matrix
- Necrosis is absent

- Epithelioid cells have eccentric moderate to abundant cytoplasm, which often contains vacuoles and may have a granular appearance, although some cells may have tapered cytoplasm
- Spindle cells may be seen, and in rare cases spindle cells may predominate
- Rare cells with intracytoplasmic lumina, which may contain red cells
- Nuclei are round to oval and mildly to moderately pleomorphic, and they occasionally have crinkled "raisinoid" nuclear envelopes, with small or inapparent nucleoli
- Multinucleated cells may be seen
- Nuclear grooves and intranuclear pseudoinclusions are common features
- Nucleoli are typically small or absent
- Minimal mitotic activity

Reference(s): {992,1441,1104,871,1335,631}

Discussion and differential diagnosis

Familiarity with the clinical, imaging, and cytomorphological features of EHE helps avoid missing this entity when developing a differential diagnosis. The differential diagnosis varies depending on the anatomical location of the neoplasm, but it generally includes other epithelioid tumours, such as adenocarcinoma, epithelioid mesothelioma, melanoma, epithelioid angiosarcoma, and epithelioid sarcoma. When a vascular neoplasm is suspected, Kaposi sarcoma may be included in the differential diagnosis. The *WWTR1::CAMTA1* gene fusion is specific for EHE and thus can help confirm the diagnosis when it is suspected. In the absence of such testing, a definitive diagnosis of EHE is likely to be challenging, although ICC studies can help to greatly narrow the differential diagnosis.

Adenocarcinoma shows cytomorphological overlap and has a higher incidence in visceral sites {1215}. In addition, EHE may stain positively, albeit weakly and focally, for epithelial markers, suggesting a diagnosis of adenocarcinoma early in the workup. EHEs do not form the 3D glandular tissue fragments seen in most adenocarcinomas. Adenocarcinomas may contain mucinous vacuoles that mimic the intracytoplasmic vacuoles seen in EHE, but the latter are mucin-negative. EHEs usually lack the pleomorphism, necrosis, and mitotic activity that may be seen in many adenocarcinomas.

Epithelioid angiosarcomas are difficult to distinguish from EHE, but they tend to be more cellular and may contain higher mitotic activity and necrosis {216,148}. Kaposi sarcoma tends to yield spindle rather than epithelioid cells.

Melanoma may be considered in the differential diagnosis given the shared characteristics of moderate to abundant often eccentric cytoplasm, cytoplasmic granularity, dispersed cell pattern, and presence of intranuclear pseudoinclusions. However, EHE lacks melanin pigment, and the intracytoplasmic lumina are not seen in melanoma {991}. Similarly, epithelioid sarcoma and mesothelioma can be excluded due to ICC differences and their lack of intracytoplasmic lumina.

Ancillary testing

EHEs express the endothelial markers CD34, CD31, podoplanin (D2-40), FLI1, and ERG, but there may be substantial variability in the degree of staining for a given marker {432,1203, 953}. The epithelial antigens CK7, CK8, CK18, and pankeratin

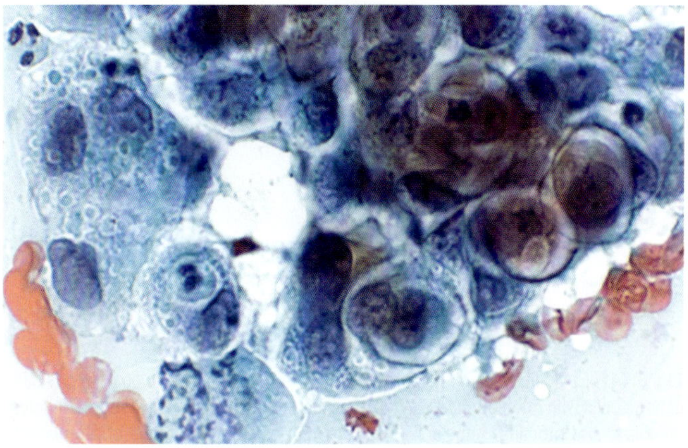

Fig. 8.138 Epithelioid haemangioendothelioma. Large tumour cells contain intracytoplasmic lumina containing red blood cells and neutrophils. A mitosis can be seen in the bottom of the field; because these are rarely seen in epithelioid haemangioendothelioma, their presence can suggest the possibility of an epithelioid angiosarcoma (Pap).

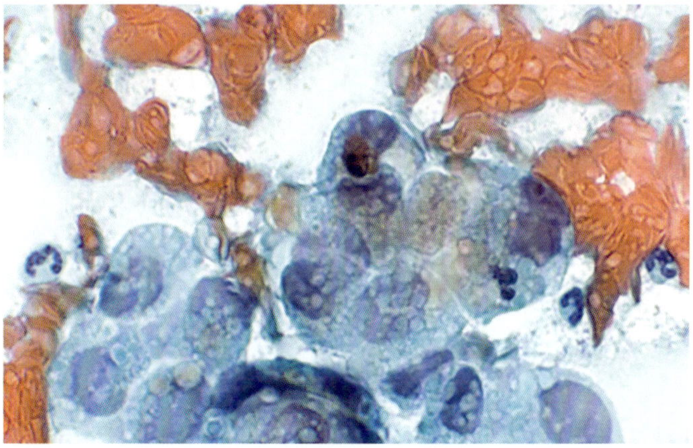

Fig. 8.137 Epithelioid haemangioendothelioma. A small tissue fragment consisting of large cells with abundant, vacuolated cytoplasm and large epithelioid nuclei with significant variation in nuclear size (Pap).

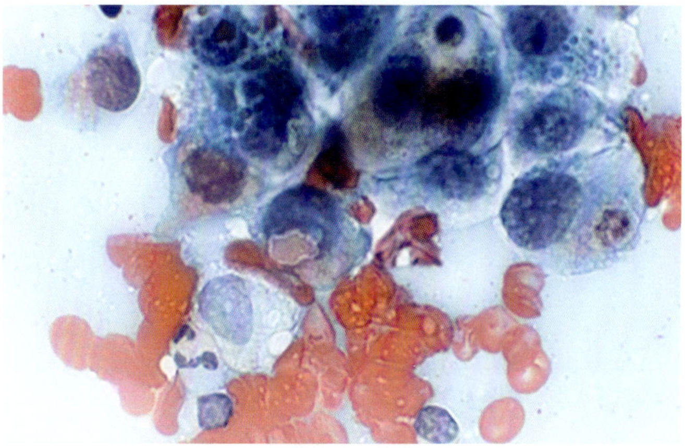

Fig. 8.139 Epithelioid haemangioendothelioma. A loosely cohesive tissue fragment consisting of epithelioid cells with abundant cytoplasm containing small vacuoles, along with red blood cells and neutrophils within intracytoplasmic lumina (Pap).

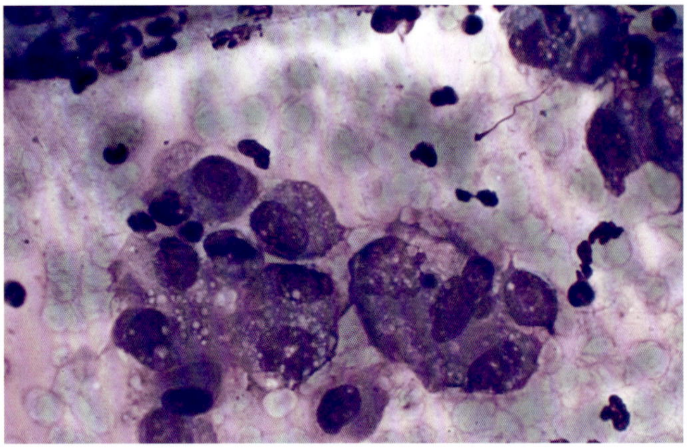

Fig. 8.140 Epithelioid haemangioendothelioma. Abundant, vacuolated cytoplasm with enlarged pleomorphic nuclei is seen. Distinct intracytoplasmic lumina are present, and the neoplastic cells on the left side of the field appear to form an intercellular lumen (Giemsa).

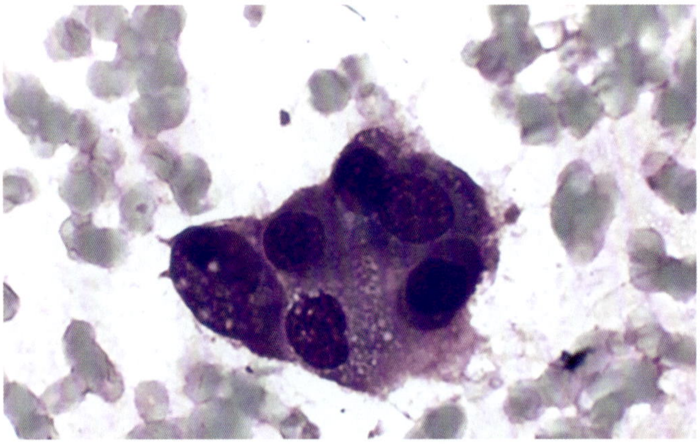

Fig. 8.141 Epithelioid haemangioendothelioma. A minute tissue fragment consisting of large cells with often abundant cytoplasm, marked anisonucleosis, irregular nuclear contours, and prominent nucleoli – features that overlap with those of adenocarcinoma, which is often in the different diagnosis (Giemsa).

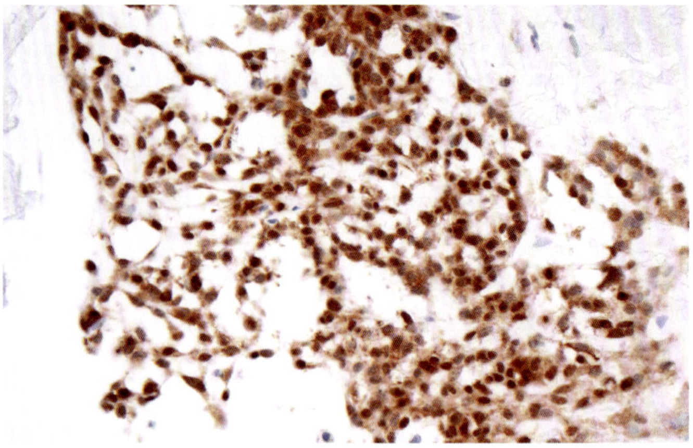

Fig. 8.142 Epithelioid haemangioendothelioma. Strong nuclear staining for CAMTA1, which is a surrogate marker for *CAMTA1::WWTR1* fusion, is a reliable diagnostic marker for epithelioid haemangioendothelioma (cell block, ICC).

are expressed in as many as 40% of cases, but expression of EMA is unusual {919,941}. SMA is expressed in approximately 50% of cases {919}. Tumours with the *WWTR1::CAMTA1* gene fusion typically show diffuse nuclear expression of CAMTA1, whereas tumours with the *YAP1::TFE3* fusion demonstrate diffuse nuclear TFE3 expression {70}. Expression of TFE3 can sometimes be seen in tumours with the *WWTR1::CAMTA1* fusion {357,429}.

Epithelioid angiosarcoma lacks the *WWTR1::CAMTA1* gene fusion seen in most EHEs. KSHV/HHV8 can be detected in Kaposi sarcoma but not EHE. Melanoma is negative for epithelial and vascular markers, whereas EHE lacks markers of melanocytic differentiation such as melan-A (MART1), SOX10, and HMB45. Epithelioid sarcoma and mesothelioma lack vascular marker expression {1119,1234}, and EHE does not express markers of mesothelial differentiation such as calretinin {1234}. Adenocarcinomas are negative for the vascular markers ERG and FLI1.

Epithelioid sarcoma

Rekhi B
Dodd LG
Klijanienko J

Definition

Epithelioid sarcoma (ES) is a malignant mesenchymal neoplasm that exhibits partial or complete epithelioid cytomorphology and immunophenotype and is characterized by loss of SMARCB1 (INI1/BAF47) in most cases.

Clinical features and imaging

Two clinicopathological subtypes are recognized. Classic or distal ES presents in the form of single or multiple, usually painless and firm, indurated superficial nodules in the upper extremities. Often, the lesions present as non-healing ulcers, mimicking inflammatory lesions of the skin. Proximal-type ES presents as a deep soft tissue mass, usually in the proximal truncal regions of the perineum and genitalia {193,518,544,766, 1168}.

There are no specific features on imaging. These tumours appear as infiltrating lesions {538}. The proximal type displays a multinodular configuration. Imaging is also useful in detecting metastatic lesions in the lymph nodes {1385}.

Histopathology

Classic-type ES is composed of nodules of atypical cells with epithelioid to fusiform shapes, variable numbers of mitotic figures, and central necrosis, leading to a granuloma-like appearance {193,1168}. Dystrophic calcification and metaplastic bone formation are uncommonly seen {193,1168}. The proximal type

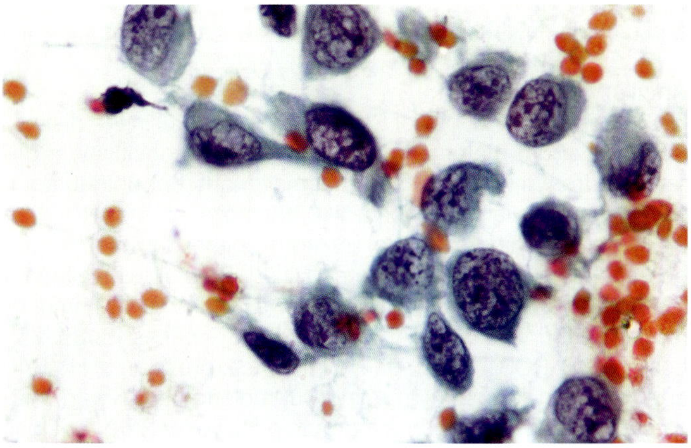

Fig. 8.143 Epithelioid sarcoma. Polygonal or epithelioid and spindle cells showing a moderate amount of cytoplasm, well-defined cellular borders, coarse chromatin with perinucleolar clearing, and distinct nucleoli (Pap).

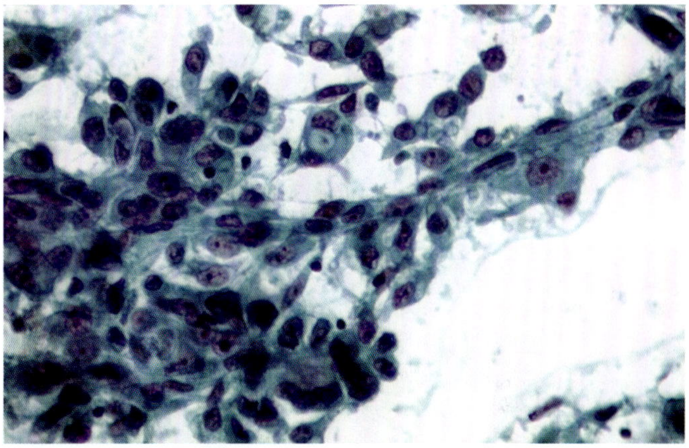

Fig. 8.145 Proximal epithelioid sarcoma. A cellular smear composed of cohesive tissue fragments of epithelioid and spindle cells containing moderate to abundant greenish cytoplasm, including a few cells with characteristic intracytoplasmic inclusions, reminiscent of rhabdoid-like morphology (Pap).

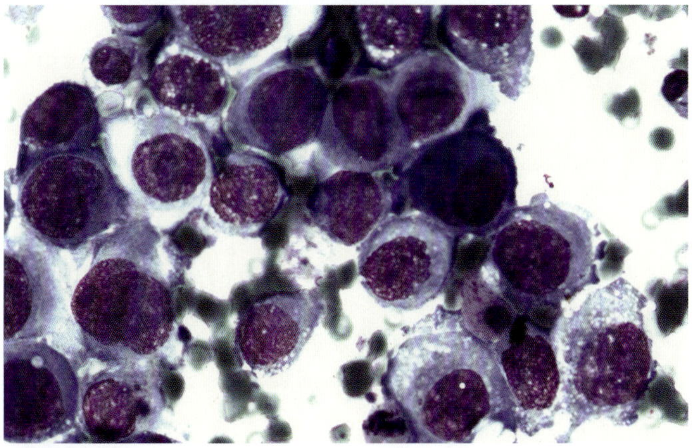

Fig. 8.144 Epithelioid sarcoma. Large, epithelioid cells showing large pleomorphic nuclei (Giemsa).

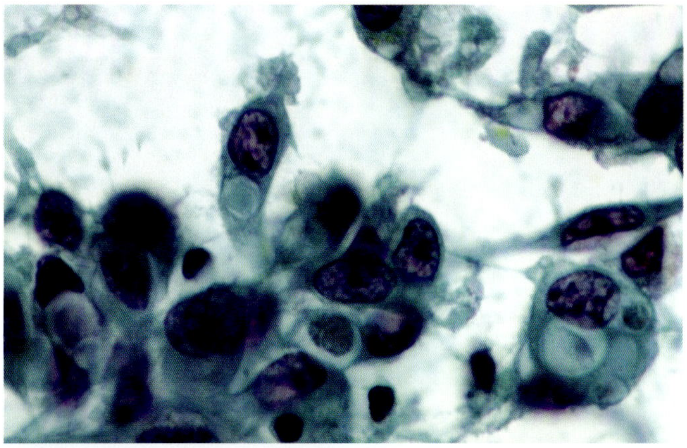

Fig. 8.146 Proximal epithelioid sarcoma. Many cells have abundant, well-defined eccentric or spindle cytoplasm and characteristic intracytoplasmic, paranuclear, rhabdoid-like inclusions, along with coarse chromatin, distinct nucleoli, and perinucleolar clearing (Pap).

displays a multinodular and diffuse arrangement of large, pleomorphic cells with rhabdoid-like morphology. Focal necrosis and haemorrhage, leading to a pseudoangiosarcomatous appearance, can be seen {518,544,1168,1167}. The hybrid form includes tumours with variable components of classic and proximal subtypes {576}.

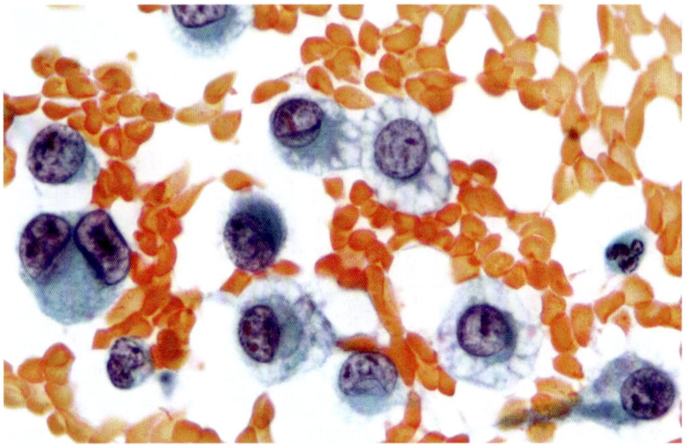

Fig. 8.147 Proximal epithelioid sarcoma. Epithelioid cells show single nuclei or binucleation and cytoplasmic vacuolization (Pap).

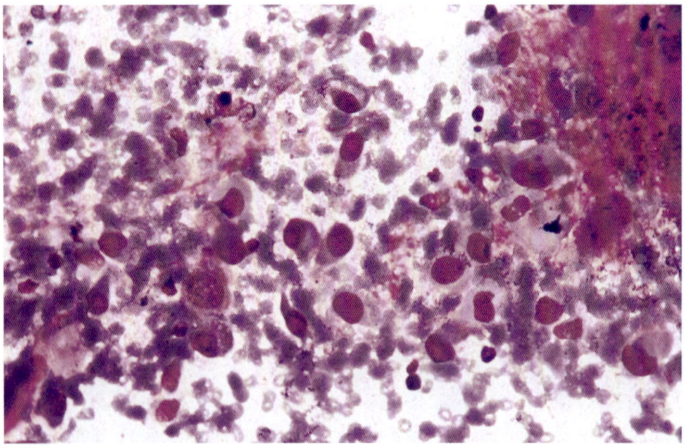

Fig. 8.148 Metastatic epithelioid sarcoma. Single scattered and loosely cohesive polygonal, epithelioid cells and rhabdoid-like cells with eccentric, abundant, well-defined cytoplasm, along with metachromatic stroma and a few lymphocytes in a bloody background (Giemsa).

Key diagnostic cytopathological features

- High cellularity
- Loosely cohesive tissue fragments and sheets and single cells
- Polygonal or epithelioid and spindle cells with moderate to abundant, well-defined cytoplasm
- Perinucleolar chromatin clearing ("vesicular" chromatin, Pap) and distinct nucleoli
- Perinuclear, intracytoplasmic inclusions, leading to a plasmacytoid or rhabdoid-like appearance, particularly in the proximal subtype
- Variable multinucleated giant cells, cytoplasmic vacuoles, and metachromatic stroma

Reference(s): {557,1553,175,608,1095,1178,461}

Discussion and differential diagnosis

The differential diagnoses include carcinoma, synovial sarcoma, epithelioid haemangioendothelioma, epithelioid angiosarcoma, epithelioid malignant peripheral nerve sheath tumour, and melanoma {1022,1178}.

Ancillary testing

CD34 positivity and loss of SMARCB1 are useful in the distinction of ES from metastatic carcinoma. CD34 positivity separates ES from a synovial sarcoma, malignant rhabdoid tumour, and myoepithelial carcinoma {1039}. Loss of SMARCB1 is also useful in differentiating ES from epithelioid haemangioendothelioma and angiosarcoma {1172}. Epithelioid malignant peripheral nerve sheath tumour shows diffuse S100 immunoreactivity and loss of SMARCB1 in 27–67% cases {648,1175}. Loss of SMARCB1 and negative immunoexpression of HMB45 and melan-A are useful in ruling out melanoma. ES and anaplastic large cell lymphoma are both positive for EMA, but loss of SMARCB1 is indicative of ES, whereas CD30, CD45 (LCA), and ALK immunoreactivity are indicative of anaplastic large cell lymphoma {1179}.

Most cases show homozygous or heterozygous deletion of *SMARCB1* (*INI1*) {1359}. ES displays immunopositivity for

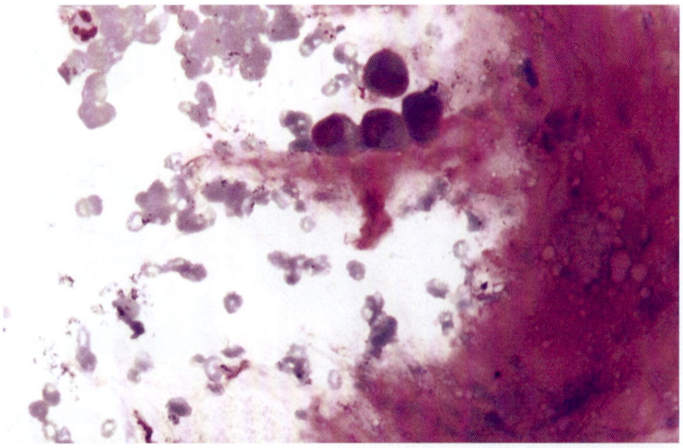

Fig. 8.149 Metastatic epithelioid sarcoma. Polygonal-shaped epithelioid cells with metachromatic stroma (Giemsa).

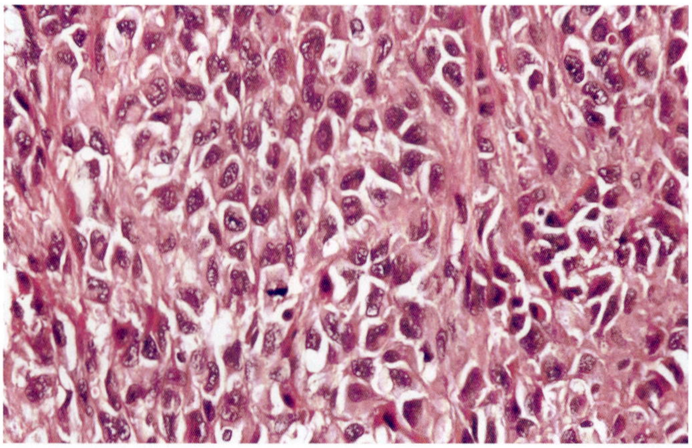

Fig. 8.150 Epithelioid sarcoma. Epithelioid and spindle cells, arranged in a diffuse pattern with scattered mitotic figures (tissue section, H&E).

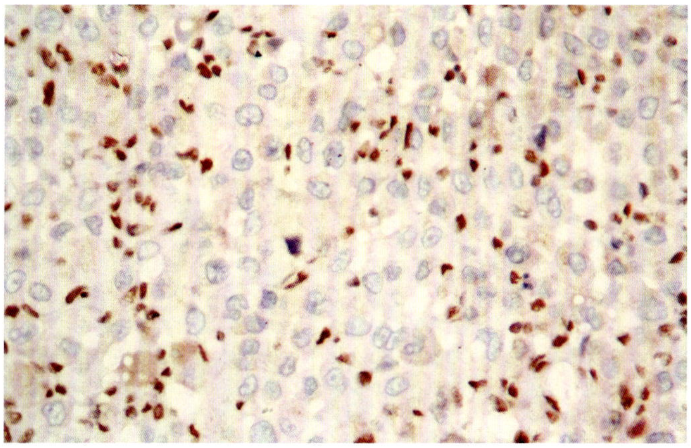

Fig. 8.151 Epithelioid sarcoma. Tumour cells displaying loss of SMARCB1 (INI1), while intervening lymphocytes and endothelial cells act as internal positive controls (cell block, ICC).

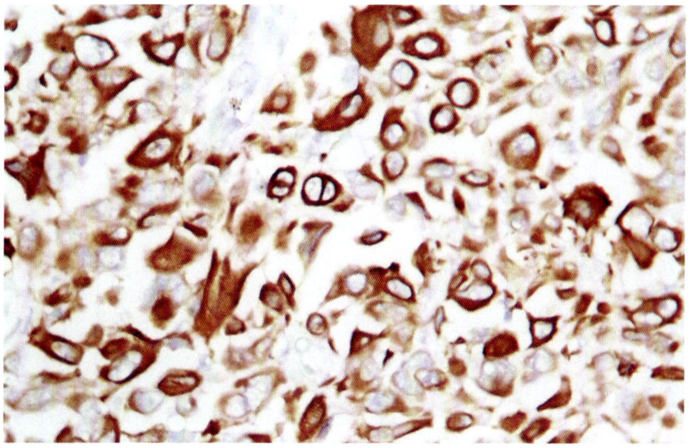

Fig. 8.152 Metastatic proximal epithelioid sarcoma. Cells displaying cytoplasmic pancytokeratin (AE1/AE3) positivity (cell block, ICC).

various epithelial markers, such as low- and high-molecular-weight cytokeratins and EMA {518,940,544,1168}. More than 50% of cases show CD34 immunopositivity {940,1167}. Loss of SMARCB1 protein is reported in > 80% cases of ES {747, 576,1172}. Certain classic-type ES cases display ERG immunopositivity {951,748}.

Chapter 8

Alveolar soft part sarcoma

Rekhi B
Klijanienko J

Definition

Alveolar soft part sarcoma (ASPS) is a rare neoplasm of uncertain histogenesis predominantly affecting the deep soft tissues of the extremities, featuring variably discohesive epithelioid cells arranged in nests resulting in a distinct alveolar appearance, with a characteristic translocation, der(17)t(X;17)(p11.2;q25) that results in *ASPSCR1::TFE3* gene fusion.

Clinical features and imaging

ASPS presents as a slowly growing, painless soft tissue mass {217}. Vaginal bleeding is common in tumours involving the female genital tract. Proptosis is a presenting condition in cases of tumours involving the orbit. The disease can be localized or metastatic. A significant percentage of patients present with or develop metastatic lesions, frequently in the lungs {1481,1171}.

On imaging, ASPS appears as a lobulated mass with flow voids, conspicuous peripheral blood vessels, and internal nodularity {900}. Hypervascularity is seen on postcontrast-enhanced CT {843}.

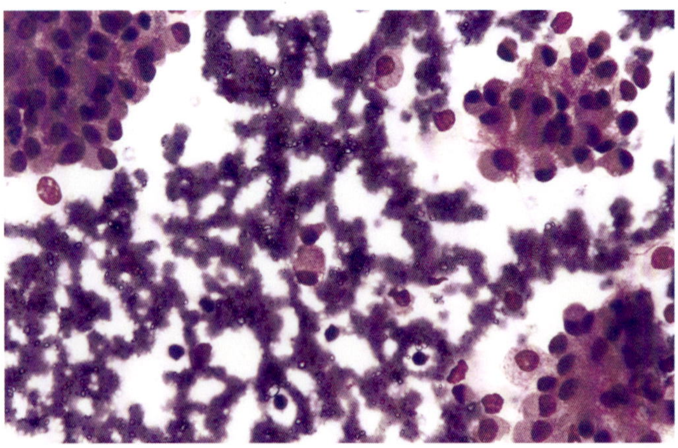

Fig. 8.153 Alveolar soft part sarcoma. Cohesive tissue fragments of cells with polygonal to plasmacytoid morphology (Giemsa).

Histopathology

ASPS is composed of large, polygonal tumour cells with well-defined cell borders, central to eccentric nuclei, and prominent nucleoli, arranged in an organoid and a uniform nesting pattern with loosely cohesive cells, imparting an alveolar growth pattern. The tumour nests are surrounded by capillary vessels, leading to a branching haemangiopericytoma-like vasculature. Variable features include cytoplasmic vacuolization, rhabdoid-like cells, multinucleation, myxoid stroma, cystic change, pleomorphic cells, xanthomatous cells, mitotic figures, and dystrophic calcification {434,1171,1521}.

The tumour cells contain DPAS-positive rhomboid or rod-shaped intracytoplasmic crystals and granules that may be focally or diffusely present {1171}. These are immunopositive for MCT1 and CD147 {771}.

Key diagnostic cytopathological features

- High cellularity
- Cohesive tissue fragments, some of which appear alveolar, and scattered cells with stripped nuclei in the clean background
- Polygonal cells with central to eccentric round nuclei, perinucleolar chromatin clearing ("vesicular", Pap), and prominent nucleoli
- Abundant, well-defined to ill-defined, granular to finely vacuolated, concentric or eccentric cytoplasm

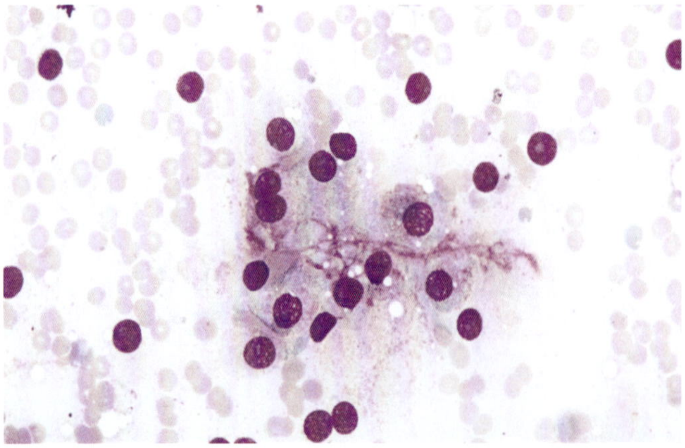

Fig. 8.154 Alveolar soft part sarcoma. A loosely cohesive minute tissue fragment and scattered cells containing abundant ill-defined granular cytoplasm, round nuclei, and prominent nucleoli, with intervening fibrillary stroma and bare nuclei (Giemsa).

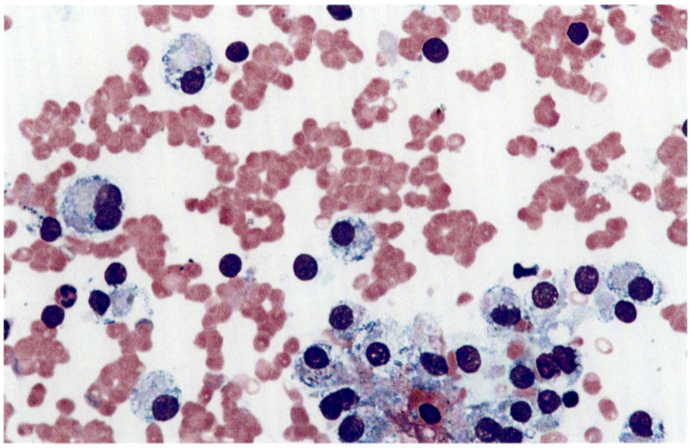

Fig. 8.155 Alveolar soft part sarcoma. A loosely cohesive tissue fragment and single scattered tumour cells with abundant, often eccentric cytoplasm containing granules and fine vacuoles, along with a few binucleate cells and bare nuclei in a bloody background (Giemsa).

- Variable papilliform tissue fragments, binucleate to multinucleate giant cells, intracytoplasmic rod-like crystals, and a thin fibrillary stroma

Reference(s): {1278,364,840,1471,1525,1176}

Discussion and differential diagnosis

The differential diagnoses include renal cell carcinoma, granular cell tumour, clear cell sarcoma, epithelioid haemangioendothelioma, epithelioid sarcoma, perivascular epithelioid cell tumour

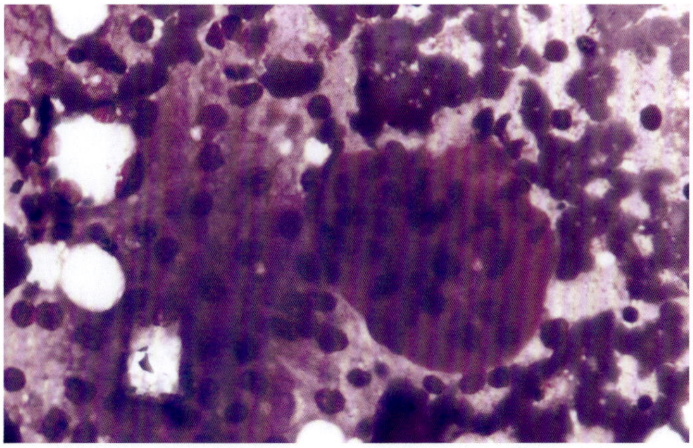

Fig. 8.156 Alveolar soft part sarcoma. A sharply contoured cohesive tissue fragment suggestive of an alveolar architecture, next to a sheet of similar cells with abundant granular cytoplasm and distinct nucleoli (Giemsa).

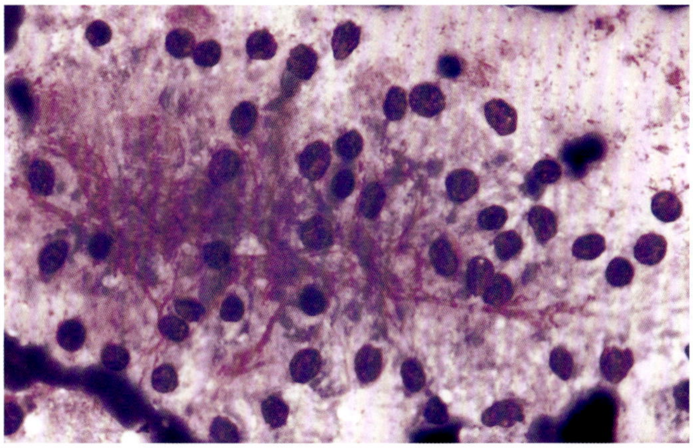

Fig. 8.157 Alveolar soft part sarcoma. A loosely cohesive tissue fragment consisting of cells with round to mildly pleomorphic nuclei, prominent nucleoli, and abundant ill-defined granular cytoplasm with intervening thin fibrillar stroma (Giemsa).

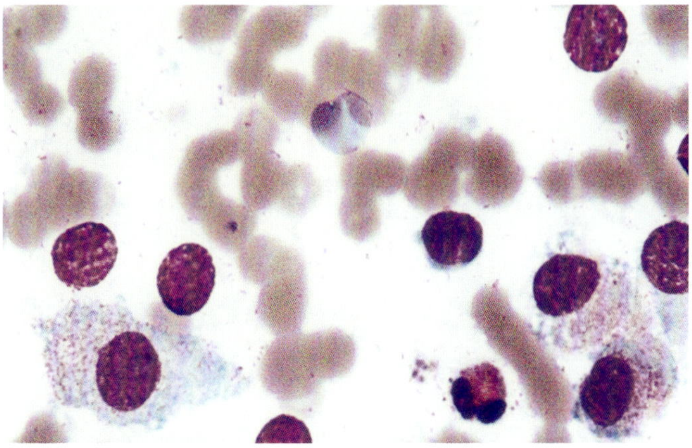

Fig. 8.158 Alveolar soft part sarcoma. Cells with abundant ill-defined cytoplasm containing granules, round nuclei, and prominent nucleoli, along with scattered bare nuclei (Giemsa).

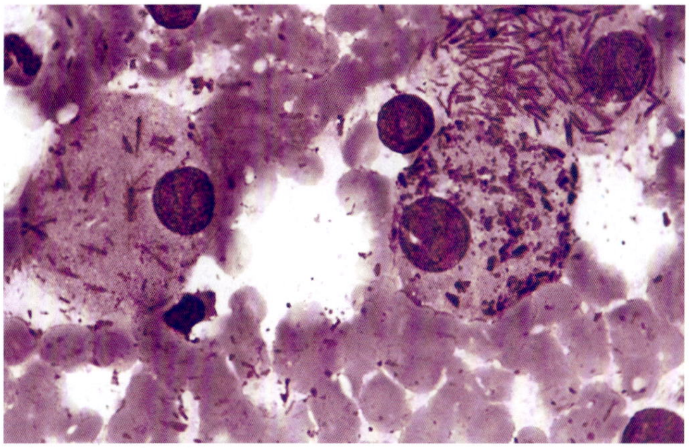

Fig. 8.159 Alveolar soft part sarcoma. On higher magnification, tumour cells contain abundant granular cytoplasm, characteristic numerous rod-like or needle crystals, and prominent nucleoli (Giemsa).

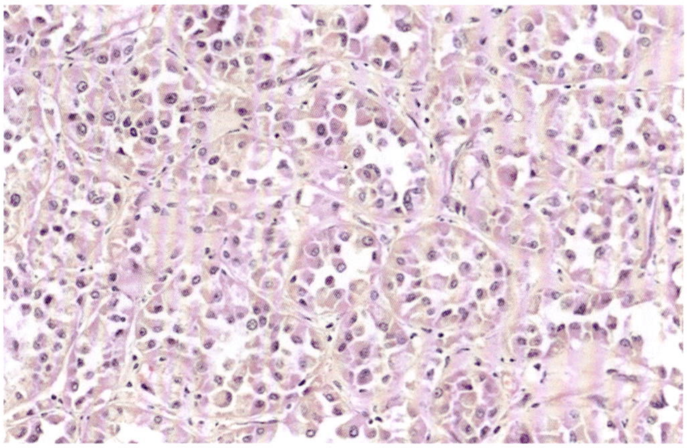

Fig. 8.160 Alveolar soft part sarcoma. Loosely cohesive polygonal cells arranged in an alveolar architecture, surrounded by thin-walled capillaries (tissue section, H&E).

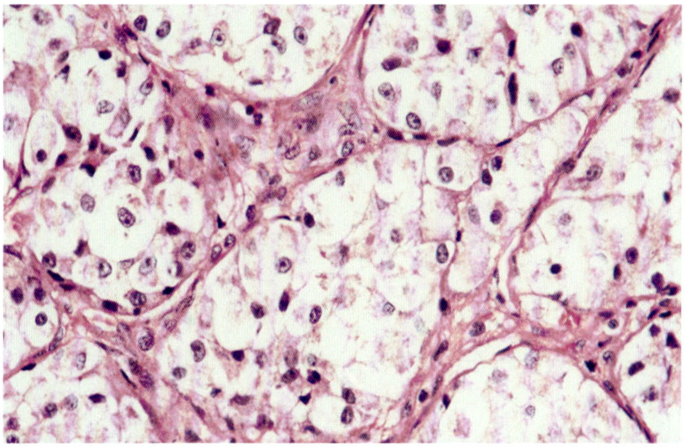

Fig. 8.161 Alveolar soft part sarcoma. Nests of tumour cells with granular to clear cytoplasm and prominent nucleoli, separated by thin fibrovascular strands (tissue section, H&E).

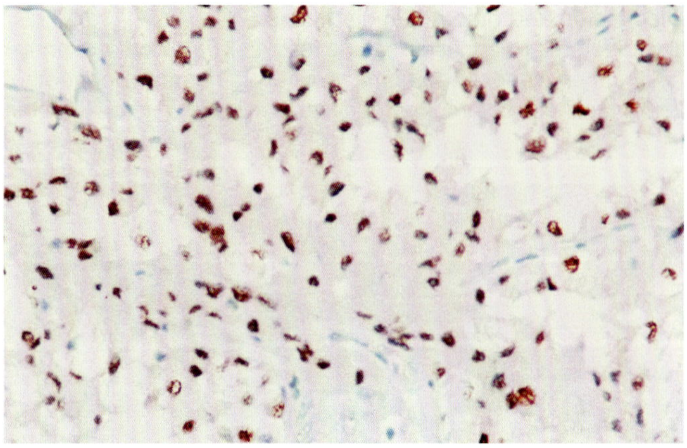

Fig. 8.162 Alveolar soft part sarcoma. Tumour cells displaying diffuse nuclear positivity for TFE3 (tissue fragment, ICC).

(PEComa), alveolar rhabdomyosarcoma, and paraganglioma {1278,1471,1171,1006,1176}.

Renal cell carcinoma displays cytomorphological features overlapping with those of ASPS, and the finding of normal kidneys on imaging is crucial in confirming a diagnosis of ASPS over metastatic renal cell carcinoma. Granular cell tumours, unless malignant, generally lack pleomorphic nuclei and prominent nucleoli, in contrast to ASPS. Similar to ASPS, epithelioid sarcoma and clear cell sarcoma of soft tissue display epithelioid or polygonal cells with moderate to abundant cytoplasm and prominent nucleoli; the prominent nucleoli are more consistently seen in clear cell sarcoma of soft tissue, which also includes some spindle cells. Plentiful intracytoplasmic granules and crystals are rarely seen within these tumours, unlike in ASPS. Epithelioid haemangioendotheliomas also have polygonal cells, but they have grooved nuclei and intracytoplasmic lumina containing red blood cells. Alveolar rhabdomyosarcomas contain epithelioid or polygonal cells with binucleate and multinucleate forms, including giant cells with a wreath-like circular arrangement of nuclei. Paragangliomas also display features overlapping with those of ASPS, including nuclear anisokaryosis with abundant granular cytoplasm and intracytoplasmic inclusions. These tumours are suspected in sites such as the abdomen and neck.

Ancillary testing

ASPS show S100 negativity, which is useful in ruling out a granular cell tumour. HMB45 and melan-A negativity rule out melanoma, clear cell sarcoma of soft parts, and PEComa {1151, 1487}. Negative immunostaining for desmin, myogenin, and MYOD1 is useful in ruling out a rhabdomyosarcoma. Synaptophysin and chromogranin negativity rules out a paraganglioma. TFE3 constitutes a highly sensitive marker for a diagnosis of ASPS; however, it is also positive in translocation-related renal cell carcinomas, neuroendocrine tumours, and granular cell tumours {1171}. PAX8 is positively expressed in most renal cell carcinomas, unlike in ASPS {108}. ASPS cells express TFE3 and cathepsin K {1069,1456,880}, but despite high sensitivity, these markers are not entirely specific, because they are also expressed in certain renal cell carcinomas {79,1171}.

ASPS has a characteristic *ASPSCR1::TFE3* gene fusion, as a result of a recurrent, non-reciprocal translocation, der(17)t(X;17)(p11.2;q25). *TFE3* gene rearrangement can be assessed by FISH, or *ASPSCR1::TFE3* fusion by RT-PCR or NGS. These are also found in certain renal cell carcinomas {78,566}.

Clear cell sarcoma of soft tissue

Domanski HA
Bui M
Rekhi B

Definition

Clear cell sarcoma (CCS) of soft tissue is a malignant mesenchymal neoplasm typically involving deep soft tissue, showing a distinctive nested growth pattern and melanocytic differentiation, and most often characterized by *EWSR1::ATF1* fusion.

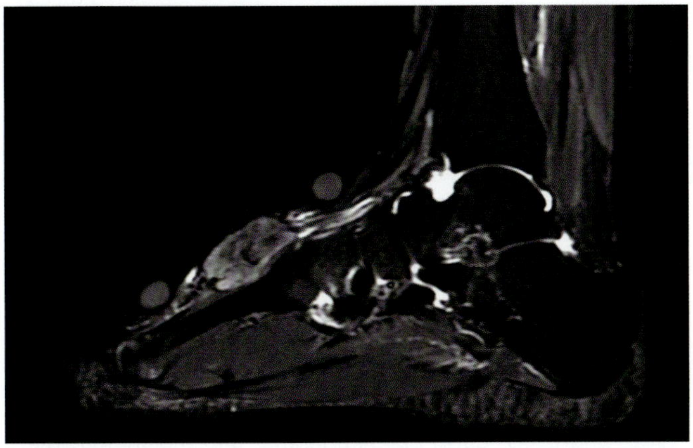

Fig. 8.163 Clear cell sarcoma. MRI shows an ill-defined soft tissue mass at the mid-dorsum of the foot.

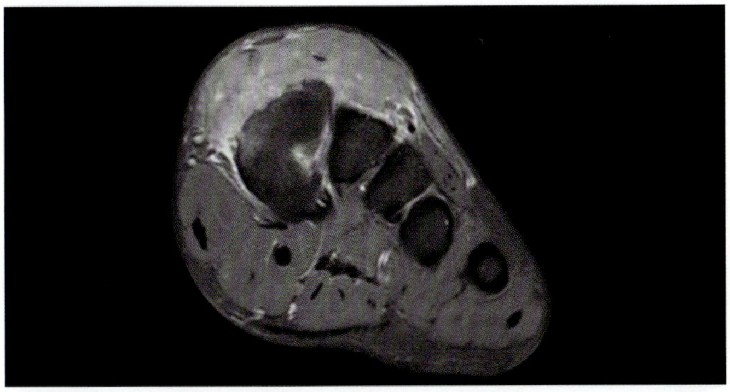

Fig. 8.164 Clear cell sarcoma. On axial T1-weighted MRI, the lesion has slightly higher signal intensity than the adjacent muscle.

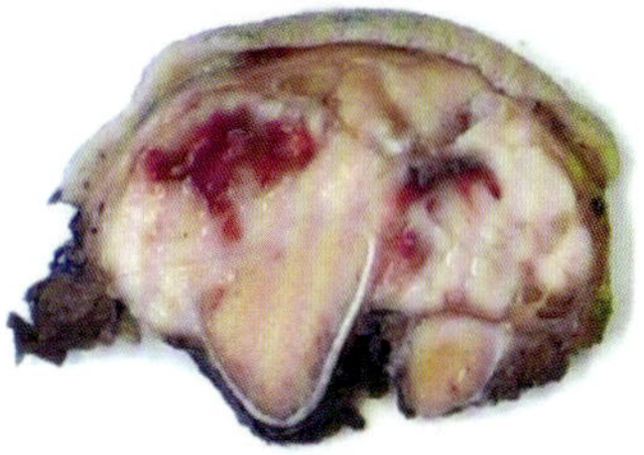

Fig. 8.165 Clear cell sarcoma. Excised tumour at the dorsum of the foot is grossly poorly circumscribed and has a tan-grey or yellow cut surface with foci of haemorrhage.

Clinical features and imaging

CCSs account for 0.8–1% of all sarcomas {328,606} and typically occur in young adults, with a peak incidence in the third decade of life; they are slightly more common in females {134, 328,606,230,299,370}. Most cases present as a slow-growing, often painful or tender soft tissue mass in the lower extremities, especially the foot and ankle, and they are often attached to aponeurotic structures and tendons {134,328,606,230,299, 370}. Rare sites include head and neck, trunk, and viscera {230, 299,370}.

MRI shows features of a non-aggressive lesion, such as well-defined margins and homogeneity on T1- and T2-weighted images, without perilesional oedema, satellite nodules, or intratumoral necrosis {486,296,1284}.

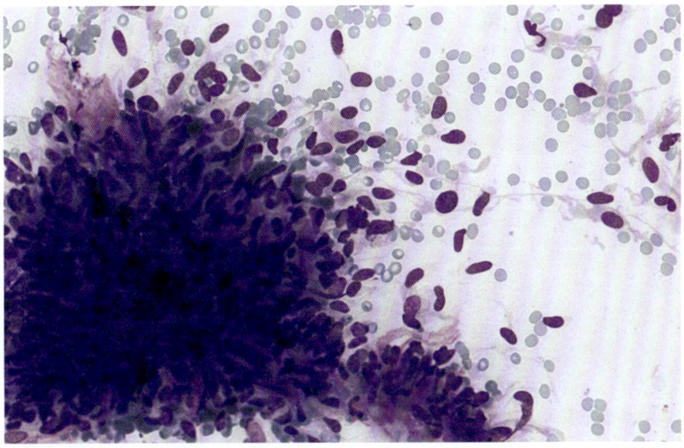

Fig. 8.166 Clear cell sarcoma. A cellular crowded tissue fragment and dispersed cells with retained or poorly preserved cytoplasm and oval to spindle hyperchromatic nuclei (Giemsa).

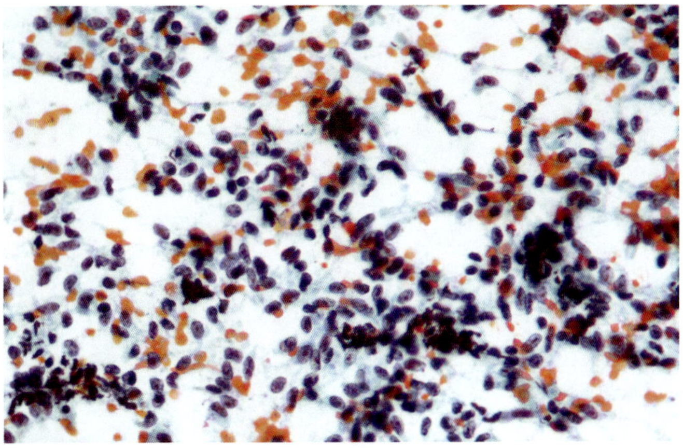

Fig. 8.167 Clear cell sarcoma of soft tissue. Small loosely cohesive tissue fragments and single round to spindle cells with oval to elongated nuclei, distinct nucleoli, and moderate to indistinct often eccentric cytoplasm (Pap).

Histopathology

There is an infiltrative growth of uniform epithelioid to fusiform cells divided into nests and fascicles by thin fibrous septa. Tumour cells display limited pleomorphism and pale eosinophilic, rarely clear cytoplasm, with centrally located round to ovoid vesicular nuclei with macronucleoli. Scattered wreath-like multinucleated tumour giant cells and melanin pigment are relatively common {505,328, 606}. Necrosis is found in one third of cases. The mitotic count is deceptively low for this highly malignant tumour.

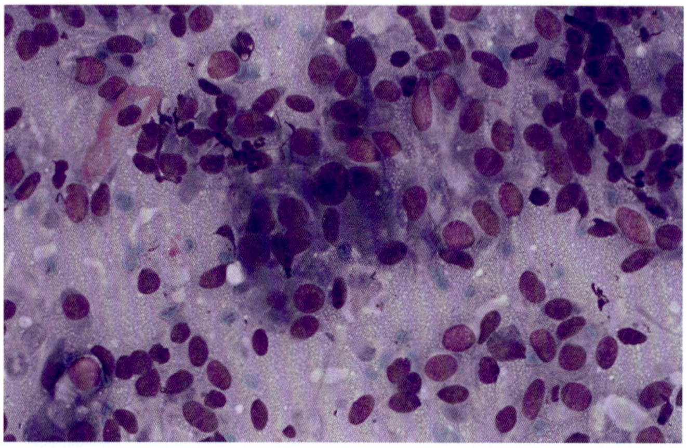

Fig. 8.168 Clear cell sarcoma. Spindle to more polygonal large cells with oval to occasionally very large and pleomorphic nuclei with macronucleoli in a finely stippled background (Giemsa).

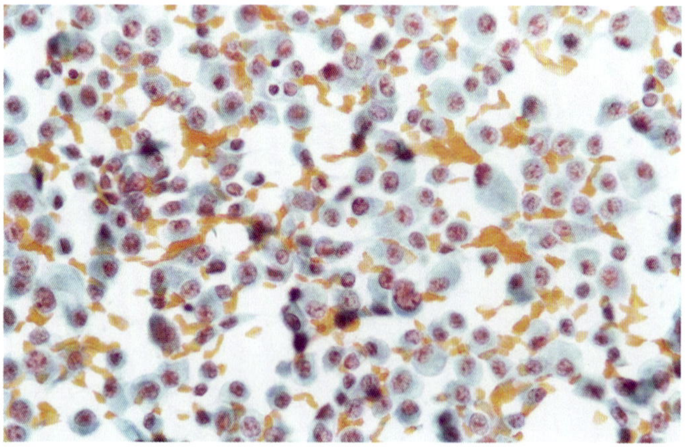

Fig. 8.169 Clear cell sarcoma of soft tissue. A hypercellular smear composed of loosely cohesive and scattered polygonal cells with round to oval nuclei, distinct nucleoli, and moderate to abundant well-defined cytoplasm (Pap).

Key diagnostic cytopathological features

- Variable but often moderate to high cellularity
- Dispersed large cells and occasional loose or cohesive tissue fragments with non-overlapping nuclei
- Finely striped ("tigroid") background
- Round, polygonal, or spindle cells with moderate to abundant clear to pale concentric or eccentric cytoplasm and central or displaced nuclei
- Round to ovoid hyperchromatic nuclei with prominent nucleoli
- Nuclei with perinucleolar chromatin clearing ("vesicular", Pap) and occasionally 2–3 smaller nucleoli
- Rare binucleated or wreath-like multinucleated cells
- Occasional microacinar tissue fragments
- Intranuclear cytoplasmic pseudoinclusions and cytoplasmic melanin may be present

Reference(s): {995,1416,1226,1152,264,761,886,173,1268,470, 53,602,619,570,275,1151}

Discussion and differential diagnosis

The differential diagnosis includes synovial sarcoma and sarcomas with epithelioid morphology (e.g. epithelioid sarcoma, Ewing sarcoma, and rhabdomyosarcoma), metastatic carcinoma, anaplastic large cell lymphoma, and melanoma. All of these tumours, like CCS, produce highly cellular smears. The tigroid background seen in CCS is also seen in Ewing sarcoma, rhabdomyosarcoma, and anaplastic large cell lymphoma {637}. Individual tumour cells of synovial sarcoma are oval to spindle, with hyperchromatic nuclei and indistinct nucleoli {709}, and single scattered epithelioid to rhabdoid-like cells are rarely seen in synovial sarcoma {1177}. Metastatic carcinoma displays crowded 3D tissue fragments and variable papillary and glandular architecture, whereas acinar formation is rarely reported in CCS {264,1151}. Prominent epithelioid differentiation is uncommon in Ewing sarcoma.

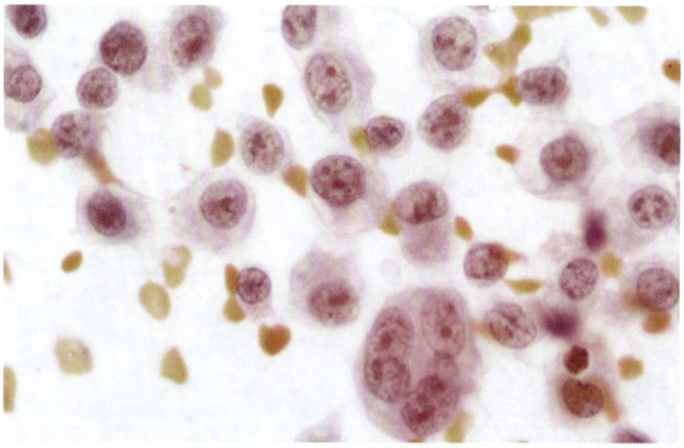

Fig. 8.170 Clear cell sarcoma of soft tissue. Individual polygonal tumour cells with round to oval nuclei, distinct single or multiple nucleoli, perinucleolar clearing, and moderate to abundant well-defined cytoplasm, including a multinucleate tumour giant cell (Pap).

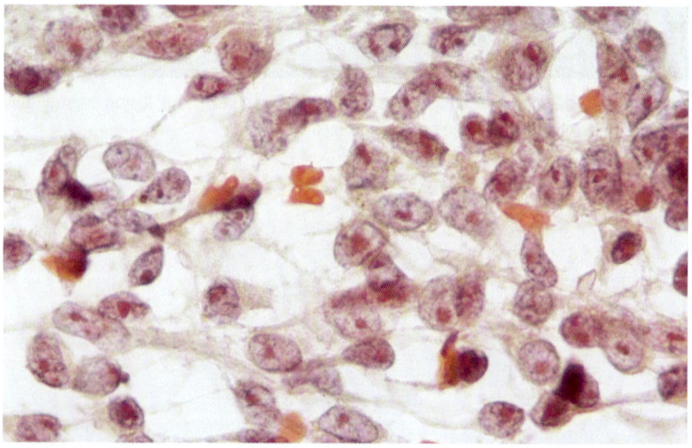

Fig. 8.171 Clear cell sarcoma of soft tissue. Loosely cohesive minute tissue fragments and single scattered polygonal to spindle tumour cells containing round to oval to spindle nuclei, distinct nucleoli, and a scant to moderate amount of often spindle cytoplasm (Pap).

Ancillary testing

Most cases of CCS of soft tissue are characterized by reciprocal translocation t(12;22)(q13;q12) resulting in an *EWSR1*::*ATF1* fusion {157,1347,1067,1094,1154,1419}. A minor subset of cases harbour translocation t(2;22)(q34;q12), which includes the *EWSR1*::*CREB1* fusion {565,1485,1151}.

CCS stains positively for S100, HMB45, melan-A, and SOX10, and it typically expresses MITF-M {506}. Synovial sarcoma displays variable keratin and EMA immunostaining. Additionally, synovial sarcoma displays *SS18*::SSX gene fusion. Epithelioid sarcoma expresses a variable number of epithelial markers and shows loss of SMARCB1 (INI1) in most instances {1178}. Anaplastic large cell lymphoma expresses CD30 and ALK. Metastatic carcinoma shows epithelial markers.

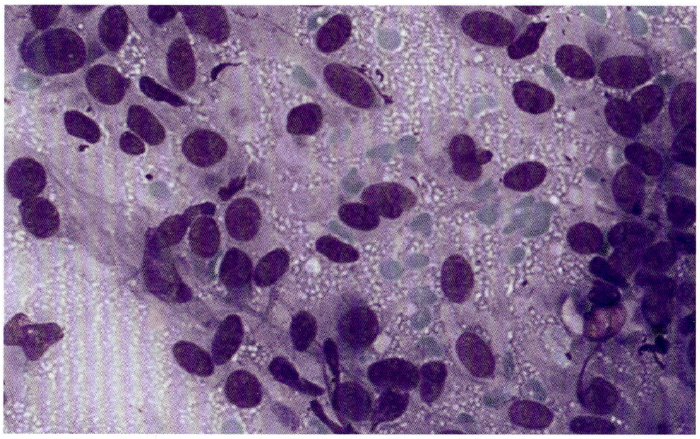

Fig. 8.172 Clear cell sarcoma. Lacy vacuolated "tigroid" background and dispersed atypical round to spindle cells with round to oval to occasionally more pleomorphic nuclei and prominent nucleoli (Giemsa).

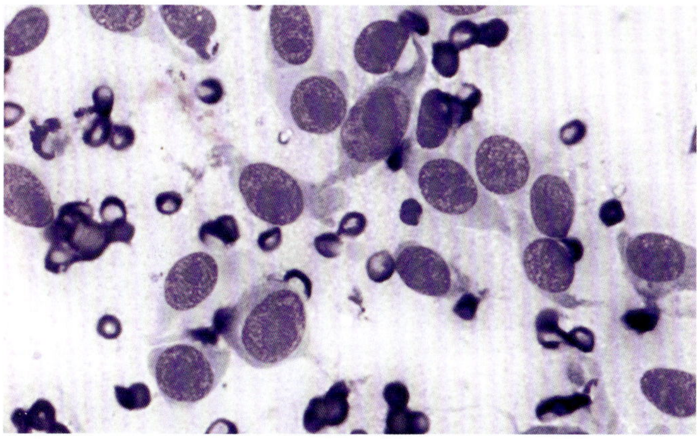

Fig. 8.173 Clear cell sarcoma. Dispersed single cells with cytoplasmic extensions and round to oval nuclei with prominent macronucleoli (Giemsa).

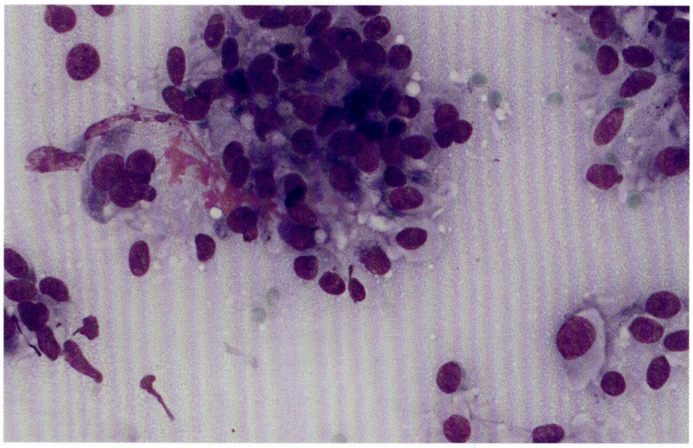

Fig. 8.174 Clear cell sarcoma. A tissue fragment showing a rare microacinar architecture (Giemsa).

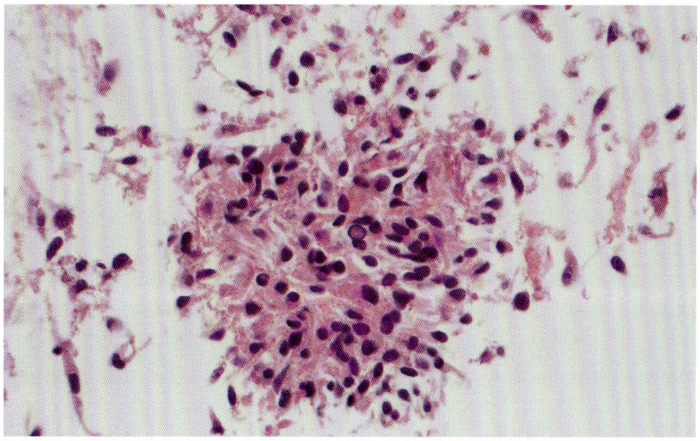

Fig. 8.175 Clear cell sarcoma. Tissue fragment of cells with round to oval or pleomorphic nuclei and an occasional intranuclear pseudoinclusion (cell block, H&E).

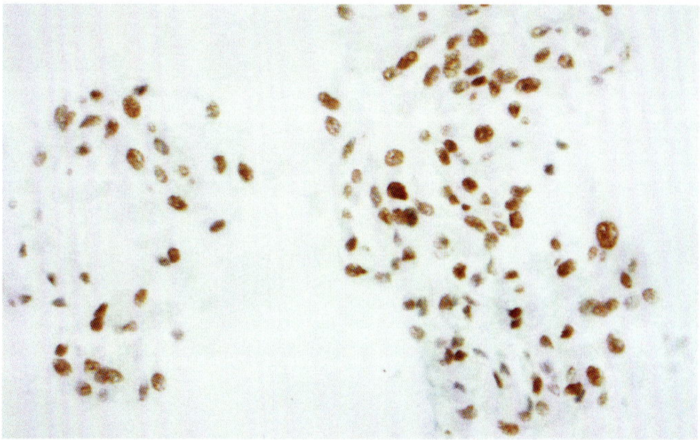

Fig. 8.176 Clear cell sarcoma. Tumour positive for SOX10 (cell block, ICC).

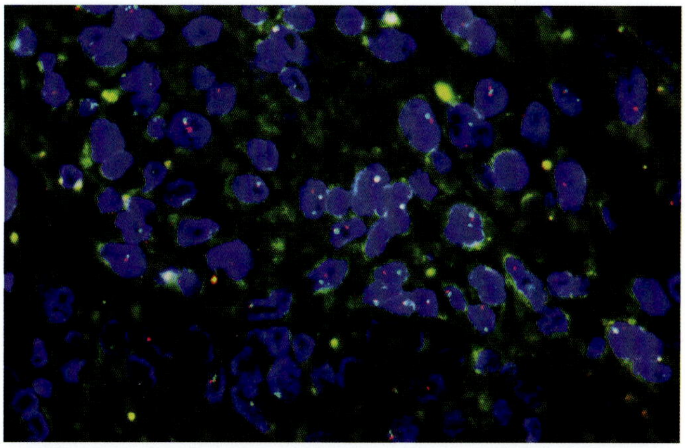

Fig. 8.177 Clear cell sarcoma of soft tissue. Tumour nuclei displaying *EWSR1* gene rearrangement in the form of single red–green split signals (FISH).

Extraskeletal osteosarcoma

Klijanienko J
Monaco SE

Definition

Extraskeletal osteosarcoma (EO) is a primary soft tissue malignant neoplasm characterized by the production of bone or osteoid matrix by neoplastic cells and arises without connection to the skeletal system.

Clinical features and imaging

EO accounts for < 1% of all soft tissue sarcomas and occurs in late adulthood, with a slight male predominance. Clinically, EO appears as a progressively enlarging, deep-seated soft tissue mass that may be associated with pain. The lower extremity is the most common site, followed by the shoulder, trunk, and retroperitoneum. About 10% of EOs may be associated with prior radiotherapy {228,101,803,821,1333,898,219,1149,838,1393,256,990,591,767, 1315}. Conventional imaging, CT, and MRI reveal a deep-seated soft tissue mass with variable mineralization, which in some cases prevents effective FNAB {1221}.

Histopathology

The osteoblastic type is composed of osteoblasts that are spindle or polygonal, with variable mitotic activity and possible necrosis {228,803,821}. Well-differentiated EO shows abundant bone formation surrounded by spindle cells {1537,6}.

Key diagnostic cytopathological features

- High cellularity
- Variably round, epithelioid, or spindle atypical osteoblasts with eccentric cytoplasm
- Benign or malignant-looking giant cells of osteoclastic type
- Eosinophilic (Pap) or orange osteoid (Giemsa)
- Magenta chondroid matrix (Giemsa)
- Frequent vessels
- Bone-producing myxoid matrix may be present
- Necrosis may be present

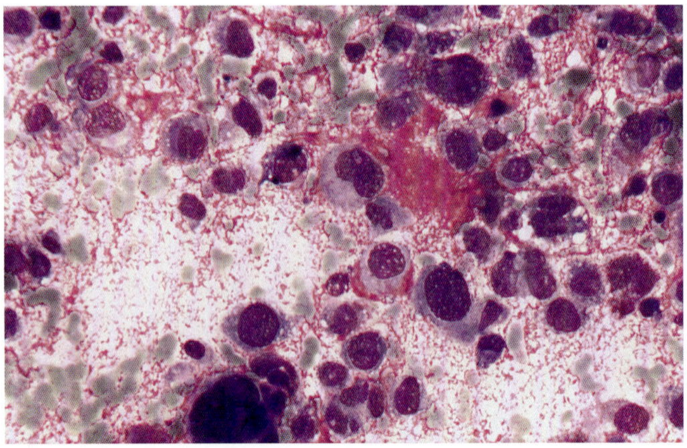

Fig. 8.178 Extraskeletal osteosarcoma. Osteoblasts and an osteoclastic giant cell with a hyperchromatic atypical nucleus and magenta osteochondroid matrix (Giemsa).

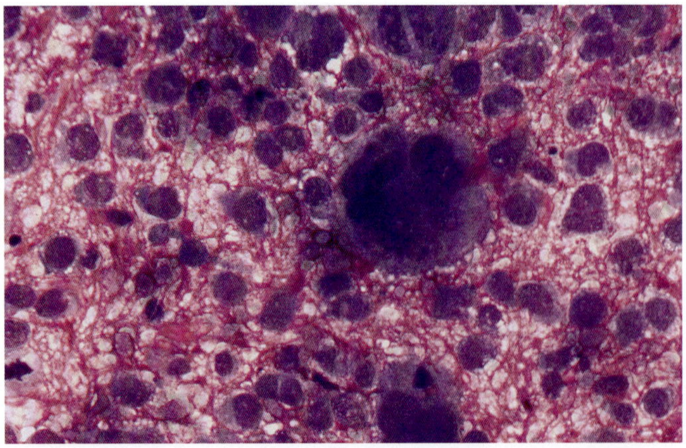

Fig. 8.179 Extraskeletal osteosarcoma. Osteoblasts, osteoclasts, and osteoid matrix (Giemsa).

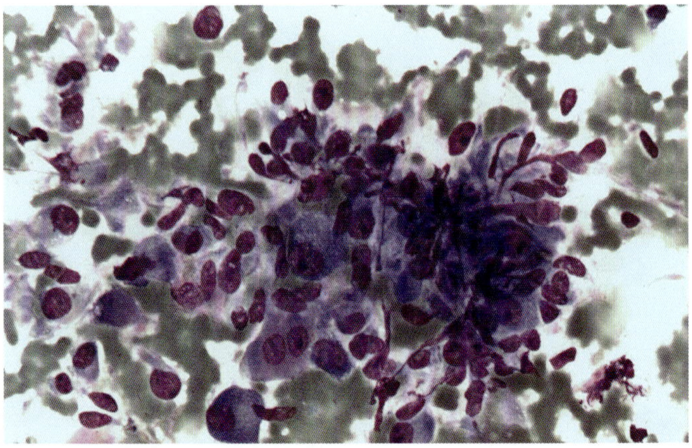

Fig. 8.180 Extraskeletal osteosarcoma. Polymorphous cells with variably enlarged and pleomorphic nuclei (Giemsa).

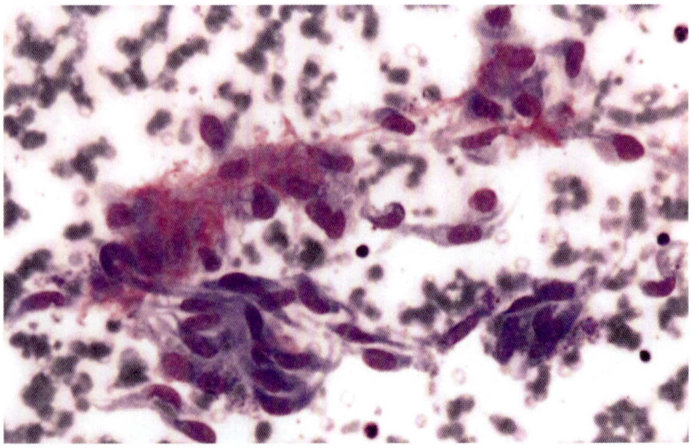

Fig. 8.181 Extraskeletal osteosarcoma. Spindle cells and osteoid matrix (Giemsa).

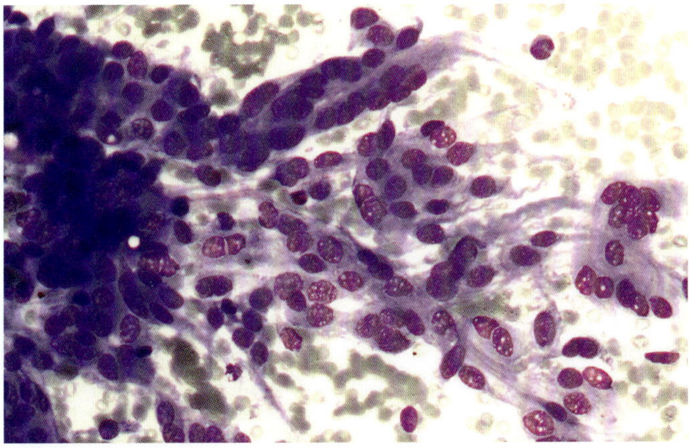

Fig. 8.182 Extraskeletal osteosarcoma. Spindle osteoblasts along with multinucleated osteoclasts (Giemsa).

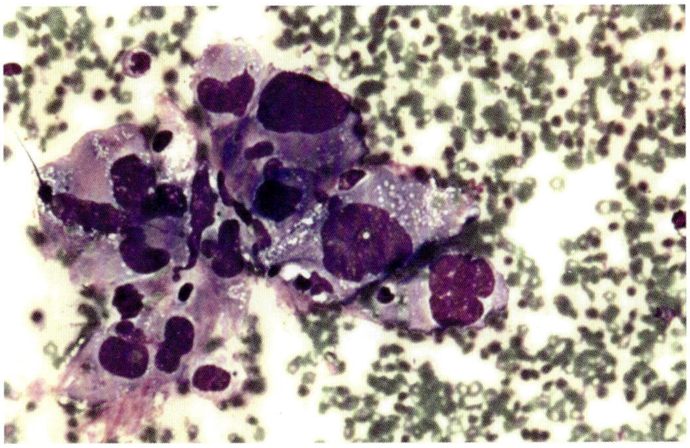

Fig. 8.183 Extraskeletal osteosarcoma. Polymorphous large malignant cells including osteoclastic cells, some showing large bizarre nuclei (Giemsa).

Discussion and differential diagnosis

An accurate diagnosis relies on the presence of the characteristic osteoblasts and osteoid or bone-producing matrix {734, 1019,1003}. Bone formation and polymorphous sarcomatous cells, including osteoblasts and osteoclasts, are indicative of EO. EO should be differentiated from skeletal osteosarcoma, chondrosarcoma, myositis ossificans, and dedifferentiated liposarcoma. The distinction between EO and bone osteosarcoma, chondrosarcoma, and myositis ossificans may be difficult. Chondrosarcomas may mimic EO, especially the chondroblastic subtype. Myositis ossificans is characterized by a zonal phenomenon, whereas EO displays an inverted zonal phenomenon, hence the importance of architectural characterization to differentiate both entities. Imaging in this context is of special value, because plain films and CT may help in the diagnosis, with a typical pattern of irregular peripheral calcification. Dedifferentiated liposarcoma is composed of pleomorphic spindle or multinucleated cells with cytoplasmic vacuolization and rare lipoblasts, but osteoblasts and bone formation are absent. A small cell EO should be differentiated from Ewing sarcoma {737,1332}.

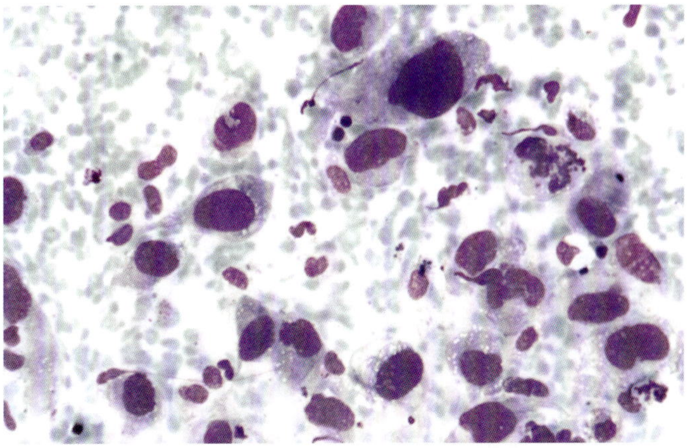

Fig. 8.184 Extraskeletal osteosarcoma. Dispersed osteoblastic cells with marked anisonucleosis and atypia (Giemsa).

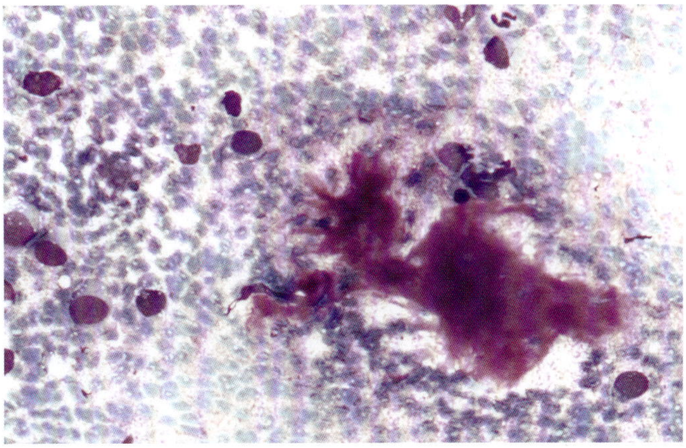

Fig. 8.185 Extraskeletal osteosarcoma. Osteoblasts and magenta bone formation (Giemsa).

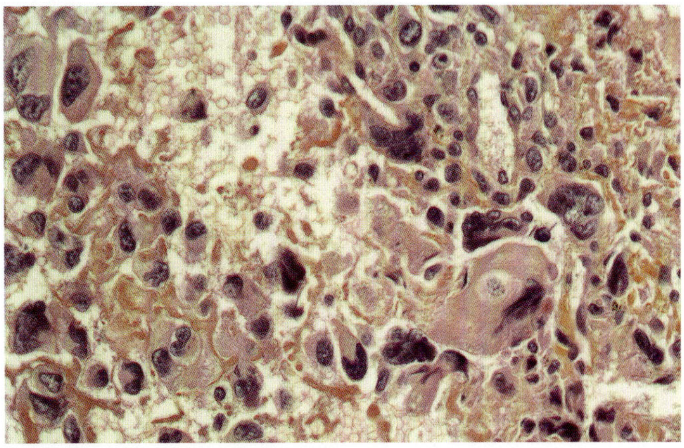

Fig. 8.186 Extraskeletal osteosarcoma. Polymorphous cells, including osteoblasts and osteoclasts, in osteoid (cell block, H&E).

Ancillary testing

No specific diagnostic molecular pathology tests are available. SATB2 immunoreactivity may be used to confirm osteoblastic differentiation {254,1530}.

Intimal sarcoma

Yang E
Dodd LG
Qian X

Definition

Intimal sarcoma (IS) is a malignant mesenchymal neoplasm arising in large blood vessels of the systemic and pulmonary circulation and also in the heart, defined by predominantly intraluminal growth with obstruction of the lumen of the vessel of origin and seeding of emboli to peripheral organs.

Clinical features and imaging

Clinical symptoms vary based on the site of origin but are often secondary to vascular occlusion or tumour emboli. Neoplasms occurring in the pulmonary artery may cause symptoms similar to those of acute or chronic pulmonary embolism {1077}. Imaging features suggestive of malignancy rather than thromboembolic disease include extravascular spread of the lesion {1536}, as well as higher FDG uptake on PET {621}. Prognosis is poor, with a rapidly progressive clinical course.

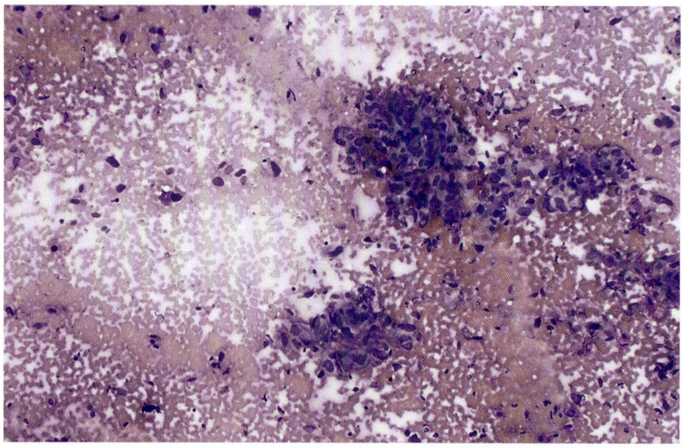

Fig. 8.187 Intimal sarcoma. Loosely cohesive tissue fragments and singly dispersed tumour cells (Giemsa).

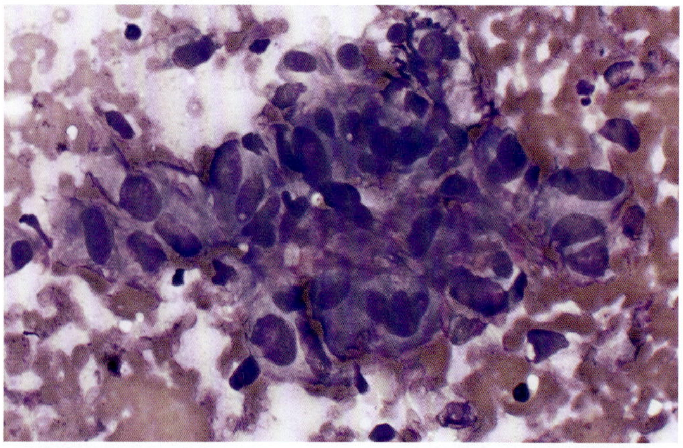

Fig. 8.188 Intimal sarcoma. A minute tissue fragment consisting of tumour cells with pleomorphic nuclei, irregular nuclear contours, variably prominent nucleoli, and moderate amounts of delicate cytoplasm with indistinct cell borders. Faint magenta stromal strands are present (Giemsa).

Histopathology

IS is a poorly differentiated malignant spindle cell neoplasm of possible fibroblastic or myofibroblastic derivation. The tumour generally does not have distinctive morphological features, with cytopathological atypia ranging from mild to severe and variable degrees of mitotic activity and necrosis. A myxoid background may be seen. Tumours may demonstrate a wide spectrum of heterologous differentiation, including rhabdomyosarcomatous, chondrosarcomatous, osteosarcomatous, and angiosarcomatous differentiation. Epithelioid morphology may also be seen.

Key diagnostic cytopathological features

- Variable cellularity
- Loosely cohesive tissue fragments and single cells
- Large pleomorphic spindle and epithelioid cells
- Varying amounts of delicate cytoplasm with ill-defined cell borders (best seen on Giemsa stain)
- Ovoid to spindle nuclei with significant anisonucleosis, irregular nuclear contours, and variably prominent nucleoli (best seen on Pap stain)
- Occasional binucleated and multinucleated cells

Reference(s): {174}

Discussion and differential diagnosis

The clinical presentation may be very similar to that of chronic pulmonary embolism or right heart failure, and diagnosis is often delayed or made at postmortem {38}. The cytomorphological differential is wide and includes primary and metastatic sarcoma, carcinoma, and melanoma. Collection of sufficient material for cell block preparation and ancillary studies is necessary.

IS is not expected to be positive for keratins or melanocytic markers, which helps in the distinction from carcinoma and melanoma. However, if cytokeratin positivity is seen, additional epithelial markers should be performed to exclude a poorly differentiated carcinoma. Angiosarcoma and leiomyosarcoma are primary sarcomas of vascular tissue origin, and their features may significantly overlap with those of IS demonstrating heterologous differentiation. Molecular analysis is critical in this situation, because demonstration of cytogenetic abnormalities commonly seen in IS (i.e. *MDM2* amplification) aids in the correct classification. Clinical and imaging correlation is required to confirm vascular origin of the tumour, as well as to exclude metastatic disease.

Ancillary testing

The most consistent cytogenetic aberrations include gains or amplifications of 12q13-q15 (*MDM2*, *CDK4*, *GLI1*) and 4q12 (*PDGFRA*) {143,319,1349}. Frequent amplifications of receptor

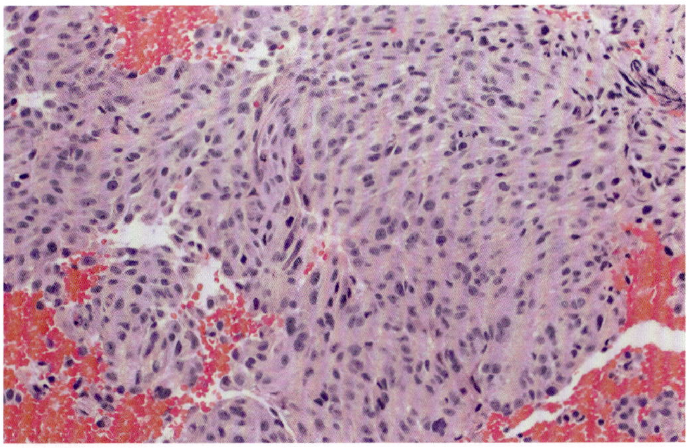

Fig. 8.189 Intimal sarcoma. A cohesive cellular tumour fragment with vaguely fascicular architecture (cell block, H&E).

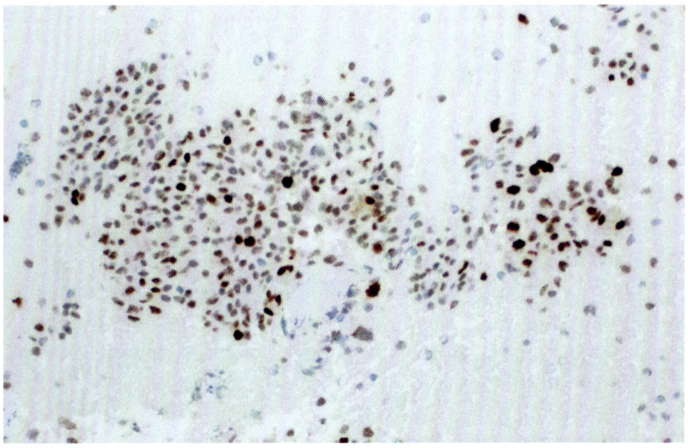

Fig. 8.190 Intimal sarcoma. MDM2-positive staining in nuclei (cell block, ICC).

tyrosine kinase genes (*PDGFRA*, *PDGFRB*, *EGFR*, *KIT*) may provide rationale for targeted therapies {1373}. IS tumour cells demonstrate variable positivity for SMA and vimentin {473}. Vascular markers tend to be negative. Myogenin and MYOD1 staining may be seen in areas of heterologous rhabdomyosarcomatous differentiation {1015}. *MDM2* amplification, which can be detected by FISH and/or NGS, is often reflected by ICC MDM2 positivity {143}. Other *MDM2*-amplified sarcomas include atypical lipomatous tumour / well-differentiated liposarcoma, dedifferentiated liposarcoma, and low-grade osteosarcoma; their distinction may be difficult in a small biopsy specimen given the protean cytomorphology of IS.

Chapter 8

Pleomorphic rhabdomyosarcoma

Agaram NP
Mito JK

Definition

Pleomorphic rhabdomyosarcoma is a high-grade pleomorphic sarcoma, usually of adults, composed of bizarre brightly eosinophilic polygonal, round, and spindle cells that display skeletal muscle differentiation.

Clinical features and imaging

These are tumours of adults and are most common in the sixth to seventh decades of life, with a mean patient age of 72 years; they occur more frequently in men than in women, with an M:F ratio of 1.8:1 {1034}. These tumours arise in the deep soft tissue. Although most often occurring in the lower extremities, they can also occur at other anatomical sites. Patients present with a rapidly growing, variably painful soft tissue mass {455}. These are highly aggressive sarcomas, with a median survival time of 7.3 months in the largest study to date, in which about 80% of patients died of disease {1034}. Patients with superficial tumours (~20%) had a favourable outcome. Metastases to lungs are common {1034,455,459}.

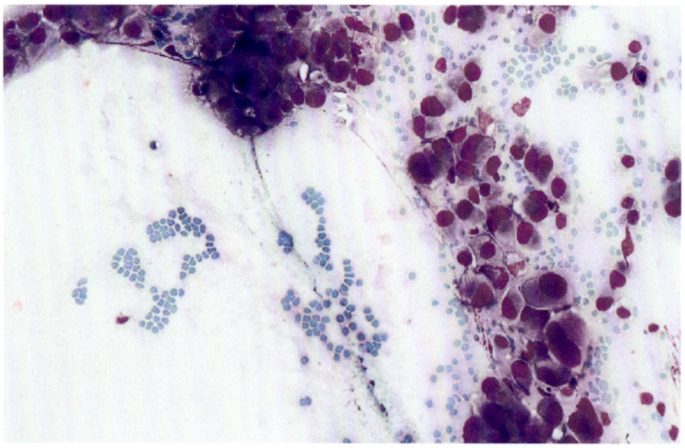

Fig. 8.191 Pleomorphic rhabdomyosarcoma. Loosely cohesive tissue fragments consisting of very large rhabdoid cells with hyperchromatic nuclei and copious, often eccentric cytoplasm (Giemsa).

Histopathology

Pleomorphic rhabdomyosarcomas are usually large, well-marginated tumours {1034} with a pseudocapsule and a whitish fleshy cut surface, often with necrosis. The tumours are composed of sheets of large, atypical and frequently multinucleated polygonal, spindle, or rhabdoid cells with eosinophilic cytoplasm. Nuclei often show marked variation in size and shape, with hyperchromasia and prominent nucleoli {459,455}.

Key diagnostic cytopathological features

- High cellularity
- Dispersed single cells and tissue fragments
- Large pleomorphic and rhabdoid cells with copious eccentric basophilic cytoplasm and round to irregular pleomorphic nuclei
- Multinucleation
- Background of haemorrhage and necrosis
- Mitoses, including atypical forms
- Evidence of skeletal muscle differentiation; cross-striations in the eccentric cytoplasm not common

Reference(s): {719,1026,394}

Discussion and differential diagnosis

The differential diagnosis includes other pleomorphic sarcomas, such as undifferentiated pleomorphic sarcoma, and other rhabdomyosarcoma subtypes with anaplasia. Non-mesenchymal neoplasms, such as sarcomatoid carcinoma, melanoma,

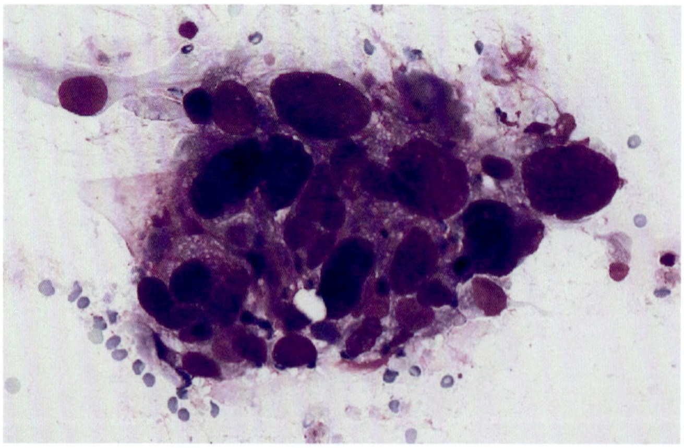

Fig. 8.192 Pleomorphic rhabdomyosarcoma. A tissue fragment consisting of very large cells with very large, highly pleomorphic nuclei. Compare to background red blood cells (Giemsa).

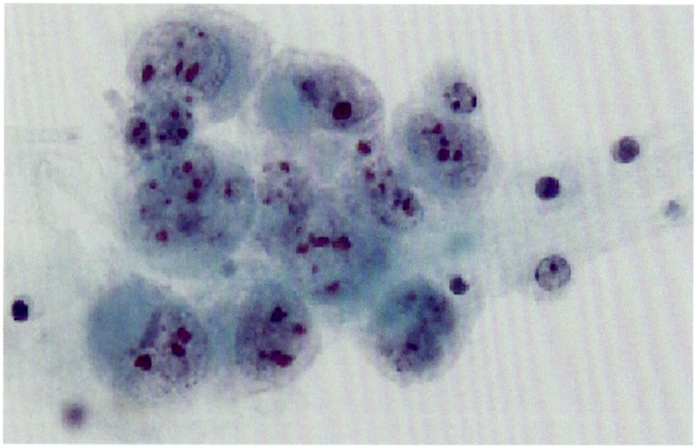

Fig. 8.193 Pleomorphic rhabdomyosarcoma. A minute tissue fragment of very large rhabdoid cells with copious eccentric cytoplasm, large pleomorphic nuclei, and prominent nucleoli (Pap).

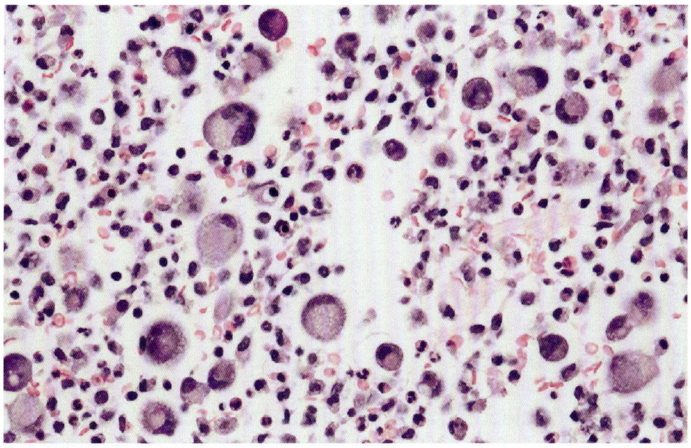

Fig. 8.194 Pleomorphic rhabdomyosarcoma. Pleural fluid showing metastatic pleomorphic rhabdomyosarcoma showing isolated very large rhabdoid cells with copious eccentric cytoplasm, large nuclei, and prominent nucleoli, amid inflammatory cells and occasional mesothelial cells (H&E).

and anaplastic large cell lymphoma, can show overlapping cytomorphology, and ICC is required.

Ancillary testing

ICC shows strong desmin expression and often limited expression of MYOD1 and myogenin. Molecular analysis has shown complex karyotypes with numerous copy-number alterations, but no specific molecular alterations have been identified {201, 503,817}.

Undifferentiated pleomorphic sarcoma

Kerr DA
Chebib I
Jo VY
Mito JK

Definition

Undifferentiated pleomorphic sarcoma (UPS) shows no identifiable line of differentiation when analysed with currently available technology. It is a heterogeneous group and a diagnosis of exclusion, although genetic subgroups (particularly in the round cell group) have emerged. Dedifferentiated types of specific soft tissue sarcomas are excluded from this category.

Clinical features and imaging

UPS predominantly affects older adults. It is common in deep somatic soft tissues but may present at any anatomical location. Frequently characterized by rapid growth, it has an otherwise non-distinctive clinical presentation. UPS was previously called undifferentiated sarcoma and was categorized as a tumour of uncertain differentiation in the fifth edition of the WHO classification of soft tissue tumours. It is now categorized as a fibroblastic and myofibroblastic neoplasm.

Histopathology

Typically, UPS is an overtly malignant, high-grade sarcoma composed of pleomorphic cells in a storiform to other non-distinctive pattern. Bizarre, multinucleated tumour giant cells are common. Tumour cell nuclei demonstrate marked variation in size and shape, hyperchromasia, and membrane irregularities {184,1405}.

Key diagnostic cytopathological features

- High cellularity
- Variable mixture of individual cells and tissue fragments
- Tissue fragments may show a storiform architecture

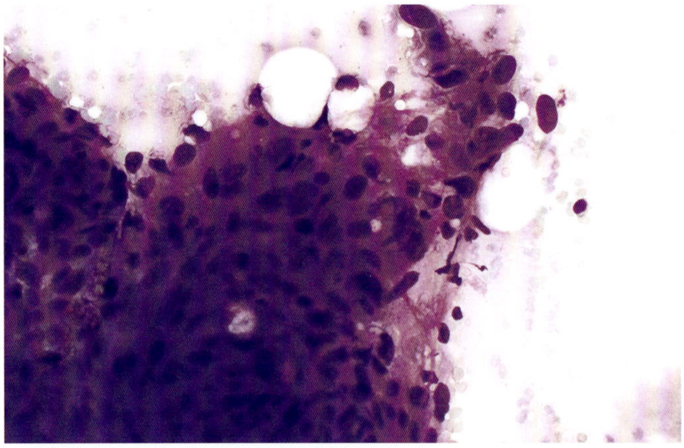

Fig. 8.195 Undifferentiated pleomorphic sarcoma. A cohesive tissue fragment consisting of spindle cells with marked nuclear enlargement and pleomorphism, as well as stroma (Giemsa).

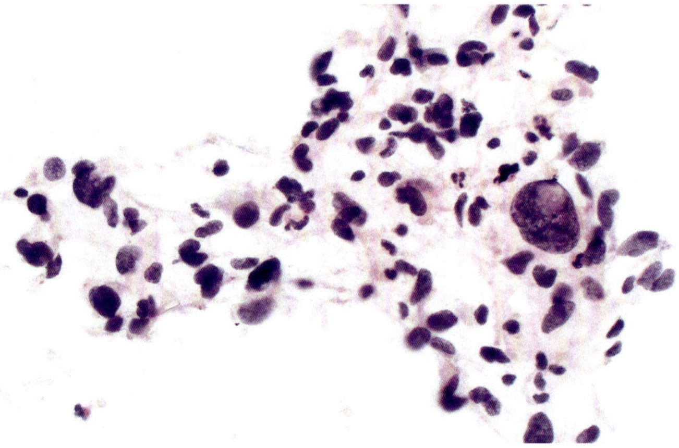

Fig. 8.197 Undifferentiated pleomorphic sarcoma. The cells are of variable size and shape, with some markedly enlarged mononucleated pleomorphic tumour cells and irregular spindle tumour cells (Pap).

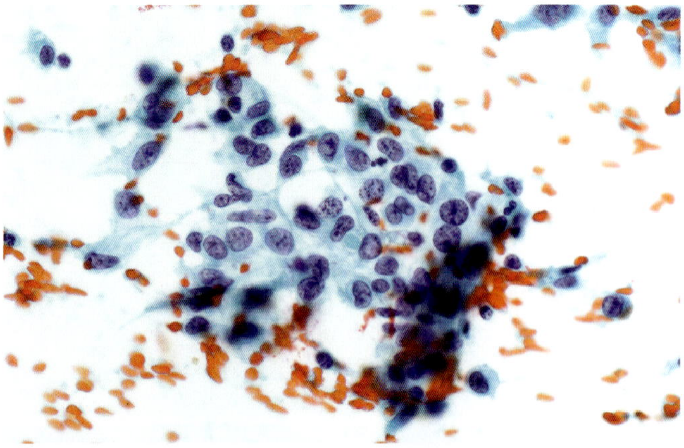

Fig. 8.196 Undifferentiated pleomorphic sarcoma. The cells show marked variability in size and shape, with large pleomorphic nuclei showing coarse, granular, irregularly distributed chromatin (Pap).

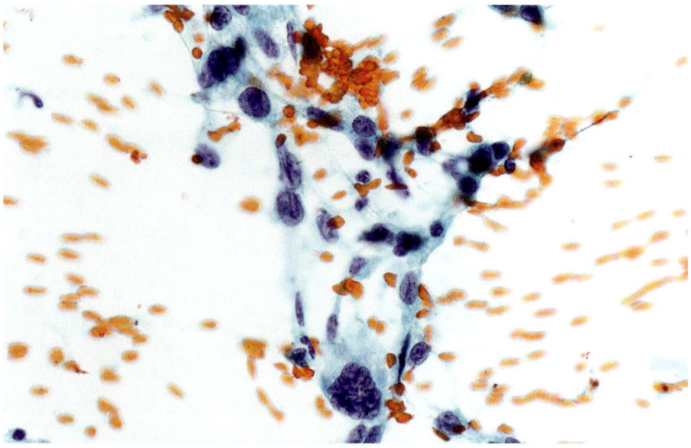

Fig. 8.198 Undifferentiated pleomorphic sarcoma. Large pleomorphic cells, some of which are spindle, with large highly pleomorphic hyperchromatic nuclei (Pap).

- Large mononucleated or frequently multinucleated pleomorphic cells
- Second population of spindle fibroblast-like cells
- Cytoplasmic vacuolization
- Tumour cells may show phagocytic activity, with cell debris or well-preserved cells within their cytoplasm
- Pronounced nuclear pleomorphism, with coarse chromatin and large nucleoli
- High mitotic rate, including atypical forms
- Background of multinucleated giant cells, haemorrhage, and necrosis

Reference(s): {1474,123,728}

Discussion and differential diagnosis

Clinical factors inform the differential diagnosis, including anatomical site {574}. Dedifferentiated liposarcoma and intimal sarcoma are considerations for retroperitoneal and great vessel tumours, respectively {248,1405}. In a patient with a history of carcinoma or melanoma, a dedifferentiated form of the prior tumour should be considered {1405,184}. A dedifferentiated component of a specific type of mesenchymal tumour, such as leiomyosarcoma, solitary fibrous tumour, or gastrointestinal stroma tumour, should be excluded. In the context of prior radiation therapy, a radiation-associated sarcoma is considered given that at least 25% of these are undifferentiated {489,777}.

For some tumours, including pleomorphic liposarcoma with its lipoblasts, extraskeletal osteosarcoma showing bone matrix, and myxofibrosarcoma with its myxoid matrix and characteristic vasculature, the characteristic diagnostic features may be limited in extent and distribution, and these cases can be problematic to distinguish with a sampling technique such as FNAB or CNB {574,184,1463}.

Although most tumours in the differential are high-grade sarcomas, cellular pleomorphism is also a feature of several benign neoplasms, such as pleomorphic lipoma and "ancient" schwannoma. Neoplasms of intermediate biological potential should also be considered {1405}, including pleomorphic dermal sarcoma and superficial CD34-positive fibroblastic tumour, which enter the differential in superficial sites {81,181}.

The diagnosis of UPS is one of exclusion, so although it can be suggested on FNAB as a diagnostic possibility, definitive diagnosis requires ICC and in many cases excision biopsy.

Ancillary testing

UPS demonstrates complex karyotypes with extensive genomic rearrangements and no specific immunophenotype or molecular signature {172}. Therefore, ICC and molecular studies are required to exclude sarcomas of specific types and lines of differentiation {184,574,1405}. *MDM2* and *CDK4* amplification or protein overexpression by ICC supports a diagnosis of intimal sarcoma or dedifferentiated liposarcoma, respectively {248,1405}.

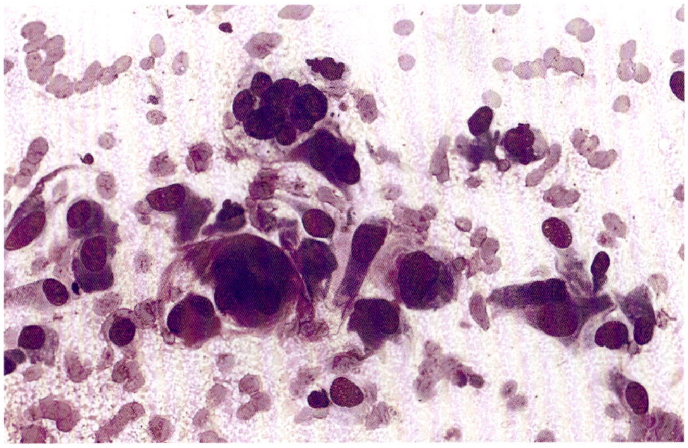

Fig. 8.199 Undifferentiated pleomorphic sarcoma. Single large mononucleated and multinucleated cells with large, often bizarre hyperchromatic nuclei (Giemsa).

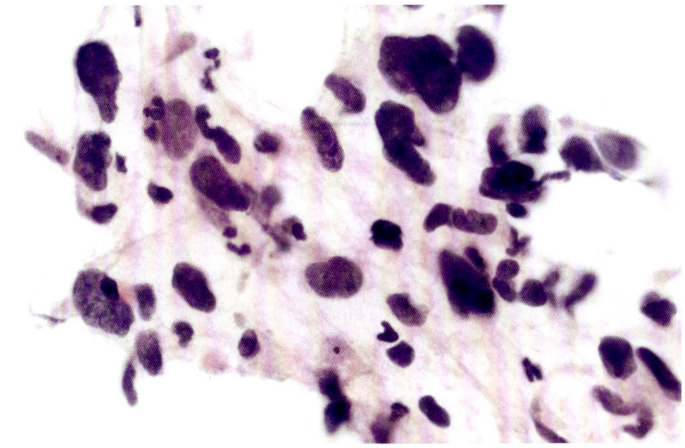

Fig. 8.200 Undifferentiated pleomorphic sarcoma. Heterogeneous pleomorphic and spindle large cells showing highly pleomorphic hyperchromatic nuclei; occasional cells contain inflammatory cells (10 o'clock) (Pap).

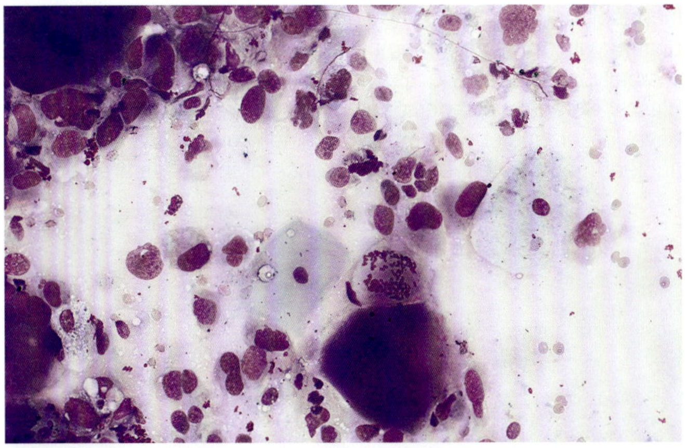

Fig. 8.201 High-grade leiomyosarcoma. Pleomorphic mononucleated and multinucleated tumour cells, osteoclast-type giant cells, and atypical mitoses can be seen in pleomorphic sarcomas, such as this high-grade leiomyosarcoma. Undifferentiated sarcoma is a diagnosis of exclusion that cannot be definitively rendered on a cytopathological specimen (Giemsa).

Chapter 8

Ewing sarcoma

Jo VY
Bui M
Klijanienko J

Definition

Ewing sarcoma is a small round cell sarcoma showing gene fusions involving a member of the FET family of genes and a member of the ETS transcription factor family, with the most common fusion being *EWSR1::FLI1*.

Clinical features and imaging

Most patients are young, with peak incidence during the second decade of life; about 80% of all patients are aged < 20 years. There is a slight male predominance (M:F ratio: 1.4:1). Ewing sarcoma is the second most common primary bone malignancy in children and young adults after osteosarcoma, arising most frequently in the long bones, pelvis, and ribs (typically in the diaphysis or diametaphysial regions). Most cases that arise in older patients (i.e. ≥ 30 years of age) are in soft tissue sites, with a wide anatomical distribution {511}. Patients with extraskeletal Ewing sarcoma present with pain and a palpable mass.

The current multimodal therapy for Ewing sarcoma has improved prognosis, with a cure rate for localized disease as high as 70%. Poorer prognosis is associated with metastatic disease, pelvic location, incomplete response to neoadjuvant chemotherapy, and early-relapsing tumours.

Histopathology

Ewing sarcoma is the prototypical round cell sarcoma. At low power, tumours are lobulated, with sheet-like growth of monotonous small round cells. Tumour cells have round nuclei with evenly distributed fine chromatin and smooth nuclear contours, inconspicuous nucleoli, and varying clear or eosinophilic cytoplasm with indistinct membranes {436,836}. There is often a small proportion of cells with darker nuclei and scant cytoplasm. Some cases designated as "atypical Ewing sarcoma" have larger nuclei with more prominent nucleoli and irregular nuclear membranes, but the presence of these features has no prognostic significance {1011}. Rarely, tumour cells can show vague rosette-like structures.

Key diagnostic cytopathological features

- High cellularity
- Predominantly single dispersed round cells, with small discohesive tissue fragments
- Admixture of "light" cells and "dark" cells, which show smaller, darker nuclei with smudged chromatin
- Nuclei are round to ovoid, with evenly distributed pale chromatin, indistinct or small nucleoli, and distinct nuclear membranes with overall smooth contours and occasional moulding
- Cytoplasm varies from scant to more abundant and pale, occasionally showing fine intracytoplasmic glycogen vacuoles and wispy cytoplasmic tags
- Numerous naked nuclei and frequent dispersal of cytoplasmic fragments, imparting a striped "tigroid" background

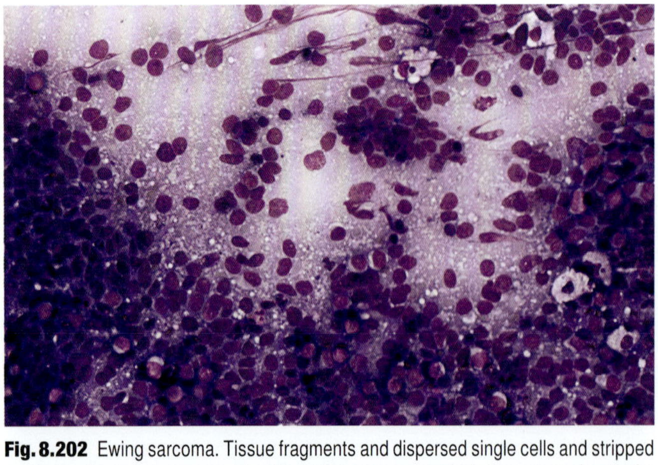

Fig. 8.202 Ewing sarcoma. Tissue fragments and dispersed single cells and stripped nuclei in a finely granular speckled "tigroid" background, which is common due to glycogen and dispersion of cytoplasmic fragments (Giemsa).

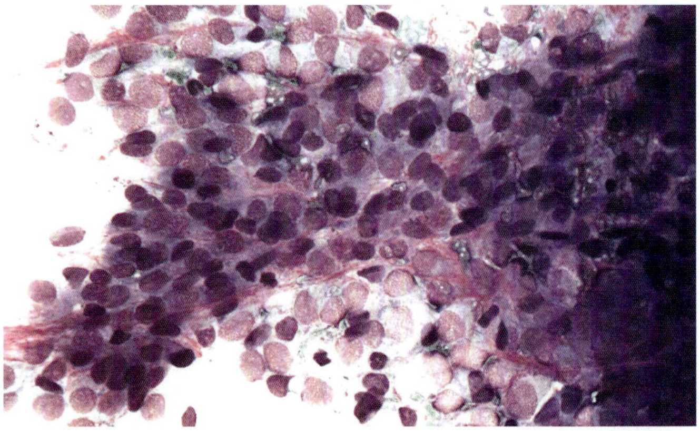

Fig. 8.203 Ewing sarcoma. A dense tissue fragment showing both light and darker cells, as well as very fine magenta stromal elements, which are rare (Giemsa).

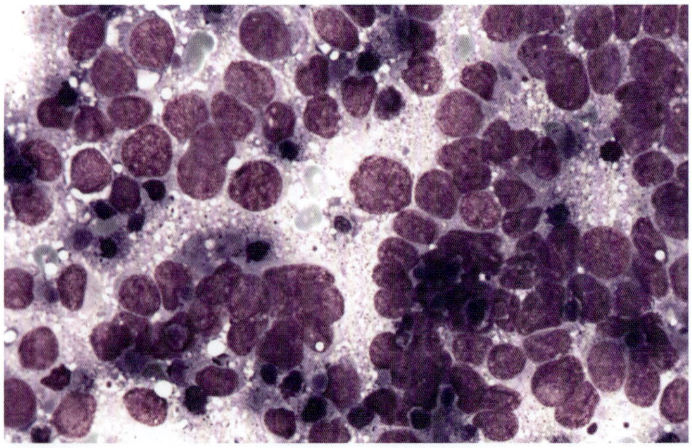

Fig. 8.204 Ewing sarcoma. Nuclei are round to pleomorphic and show focal nuclear moulding, with single-cell necrosis in the granular background (Giemsa).

- Some cases may show atypical features such as abundant cytoplasm, enlarged nuclei, nuclear grooves and pronounced nuclear membrane irregularity, coarser chromatin, and more prominent nucleoli
- Vague rosette formation may be seen in small tissue fragments

Reference(s): {519,737,1183}

Discussion and differential diagnosis

The differential diagnosis of small round cell tumours requires ancillary testing, and in most laboratories it is more efficient to use ICC panels before undertaking molecular testing. Ewing sarcoma has a broad and varied list of cytomorphological mimics. Chief considerations among other sarcomas are alveolar rhabdomyosarcoma, poorly differentiated synovial sarcoma, and desmoplastic small round cell tumour, as well as molecularly defined subsets of undifferentiated round cell sarcomas, such as *CIC*-rearranged sarcoma. Alveolar rhabdomyosarcoma usually shows larger, more atypical nuclei and multinucleated wreath-like giant cells. Poorly differentiated synovial sarcoma can show a predominant round cell morphology, but foci of conventional spindle morphology and large tissue fragments may be present. Most cases of desmoplastic small round cell tumour arise in the abdominal cavity of young men, and smears show more cohesive tissue fragments of small round cells and a frequent desmoplastic stroma.

Ancillary testing

ICC is useful and efficient for the diagnosis of Ewing sarcoma and to exclude cytomorphological mimics, facilitating the identification of cases for molecular confirmation. The vast majority of Ewing sarcomas show strong, diffuse membranous staining for CD99 {859,436}. NKX2-2 has high sensitivity for Ewing sarcoma and higher specificity than CD99, although staining may also be seen in subsets of other tumour types, including small cell carcinoma, synovial sarcoma, melanoma, and mesenchymal chondrosarcoma {600,1541,903}. Up to one third of cases can show staining for keratin {436} and the neuroendocrine markers synaptophysin, chromogranin, CD56, and INSM1 {858,1424}.

Many cases previously considered to be atypical Ewing sarcoma are now known to represent molecularly distinct groups of undifferentiated round cell sarcomas (see Table 8.01, p. 218), the most notable being round cell sarcomas with *EWSR1* fusions to non-ETS partners, which have been renamed "sarcomas with *EWSR1::NFATC2* fusions", as well as *CIC*-rearranged sarcomas and sarcomas with *BCOR* genetic alterations {65}. The distinction depends on some cytopathological nuances and clinical features, but ancillary tests are required in most cases. These tumours often show less consistent CD99 staining than

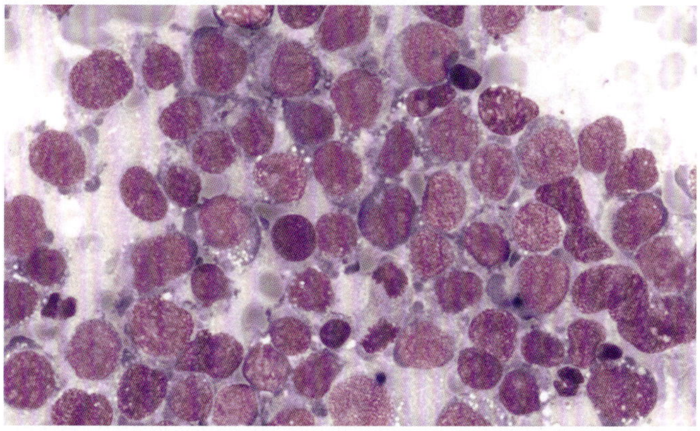

Fig. 8.205 Ewing sarcoma. Single cells with round to oval nuclei and a small amount of cytoplasm, commonly containing minute vacuoles (Giemsa).

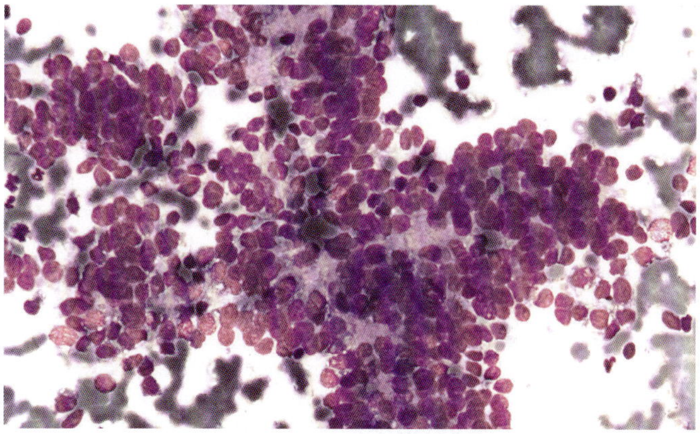

Fig. 8.207 Ewing sarcoma. Tissue fragments showing rosette formation (Giemsa).

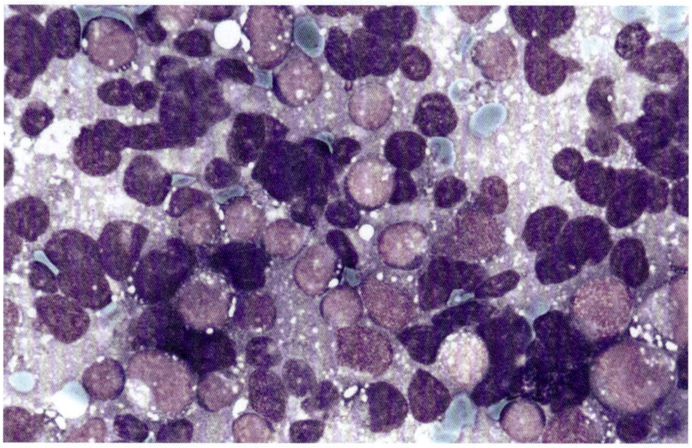

Fig. 8.206 Ewing sarcoma. Sheets of cells in a large tissue fragment with round nuclei and indistinct cytoplasmic margins (cell block, H&E).

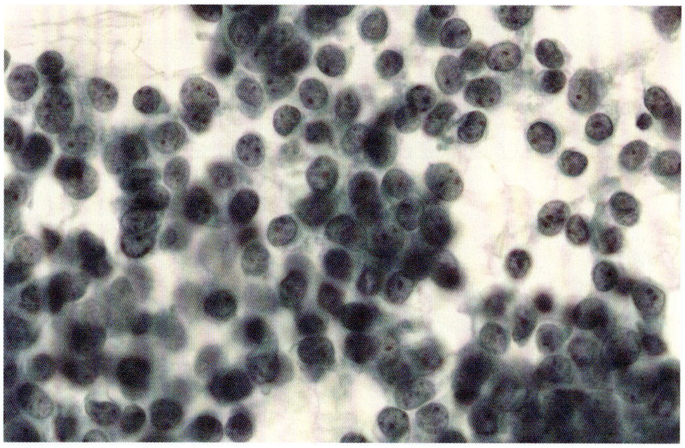

Fig. 8.208 Ewing sarcoma. Cells have fine, evenly dispersed nuclear chromatin and small nucleoli (Pap).

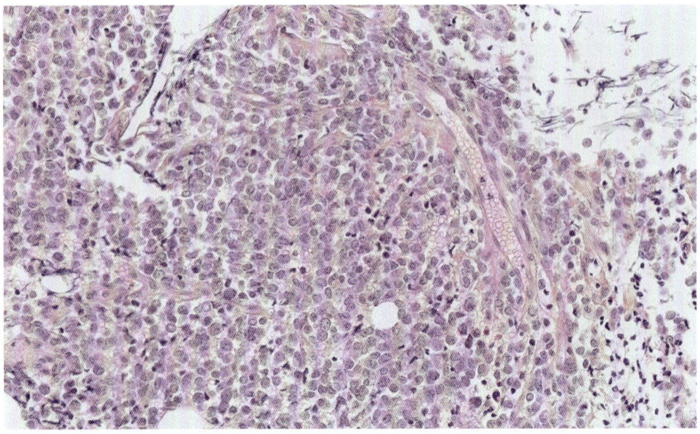

Fig. 8.209 Ewing sarcoma. The round cell population is often composed of a dual population of light cells and smaller dark cells (Giemsa).

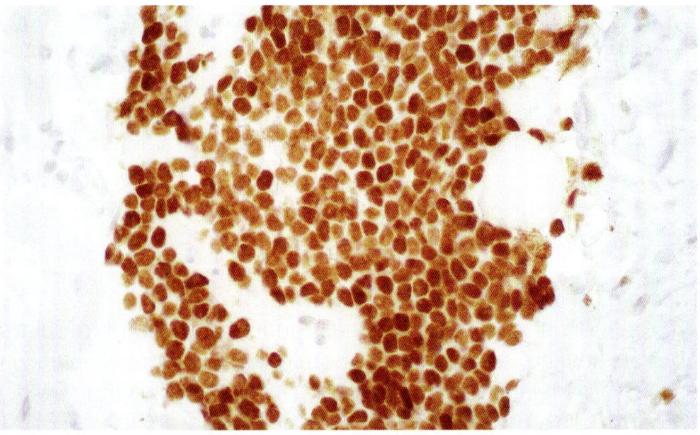

Fig. 8.210 Ewing sarcoma. Nuclear staining for NKX2-2 is highly sensitive and specific for Ewing sarcoma (cell block, ICC).

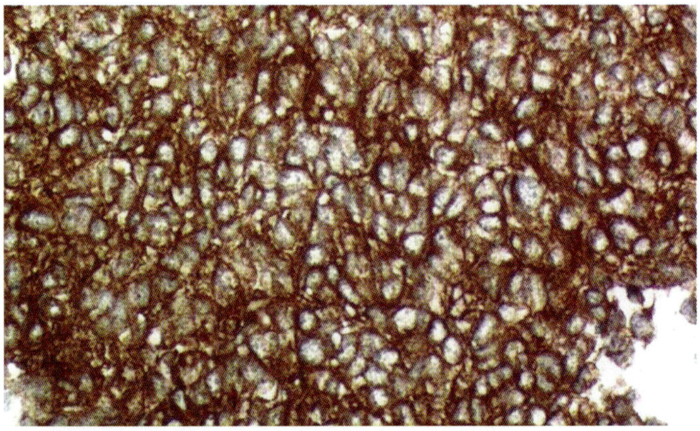

Fig. 8.211 Ewing sarcoma. Diffuse membranous staining in CD99 (cell block, ICC).

Ewing sarcoma, often with only focal or even negative staining. Most round cell sarcomas with *ESWR1::NFATC2* fusions cannot be distinguished from Ewing sarcoma on cytomorphological grounds and can only be identified by molecular sequencing, although some cases show pseudoacinar structures, fibrous or myxoid stroma, and spindle cell morphology. *PATZ1*-rearranged sarcomas, previously included in the "*EWSR1* fusions to non-ETS partners" group, are now grouped with the tumours of uncertain differentiation, in light of the variable immunohistochemical expression of myogenic and neurogenic markers by the tumours cells {222}.

CIC-rearranged sarcoma and round cell sarcoma with *BCOR* alterations frequently show increased nuclear size and pleomorphism, more prominent nucleoli, spindle cells, myxoid or fibrotic stroma, and necrosis. Most cases of *CIC*-rearranged sarcoma are positive for WT1 and ETV4; the diagnosis should be confirmed by molecular testing using either FISH for *CIC* rearrangement or sequencing. Sarcomas with *BCOR* alterations include tumours with *BCOR* fusions (most commonly *BCOR::CCNB3*) or internal tandem duplication (ITD) of the *BCOR* gene. ICC for BCOR is positive, and cyclin B3 (CCNB3) is positive in cases harbouring *BCOR::CCNB3*, which show more varied and nonspecific ICC, with frequent staining for SATB2, TLE1, and cyclin D1.

Table 8.01 Undifferentiated spindle, round, and epithelioid cell sarcomas

Tumour type	Immunocytochemistry (positive)	Molecular genetics
Ewing sarcoma	CD99, NKX2-2	FET::ETS fusions: *EWSR1::FLI1* (85%); *EWSR1::ERG* (10%); *FUS::FLI1*, *FUS::ERG*, and other (rare) FET::ETS fusions (5%)
***NFATC2*-rearranged sarcoma**	CD99 diffusely positive (~50%); keratin, EMA, NKX2-2, and NKX3-1 (variably positive)	*EWSR1::NFATC2*, *FUS::NFATC2*; *EWSR1* break-apart FISH shows amplification of 5′ probe
***CIC*-rearranged sarcoma**	CD99 variable (~85%), ETV4, WT1	*CIC::DUX4L8* (*DUX2*) (95%), *CIC::FOXO4*, *CIC::LEUTX*, *CIC::NUTM1*, *CIC::NUTM2A*
Sarcoma with *BCOR* alterations	CD99 variable (~50%), BCOR, cyclin B3 (CCNB3), SATB2, cyclin D1, TLE1	*BCOR::CCNB3* (90%), *BCOR::MAML3*, *BCOR* internal tandem duplication (ITD)

Alveolar rhabdomyosarcoma is positive for desmin and MYOD1, showing a characteristic diffuse nuclear staining pattern, and *FOXO1* rearrangement defines this tumour. Poorly differentiated synovial sarcoma is positive in ICC for SS18::SSX and SSX, and *SS18* rearrangement can be confirmed by FISH. Desmoplastic small round cell tumour has a distinctive immunophenotype of staining for keratin, EMA, and desmin, as well as nuclear staining for antibodies against the C-terminus of WT1; it is also characterized by an *EWSR1* rearrangement, but the defining fusion is *EWSR1::WT1*.

Non-mesenchymal tumours frequently enter the differential diagnosis and include lymphoblastic lymphoma, which also shows diffuse CD99 staining, but lymphoid markers, including TdT, make the diagnosis. Malignant melanoma can be excluded by S100 or SOX10, as well as HMB45 and melan-A (MART1). Given that Ewing sarcomas can show staining for keratin and neuroendocrine markers, exclusion of neuroendocrine tumours is often necessary, such as in the lung, where Ewing sarcoma may be mistaken for carcinoid or atypical carcinoid tumour {363}.

FISH is commonly employed to detect *EWSR1* rearrangement, and it is considered diagnostic in the setting of appropriate clinical, cytomorphological, and ICC features. However, some cases have variant fusions involving *FUS* in lieu of *EWSR1*, which can be identified by FISH for *FUS*. Given that *EWSR1* fusions are common in many neoplasms, including other round cell sarcomas, sequencing-specific studies may be necessary to detect the specific *EWSR1::FLI1* fusion or the rare *EWSR1::ERG* variant {644}.

CIC-rearranged sarcoma

Teot LA
Chebib I

Definition

CIC-rearranged sarcoma is a high-grade round cell undifferentiated sarcoma defined by *CIC*-related gene fusions, most often *CIC::DUX4*.

Clinical features and imaging

CIC-rearranged sarcomas present as mass lesions and have been described in most sites, including the soft tissue of the extremities, head and neck, and retroperitoneum (80–85% of cases), visceral organs (10–15%), and rarely bone (< 5%). There is a wide age range, with a median patient age of 25–35 years, and a slight male predominance {1540,465,71}. Imaging shows aggressive mass lesions but nonspecific imaging characteristics. By CT, tumours show isodense to hypodense attenuation, and they are metabolically active by FDG PET. MRI shows mass contrast enhancement, necrosis, perilesional oedema, and fluid-fluid level {154}.

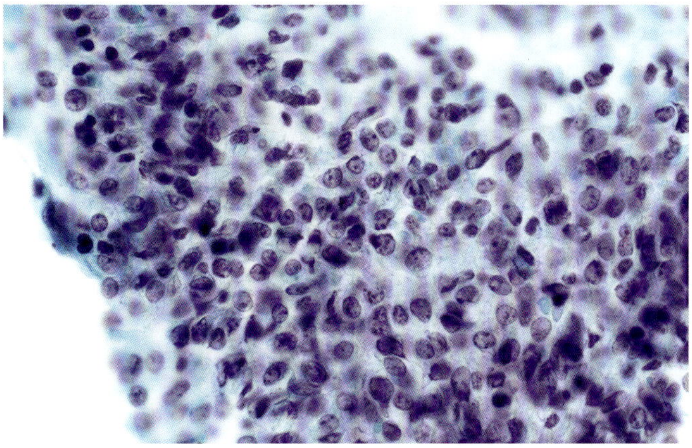

Fig. 8.212 *CIC*-rearranged sarcoma. The tumour cells have scant to moderate pale to vacuolated cytoplasm; indistinct cell borders; and round, ovoid, elongate, or spindle nuclei with irregular membranes, evenly dispersed chromatin, and conspicuous nucleoli (Pap).

Histopathology

Tumours are composed of sheets of uniform undifferentiated small round cells with areas of lobular growth separated by fibrous stroma. Variant morphologies, such as epithelioid, rhabdoid, and spindle, can be seen in 10–20% of cases. Necrosis is common, and a subset of cases show myxoid stroma {1540, 465,71}.

Key diagnostic cytopathological features

- High cellularity
- Sheets, large tissue fragments, and single cells
- Syncytial tissue fragments containing delicate vessels, with tumour cells showing poorly defined borders and occasional nuclear moulding
- Round cells with scant to moderate, often vacuolated cytoplasm, which can be concentric or eccentric
- Nuclei showing mild anisonucleosis, pleomorphism, and atypia
- Nuclei round to ovoid with fine and evenly dispersed dark chromatin, irregular membranes, and often prominent nucleoli
- Occasional elongate, spindle, pencillate, or angulated nuclei
- Variable mitotic figures, necrosis, myxoid matrix, and striped or "tigroid" background

Reference(s): {665,199,1174}

Discussion and differential diagnosis

The differential diagnosis of *CIC*-rearranged sarcoma includes Ewing sarcoma, *BCOR::CCNB3* sarcoma, alveolar

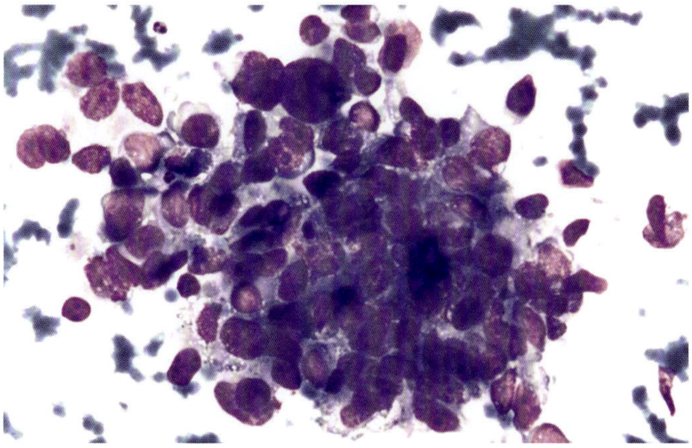

Fig. 8.213 *CIC*-rearranged sarcoma. The cells in this cohesive tissue fragment have scant, vacuolated, grey-blue cytoplasm and round to ovoid nuclei with evenly dispersed chromatin and prominent nucleoli. Cell borders are indistinct and nuclear moulding is present (Giemsa).

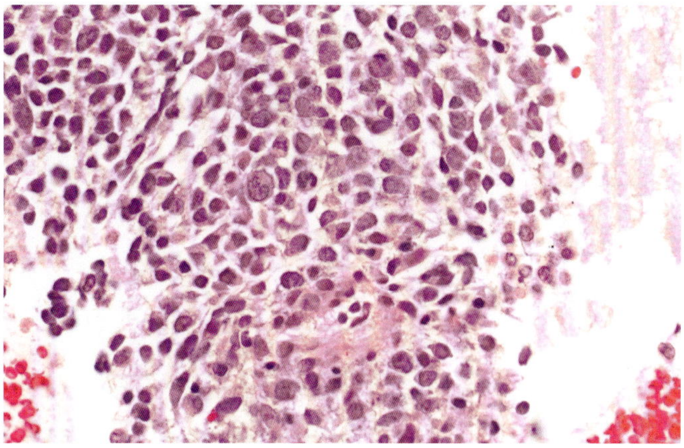

Fig. 8.214 *CIC*-rearranged sarcoma. A tissue fragment consisting of cells with scant to mildly abundant, eosinophilic to vacuolated cytoplasm and round, ovoid, or spindle nuclei showing mild anisocytosis, pleomorphism, and atypia, as well as prominent nucleoli (cell block, H&E).

Chapter 8

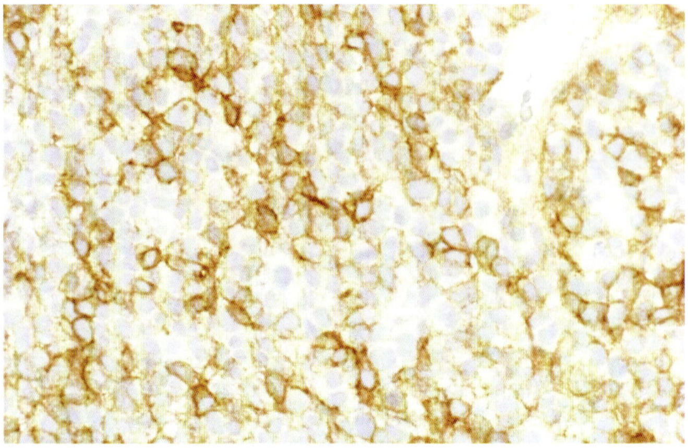

Fig. 8.215 *CIC*-rearranged sarcoma. Patchy, variable membranous staining for CD99 (cell block, ICC).

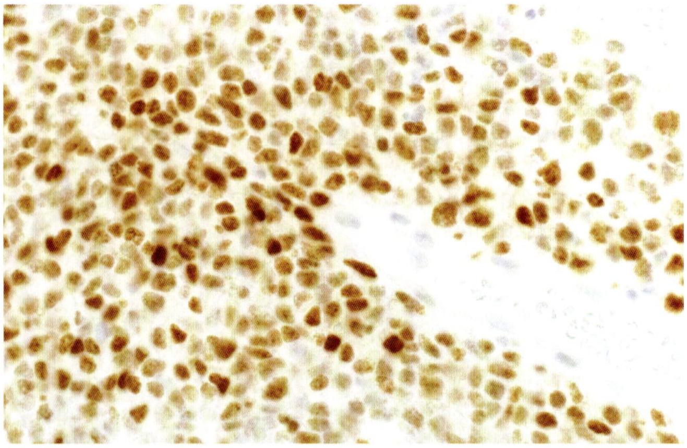

Fig. 8.216 *CIC*-rearranged sarcoma. Diffuse nuclear staining for WT1 (cell block, ICC).

rhabdomyosarcoma, poorly differentiated synovial sarcoma, and desmoplastic round cell tumour, as well as carcinomas and lymphomas. The cells in Ewing sarcoma are usually singly dispersed or in small tissue fragments, and they are uniform with scant cytoplasm, round nuclei, fine pale chromatin, and inconspicuous nucleoli {199}. Giemsa smears may have a striped or "tigroid" background. *BCOR*::*CCNB3* sarcomas tend to be more pleomorphic and may have spindle cells and myxoid stroma {672,462,1490}. Alveolar rhabdomyosarcomas have atypical, hyperchromatic nuclei with coarse chromatin and prominent nucleoli; large, multinucleated wreath-like cells with abundant cytoplasm may also be present {199}. Poorly differentiated round cell synovial sarcomas have round to short spindle cells with hyperchromatic nuclei with granular chromatin, and nuclear moulding may be present {1306,199}. Desmoplastic round cell tumour is characterized by granular chromatin and nuclear moulding, and pseudorosettes and fragments of metachromatic stroma may be present {199}. Given the cytomorphological overlap between these tumours, definitive diagnosis requires ICC and molecular testing {665,199,1440,1174}.

Ancillary testing

CIC-rearranged sarcomas show strong, diffuse nuclear staining for ETV4 and WT1 {1336,1540,793}. Most show patchy, variable staining for CD99, although diffuse membranous staining is present in some tumours {71}. They are usually negative for NKX2-2, S100, cytokeratin, EMA, and desmin, although rare tumours are focally positive for one or more of these markers {1336,1540,793}. SMARCB1 (INI1) is retained. Nuclear staining for NUT is present in tumours with *CIC*::*NUTM1* rearrangements {796}. *CIC* rearrangements can be demonstrated by FISH and other molecular genetic techniques {620,673,1539}.

Sarcomas with *BCOR* genetic alterations

Teot LA
Agaram NP
Silverman J

Definition

Several groups of primitive round cell sarcomas show *BCOR* genetic alterations, resulting in oncogenic activation and BCOR overexpression. Although these pathological entities show distinct clinical presentations, there is overlap with regard to morphology, immunoprofile, and gene expression, suggesting a shared pathogenesis. The first group is characterized by sarcomas with *BCOR*-related gene fusions, most frequently *BCOR::CCNB3*. The second group shows *BCOR* internal tandem duplication (ITD), which has been described in infantile undifferentiated round cell sarcomas and primitive myxoid mesenchymal tumours of infancy.

Clinical features and imaging

BCOR::CCNB3 sarcomas have a striking predilection for children, with > 90% of patients aged < 20 years {672,891}, and a male predominance, with an M:F ratio of 4.5:1 {850,1527, 1134}. They arise more often in bone than in soft tissue (ratio: 1.5:1), with a predilection for the pelvis, lower extremities, and paraspinal region {1107,1134}. Sarcomas with alternative *BCOR* gene rearrangements occur in a wider age range {1337}. Sarcomas with *BCOR* ITD and primitive myxoid mesenchymal tumour of infancy occur in the first year of life or are present at birth {43,674}, and they usually arise in the soft tissues of the trunk, retroperitoneum, or head and neck {674}. Osseous lesions often show cortical destruction and extension into the soft tissues {244,1134}.

Histopathology

BCOR family tumours show considerable morphological overlap. Patterns include sheets or vague nests of uniform round to ovoid cells, solid areas with plump spindle cells arrayed in short fascicles, and hypocellular areas with short spindle cells in a myxoid matrix {891,672,1134,819,1102,43,1229,674}. A rich network of delicate vessels is typically present. Cells are deceptively bland, with fine chromatin and inconspicuous nucleoli. Mitoses are variable.

Key diagnostic cytopathological features

- High cellularity
- Single cells and pseudopapillary tissue fragments with vascular cores
- "Light and dark cell pattern" similar to Ewing sarcoma
- Round cells with variable numbers of spindle cells and rare single rhabdoid-like cells

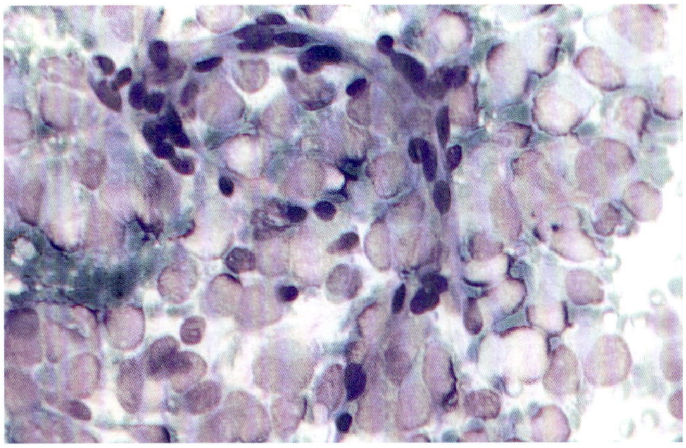

Fig. 8.218 Sarcoma with *BCOR* genetic alterations. A delicate vessel is present within this loosely cohesive tissue fragment consisting of round to short spindle tumour cells, which have scant to moderate cytoplasm and round to ovoid to elongate and pleomorphic nuclei with pale, fine chromatin and inconspicuous nucleoli (Giemsa).

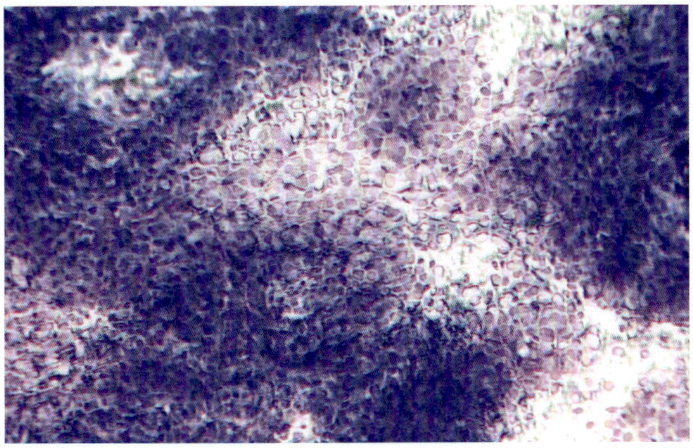

Fig. 8.217 Sarcoma with *BCOR* genetic alterations. High cellularity with crowded tissue fragments and dispersed cells, which are predominantly round cells (Giemsa).

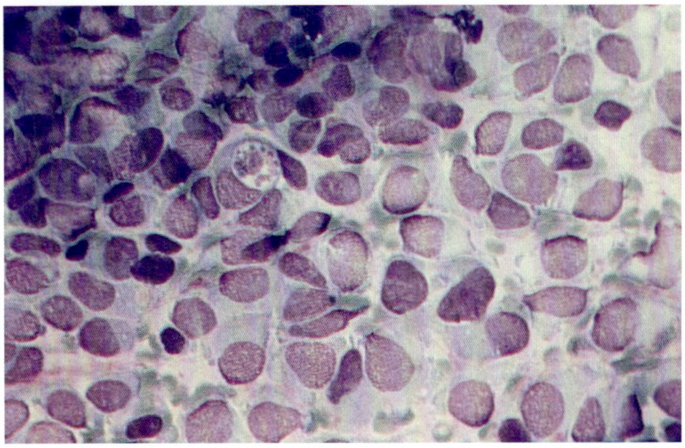

Fig. 8.219 Sarcoma with *BCOR* genetic alterations. Dispersed cells have scant to moderate cytoplasm and round to ovoid to elongate or pleomorphic nuclei with fine, evenly dispersed chromatin and inconspicuous nucleoli (Giemsa).

- Scant to abundant cytoplasm, pale nuclei with fine chromatin, and inconspicuous nucleoli
- Variable pleomorphism
- Variable stromal and delicate vascular fragments, myxoid matrix, and necrosis

Reference(s): {462,1490}

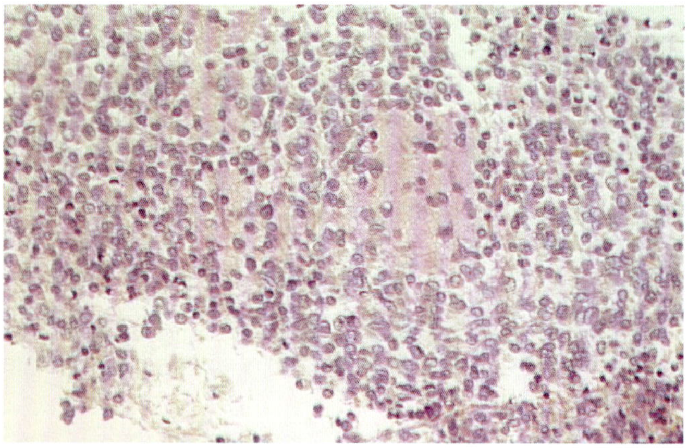

Fig. 8.220 Sarcoma with *BCOR* genetic alterations. A dense sheet of round to spindle cells with scant to moderate eosinophilic cytoplasm and pale, round to ovoid to elongate and pleomorphic nuclei with fine chromatin and inconspicuous nucleoli, with foci of pale eosinophilic matrix (cell block, H&E).

Discussion and differential diagnosis

The differential diagnosis of *BCOR* family tumours includes various primitive round and spindle cell mesenchymal tumours. In Ewing sarcoma, cells are usually more monotonous, pseudorosettes may be present, spindle cells are rare or absent, and myxoid matrix is absent {672,462,1490}. Although synovial sarcoma can closely mimic *BCOR* family tumours cytopathologically, both Ewing sarcoma and synovial sarcoma lack the small, delicate vascular fragments seen in *BCOR* family tumours {1490}. *CIC*-rearranged sarcomas often have prominent nucleoli and more pronounced anisonucleosis {665,199,672,1174}. Alveolar rhabdomyosarcoma comprises predominantly single cells with atypical, hyperchromatic nuclei with coarse chromatin and prominent nucleoli; large, multinucleated wreath-like cells with abundant cytoplasm may also be present {199,462}. Given the cytomorphological overlap between *BCOR* family tumours and other mesenchymal tumours, definitive diagnosis requires ICC and/or molecular studies.

Ancillary testing

Tumours with *BCOR* gene alterations show strong, diffuse nuclear staining for BCOR in ICC, and most are positive for SATB2, TLE1, and cyclin D1. In contrast to other *BCOR* family tumours, *BCOR::CCNB3* sarcomas also express cyclin B3 {1134,891,1288}, and CD99 is positive in approximately 50% of cases {672}. Various molecular techniques can be used to detect *BCOR* rearrangements and *BCOR* ITD.

Desmoplastic small round cell tumour

Monaco SE
Silverman J
Teot LA

Definition

Desmoplastic small round cell tumour (DSRCT) is a malignant mesenchymal neoplasm composed of small round tumour cells, associated with prominent stromal desmoplasia, polyphenotypic differentiation, and *EWSR1::WT1* gene fusion.

Clinical features and imaging

DSRCTs are aggressive tumours occurring in adolescents and young adults, with a peak incidence in the third decade of life. These tumours usually occur in the abdomen of male patients, with peritoneal seeding, and they can rarely occur in the thoracic, sinonasal, intraosseous, or paratesticular regions {1408,464}. Patients typically present with extensive tumour involvement at diagnosis, sometimes with ascites or bowel obstruction, progressing to lymph node, liver, lung, and bone metastases in later stages. On abdominal imaging, numerous omental and mesenteric implants are seen, without a primary solid organ mass {622}. These tumours have a poor prognosis, with death usually within 2 years of diagnosis and a 5-year survival rate of < 30%, even with multimodality treatment options such as neoadjuvant chemotherapy and aggressive surgery with postoperative chemoradiation. Hyperthermic intraperitoneal chemotherapy and immunotherapy have been attempted in these patients, but prognosis remains poor {551,388,1522}.

Histopathology

DSRCTs show nests of uniform small cells with round to oval nuclei, inconspicuous nucleoli, and scant cytoplasm within a prominent fibroblastic stroma. These lesions tend to be nodular, ranging from 1–2 mm micronodules up to large 400 mm masses {190}. Apoptotic debris, rosettes, eosinophilic cytoplasmic inclusions, and nuclear moulding can be seen to varying degrees. Variants include rhabdoid, epithelioid, and small cell morphologies.

Key diagnostic cytopathological features

- High cellularity
- Loosely cohesive, hyperchromatic round cells with scant to moderate cytoplasm and variable nuclear moulding
- Metachromatic stromal material in the background of smears and cell block material, but rare in body fluids and liquid based preparations
- Occasional pseudorosettes
- Paranuclear cytoplasmic densities, heart/kidney-shaped nuclei, and cytoplasmic vacuolization can be seen

Reference(s): {190,133,218,36,263,736,49}

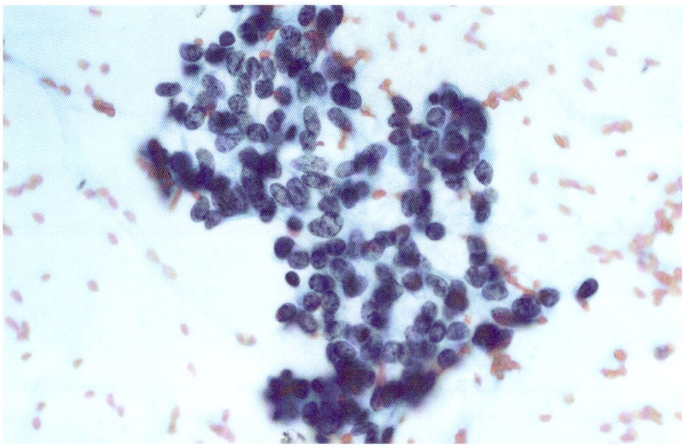

Fig. 8.222 Desmoplastic small round cell tumour. A loosely cohesive tissue fragment consisting of round cells with round or indented nuclei and scant cytoplasm (Pap).

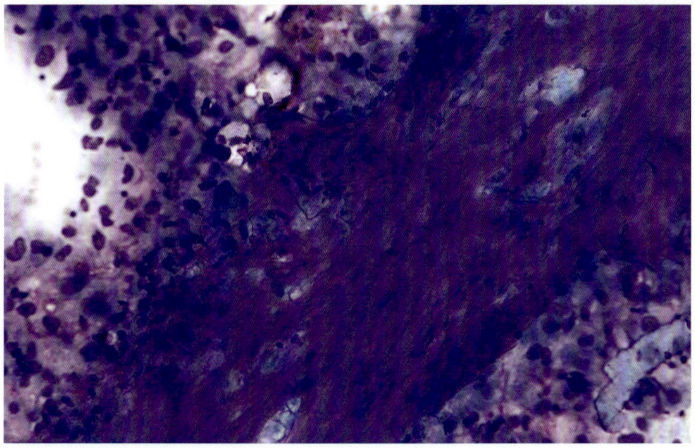

Fig. 8.221 Desmoplastic small round cell tumour. A large tissue fragment with dense magenta stromal material and round cells with light blue cytoplasm (Giemsa).

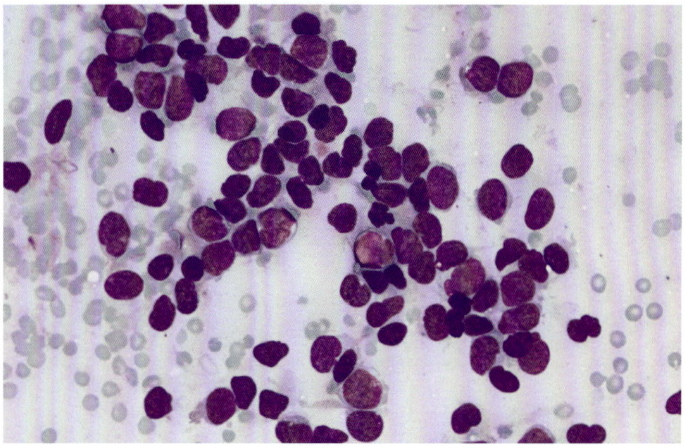

Fig. 8.223 Desmoplastic small round cell tumour. Loosely cohesive tissue fragments consisting of cells with round or indented heart-shaped nuclei and scant cytoplasm (Giemsa).

Chapter 8

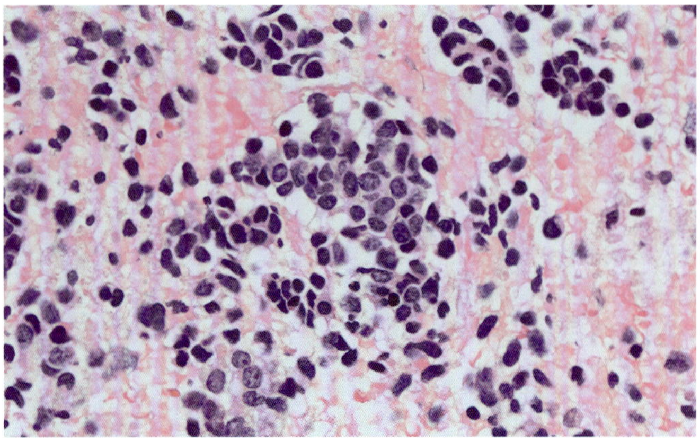

Fig. 8.224 Desmoplastic small round cell tumour. Round cells with mildly pleomorphic nuclei, granular chromatin, variably prominent nucleoli, and scant cytoplasm in small sheets, separated by fibrotic stroma (CNB, H&E).

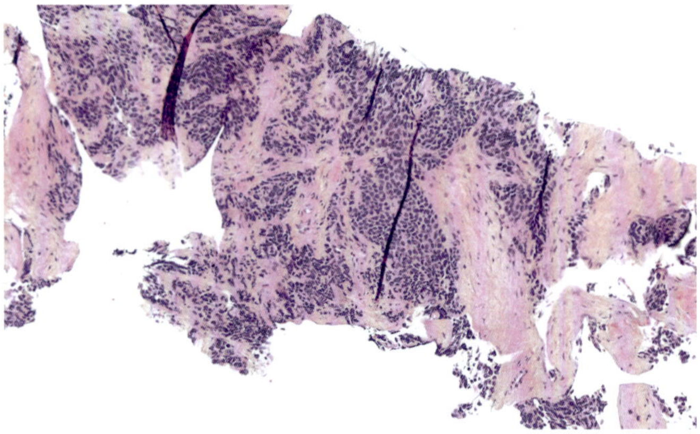

Fig. 8.225 Desmoplastic small round cell tumour. Round cells in sheets separated by broad fibrotic stroma (CNB, H&E).

Discussion and differential diagnosis

DSRCT overlaps morphologically with a variety of epithelial, mesenchymal, and lymphoproliferative tumours. The diagnosis can be established on small biopsy, with sufficient cell block material showing the multiphenotypic differentiation, exclusion of other small round cell tumours, and confirmation of the pathognomonic *EWSR1::WT1* translocation {290,736}. The differential diagnosis includes rhabdomyosarcoma, synovial sarcoma, small cell osteosarcoma, mesenchymal chondrosarcoma, neuroblastoma, rhabdoid tumours, Wilms tumour, round cell sarcomas (including *CIC*-rearranged sarcomas), and Ewing sarcoma.

Ancillary testing

DSRCTs have unique ICC, showing positivity for epithelial markers (cytokeratins, EMA), myogenic markers (desmin in a punctate perinuclear staining pattern), and neural markers (S100, NSE). CD99 can show cytoplasmic staining that differs from the membranous staining in Ewing sarcoma {773}. SALL4 positivity has also been reported in occasional DSRCTs {950}. The WT1 (C19) stain is also positive if it detects the C-terminus, due to the in-frame translocation t(11;22)(p13;q12) in these tumours resulting in an *EWSR1::WT1* fusion gene, in which the N-terminal region of *EWSR1* is fused with the C-terminal region of *WT1* {1408,562}. Wilms tumour is differentiated by showing positive nuclear staining for the WT1 N-terminus. Ewing sarcoma shares the feature of *EWSR1* rearrangements, but typically involving other genes (*FLI1*, *ERG*, others) {1248}. The *EWSR1::WT1* fusion results in upregulation of the expression of PDGFRA, VEGF, and other proteins related to proliferation {917}. NGS has shown rare mutations in *TERT*, *ARID1A*, *HRAS*, and *TP53*, in addition to overexpression of *FGFR4* {1322}.

Embryonal rhabdomyosarcoma

Teot LA
Agaram NP
Silverman J

Definition

Embryonal rhabdomyosarcoma (ERMS) is a malignant soft tissue tumour with morphological and immunophenotypic features of embryonic skeletal muscle.

Clinical features and imaging

Rhabdomyosarcoma is the most common paediatric soft tissue sarcoma, with 4.5 cases per 1 million people aged 0–20 years {1318}. The most common subtype is ERMS, with one third of cases presenting in children aged < 5 years. Tumours most often arise in the head and neck (including the orbit) and the genitourinary system {1477,547}, and less frequently in the biliary tract, retroperitoneum, and abdomen. They rarely involve the extremities. The clinical presentation depends on location. Although most ERMSs are sporadic, some are associated with genetic susceptibility syndromes such as Costello syndrome (*HRAS* mutations), neurofibromatosis type 1 (*NF1* mutations), Noonan syndrome (mutations in several genes), Beckwith–Wiedemann syndrome (dysregulation of imprinting in the 11p15.5 region), *DICER1*-related tumour predisposition syndrome, and Li–Fraumeni syndrome (*TP53* mutations) {1318}.

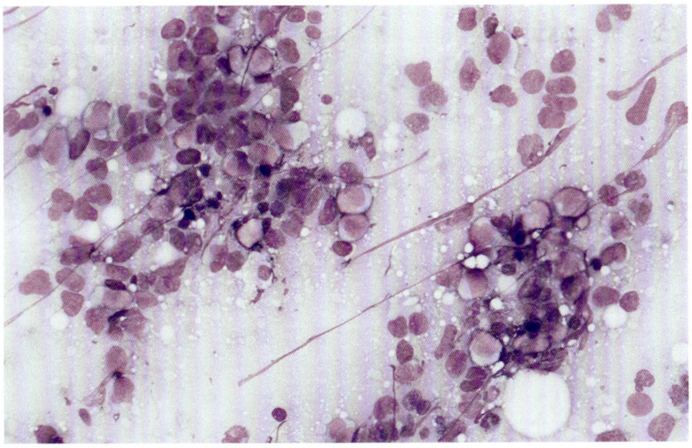

Fig. 8.226 Embryonal rhabdomyosarcoma. Loosely cohesive and single dispersed round and spindle cells showing nuclear pleomorphism and in some cells eccentric cytoplasm. Chromatin smearing is present (Giemsa).

Histopathology

ERMS is composed of primitive mesenchymal cells in various stages of myogenesis. Typical ERMS is made up of primitive stellate to short spindle cells in a loose myxoid matrix, with a pattern of alternating dense and loose cellularity. Differentiating rhabdomyoblasts may be absent or numerous and are characterized by eosinophilic and elongated cytoplasm, or differentiated cells with cross-striations. Differentiation is often more evident after therapy {82}. A subset of ERMS cases consist predominantly of primitive round cells, simulating alveolar rhabdomyosarcoma (ARMS) in the so-called "dense pattern" {1212}. Botryoid ERMS is characterized by polypoid architecture with linear condensations of tumour cells in the "cambium layer" abutting an epithelial surface with underlying hypocellular areas. A subset of ERMS cases exhibit anaplasia, defined as the presence of cells with markedly enlarged, hyperchromatic nuclei, often with bizarre, multipolar mitotic figures {1139}.

Key diagnostic cytopathological features

- High cellularity
- Single cells, small loosely cohesive tissue fragments, and large tissue fragments with tightly packed cells

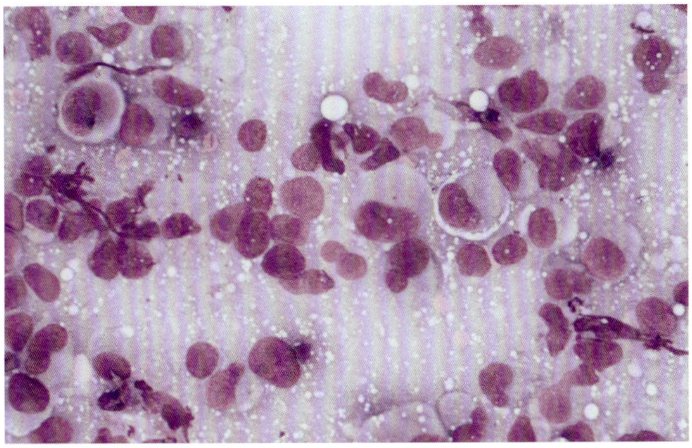

Fig. 8.227 Embryonal rhabdomyosarcoma. Large cells are round to spindle, with abundant eccentric cytoplasm, indicative of rhabdomyoblastic differentiation, and round, ovoid, or irregular nuclei with granular chromatin and inconspicuous nucleoli. Plentiful stripped nuclei are present (Giemsa).

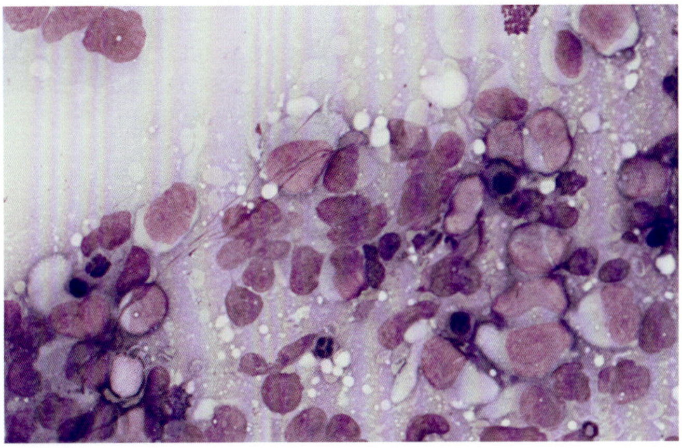

Fig. 8.228 Embryonal rhabdomyosarcoma. Single or loosely cohesive minute tissue fragments consisting of round cells with a high N:C ratio and scant cytoplasm, with round and often pleomorphic nuclei with granular chromatin and inconspicuous nucleoli. Occasional cells have more abundant, often eccentric cytoplasm. Mitotic figures and single necrotic cells are present (Giemsa).

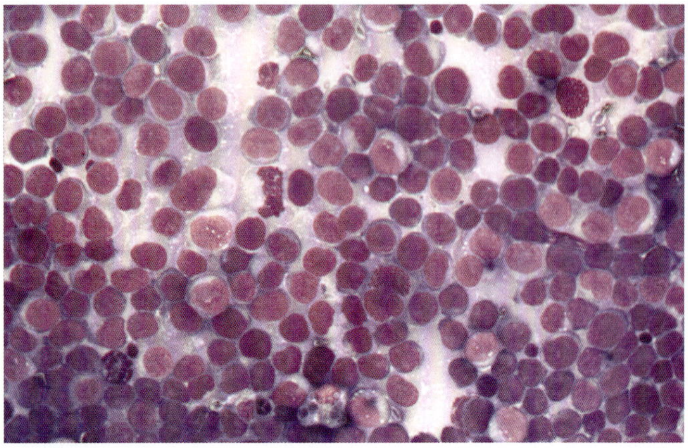

Fig. 8.229 Embryonal rhabdomyosarcoma. Highly cellular tumour with largely single dispersed cells, which are predominantly round with scant cytoplasm and round, ovoid, or more pleomorphic hyperchromatic nuclei with granular chromatin and inconspicuous nucleoli. Mitotic figures and single necrotic cells are present (Giemsa).

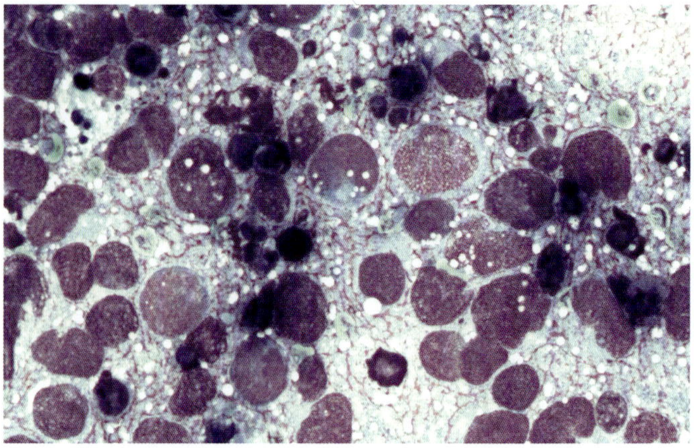

Fig. 8.230 Embryonal rhabdomyosarcoma. Large round cells with pleomorphic nuclei showing marked variation in size and granular chromatin and inconspicuous nucleoli. Very occasional cells show rhabdomyoblastic differentiation with more abundant eccentric cytoplasm (Giemsa).

- Primitive small round, stellate, and short spindle cells with scant cytoplasm and hyperchromatic nuclei with granular chromatin
- Variable numbers of cells with rhabdomyoblastic differentiation consisting of larger round, tadpole, or ribbon-like cells with greyish blue (Giemsa) cytoplasm, rarely with cross-striations
- Binucleate and multinucleate cells variably present
- Variably prominent loose myxoid matrix

Reference(s): {1274,87,37,1117,733}

Discussion and differential diagnosis

The principal differential diagnostic considerations include ARMS and other round cell mesenchymal tumours. With the exception of ARMS, these tumours lack cells with rhabdomyoblastic differentiation. ARMS is composed predominantly of singly dispersed or loose tissue fragments of round cells with enlarged, round nuclei. Cells with a wreath-like arrangement of their multiple nuclei may be present, and spindle cells and large tissue fragments of densely packed cells are usually absent {87,1117}. Ewing sarcoma shows monomorphic round cells with scant cytoplasm and round to ovoid pale nuclei with fine chromatin and inconspicuous nucleoli. Pseudorosettes may be present, and myxoid matrix is usually absent {37,1117,733}. The primitive round and spindle cells in *CIC*-rearranged and *BCOR* family tumours are larger and have a greater degree of anisonucleosis and pleomorphism than those in ERMS. *BCOR* family tumours also have delicate vascular fragments that are absent in ERMS {672,462,1490}. The cells in poorly differentiated synovial sarcoma are relatively uniform and larger, and they have irregular hyperchromatic nuclei with one or more nucleoli {1306,199}. Rhabdoid cells in malignant rhabdoid tumour have distinct cytoplasmic inclusions and round nuclei with prominent nucleoli and perinucleolar chromatin clearing ("vesicular" in the Pap stain), and they are often larger than round differentiating rhabdomyoblasts. Given the overlap in cytomorphological features between these tumours, definitive diagnosis requires ICC and/or molecular studies {37,1117,733,665,199,1440,1174}.

Ancillary testing

By ICC, ERMSs are positive for desmin, myogenin (MYF4), and MYOD1, although the extent of immunoreactivity is variable {977}. ERMS usually shows patchy variable staining for myogenin in < 50% of nuclei, which helps to distinguish it from ARMS, in which nuclear staining for myogenin is usually strong and diffuse. ERMS is often positive for MSA and SMA, and aberrant expression of keratins, S100, and NFP may also be seen {247}. *FOXO1* gene fusion is absent in ERMS, whereas it is present in the majority of ARMS tumours {291}. Assessment of fusion status using FISH or other molecular techniques is critical, because cytopathological and histopathological distinction between these tumours is sometimes difficult, and current treatment is in part determined by fusion status {560,483}.

Alveolar rhabdomyosarcoma

Rekhi B
Agaram NP
Teot LA

Definition

Alveolar rhabdomyosarcoma (ARMS) is a malignant neoplasm composed of a monomorphic population of primitive round cells showing skeletal muscle differentiation. The presence of either a *PAX3::FOXO1* or a *PAX7::FOXO1* fusion gene is detected in the majority of cases.

Clinical features and imaging

ARMS occurs across all ages, with a peak incidence in people aged 10–25 years; it arises most commonly in the deep soft tissue of extremities, followed by head and neck, paraspinal, and perineal regions, and rarely in the breast {552,1145,83, 1421}. Patients present with a rapidly growing malignant soft tissue mass. Nearly 30% of patients present with locoregional or distant metastasis {1036,867,1211}. Tumours occurring in the head and neck region involving the meninges lead to cranial nerve defects {1430}; those in the paraspinal region can cause compression of the spinal nerves {1237}, and those occurring in the pelvis result in symptoms related to bowel obstruction {450}.

Histopathology

ARMS is a cellular tumour composed of primitive small round cells, arranged in nests, with intervening fibrovascular septa. Loss of cohesion of the cells in the centre creates an alveolar growth pattern. Some cases show a compact arrangement of tumour cells leading to a solid-type growth pattern with pseudocystic spaces and interspersed mitotic figures. Individual tumour cells contain scant cytoplasm and hyperchromatic nuclei; there is a variable number of cells with rhabdomyoblastic differentiation, and wreath-like multinucleated giant cells may be present. Rarely, cells with vacuolated cytoplasm due to intracytoplasmic glycogen are noted {1074,1211,83,1210,1075}.

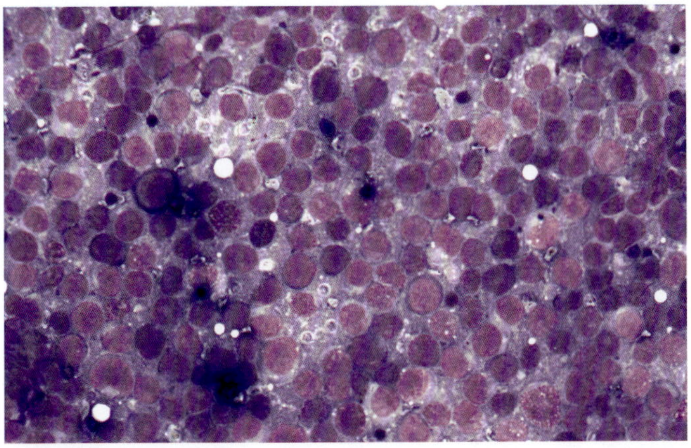

Fig. 8.231 Alveolar rhabdomyosarcoma. Highly cellular tumour showing round and polymorphous cells with a high N:C ratio, large central nuclei, and scant basophilic cytoplasm with mitotic figures and necrosis of single cells (Giemsa).

Key diagnostic cytopathological features

- High cellularity
- Single scattered intact cells and loosely cohesive tissue fragments
- Monomorphic round cells, with scant to moderate, blue to finely vacuolated cytoplasm (Giemsa) and hyperchromatic nuclei
- Variable numbers of rhabdomyoblastic cells may be present, showing large round to oval nuclei and moderate to abundant blue cytoplasm (Giemsa) or greenish cytoplasm (Pap)
- Binucleate and multinucleated forms, including with wreath-like circular arrangement of nuclei, are frequently seen
- Scattered mitotic figures and bare nuclei are often present

Reference(s): {35,294,87,733,1169}

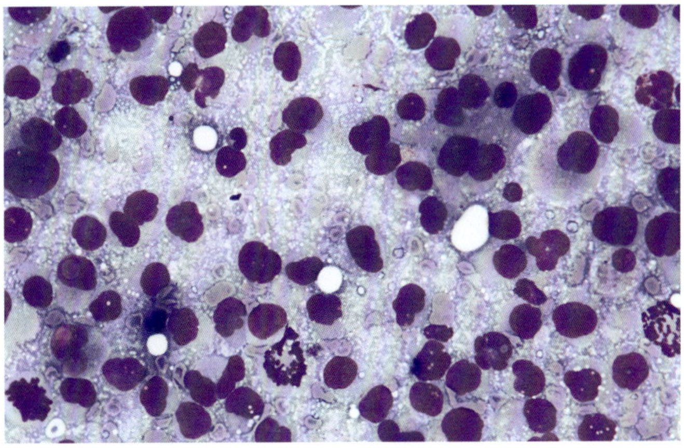

Fig. 8.232 Alveolar rhabdomyosarcoma. Predominantly round cells with moderate to abundant bluish cytoplasm, including multinucleated giant cells with a wreath-like, circular arrangement of nuclei and scattered mitotic figures, in a lacy tigroid background due to cytoplasmic glycogen (Giemsa).

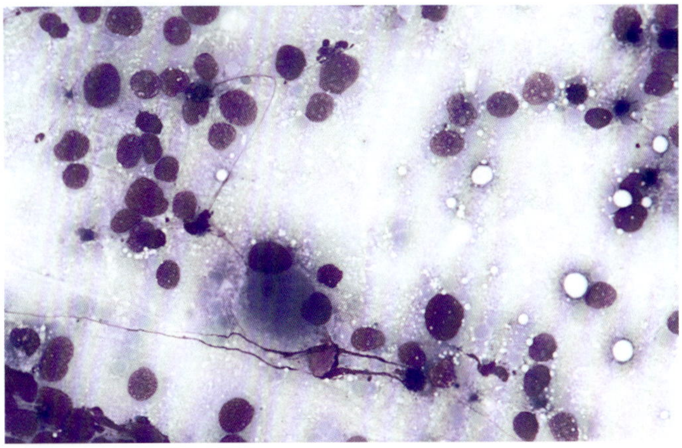

Fig. 8.233 Alveolar rhabdomyosarcoma. Round to elongated cells, including a binucleated cell containing abundant bluish cytoplasm (a rhabdomyoblast) (Giemsa).

Discussion and differential diagnosis

Various round cell tumours constitute the differential diagnoses. Ewing sarcomas show a dual population of poorly differentiated round cells, including small, dark cells and large, sometimes finely vacuolated cells. Rhabdoid tumours show features overlapping those of ARMS, with individual tumour cells displaying characteristic perinuclear intracytoplasmic globular inclusions. Poorly differentiated synovial sarcomas are composed of round to ovoid cells with tapering cytoplasm, seen individually and in tissue fragments. Rarely, anaplastic large cell lymphoma can be misdiagnosed as ARMS, and ICC greatly assists. Differentiating ARMS from embryonal rhabdomyosarcoma (ERMS) can be difficult on smears, but ARMS is characterized by relative hypercellularity and monomorphic small round cells in discohesive tissue fragments, with a variable number of multinucleated giant cells. On the other hand, smears of ERMS display large tissue fragments with eosinophilic material and scattered cells, including round, tadpole, and ribbon forms {87,1117,733,1169}.

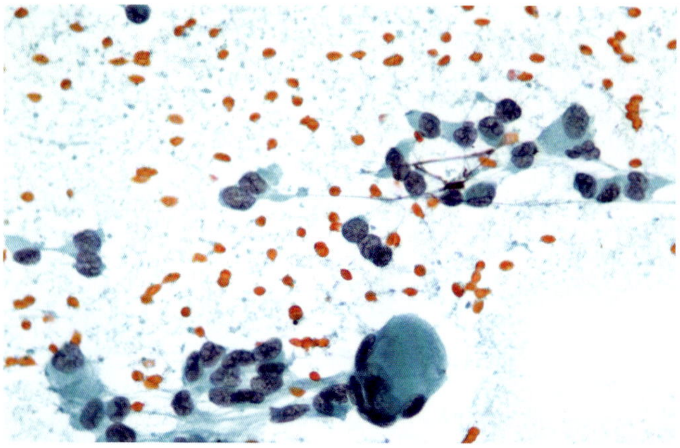

Fig. 8.234 Alveolar rhabdomyosarcoma. Scattered tumour cells containing moderate to abundant, often eccentric cytoplasm and multinucleated giant cells (rhabdomyoblasts) (Pap).

Ancillary testing

ARMS is positive for desmin, myogenin, and MYOD1, indicative of skeletal muscle differentiation. Myogenin expression is typically diffuse and strong in ARMS, unlike in ERMS {326,585, 1170}. Certain cases of ARMS show aberrant immunoexpression of epithelial and neuroendocrine markers {94,1170}.

Ewing sarcomas are positive for CD99 (MIC2) (membranous) and NKX2-2, and negative for desmin, myogenin, and MYOD1.

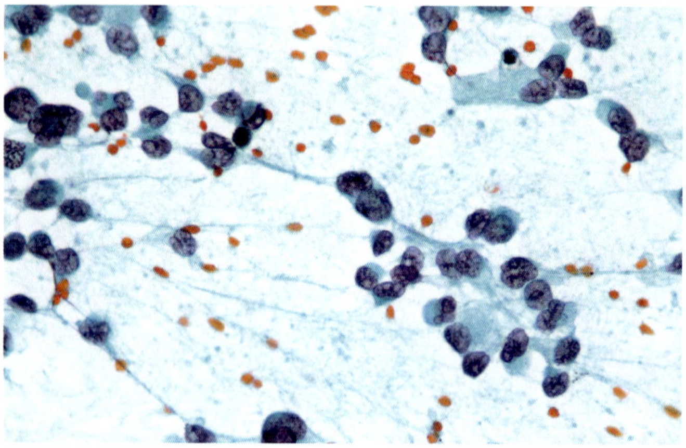

Fig. 8.235 Alveolar rhabdomyosarcoma. Loosely cohesive tissue fragments and individual cells, which are round cells with moderate to abundant, often eccentric cytoplasm and highly irregular nuclei, including binucleate and multinucleated forms (Pap).

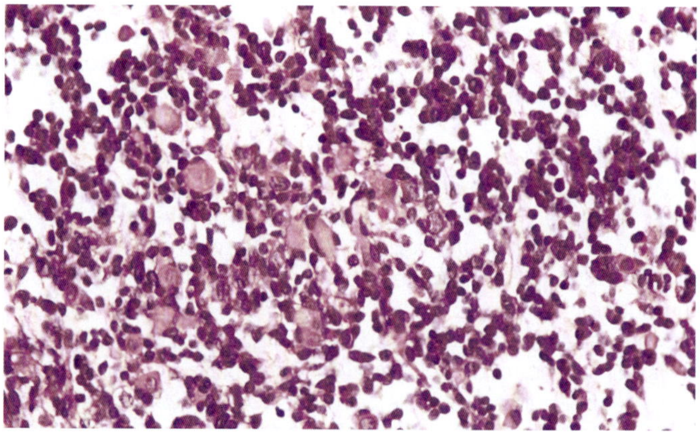

Fig. 8.237 Alveolar rhabdomyosarcoma. Malignant round cells showing a high N:C ratio and scant cytoplasm, arranged in discohesive sheets, with interspersed cells containing abundant cytoplasm and multinucleated forms, including a wreath-like, peripheral circular arrangement of tumour nuclei (cell block, H&E).

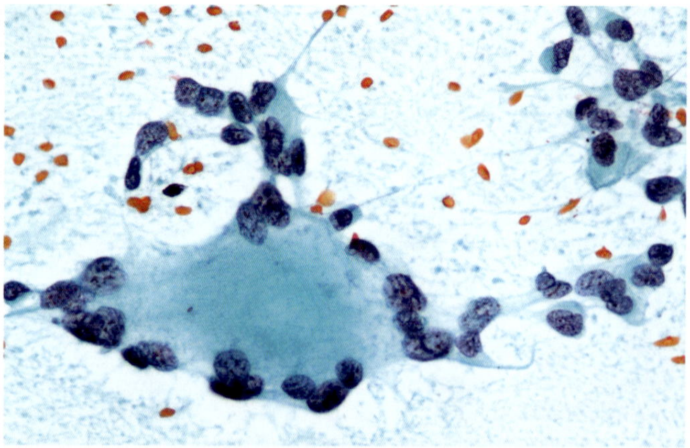

Fig. 8.236 Alveolar rhabdomyosarcoma. A multinucleate giant cell with a wreath-like, peripheral circular arrangement of tumour nuclei in a rhabdomyoblast (Pap).

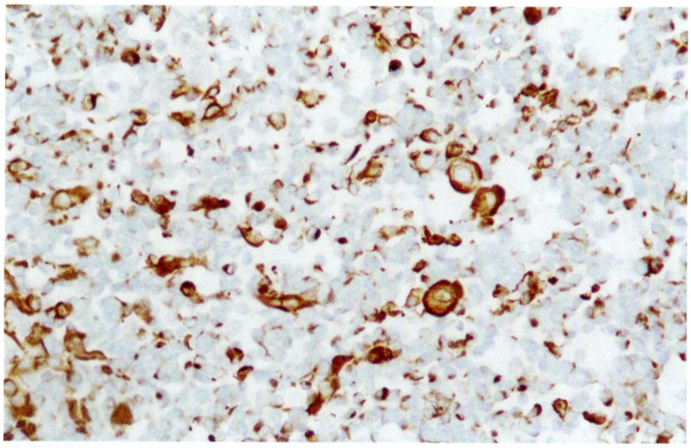

Fig. 8.238 Alveolar rhabdomyosarcoma. Positive cytoplasmic desmin (cell block, ICC).

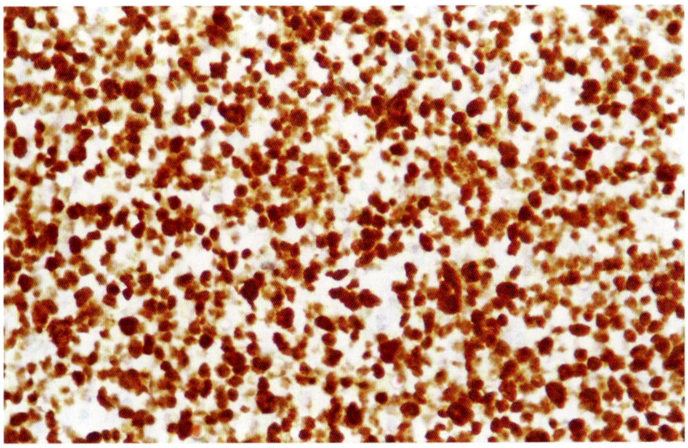

Fig. 8.239 Alveolar rhabdomyosarcoma. Diffuse nuclear positivity for MYOD1 (cell block, ICC).

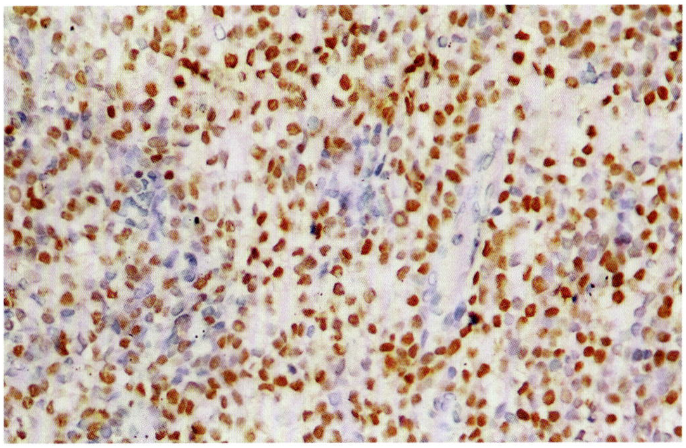

Fig. 8.240 Alveolar rhabdomyosarcoma. Nuclear positivity for myogenin (cell block, ICC).

Ewing sarcoma is characterized by t(11;22)(q24;q12) and t(21;22)(q22;q12) translocations in most cases, unlike ARMS {733,1169, 600}. Rhabdoid tumours display loss of SMARCB1 (INI1) {572}. Poorly differentiated synovial sarcomas invariably display characteristic t(X;18)(p11.2;q11.2) translocation {729}. Desmoplastic small round cell tumour and lymphoblastic lymphoma can be differentiated with specific immunostains. CD45 (LCA), CD30, and ALK are useful in separating ARMS from anaplastic large cell lymphoma {1179}.

ARMS is characterized by t(2;13)(q35;q14) and t(1;13)(p36;q14) chromosomal translocations, leading to *PAX3::FOXO1* and *PAX7::FOXO1* fusions, respectively, in 50–88.8% of cases {107,686}. The translocation t(2;13) is relatively more common than t(1;13) translocation and has been reported to have a poorer prognosis in some studies {1334}. However, in a subsequent study, the *PAX::FKHR* fusion type was not found to be a significant predictor for survival {1344}. FISH can be used for the detection of *FOXO1*, using a break-apart probe {356}. RNA sequencing can be used to determine the gene fusions.

Neuroblastic tumours

Teot LA
Silverman J

Definition

Neuroblastic tumours comprise a group of tumours of neural crest origin spanning a continuum of maturation and including ganglioneuroma, ganglioneuroblastoma, and neuroblastoma.

Clinical features and imaging

Neuroblastoma is the most common extracranial malignancy of childhood, with the majority of cases diagnosed before 5 years of age and approximately 50% presenting clinically before the age of 2 years, with a median age of 23 months. Neuroblastomas can arise from any site containing sympathetic neural tissue; they most commonly occur in the adrenal gland (~40% of cases), followed by the retroperitoneal, thoracopulmonary, mediastinal, cervical, and pelvic regions. Approximately 70% of patients present with metastatic disease to regional lymph nodes, liver, bones, and lungs. The prognosis of neuroblastoma is correlated with patient age at diagnosis, primary site, histopathology, and grade. In general, children under 1 year of age have the best prognosis {658,1295,1294,160,245}.

The International Neuroblastoma Pathology Classification (INPC) categorizes clinically aggressive and non-aggressive groups of neuroblastomas on the basis of unfavourable and favourable histopathology, respectively, as defined by the presence or absence of Schwannian stroma, differentiating neuroblasts, and maturing and mature ganglion cells {1295,1294,160}. Other prognostic indicators are the mitosis-karyorrhexis index (MKI) for the Schwannian stroma–poor neuroblastoma category and molecular and ploidy findings {1545,617}. There are multiple systems for staging neuroblastoma: the International Neuroblastoma Staging System (INSS) is based on surgical resection findings, and the International Neuroblastoma Risk Group Staging System (INRGSS) is based on postsurgical findings, pretreatment imaging, the patient's age, and the clinical extent of disease {1295,245}. CT or MRI is used to evaluate the extent of disease {687}. Neuroblastoma often presents as a large, nodular, heterogeneous, solid mass involving the adrenal gland or occurring anywhere along the sympathetic chain. The presence of stippled calcification and/or intraspinal extension is useful in differentiating neuroblastoma from other small round cell tumours. Nuclear medicine studies (e.g. MIBG scintigraphy) are also used to detect occult disease and bony metastasis.

Histopathology

By definition, neuroblastomas are composed of > 50% neuroblasts, and ganglioneuromas are composed exclusively of mature ganglion cells, neurites, Schwann cells, and fibrous tissue. Ganglioneuroblastoma contains > 50% ganglioneuromatous elements, with a relatively small neuroblastic component. Neuroblasts are small to medium-sized cells with scant cytoplasm and ill-defined cell borders. The nuclei are round to oval, with fine granular chromatin and indistinct to small nucleoli. The neuroblasts are arranged diffusely or in nests separated by thin fibrovascular septa, with variable amounts of fibrillary neuropil. As cells differentiate towards ganglion cells, the nuclei enlarge and acquire vesicular chromatin and a single prominent nucleolus, with characteristic abundant, largely eccentric eosinophilic amphophilic cytoplasm. Other features of neuroblastoma include variable amounts of neuropil and Schwannian stroma, Homer Wright pseudorosettes, necrosis, and lymphoid cells {658,657,1043}.

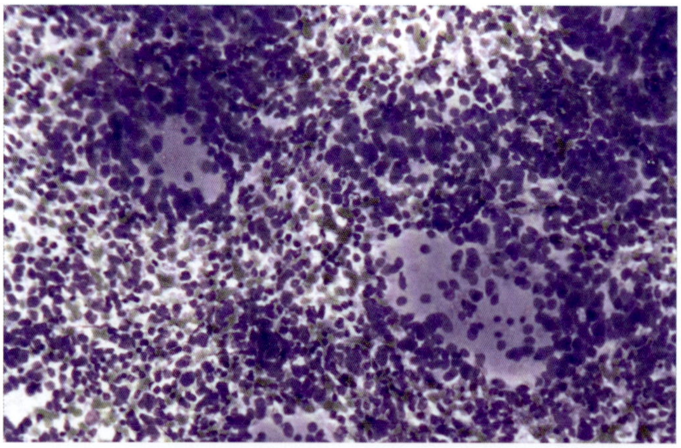

Fig. 8.241 Neuroblastoma. Highly cellular tumour with neuroblasts seen singly and in tissue fragments admixed with neuropil, and occasionally in pseudorosettes. The neuroblasts have scant, indistinct cytoplasm and round, ovoid, or angulated, mildly pleomorphic nuclei (Giemsa).

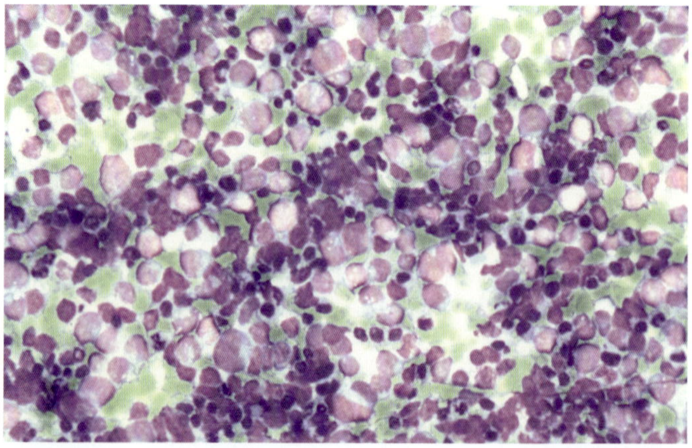

Fig. 8.242 Neuroblastoma. Dispersed neuroblasts with round, ovoid, angular, or irregular nuclei and scant cytoplasm, admixed with larger cells with scant or more abundant eccentric cytoplasm, suggesting early ganglionic differentiation; however, recognizable ganglion cells are not present, and neuropil is absent. Small lymphocytes are present in the background (Giemsa).

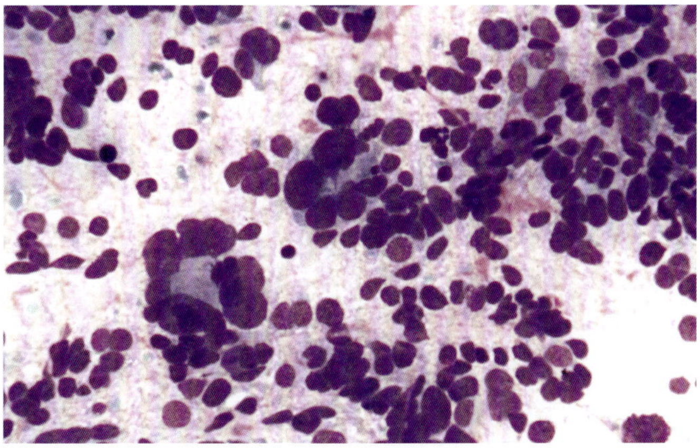

Fig. 8.243 Neuroblastoma. Pleomorphic cells including neuroblasts with scant cytoplasm admixed with larger cells showing ganglionic differentiation in the form of abundant, eccentric cytoplasm and enlarged, round nuclei; binucleate forms are present. Delicate fibrillar matrix is present in the background (Giemsa).

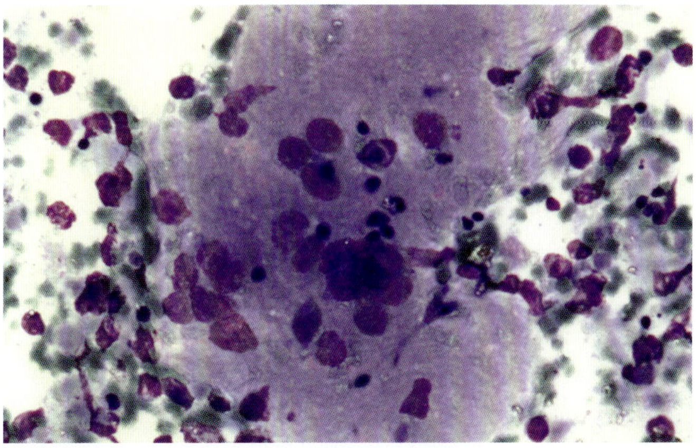

Fig. 8.244 Neuroblastoma. Neuroblasts within this fragment of fibrillar neuropil have indistinct cytoplasmic borders and round, oval, or angulated nuclei with finely granular chromatin. Single neuroblasts are present in the background (Giemsa).

Key diagnostic cytopathological features

- High cellularity (neuroblastoma) to moderate or low cellularity (ganglioneuroblastoma, ganglioneuroma)
- Neuroblasts arrayed singly, in small tissue fragments and sheets, and admixed with fibrillary neuropil
- Neuroblasts have a high N:C ratio, with scant cytoplasm with indistinct borders and round, oval, or angulated nuclei with granular chromatin and inconspicuous or small nucleoli
- Pseudorosettes inconspicuous to prominent
- Fibrillary neuropil is scant to abundant, with fine fibrillary strands or in larger fragments with admixed neuroblasts
- Variable pleomorphism
- Variable mitotic figures, karyorrhectic debris, necrosis, calcification, and small lymphocytes
- Variable numbers of immature, maturing, and/or mature ganglion cells
- Schwann cells vary from absent to the predominant cell type
- Schwann cells are arrayed in syncytial sheets, large tissue fragments, or singly; they are spindle cells with modest pale to bubbly cytoplasm, indistinct cell borders, elongate to curved nuclei, pale chromatin, and indistinct nucleoli

Reference(s): {468,449,448,37,1395,738,752,131}

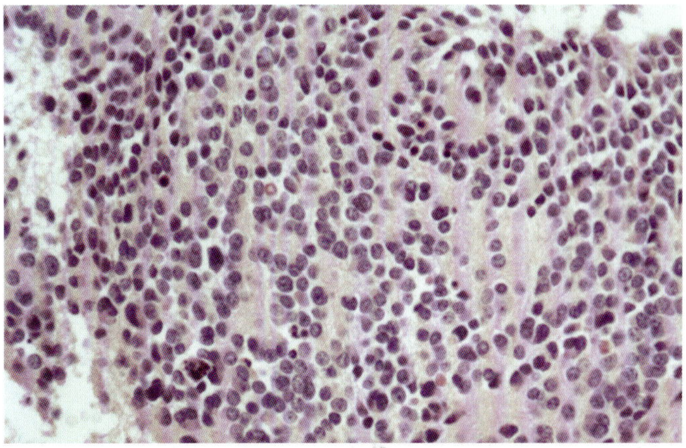

Fig. 8.245 Neuroblastoma. Sheets of neuroblasts admixed with variable amounts of neuropil. The cells in this field are relatively uniform, with scant cytoplasm and round, ovoid, or angulated nuclei with fine chromatin. Pseudorosettes are evident. Cells with ganglionic differentiation are absent. A few mitotic figures and karyorrhectic cells are present (cell block, H&E).

Discussion and differential diagnosis

The differential diagnosis of neuroblastoma includes other paediatric round cell tumours. With the exception of Ewing sarcoma, these tumours lack Homer Wright pseudorosettes and neuropil. When present in Ewing sarcoma, neuropil is predominantly associated with pseudorosettes and is otherwise scant, and the cells are more monomorphic than those in neuroblastoma. The cells in lymphoblastic lymphoma are intermediate in size, with scant cytoplasm, and they have distinct cellular borders and round, ovoid, or indented nuclei with finely dispersed chromatin and one or more nucleoli. Of note, cytoplasmic fragments in neuroblastoma may mimic the cytoplasmic fragments ("lymphoglandular bodies") seen in lymphoblastic lymphoma, although these are usually more numerous. In rhabdomyosarcoma, the nuclei of both the primitive cells and those with rhabdomyoblastic differentiation are more hyperchromatic; if present, tadpole and ribbon-like rhabdomyoblasts help to distinguish rhabdomyosarcoma from neuroblastoma. In contrast to neuroblastoma, *CIC*-rearranged and *BCOR* family tumours may have spindle cells, and the round cells are larger and have a greater degree of pleomorphism than those in embryonal rhabdomyosarcoma. *BCOR* family tumours also have delicate vascular fragments that are absent in neuroblastoma {672,462}. The cells in poorly differentiated synovial sarcoma are relatively uniform, larger, and have irregular hyperchromatic nuclei with one or more nucleoli {1306, 199}. In contrast to immature, maturing, and mature ganglion cells, the rhabdoid cells in malignant rhabdoid tumour have distinct cytoplasmic inclusions and round nuclei with macronucleoli and perinucleolar clearing. The presence of maturing and mature ganglion cells and Schwann cells distinguishes ganglioneuroblastoma and ganglioneuroma from other diagnostic considerations. Undifferentiated neuroblastoma lacks pseudorosettes and neuropil, and the distinction of this entity from other paediatric round cell tumours requires ICC and/or molecular studies {37,1117,733,199,1440,1174}.

Ancillary testing

By ICC, neuroblastic cells are positive for PHOX2B, NSE, synaptophysin, chromogranin, neurofilament, CD57, and CD56, and they are negative for epithelial markers (EMA and cytokeratin), WT1, CD99, CD45, and muscle markers {146,1078}. PHOX2B is highly specific and is especially helpful for distinguishing undifferentiated neuroblastoma, in which staining for other neural markers may be lost or focal, from other round cell tumours {856}. Schwann cells are positive for S100 and SOX10. Flow cytometric analysis for DNA ploidy and molecular studies for *MYCN* amplification, 1p deletion, 11q deletion, 17q gain, and abnormalities in *ALK* and *ATRX* have prognostic and therapeutic implications {1545,617,844,1340,1258,211,180,982,1188,1395,738,869,131}.

Soft tissue metastases

Bode-Lesniewska B
Domanski HA
Silverman J

Definition

Metastases in the soft tissue are malignant neoplasms originating from another organ, metastatic to the soft tissues.

Clinical features and imaging

Soft tissue metastases occur mostly in known and advanced aggressive malignancies and are reported in 1–10% of such cases {112,283,4,1116,1361}. The primary tumour is clinically known in most cases; however, soft tissue metastasis may present as a primary manifestation of a metastatic disease {1304,27,654,660,4}. Only 1% of soft tissue masses turn out to be a metastasis of a primary from another site: lung, melanoma, kidney, breast, gastrointestinal, and bladder metastases are most common {4}. Distant soft tissue metastases from primary sarcomas are rare and usually a late event in aggressive sarcoma types {1150}. Umbilical metastases, the so-called "Sister Mary Joseph's nodule", are signs of intra-abdominal or pelvic malignancy, mostly from the female genital tract, including ovary and fallopian tube, or from the stomach {717,34,1262}.

In most cases, the clinical presentation and the imaging are similar to those of a primary soft tissue tumour. It is clinically important to differentiate between a metastasis and a second primary tumour, and the confirmation of a metastasis and exclusion of a second primary in the soft tissue is the main goal of the FNAB. The acquisition of an adequate tumour sample for ancillary testing of therapeutic targets is another important objective.

Histopathology

The histopathological features of the soft tissue metastasis correspond to the appearance of the primary tumour, including histopathological subtype, and the degree of differentiation.

Key diagnostic cytopathological features

- High cellularity
- Variable number of cohesive tissue fragments and single intact cells
- Necrotic debris may be observed in the background
- Abundant cytoplasm and nuclei with irregular, coarse chromatin and prominent nucleoli and perinucleolar clearing are seen in cases of metastatic carcinoma or melanoma
- Adenocarcinoma cells may show intracellular or extracellular mucin
- Metastatic squamous cell carcinoma shows variable keratinization
- Melanin in pigmented malignant melanoma

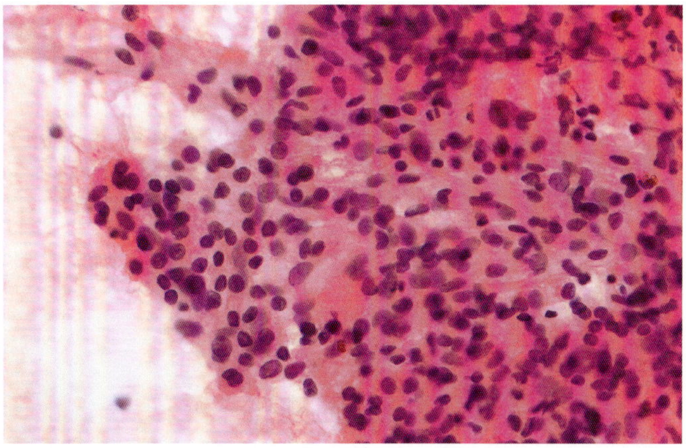

Fig. 8.247 Metastasis of a renal cell carcinoma to skeletal muscle. A tissue fragment consisting of cells with pale, poorly defined cytoplasm and round to mildly pleomorphic nuclei, in a nested pattern separated by thin vessels (H&E).

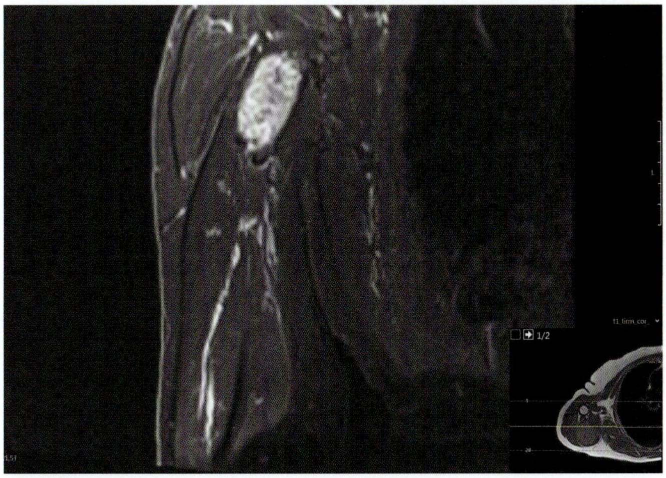

Fig. 8.246 Metastasis of a renal cell carcinoma to skeletal muscle. MRI of a mass in the right triceps muscle.

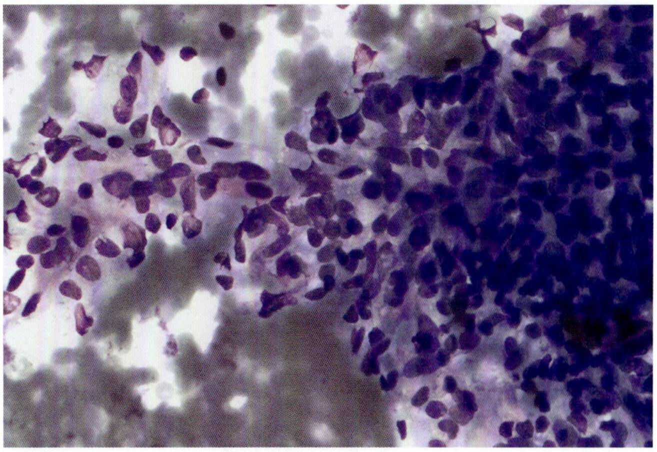

Fig. 8.248 Metastasis of a renal cell carcinoma to skeletal muscle. A tissue fragment of crowded cells with mild to moderately pleomorphic nuclei and considerable cytoplasm, separated by thin vessels (Giemsa).

- Spindle cells can be observed in metastatic sarcomatoid carcinomas, such as primary kidney or lung carcinomas, or in malignant melanomas

Discussion and differential diagnosis

Close correlation with the patient history of known malignant diseases and imaging is a necessary requirement for the efficient evaluation of an FNAB of a potential metastasis. The microscopic features of carcinomas and melanomas are in most cases easy to differentiate from those of most mesenchymal neoplasms, especially those showing spindle or myxoid features. Difficulties may be encountered in cases of soft tissue metastases of sarcomatoid carcinomas, where both microscopy and ICC show features overlapping those of undifferentiated pleomorphic sarcoma. Metastases of sarcomatoid carcinomas may contain heterologous elements such as chondrosarcomatous or osteosarcomatous areas and must be differentiated from rare cases of much less common extraskeletal osteosarcoma. On the other hand, more typical carcinomas must be differentiated from mesenchymal tumours showing epithelioid features, such as granular cell tumour, epithelioid sarcoma, epithelioid angiosarcoma, alveolar soft part sarcoma, and epithelioid malignant peripheral nerve sheath tumour. Soft tissue involvement by haematological malignancy is rarely observed in myeloid sarcoma, plasmacytoma, or non-Hodgkin lymphoma, requiring the differential diagnosis with round cell sarcomas.

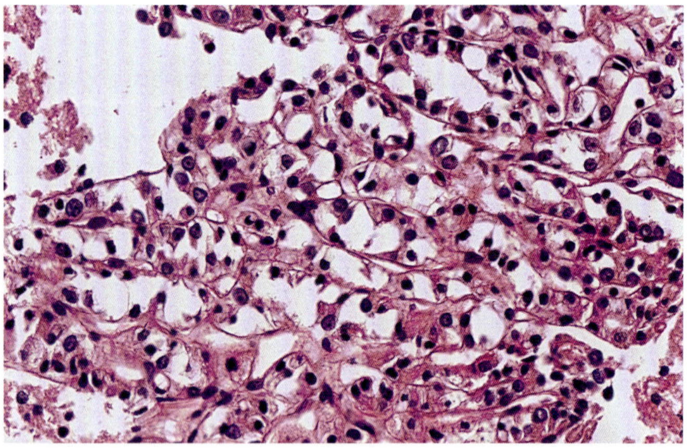

Fig. 8.249 Metastasis of a renal cell carcinoma to skeletal muscle. Carcinoma with clear cell features and thin vessels separating nests of tumour cells (cell block, H&E).

Ancillary testing

ICC, preferably on cell blocks and combined with microscopic appearance and clinical history, is the most important ancillary method to establish the diagnosis of a metastasis in the

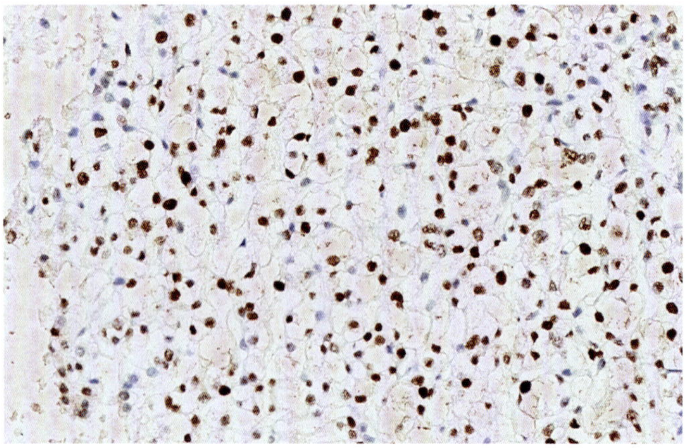

Fig. 8.250 Metastasis of a renal cell carcinoma to skeletal muscle. Nuclear positivity for PAX8 (cell block, ICC).

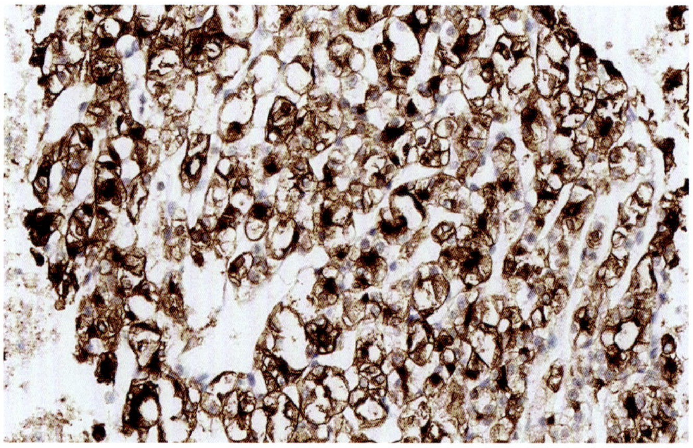

Fig. 8.252 Metastasis of a renal cell carcinoma to skeletal muscle. Diffuse and strong CD10 cytoplasmic positivity (cell block, ICC).

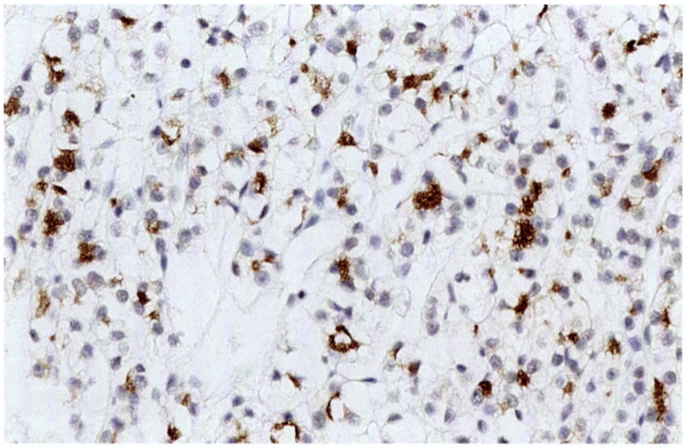

Fig. 8.251 Metastasis of a renal cell carcinoma to skeletal muscle. Cytoplasmatic positivity of RCCm (cell block, ICC).

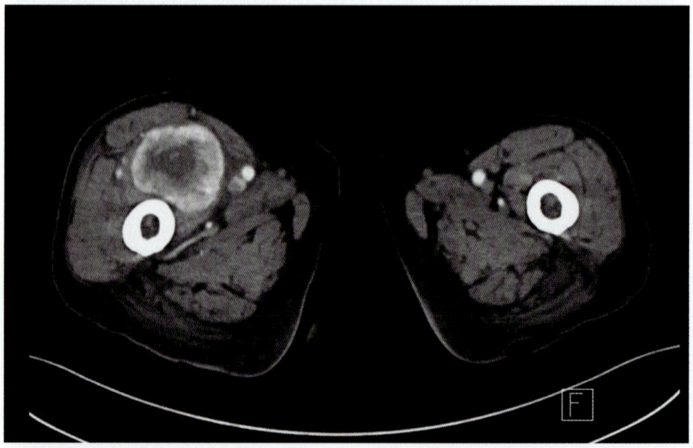

Fig. 8.253 Metastasis of a lung squamous cell carcinoma to skeletal muscle. CT demonstrating a large mass deeply located in the muscle of the right thigh.

soft tissues {1116}. Strong cytokeratin expression in the proper microscopic context supports the diagnosis of a metastatic carcinoma, and the additional expression of organ-specific markers helps to identify the primary site of origin: for example, TTF1 for lung carcinoma, GATA3 and hormone receptors for breast carcinoma, GATA3 and p63 for urothelial carcinoma, PAX8 for kidney or gynaecological primaries, and CDX2 for gastrointestinal tract primaries. Metastases of sarcomatoid carcinoma may totally lack or show only very limited cytokeratin expression. On the other hand, several sarcoma types, including synovial sarcoma, epithelioid sarcoma, Ewing sarcoma, and epithelioid angiosarcoma, may be positive for cytokeratin. The expression

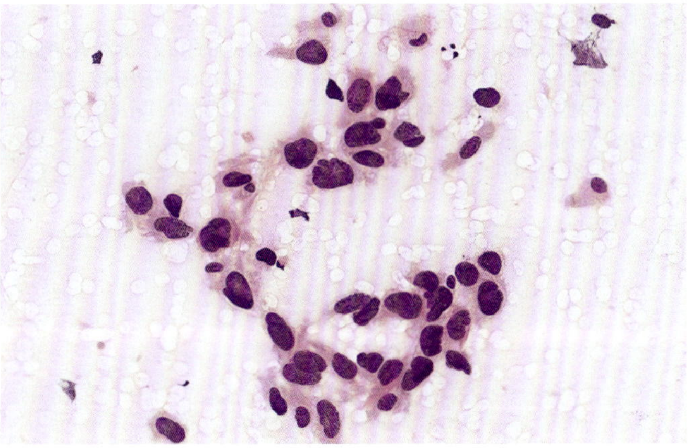

Fig. 8.254 Metastasis of a lung squamous cell carcinoma to skeletal muscle. A loosely cohesive tissue fragment of cells with dense, often spindle cytoplasm and hyperchromatic irregular nuclei (H&E).

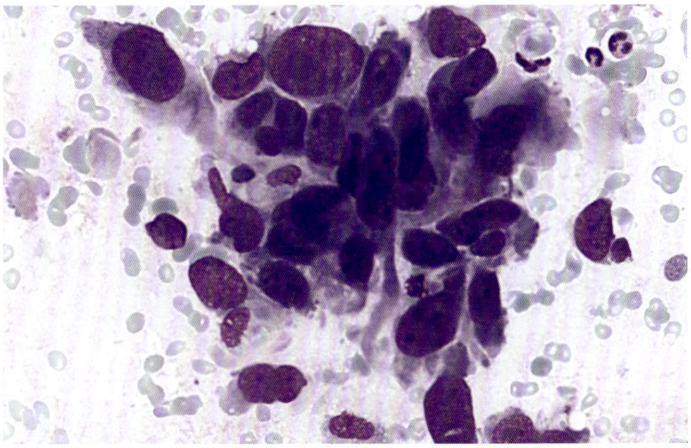

Fig. 8.255 Metastasis of a lung squamous cell carcinoma to skeletal muscle. A cohesive tissue fragment consisting of cells with well-defined, sometimes spindle cytoplasm and hyperchromatic pleomorphic nuclei (Giemsa).

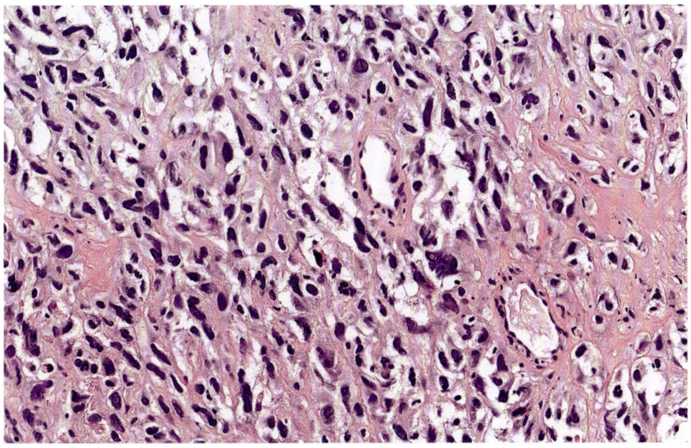

Fig. 8.256 Metastasis of a lung squamous cell carcinoma to skeletal muscle. Poorly differentiated malignant tumour in finely reticular sclerotic background (CNB, H&E).

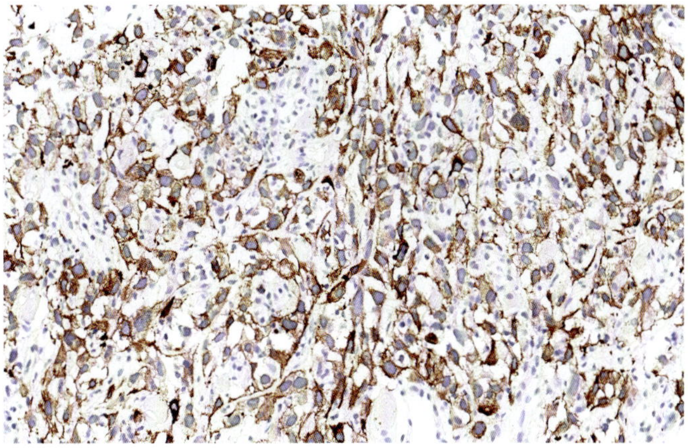

Fig. 8.257 Metastasis of a lung squamous cell carcinoma to skeletal muscle. Diffuse and strong cytoplasmic expression of cytokeratin AE1/AE3 (CNB, ICC).

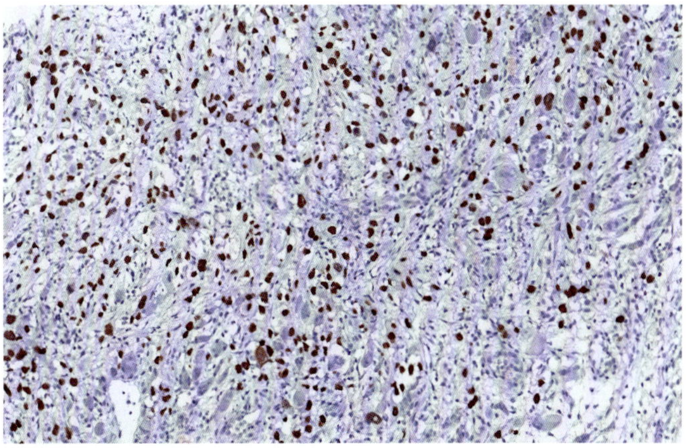

Fig. 8.258 Metastasis of a lung squamous cell carcinoma to skeletal muscle. Nuclear expression of p40 (CNB, ICC).

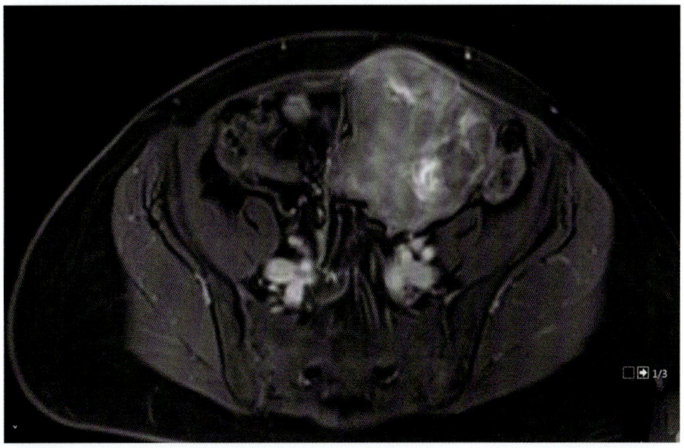

Fig. 8.259 Metastasis of a malignant melanoma to abdominal wall. MRI of a large tumour mass in the abdominal wall, corresponding to a metastasis of a malignant melanoma.

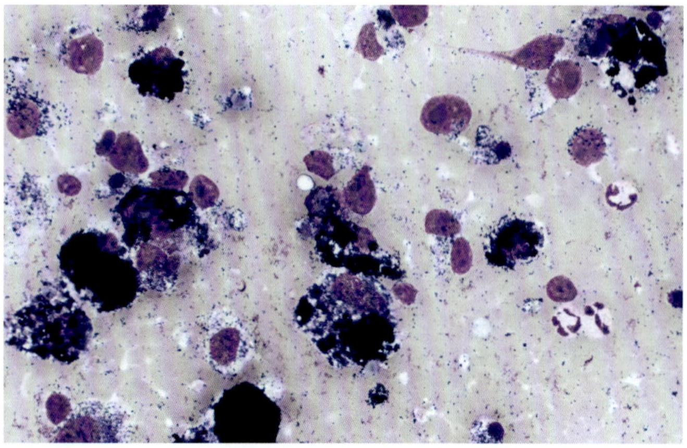

Fig. 8.260 Metastasis of a malignant melanoma to abdominal wall. Minute tissue fragments and single cells showing marked nuclear pleomorphism, macronucleoli, and bluish-black melanin pigment (Giemsa).

of melanocytic markers suggests the diagnosis of metastatic melanoma in the vast majority of cases, but the immunoprofile of a clear cell sarcoma is indistinguishable, and the application of molecular testing (FISH, PCR, NGS) to demonstrate the presence of the rearrangement of the *EWSR1* gene is necessary to diagnose clear cell sarcoma. Unlike round cell sarcomas, plasma cell neoplasms express CD138, and non-Hodgkin lymphoma express lymphatic markers.

FNAB can provide a cell block for targetable predictive markers {271,1206}, such as ER or PR; for FISH for *ERBB2* (*HER2*); and for NGS panels including *ALK*, *ROS1*, *NTRK1*, *NTRK2*, *NTRK3*, *BRAF*, and other genes.

Sample reports: Malignant

Rekhi B
Field AS
Qian X

The sample reports provided here are based on the standardized cytopathology report in the *Diagnostic categories and report structure* section of the first chapter. See that section for a discussion on the structure and components.

These are sample reports that include the components required in one possible format; the final report format depends on local practice and local laboratory information system requirements. For brevity, demographics and ROSE are not presented here.

Each institution should select a term for the main heading of the diagnostic summary, such as "Diagnostic summary" (as used in the examples below), "Diagnosis", or "Final diagnosis", and use it consistently.

Sample report 1

Specimen type:
Ultrasound-guided FNAB
Clinical and imaging information:
37-year-old female with a left medial thigh mass. MRI shows a 32 mm soft tissue mass deep to the superficial fascia in the posteromedial aspect of semi-membranous muscle, with diffuse homogeneous enhancement.

Diagnostic summary:
Site: Medial mid left thigh
Category: Malignant
Diagnosis: Myxoid liposarcoma, provisionally low-grade (see comment below)

Material received:
Six air-dried slides and two alcohol-fixed slides. 3 mL bloodstained fluid for cell block.

Microscopic description:
These moderately cellular smears show tissue fragments of myxoid stroma containing small capillaries branching and anastomosing in a plexiform pattern, with scattered lipoblasts featuring one or more eccentric clear vacuoles that displace and indent the nucleus, and with small spindle cells with mildly irregular nuclei. In the cell block there is considerable material, and the tumour cells are positive in immunocytochemistry for DDIT3. Confirmatory FISH is underway.

Comment: The features of this malignant neoplasm are those of myxoid liposarcoma. High-grade features such as hypercellularity or a significant round cell component are not identified in this limited sample. Clinical and imaging correlation is recommended.

Supplementary report 1:
FISH demonstrates *DDIT3* gene rearrangement, confirming the diagnosis of myxoid liposarcoma.

(Editor's note: The cytopathologist has issued a report based on the cytopathology and ICC, and then provided a final integrated report with the FISH.)

Sample report 2

Specimen type:
Ultrasound-guided FNAB
Clinical and imaging information:
40-year-old male with a 65 mm right levator scapulae intramuscular neoplastic mass suggestive of sarcoma on CT and MRI.

Diagnostic summary:
Site: Right levator scapulae mass
Category: Malignant
Diagnosis: Synovial sarcoma (see comment and supplementary report below)

Material received:
Six air-dried Giemsa-stained smears from ROSE, two alcohol-fixed smears. 4 mL pink fluid for cell block.

Microscopic description:
These highly cellular smears show branching tissue fragments (some containing capillaries); loosely cohesive small tissue fragments; and single cells, which are uniform spindle cells with poorly defined scant cytoplasm, hyperchromatic oval nuclei, and inconspicuous nucleoli. There are no epithelioid cells, glandular structures, round cells, or marked atypia. Occasional mitoses are present. There is no necrosis. Cell block shows spindle cells positive for SS18::SSX and TLE1, supporting a diagnosis of synovial sarcoma. S100 and SOX10 are negative, arguing against neural differentiation, and desmin is negative, arguing against muscle differentiation. CK7 shows patchy positivity, and CD34 is negative.

Comment: The overall features of this malignant spindle cell neoplasm support a diagnosis of synovial sarcoma. Molecular testing is underway.

Supplementary report 1:
This neoplasm is positive for *SS18::SSX1* by NGS, confirming synovial sarcoma.

(Editor's note: The cytopathologist could have issued a report categorizing the lesion as malignant, and then followed up with a supplementary report with the ICC, but has instead decided to wait for the ICC on the cell block. The confirmatory NGS has confirmed the diagnosis, and this is presented in the final integrated report.)

Sample report 3

Specimen type:
FNAB
Clinical and imaging information:
51-year-old male patient with a firm, palpable 60 mm mass in his right medial lower thigh, of 7 months' duration. No other lesion elsewhere in his body. CT shows a large, 70 mm heterogeneous mass infiltrating the muscles, with adjacent oedema.

Diagnostic summary:
Site: Right medial lower thigh
Category: Malignant
Diagnosis: Suggestive of high-grade sarcoma (see comment below)

Material received:
Five air-dried smears, two alcohol-fixed smears. 2 mL bloodstained fluid.

Microscopic description:
These highly cellular smears show poorly cohesive tissue fragments and single scattered plump spindle and pleomorphic cells exhibiting marked nuclear enlargement, hyperchromasia, and variation in shape, with prominent nucleoli and scattered mitotic figures, including atypical forms, in a background of inflammatory cells and necrosis. There is no diagnostic material in the cell block.

Comment: The features of this malignancy suggest a high-grade sarcoma. Correlation with clinical history and imaging is required. Repeat study (to obtain material for immunocytochemistry) and/or CNB is recommended.

Sample report 4

Specimen type:
CT-guided FNAB
Clinical and imaging information:
55-year-old female with pain and lump in central lower back. CT shows large destructive tumour in sacrum with adjacent soft tissue component. MRI shows lobulated mass, hypointense on T1-weighted and heterogeneously hyperintense on T2-weighed images, including postcontrast sequence.

Diagnostic summary:
Site: Central lower back
Category: Malignant
Diagnosis: Chordoma

Material received:
Six air-dried Giemsa-stained smears from ROSE, two alcohol-fixed smears. 4 mL bloody fluid for cell block.

Microscopic description:
Moderately cellular smears composed of round to epithelioid cells arranged in minute tissue fragments and cords with abundant fibrillary myxoid matrix. The tumour cells have moderate to abundant granular to vacuolated cytoplasm, and the vacuolated cells are consistent with physaliphorous cells. There is a background of blood.

Comment: The features are those of a chordoma. Correlation with the imaging findings at a multidisciplinary meeting has taken place. Confirmatory immunocytochemistry stains are underway on the cell block.

Supplementary report 1:
There is considerable material in the cell block, which is positive for pancytokeratin (AE1/AE3) and positive in nuclei for brachyury. There is patchy staining for S100, whereas SOX10, GFAP, and PAX8 are negative.

(Editor's note: In this case, the cytopathologist has provided a categorization and diagnosis based on the cytomorphology and then issued a final report incorporating ICC.)

Sample report 5

Specimen type:
CT-guided FNAB
Clinical and imaging information:
11-year-old boy, slow-growing soft tissue mass in left upper arm. Plain radiograph shows a large mass involving muscles and infiltrating humerus. MRI shows 80 mm soft tissue mass isointense on T1-weighted and heterogeneous on T2-weighted images with postcontrast enhancement.

Diagnostic summary:
Site: Left upper arm
Category: Malignant
Diagnosis: Ewing sarcoma

Material received:
Four air-dried Giemsa-stained smears from ROSE, two alcohol-fixed smears. 3 mL bloody fluid for cell block.

Microscopic description:
Highly cellular smears with loosely cohesive round cells, including light and dark cells, with a high N:C ratio, against a granular proteinaceous background that appears "tigroid" in the Giemsa smears. The cells show focal rosette formation and contain a scant to moderate amount of cytoplasm with fine cytoplasmic vacuoles in Giemsa-stained smears. Cell block immunocytochemistry shows tumour diffusely positive for NKX2-2 and CD99 (MIC2) (cytoplasmic and membranous) and negative for SATB2.

Comment: The cytopathology and immunocytochemistry are diagnostic of Ewing sarcoma.

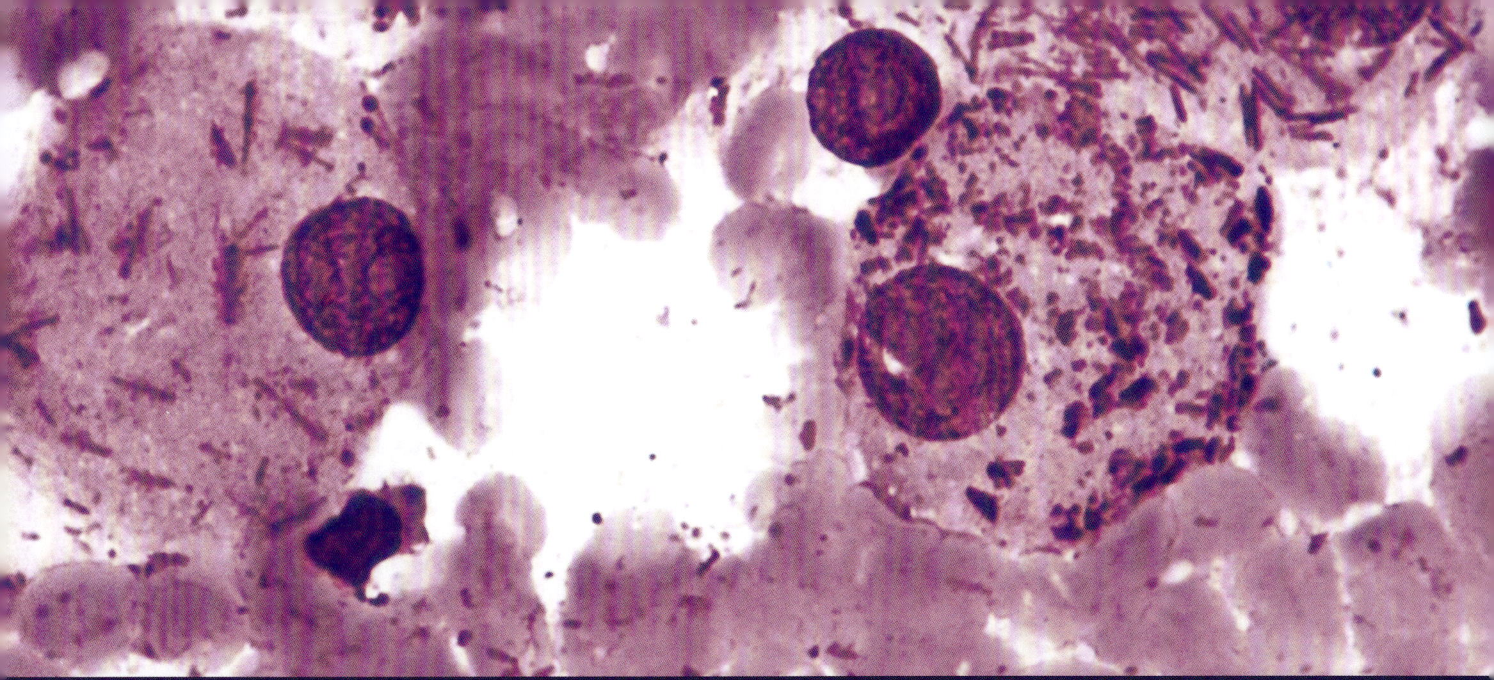

9

Diagnostic management recommendations for each diagnostic category

Edited by: Rekhi B

Insufficient/Inadequate/Non-diagnostic
Benign
Atypical
Soft tissue neoplasm of uncertain malignant potential
Suspicious for malignancy
Malignant

Category: Insufficient/Inadequate/ Non-diagnostic

Raymond WA
Bode-Lesniewska B
Field AS
Monaco SE

Definition: A specimen categorized as "Inadequate/Insufficient/Non-diagnostic" lacks sufficient material, in quantity or quality, for a reliable diagnosis.

An "Insufficient/Inadequate/Non-diagnostic" categorization may result from a variety of technical, preparation, and sampling issues and is defined in relation to the clinical history, physical examination and imaging findings, and fundamentally the material for assessment on the direct smears or in LBC preparation. The reasons why an FNAB is categorized as "Insufficient" should be stated in the report, such as obscuring blood or ultrasound gel, slow drying artefact in Giemsa stains, air-drying artefact in alcohol-fixed Pap-stained slides, crush artefact, lysis of cells due to contamination with local anaesthetic, formalin vapour effect, low cellularity of the sample due to technical difficulties in obtaining material or the nature of the specimen, or poor FNAB technique.

Some soft tissue tumours have abundant collagen, for example desmoid fibromatosis or low-grade fibromyxoid sarcoma; this may produce low cellularity {282,1058}, and CNB is required {80,344}. Superficial fat tumours may yield only fat, and myxoid lesions only acellular or paucicellular myxoid background, and correlation with clinical and imaging findings is required.

In contradistinction to an "Insufficient" categorization, any FNAB is adequate if it is diagnostic of a neoplasm or lesion consistent with the clinical setting and imaging findings. If there are any atypical features, even if smears are technically suboptimal, the case is categorized as "Atypical" rather than "Insufficient". When only benign cells are present, such as fat or skeletal muscle, some cytopathologists categorize this as "Non-diagnostic" if the FNAB target was regarded as a suspicious mass or lesion; others describe and categorize the material on the smears as "Benign" and add a mandatory caveat that "the material may not represent the targeted lesion". In this the first edition of the WHO Reporting System for Soft Tissue Cytopathology (WHO System), both approaches are acceptable; an institution or cytopathologist should clearly communicate with their clinicians, choose which approach to take, and stick to it. In both scenarios, a repeat biopsy, most commonly repeat FNAB or CNB, is required. Site also influences concepts of adequacy; for example, the differential diagnosis of deeply located, intramuscular, and especially large fatty tumours includes lipoma-like atypical lipomatous tumour / well-differentiated liposarcoma, and the requirement for adequate material shifts not only in regard to the amount and features of the material on the FNAB smears, but also as to the availability of material for studies to determine *MDM2* amplification status {753}.

The FNAB sample may be "Insufficient", but a later cell block or other ancillary test may provide sufficient material for a diagnosis. An institution or cytopathologist can decide whether to issue the FNAB report including a statement that ancillary tests are to follow, and then later a supplementary report where the diagnostic category may be changed, or to report the FNAB only once all cell block and ancillary tests are available.

Reported rates of the "Insufficient/Inadequate/Non-diagnostic" category vary widely {1001,753,720,188}, influenced by the criteria used to define adequacy, the type of procedure, imaging and clinical findings, and the expertise of the person performing the procedure. In a meta-analysis of 13 reports on the adequacy of bone and soft tissue FNAB, the range of adequate specimens for soft tissue lesions was 39–95% {188}.

Reports on the ROM for soft tissue FNAB are limited, but the ROM for the "Insufficient/Inadequate/Non-diagnostic" category is often reported as high, most likely due to sampling error. A recent large single-institution retrospective study of 2214 cases showed a ROM of 29.87% for the "Insufficient" category, but it also showed that the ROM for all categories varied with the FNAB cytopathological pattern, from low for lipomatous tumours; to higher for spindle cell, epithelioid, and myxoid tumours; to very high for pleomorphic and round cell tumours {460}.

Management of a patient with an "Inadequate/Insufficient/Non-diagnostic" FNAB report requires correlation with the clinical and imaging findings, and repeat FNAB, ideally with ROSE, is required in almost all cases, with or without CNB if available. If the repeat procedures do not yield a diagnosis in cases of clinical and/or imaging suspicion, then CNB (if it has not been performed up to this point) or incisional or excisional biopsy should be recommended. Imaging guidance, which decreases the sampling error, is recommended for all impalpable or difficult to access lesions {80}.

Category: Benign

Dodd LG
Field AS
Kerr DA

Definition: A specimen categorized as "Benign" demonstrates unequivocal benign cytopathological features, which may or may not be diagnostic of a specific process or benign neoplasm.

A "Benign" categorization is applied when a sample is adequate for interpretation and shows unequivocal features of a benign lesion. This may represent a specific benign neoplasm or process that is subclassified based on its distinctive cytomorphological pattern, such as a specific type of stroma or matrix constituting adipocytic, myxoid, and chondro-osseous patterns; a prominent cellular feature such as inflammation or multinucleate giant cells; or a specific cell shape, as in spindle or epithelioid patterns.

In this WHO Reporting System for Soft Tissue Cytopathology (WHO System), the "intermediate" lesions of the WHO classification of soft tissue and bone tumours are divided and categorized into two distinct categories: "locally aggressive" lesions, such as fibromatosis, are categorized into the "Benign" category; and "rarely metastasizing" tumours, such as angiomatoid fibrous histiocytoma, are categorized into the "Soft tissue neoplasm of uncertain malignant potential" ("STNUMP") category. The "STNUMP" category includes neoplasms whose cytopathological and often histopathological and ICC features are not always a reliable predictor of the behaviour of the neoplasm, as well as some unpredictable neoplasms that most commonly behave in a benign fashion but have a small potential for malignant behaviour.

Benign soft tissue lesions greatly outnumber aggressive or malignant tumours, including sarcomas, by an estimated factor of 100 to 1 {1214}. Many of the lesions included in this FNAB category are not neoplastic, such as focal fat necrosis, mass-forming inflammatory processes, and ganglion cysts, but they are included because they fall into the differential diagnosis of neoplastic lesions clinically and on imaging and are frequently sampled by FNAB.

Benign lesions can cause significant morbidity by obstruction, impingement, or other physical mechanisms, and they may be difficult to remove; for example, vascular neoplasms and malformations can be large and infiltrative, necessitating difficult and often multistage removal; fibromatosis, a locally aggressive tumour, is also difficult to excise {884}. In addition, some benign lesions may be transient or self-limited, such as nodular fasciitis {385}.

Overall accuracy in FNAB of soft tissue is affected by individual cytopathologists' experience, which can be limited other than in specialist orthopaedic and oncological institutions where relatively rare soft tissue neoplasms tend to be seen more frequently, and by the use of a multidisciplinary approach, which is highly recommended {832}.

The sensitivity and specificity of FNAB for separating benign from malignant soft tissue lesions ranges depending on various study parameters, with an overall sensitivity of 97.4% and specificity of 98.2% in a large meta-analysis {188}. Studies vary in requiring surgical pathology follow-up or accepting that clinical and imaging follow-up suffices to confirm the "Benign" FNAB. The negative predictive value for a benign lesion ranges from 94% to 98% {763,696,33,1470,681,1017,753}, and the ROM for the "Benign" category can be conservatively estimated to be 5% or less. In a recently published single-institution retrospective review, the ROM was 2.49% {460}, although this same review showed that the overall ROM across the categories varied with the cytomorphological pattern, from 3% for lipomatous tumours reported on FNAB to 62.78% for spindle cell, 78.15% for epithelioid, 84.58% for myxoid, 94.26% for pleomorphic, and 100% for round cell tumours.

A "Benign" soft tissue FNAB should be correlated with the clinical and imaging findings and with ancillary testing, such as ICC for MDM2 in fat neoplasms. Any discrepancy in this triple approach should lead to consideration of repeat FNAB with ROSE and cell block, and potentially CNB if available. CT scans, ultrasound, and particularly MRI are all useful in assessing soft tissue neoplasms {471,1016}, and ultrasound is recommended in assessing superficial lesions and for FNAB guidance. The management of soft tissue lesions categorized as "Benign" depends on many factors, including lesion size, depth, and location, as well as patient comfort and preference. Some benign lesions are removed for cosmetic purposes only, and some can be monitored clinically for signs of growth or change. Surgical removal is best accomplished with thoughtful preoperative planning and assessment. With some benign or locally aggressive lesions, such as desmoid fibromatosis, active surveillance is the current preferred approach in most clinical scenarios {884}.

Category: Atypical

Raymond WA
Field AS

Definition: A specimen categorized as "Atypical" demonstrates features predominantly seen in benign lesions and minimal features that may raise the possibility of a malignant lesion, but with features insufficient, in either number or quality, to diagnose a benign or malignant process or lesion.

The "Atypical" category is used when there are cytopathological features present that are essentially benign, but with occasional features uncommon in benign lesions that raise the remote possibility of a malignancy and thus cannot be ignored. This indeterminate category is included to increase the negative predictive value of a "Benign" categorization. Whenever atypical features are present, the FNAB is categorized as "Atypical", even if the overall material shows technical faults and would otherwise be categorized as "Insufficient', or when suboptimal preparation has resulted in a degree of artefactual or degenerative change but sufficient atypical cytomorphological features are present and a malignancy cannot be entirely excluded. Most of the specimens in this category are likely to be from reactive, inflammatory, or reparative processes, but specific features sufficient for a definitive benign diagnosis are lacking.

The WHO Reporting System for Soft Tissue Cytopathology (WHO System) uses the term "Atypical", consistent with the other WHO Reporting Systems, to separate FNAB samples that are considered more likely to be benign from those that are more likely to be malignant and categorized as "Suspicious for malignancy". The ROM increases from the "Atypical" category to the "Suspicious for malignancy" category, assisting clinicians in the further diagnostic management of their patients.

Categorization of a soft tissue FNAB as "Atypical" may be based on the cellular pattern, high cellularity, the stromal component, and nuclear features such as variable nuclear enlargement and pleomorphism. Nuclear enlargement, hyperchromasia, and pleomorphism can also be seen as part of the spectrum of degeneration, for example in ancient change in a schwannoma. Potential problems arise due to cytomorphological overlap between different tumour types, in particular low-grade spindle cell tumours {753}.

Soft tissue inflammatory lesions may have nuclear pleomorphism and atypia, such as ganglion-like cells in nodular fasciitis, or fibroblastic proliferation after infarction or reparative changes after biopsy, traumatic haematoma, or radiotherapy, and the features may overlap with those of a neoplastic process. A specimen may also be rendered "Atypical" for technical reasons related to the expertise of the operator performing the FNAB, the quality of smear preparation and staining, the nature and accessibility of the site of the lesion, and the experience of the cytopathologist interpreting the specimen.

This category is not a "wastebasket" for unknown diagnoses, and the atypical features should always be specified in the microscopic description and the differential diagnosis discussed, with a favoured diagnosis provided if possible. Several studies have reported the proportion of cases in the atypical/suspicious category as 1–2% {1330,1470}.

The ROM has been reported as 46% in one study of soft tissue and bone lesions {753}. A recent single-institution retrospective review of more than 2200 cases categorized using the WHO System reported a ROM of 39.62%, and it was observed that the ROM varied across all categories when the pattern was taken into account, from 3% for lipomatous tumours to 62.78% for spindle cell, 78.15% for epithelioid, 84.58% for myxoid, 94.26% for pleomorphic, and 100% for round cell tumours {460}.

Correlation with clinical findings, imaging, and any available ancillary tests on FNAB material are essential once a soft tissue FNAB is categorized as "Atypical", and discussion by a multidisciplinary team is recommended. If the findings indicate that the lesion is highly likely to be a benign neoplasm or a reactive or inflammatory process, then observation and clinical follow-up may be considered, but if the findings are discrepant or clinical and imaging findings suggest malignancy, a repeat FNAB should be recommended, ideally with ROSE and where available CNB, and incisional biopsy with or without frozen section or excisional biopsy could be considered.

Category: Soft tissue neoplasm of uncertain malignant potential

Layfield LJ
Field AS

Definition: Neoplasms in the "Soft tissue neoplasm of uncertain malignant potential" ("STNUMP") category are mesenchymal neoplasms that cannot be unequivocally diagnosed as benign or malignant on cytopathological analysis and ancillary testing, including tumours with intermediate biological potential and tumours requiring the application of histopathological criteria to determine whether they are benign or malignant.

The category of "Soft tissue neoplasm of uncertain malignant potential" ("STNUMP") represents a diverse group of neoplasms whose biological behaviour cannot be predicted on an FNAB or CNB, or in some cases on histopathology, even if a definitive diagnosis of a specific tumour type can be made by routine FNAB cytopathology and ancillary testing.

The WHO classification of soft tissue and bone tumours has an "indeterminate" group of neoplasms, which comprises "intermediate (locally aggressive)" neoplasms, such as fibromatosis, which are categorized in the WHO Reporting System for Soft Tissue Cytopathology (WHO System) into the "Benign" category, and "intermediate (rarely metastasizing)" neoplasms, which are categorized into the "STNUMP" category, along with tumours whose criteria for risk stratification for malignancy are based on histopathological parameters that can be applied only to resected specimens.

The categories "Atypical" and "STNUMP" address two fundamentally different diagnostic issues. The category "Atypical" is used when the cytopathologist cannot recognize a specific type of soft tissue neoplasm and so cannot definitively assign the specimen to the "Benign" or "Malignant" category, or when a specific line of differentiation is identified but there are insufficient cytopathological features to warrant categorization as "Suspicious for malignancy". The category "STNUMP" is used when the cytopathologist is able to diagnose a specific neoplasm, but either definitive criteria cannot be applied for risk stratification and ROM, or the specific tumour type has an inherent but unpredictable risk of metastasis.

Neoplasms in the "STNUMP" category include the following:

First, three tumours of intermediate biological risk: dermatofibrosarcoma protuberans, a locally aggressive, frequently recurring fibroblastic neoplasm with a small risk of high-grade fibrosarcomatous transformation; inflammatory myofibroblastic tumour, a locally aggressive, rarely metastasizing neoplasm; and angiomatoid fibrous histiocytoma, another locally aggressive, rarely metastasizing neoplasm.

Second, myoepithelial neoplasms of soft tissue and perivascular epithelioid cell tumour (PEComa), whose criteria for malignancy are best assessed on histopathological features {579, 439,358,121}.

Third, solitary fibrous tumour, whose risk stratification schemes predicting its risk of malignant behaviour are best applied to CNB and excision specimens rather than to FNAB material {306,310}.

Currently, there is insufficient published data associated with the "STNUMP" category to establish a ROM, and estimates of ROM for each of the diverse tumour types based on histopathology have been proposed. A recent single-institution retrospective study of more than 2200 FNAB samples using the WHO System categories showed a ROM of 51.43% {460}. Specific FNAB diagnoses with appropriate ancillary testing can establish appropriate management for the patients.

An "STNUMP" categorization requires correlation of the clinical, imaging, cytopathological, and any ancillary test findings. If ancillary testing is not available on the original FNAB, repeat FNAB with CNB, if available, to obtain material for confirmatory ICC, FISH, or NGS is recommended. In most cases, complete resection is usually performed for definitive treatment, and the excised specimen can be assessed for histopathological features that enable risk stratification to be carried out.

Category: Suspicious for malignancy

Klijanienko J
Field AS
Raymond WA

Definition: A specimen categorized as "Suspicious for malignancy" demonstrates some cytopathological features suggestive of malignancy, but with features insufficient, in either number or quality, for an unequivocal diagnosis of malignancy.

There is likely to be wide interobserver variability in this category, dependent on the expertise of the FNAB operator, the quality of material provided, the quality of the smear preparation, the availability of material for cell block and ancillary testing, the inherent nature of the lesion, and the cytopathologist's experience and confidence in rendering a malignant diagnosis.

The "Suspicious for malignancy" category should have a high positive predictive value for malignancy, because the WHO Reporting System for Soft Tissue Cytopathology (WHO System) includes a separate "Atypical" category for atypical FNAB samples, which are most likely benign, with a lower ROM. The "Suspicious for malignancy" category also functions to avoid false positive diagnoses and ensure a positive predictive value, close to 100%, in the "Malignant" category.

The "Suspicious for malignancy" category includes cases producing cellular smears in which there is significant nuclear enlargement, anisonucleosis, irregularity of nuclear membranes, and coarse chromatin, possibly with prominent nucleoli and mitotic figures, in particular because soft tissue neoplasms may show considerable intratumoural cytomorphological heterogeneity and overlap between lesions, and none of these features is diagnostic of malignancy. It also includes cases that produce low cellularity, such as lipomatous tumours, where it may be difficult to obtain sufficient atypical cells in a cytopathology preparation to allow for a diagnosis of malignancy, as well as cases where there are atypical cells showing features suggestive of malignancy but a confident diagnosis of malignancy cannot be made due to suboptimal preparation, preservation, or staining. Such specimens cannot be regarded as "Inadequate/Insufficient/Non-diagnostic". The background features may include necrosis, myxoid material, and inflammatory cells.

Ancillary techniques, such as ICC on cell block material, can assist in confirming a specific tumour type, but the inherent features of some soft tissue tumours produce low cellularity, insufficient for definitive assessment, or the ICC may suggest a cell lineage but not a malignant diagnosis. Molecular studies in an increasing number of specific tumours, such as *MDM2* FISH analysis for liposarcoma, may allow a definitive diagnosis where the cytomorphological categorization was "Suspicious for malignancy"; if one of these tumours is suspected on the FNAB, such ancillary tests can be requested. In all cases, the tumour type suspected, or a differential diagnosis, should be stated in the cytopathology report.

The rate of "Suspicious for malignancy" cases varies. In a review of 1114 bone and soft tissue lesions, 1% showed cells suspicious for malignancy, of which 5 of the 7 with follow-up (71%) were confirmed as malignant on histopathology {696}. One text {233} suggests using atypical and suspicious categories for FNAB, but most studies do not provide ROM for atypical/suspicious FNAB and only indicate overall sensitivity and specificity in distinguishing benign from malignant. Several other studies reported the proportion of cases in the atypical/suspicious category as 1–2%, usually representing only 1 or 2 cases {1330,1470}.

The category has a high positive predictive value for malignancy, with a reported ROM of 71–80% {696,753}, and in one recent retrospective single-institution study of more than 2200 cases, the ROM was 68.42% based on using the WHO System's six categories {460}. The authors of the study made the interesting observation that the ROM varies not only with categorization into the six categories but also with the FNAB pattern seen, from 3% for lipomatous tumours, which include one of the most common FNAB targets (superficial lipoma), to 62.78% for spindle cell, 78.15% for epithelioid, 84.58% for myxoid, 94.26% for pleomorphic, and 100% for round cell tumours. The WHO System approach to diagnosis is based on these cytopathological patterns, which have been previously detailed {413}. Further research around this finding will be worthwhile to guide cytopathologists and clinicians.

It is essential that clinical, imaging, cytopathological, and any ancillary findings available should be correlated, ideally in a multidisciplinary meeting. If there are discrepancies, repeat FNAB should be recommended to confirm the malignancy, preferably with ROSE to effectively triage material for cell block, ICC, FISH, or NGS, along with CNB whenever available. In some situations, incisional biopsy with or without frozen section or a surgical excision biopsy may be required.

Category: Malignant

Domanski HA
Field AS

Definition: A specimen categorized as "Malignant" demonstrates unequivocal cytopathological features of malignancy.

The "Malignant" category is used when unequivocal cytomorphological features of malignancy are present. No single cytopathological feature is diagnostic of malignancy, but the presence of round cells, prominent nuclear atypia, marked abnormalities of N:C ratio, atypical mitotic figures, marked variability in cell size and shape, necrosis, and hypercellularity are highly suggestive of malignancy.

After confirmation of malignancy, cytopathological examination should establish the type of malignancy by differentiating between sarcomas, metastatic carcinomas, melanoma, and lymphomas. Whenever possible, further subtyping into a specific sarcoma type or at least designation of the sarcoma as low-grade or high-grade should be performed, and ICC, FISH, and molecular analysis can aid in the specific identification of many sarcoma types. Some soft tissue malignancies have characteristic molecular features; for example, *MDM2* amplification is particularly helpful in establishing malignancy in fat tumours. Other sarcomas are associated with specific translocations, such as *ASPSCR1*::*TFE3* in clear cell sarcoma, *FUS*::*CREB3L2* in low-grade fibromyxoid sarcoma, and *FUS*::*DDIT3* in myxoid liposarcoma {404,111}. Correlation with histopathological features in CNB is almost always helpful in achieving a precise diagnosis.

The "Malignant" category must be used in conjunction with clinical history, physical examination, and imaging findings. The report should almost always state that "correlation with clinical and imaging findings is required". The diagnosis of malignancy is dependent in part on the quality of the material provided for assessment and in part on the cytopathologist's experience and confidence.

This category includes both primary low- or high-grade sarcomas and secondary tumours occurring in the soft tissues, and distinguishing metastases has significant impact on further clinical management. Clinical data and information about previous malignancies, together with the cytopathological features of the FNAB smears, are usually sufficient to render a correct diagnosis in many cases of secondary malignancies {342,1423, 1017}. However, when a mass in soft tissue is the first manifestation of a carcinoma, melanoma, or lymphoma, ancillary tests are often necessary to determine the site of the primary malignant lesion and to assist with potential treatment targets.

If the tumour is a primary malignant soft tissue neoplasm but a specific tumour cannot be diagnosed, it is categorized as "Malignant", and a differential diagnosis is provided. In some cases, a diagnosis of high-grade or low-grade sarcoma can allow for planning surgical treatment and further management. However, ideally as specific a diagnosis as possible should be made in all cases, and this is required in those types of sarcomas where optimal treatment includes neoadjuvant or adjuvant therapy and a precise diagnosis is required prior to excision biopsy. Ancillary testing of FNAB material and CNB is often essential to achieve this precise histopathological diagnosis {783,1062,342,198,22, 463,343}; for example, "small round cell neoplasms" can be categorized as "Malignant" routinely on FNAB, but the required specific diagnosis is difficult on the basis of cytomorphology alone {343,463}, and ancillary tests are often essential to reach a specific histopathological diagnosis. Similarly, the myxoid soft tissue neoplasms have overlapping cytopathological features {1231, 1463}, and although the sensitivity and specificity for detecting malignancy in this group of neoplasms is high {1231}, additional ICC, FISH, or molecular tests are usually required to make definitive diagnoses {785,1241}.

The ROM for the "Malignant" category ranges from 91% to 100% based on several retrospective studies {753,1001,176,1017, 705,1231}. A more recent large retrospective study reported a ROM of 97.69%, noting that the ROM varies depending on both the cytomorphological pattern and the WHO Reporting System for Soft Tissue Cytopathology (WHO System) categorization {460}.

Clinical and imaging correlation is always necessary in evaluating neoplasms within the "Malignant" category {289,158}, and management decisions as to any further diagnostic workup and definitive management should be made by a multidisciplinary team. If FNAB does not provide enough material for diagnosis, or if the cytopathological findings are inconsistent with clinical and imaging assessments, the imaging findings should be carefully reviewed and correlated. If suspicion remains high, repeat FNAB should be conducted – preferably with ROSE and triaging of material for appropriate ancillary tests, or CNB, or simple excision biopsy – before proceeding with any major surgical or oncological interventions.

Contributors

AGARAM, Narasimhan P.
Memorial Sloan Kettering Cancer Center
1275 York Ave
New York NY 10065

BODE-LESNIEWSKA, Beata
Institute of Pathology
Lucerne Cantonal Hospital
Spitalstrasse
6000 Lucerne

BONGIOVANNI, Massimo
Unilabs
Biopole 3, Rte de la Corniche 9A
1066 Epalinges

BUI, Marilyn M.
Moffitt Cancer Center
12902 Magnolia Dr
Tampa FL 33612

CARRILHO, Carla
Faculty of Medicine
Eduardo Mondlane University
Avenida Agostinho Neto, 679, 3 Esquerdo
1164 Maputo

CHEBIB, Ivan
Massachusetts General Hospital and
Harvard Medical School
55 Fruit St WRN2
Boston MA 02114

CREE, Ian A.
International Agency for Research on Cancer
25 Av. Tony Garnier, CS 90627
69366 Lyon, CEDEX 07

DODD, Leslie G.
University of North Carolina
101 Manning Dr
Chapel Hill NC 27514

DOMANSKI, Henryk A.
Skåne University Hospital
Sölvegatan 25B
22185 Lund

FIELD, Andrew S.
University of NSW Sydney and
University of Notre Dame Medical Schools
Department of Anatomical Pathology
St Vincent's Hospital Sydney
Victoria St
Darlinghurst, Sydney NSW 2010

FONSECA, Anil Felix Angelo
Gandhi Medical College/TIMS
Hyderabad, Telangana

GAJDZIS, Pawel
Wroclaw Medical University
Borowska 213
50-556 Wrocław

GEIJER, Mats
University of Gothenburg
Sahlgrenska Academy
Clinical Sciences, Radiology
41345 Gothenburg

GRAYSON, Wayne
Ampath Laboratories, Johannesburg, and
School of Pathology, University of the
Witwatersrand
7 York Rd, Parktown
Johannesburg 2193

HIROSHIMA, Kenzo
Chiba University Graduate School of
Medicine
1-8-1 Inohana, Chuo-ku
Chiba 260-8670

HOLMES, Brittany J.
Stanford University School of Medicine
300 Pasteur Dr, Lane Building, L235
Stanford CA 94305

JAIN, Deepali
All India Institute of Medical Sciences
Ansari Nagar, New Delhi, and
University of Pittsburgh Medical Center
Pittsburgh PA 15261

JO, Vickie Y.*
Brigham and Women's Hospital and
Harvard Medical School
75 Francis St
Boston MA 02115

KERR, Darcy A.
Dartmouth Health
1 Medical Center Dr
Lebanon NH 03756

KILPATRICK, Scott E.
Cleveland Clinic Administrative Campus
Laboratory
3050 Science Park Dr, ACIII-4
Beachwood OH 44122-7355

KLIJANIENKO, Jerzy
Institut Curie
26 Rue d'Ulm
75248 Paris

LAYFIELD, Lester J.
University of Missouri
1 Hospital Dr
Columbia MO 65212

LAZAR, Alexander J.
University of Texas
MD Anderson Cancer Center
1515 Holcombe Blvd, Unit 85
Houston TX 77030

LOKUHETTY, Dilani
International Agency for Research on Cancer
25 Av. Tony Garnier, CS 90627
69366 Lyon, CEDEX 07

MEHROTRA, Ravi
Centre for Health Innovation and Policy
361, Sector 15A
Noida 20301

MICHELOW, Pamela
University of the Witwatersrand and
National Health Laboratory Service
PO Box 1038
Johannesburg 2000

MITO, Jeffrey K.
Brigham and Women's Hospital
75 Francis St, Dept. of Pathology, Amory 3
Boston MA 02115

MONACO, Sara E.
Geisinger Medical Center
100 N Academy Ave, MC 19-20
Danville PA 17822

OZAWA, Michael
Stanford University
300 Pasteur Dr
Stanford CA 94304

PANTANOWITZ, Liron
University of Pittsburgh
UPMC Shadyside, Cancer Pavilion
5230 Centre Ave
Pittsburgh PA 15232

---

* Indicates disclosure of interests (see p. 251).

PITMAN, Martha Bishop
Harvard Medical School
Massachusetts General Hospital
55 Fruit St
Boston MA 02114

QIAN, Xiaohua
Stanford University School of Medicine
300 Pasteur Dr, Room H2110, MC 5324
Stanford CA 94305

RAJWANSHI, Arvind
All India Institute of Medical Sciences
Raebareli 229401

RAYMOND, Wendy A.
Department of Surgical Pathology, Flinders Medical Centre and Flinders University; and Clinpath Pathology
Flinders Dr
Bedford Park
Adelaide SA 5042

REKHI, Bharat
Tata Memorial Centre, HBNI University
Dr Ernest Borges Rd, Parel
Mumbai, Maharashtra 400012

SCHAEFER, Inga-Marie
Brigham and Women's Hospital and Harvard Medical School
75 Francis St
Boston MA 02115

SCHMITT, Fernando
RISE (Health Research Network);
Medical Faculty of the University of Porto;
Molecular Pathology Unit, Ipatimup
Rua Júlio Amaral de Carvalho 45
4200-135 Porto

SEWELL, William Arthur
University of NSW Sydney and
St Vincent's Hospital Sydney
Victoria St
Darlinghurst NSW 2010

SILVERMAN, Jan
University of North Carolina School of Medicine
101 Manning Dr
Chapel Hill NC 27514

STELOW, Edward B.
University of Virginia School of Medicine
PO Box 800214
Charlottesville VA 22908-0214

TEOT, Lisa Anne
Boston Children's Hospital and
Harvard Medical School
300 Longwood Ave
Boston MA 02115

VANDENBUSSCHE, Christopher J.
Johns Hopkins Hospital
600 N Wolfe St, Pathology 406
Baltimore MD 21287

YANG, Eric
Stanford University School of Medicine
300 Pasteur Dr, H2128B
Stanford CA 94305

ZARKA, Matthew A.
Mayo Clinic Arizona
13400 E Shea Blvd
Scottsdale AZ 85259

Declaration of interests

Dr Jo reports that her spouse is a salaried employee of, and holds stocks in, Merck & Co.

Sources

Note: For any figure, table, or box not listed below, the original source is this volume; the suggested source citation is

International Academy of Cytology – International Agency for Research on Cancer – World Health Organization Joint Editorial Board. WHO Reporting System for Soft Tissue Cytopathology. Lyon (France): International Agency for Research on Cancer; 2026. (IAC-IARC-WHO cytopathology reporting systems series, 1st ed.; vol. 4). https://publications.iarc.fr/651.

Figures

2.01	Klijanienko J
2.02	Klijanienko J
2.03	Klijanienko J
2.04	Klijanienko J
2.05	Klijanienko J
2.06	Klijanienko J
2.07	Klijanienko J
2.08	Klijanienko J
2.09	Klijanienko J
2.10	Klijanienko J
2.11	Jain D
2.12	Chebib I
2.13	Chebib I
2.14	Chebib I
2.15	Rekhi B
2.16	Bode-Lesniewska B
2.17	Bode-Lesniewska B
2.18	Bode-Lesniewska B
2.19	Bode-Lesniewska B
4.01	Dodd LG
4.02	Dodd LG
4.03	Kerr DA
4.04	Kerr DA
4.05	Kerr DA
4.06	Dodd LG
4.07	Michelow P
4.08	Michelow P
4.09	Michelow P
4.10	Michelow P
4.11	Michelow P
4.12	Michelow P
4.13	Michelow P
4.14	Michelow P
4.15	Chebib I
4.16	Chebib I
4.17	Chebib I
4.18	Kerr DA
4.19	Kerr DA
4.20A–C	Kathryn Stevens, Department of Radiology, Stanford Center for Academic Medicine, Palo Alto, CA
4.21	Holmes BJ
4.22	Holmes BJ
4.23	Holmes BJ
4.24	Holmes BJ
4.25	Holmes BJ
4.26	Pantanowitz L
4.27	Monaco SE
4.28	Monaco SE
4.29	Pantanowitz L
4.30	Pantanowitz L
4.31	Domanski HA
4.32	Domanski HA
4.33	Bui M
4.34	Domanski HA
4.35	Domanski HA
4.36	Domanski HA
4.37	Domanski HA
4.38	Domanski HA
4.39	Domanski HA
4.40	Domanski HA
4.41	Domanski HA
4.42	Domanski HA
4.43	Domanski HA
4.44	Domanski HA
4.45	Domanski HA
4.46	Domanski HA
4.47	Domanski HA
4.48	Domanski HA
4.49	Domanski HA
4.50	Domanski HA
4.51	Domanski HA
4.52	Domanski HA
4.53	Domanski HA
4.54	Qian X
4.55	Qian X
4.56	Qian X
4.57A–C	Field AS
4.58	Domanski HA
4.59	Domanski HA
4.60	Klijanienko J
4.61	Domanski HA
4.62	Domanski HA
4.63	Domanski HA
4.64	Domanski HA
4.65	Domanski HA
4.66	Domanski HA
4.67	Dodd LG
4.68	Dodd LG
4.69	Dodd LG
4.70	Domanski HA
4.71	Domanski HA
4.72	Domanski HA
4.73	Domanski HA
4.74	Domanski HA
4.75	Domanski HA
4.76	Domanski HA
4.77	Domanski HA
4.78	Domanski HA
4.79	Domanski HA
4.80	Domanski HA
4.81	Domanski HA
4.82	Domanski HA
4.83	Domanski HA
4.84A,B	Domanski HA
4.85	Domanski HA
4.86	Domanski HA
4.87	Domanski HA
4.88	Domanski HA
4.89	Domanski HA
4.90	Domanski HA
4.91A–D	Monaco SE
4.92	Domanski HA
4.93	Domanski HA
4.94	Domanski HA
4.95	Domanski HA
4.96	Domanski HA
4.97	Domanski HA
4.98	Domanski HA
4.99	Klijanienko J
4.100	Klijanienko J
4.101	Klijanienko J
4.102	Klijanienko J
4.103	Gajdzis P
4.104	Jo VY
4.105	Gajdzis P
4.106	Klijanienko J
4.107	Klijanienko J
4.108	Klijanienko J
4.109	Jo VY
4.110	Klijanienko J
4.111	Klijanienko J
4.112	Domanski HA
4.113	Domanski HA
4.114	Domanski HA
4.115	Domanski HA
4.116	Domanski HA

4.117	Domanski HA
4.118	Klijanienko J
4.119	Klijanienko J
4.120	Klijanienko J
4.121A–D	Kathryn Stevens, Department of Radiology, Stanford Center for Academic Medicine, Palo Alto, CA
4.122	Holmes BJ
4.123	Holmes BJ
4.124	Holmes BJ
4.125	Holmes BJ
4.126	Holmes BJ
4.127	Holmes BJ
4.128	Holmes BJ
4.129	Kilpatrick SE
4.130	Holmes BJ
4.131	Dodd LG
4.132	Dodd LG
4.133	Monaco SE
4.134	Monaco SE
4.135	Domanski HA
4.136	Domanski HA
4.137	Domanski HA
4.138	Domanski HA
4.139	Rekhi B
4.140	Dodd LG
4.141	Dodd LG
4.142	Dodd LG
4.143	Dodd LG
4.144	Dodd LG
4.145	Klijanienko J
4.146	Dodd LG
4.147	Dodd LG
4.148	Dodd LG
4.149	Dodd LG
4.150	Pitman MB
4.151	Pitman MB
4.152	Kilpatrick SE
4.153	Kilpatrick SE

5.01	Raymond WA
5.02	Raymond WA
5.03	Raymond WA
5.04	Raymond WA
5.05	Raymond WA

6.01	Domanski HA
6.02	Domanski HA
6.03	Domanski HA
6.04	Domanski HA
6.05	Domanski HA
6.06	Domanski HA
6.07	Domanski HA
6.08	Domanski HA
6.09	Domanski HA
6.10	Domanski HA
6.11	Domanski HA
6.12	Chebib I
6.13	Chebib I
6.14	Chebib I
6.15	Chebib I
6.16	Chebib I
6.17	Chebib I
6.18	Chebib I
6.19	Ozawa M
6.20	Jo VY
6.21	Jo VY
6.22	Jo VY
6.23	Ozawa M
6.24	Susan Shyu, York Laboratory Services, York, PA
6.25	Chebib I
6.26	Chebib I
6.27	Ozawa M
6.28	Ozawa M
6.29	Domanski HA
6.30	Rekhi B
6.31	Domanski HA
6.32	Domanski HA
6.33	Domanski HA
6.34	Rekhi B
6.35	Rekhi B
6.36	Rekhi B
6.37	Jo VY
6.38	Jo VY
6.39	Jo VY
6.40	Domanski HA
6.41	Domanski HA
6.42	Domanski HA
6.43	Domanski HA
6.44	Klijanienko J
6.45	Klijanienko J
6.46	Qian X
6.47	Klijanienko J
6.48	Domanski HA

7.01	Klijanienko J
7.02	Klijanienko J
7.03	Klijanienko J
7.04	Klijanienko J
7.05	Raymond WA
7.06	Raymond WA
7.07	Raymond WA

8.01	Klijanienko J
8.02	Klijanienko J
8.03	Klijanienko J
8.04	Klijanienko J
8.05	Klijanienko J
8.06	Klijanienko J
8.07	Klijanienko J
8.08	Bode-Lesniewska B
8.09	Bode-Lesniewska B
8.10	Bode-Lesniewska B
8.11	Bode-Lesniewska B
8.12	Jo VY
8.13	Dodd LG
8.14	Bode-Lesniewska B
8.15	Jo VY
8.16	Bode-Lesniewska B
8.17	Klijanienko J
8.18	Klijanienko J
8.19	Klijanienko J
8.20	Klijanienko J
8.21	Klijanienko J
8.22	Rekhi B
8.23	Rekhi B
8.24	Rekhi B
8.25	Rekhi B
8.26	Rekhi B
8.27	Rekhi B
8.28	Rekhi B
8.29	Rekhi B
8.30	Klijanienko J
8.31	Dodd LG
8.32	Klijanienko J
8.33	Dodd LG
8.34	Klijanienko J
8.35	Dodd LG
8.36	Dodd LG
8.37	Dodd LG
8.38	Dodd LG
8.39	Klijanienko J
8.40	Klijanienko J
8.41	Klijanienko J
8.42	Klijanienko J
8.43	Klijanienko J
8.44	Klijanienko J
8.45	Klijanienko J
8.46	Klijanienko J
8.47	Klijanienko J
8.48	Rekhi B
8.49	Rekhi B
8.50	Rekhi B
8.51	Rekhi B
8.52	Rekhi B
8.53	Rekhi B
8.54	Rekhi B
8.55	Rekhi B
8.56	Rekhi B
8.57	Rekhi B
8.58	Rekhi B
8.59	Klijanienko J
8.60	Rekhi B
8.61	Klijanienko J
8.62	Rekhi B
8.63	Klijanienko J
8.64	Rekhi B
8.65	Rekhi B
8.66	Rekhi B
8.67	Rekhi B
8.68	Chebib I
8.69	Chebib I
8.70	Chebib I
8.71	Chebib I
8.72	Chebib I
8.73	Pitman MB
8.74	Pitman MB
8.75	Pitman MB

8.76	Pitman MB
8.77	Pitman MB
8.78	Pitman MB
8.79	Pitman MB
8.80	Pitman MB
8.81	Pitman MB
8.82	Pitman MB
8.83	Pitman MB
8.84	Klijanienko J
8.85	Domanski HA
8.86	Domanski HA
8.87	Domanski HA
8.88	Domanski HA
8.89	Klijanienko J
8.90	Klijanienko J
8.91	Klijanienko J
8.92	Klijanienko J
8.93	Domanski HA
8.94	Domanski HA
8.95	Domanski HA
8.96	Chebib I
8.97	Chebib I
8.98	Rekhi B
8.99	Chebib I
8.100	Chebib I
8.101	Rekhi B
8.102	Chebib I
8.103	Pantanowitz L
8.104	Klijanienko J
8.105	Jo VY
8.106	Jo VY
8.107	Jo VY
8.108	Jo VY
8.109	Jo VY
8.110	Klijanienko J
8.111	Klijanienko J
8.112	Jo VY
8.113	Jo VY
8.114	Klijanienko J
8.115	Klijanienko J
8.116	Jo VY
8.117	Klijanienko J
8.118	Jo VY
8.119	Domanski HA
8.120	Klijanienko J
8.121	Domanski HA
8.122	Klijanienko J
8.123	Klijanienko J
8.124	Agaram NP
8.125	Agaram NP
8.126	Rekhi B
8.127	Rekhi B
8.128	Rekhi B
8.129	Rekhi B
8.130	Klijanienko J
8.131	Klijanienko J
8.132	Klijanienko J
8.133	Klijanienko J
8.134	Klijanienko J
8.135	VandenBussche CJ
8.136	VandenBussche CJ
8.137	VandenBussche CJ
8.138	VandenBussche CJ
8.139	VandenBussche CJ
8.140	VandenBussche CJ
8.141	VandenBussche CJ
8.142	Jo VY
8.143	Rekhi B
8.144	Klijanienko J
8.145	Rekhi B
8.146	Rekhi B
8.147	Rekhi B
8.148	Rekhi B
8.149	Rekhi B
8.150	Rekhi B
8.151	Rekhi B
8.152	Rekhi B
8.153	Rekhi B
8.154	Rekhi B
8.155	Rekhi B
8.156	Rekhi B
8.157	Rekhi B
8.158	Rekhi B
8.159	Rekhi B
8.160	Rekhi B
8.161	Rekhi B
8.162	Rekhi B
8.163	Domanski HA
8.164	Domanski HA
8.165	Domanski HA
8.166	Domanski HA
8.167	Rekhi B
8.168	Domanski HA
8.169	Rekhi B
8.170	Rekhi B
8.171	Rekhi B
8.172	Domanski HA
8.173	Domanski HA
8.174	Domanski HA
8.175	Domanski HA
8.176	Domanski HA
8.177	Rekhi B
8.178	Klijanienko J
8.179	Klijanienko J
8.180	Klijanienko J
8.181	Klijanienko J
8.182	Klijanienko J
8.183	Klijanienko J
8.184	Klijanienko J
8.185	Klijanienko J
8.186	Klijanienko J
8.187	Yang E
8.188	Yang E
8.189	Yang E
8.190	Yang E
8.191	Agaram NP
8.192	Agaram NP
8.193	Agaram NP
8.194	Agaram NP
8.195	Kerr DA
8.196	Chebib I
8.197	Mito JK
8.198	Chebib I
8.199	Kerr DA
8.200	Mito JK
8.201	Kerr DA
8.202	Bui M
8.203	Klijanienko J
8.204	Klijanienko J
8.205	Klijanienko J
8.206	Klijanienko J
8.207	Klijanienko J
8.208	Klijanienko J
8.209	Klijanienko J
8.210	Jo VY
8.211	Klijanienko J
8.212	Chebib I
8.213	Klijanienko J
8.214	Chebib I
8.215	Chebib I
8.216	Chebib I
8.217	Klijanienko J
8.218	Klijanienko J
8.219	Klijanienko J
8.220	Klijanienko J
8.221	Monaco SE
8.222	Anjali Saqi, Department of Pathology, Columbia University Medical Center, New York, NY
8.223	Anjali Saqi, Department of Pathology, Columbia University Medical Center, New York, NY
8.224	Anjali Saqi, Department of Pathology, Columbia University Medical Center, New York, NY
8.225	Monaco SE
8.226	Domanski HA
8.227	Domanski HA
8.228	Domanski HA
8.229	Klijanienko J
8.230	Klijanienko J
8.231	Klijanienko J
8.232	Rekhi B
8.233	Rekhi B
8.234	Rekhi B
8.235	Rekhi B
8.236	Rekhi B
8.237	Rekhi B
8.238	Rekhi B
8.239	Rekhi B
8.240	Rekhi B
8.241	Klijanienko J
8.242	Klijanienko J
8.243	Klijanienko J
8.244	Klijanienko J
8.245	Klijanienko J
8.246	Domanski HA
8.247	Domanski HA
8.248	Domanski HA
8.249	Domanski HA

8.250	Domanski HA
8.251	Domanski HA
8.252	Domanski HA
8.253	Domanski HA
8.254	Domanski HA
8.255	Domanski HA
8.256	Domanski HA
8.257	Domanski HA
8.258	Domanski HA
8.259	Domanski HA
8.260	Domanski HA

Tables

1.01	Domanski HA
2.01	Sewell WA
2.02	Chebib I
2.03	Chebib I
2.04	Chebib I
2.05	Bode-Lesniewska B
2.06	Bode-Lesniewska B
4.01	Holmes BJ
8.01	Jo VY

Images on the cover

Top left	Fig. 4.74: Domanski HA
Bottom left	Fig. 8.79: Pitman MB
Top centre	Fig. 6.14: Chebib I
Bottom centre	Fig. 8.16: Bode-Lesniewska B
Top right	Fig. 8.31: Dodd LG
Bottom right	Fig. 8.236: Rekhi B

Images on the chapter title pages

Chapter 1	Fig. 2.16: Bode-Lesniewska B
Chapter 2	Fig. 2.15: Rekhi B
Chapter 3	Fig. 4.122: Holmes BJ
Chapter 4	Fig. 4.127: Holmes BJ
Chapter 5	Fig. 5.01: Raymond WA
Chapter 6	Fig. 6.04: Domanski HA
Chapter 7	Fig. 7.01: Klijanienko J
Chapter 8	Fig. 8.167: Rekhi B
Chapter 9	Fig. 8.159: Rekhi B

References

1. Abad-Licham M, Galvez-Olortegui J, Astigueta J, et al. Diagnostic validity of fine-needle capillary cytology in palpable tumours at the Oncology Institute of Peru. Ecancermedicalscience. 201812:805. Cited in: PubMed; PMID 29492099.
2. Abbott JJ, Oliveira AM, Nascimento AG. The prognostic significance of fibrosarcomatous transformation in dermatofibrosarcoma protuberans. Am J Surg Pathol. 2006 Apr;30(4):436-43. Cited in: PubMed; PMID 16625088.
3. Abdou AG, Aiad H, Youssef Asaad N. Fine Needle Aspiration Cytology of Chondroid Tenosynovial Giant Cell Tumor of the Hand. Rare Tumors. 2015 May;7(2):5814. Cited in: PubMed; PMID 26266013.
4. Abed R, Grimer RJ, Carter SR, et al. Soft-tissue metastases: their presentation and origin. J Bone Joint Surg Br. 2009 Aug;91(8):1083-5. Cited in: PubMed; PMID 19651839.
5. Abendroth CS, Dabbs DJ. Immunocytochemical staining of unstained versus previously stained cytologic preparations. Acta Cytol. 199539(3):379-86. Cited in: PubMed; PMID 7539200.
6. Abramovici LC, Hytiroglou P, Klein RM, et al. Well-differentiated extraskeletal osteosarcoma: report of 2 cases, 1 with dedifferentiation. Hum Pathol. 2005 Apr;36(4):439-43. Cited in: PubMed; PMID 15892008.
7. ACKERMAN LV. Extra-osseous localized non-neoplastic bone and cartilage formation (so-called myositis ossificans): clinical and pathological confusion with malignant neoplasms. J Bone Joint Surg Am. 1958 Apr;40-A(2):279-98. Cited in: PubMed; PMID 13539055.
8. Adan A, Alizada G, Kiraz Y, et al. Flow cytometry: basic principles and applications. Crit Rev Biotechnol. 2017 Mar;37(2):163-176. Cited in: PubMed; PMID 26767547.
9. Agaimy A, Blakely M, Breimer GE, et al. Extra-abdominal and intra-abdominal FET::CREM fusion mesenchymal neoplasms: comparative clinicopathological study of 9 new cases further supporting a distinct potentially aggressive sarcoma and report of novel sites. Virchows Arch. 2024 Dec;485(6):1007-1019. Cited in: PubMed; PMID 39249507.
10. Agaimy A, Foulkes WD. Hereditary SWI/SNF complex deficiency syndromes. Semin Diagn Pathol. 2018 May;35(3):193-198. Cited in: PubMed; PMID 29397238.
11. Agaimy A, Kirsche H, Semrau S, et al. Cytokeratin-positive epithelioid angiosarcoma presenting in the tonsil: a diagnostic challenge. Hum Pathol. 2012 Jul;43(7):1142-7. Cited in: PubMed; PMID 22406364.
12. Agaimy A, Michal M, Stoehr R, et al. Recurrent novel HMGA2-NCOR2 fusions characterize a subset of keratin-positive giant cell-rich soft tissue tumors. Mod Pathol. 2021 Aug;34(8):1507-1520. Cited in: PubMed; PMID 33742141.
13. Agaram NP, Chen HW, Zhang L, et al. EWSR1-PBX3: a novel gene fusion in myoepithelial tumors. Genes Chromosomes Cancer. 2015 Feb;54(2):63-71. Cited in: PubMed; PMID 25231231.
14. Agaram NP, LaQuaglia MP, Alaggio R, et al. MYOD1-mutant spindle cell and sclerosing rhabdomyosarcoma: an aggressive subtype irrespective of age. A reappraisal for molecular classification and risk stratification. Mod Pathol. 2019 Jan;32(1):27-36. Cited in: PubMed; PMID 30181563.
15. Agaram NP, Sung YS, Zhang L, et al. Dichotomy of Genetic Abnormalities in PEComas With Therapeutic Implications. Am J Surg Pathol. 2015 Jun;39(6):813-25. Cited in: PubMed; PMID 25651471.
16. Agaram NP, Zhang L, Sung YS, et al. Expanding the Spectrum of Intraosseous Rhabdomyosarcoma: Correlation Between 2 Distinct Gene Fusions and Phenotype. Am J Surg Pathol. 2019 May;43(5):695-702. Cited in: PubMed; PMID 30720533.
17. Agarwal P, Toi PC, Subramaniam H, et al. Prospective comparison of cytological specimen adequacy assessment by different rapid staining techniques for rapid on-site evaluation in fine needle aspiration cytology and their cost-effectiveness. Diagn Cytopathol. 2019 May;47(5):469-474. Cited in: PubMed; PMID 30585436.
18. Agarwal S, Nangia A, Jyotsna PL, et al. Spindle cell lipoma masquerading as lipomatous pleomorphic adenoma: A diagnostic dilemma on fine needle aspiration cytology. J Cytol. 2013 Jan;30(1):55-7. Cited in: PubMed; PMID 23661944.
19. Agnihotri MA, Kothari KS, Naik LP. Fat Necrosis of the Breast Masquerading as Malignancy Diagnosed on Fine-Needle Aspiration Cytology. J Midlife Health. 2020 Jan-Mar;11(1):49-50. Cited in: PubMed; PMID 32684729.
20. Agoff SN, Folpe AL, Grieco VS, et al. Spindle cell lipoma of the oral cavity. Report of a rare intramuscular case with fine needle aspiration findings. Acta Cytol. 200145(1):93-8. Cited in: PubMed; PMID 11213514.
21. Agrawal P, Srinivasan R, Rajwanshi A, et al. Fine needle aspiration cytology of paediatric soft tissue tumours highlighting challenges in diagnosis of benign lesions and unusual malignant tumours. Cytopathology. 2019 May;30(3):301-308. Cited in: PubMed; PMID 30848523.
22. Agrawal T, Monaco SE. Musculoskeletal small biopsies from small patients: current status in 2 academic hospitals. J Am Soc Cytopathol. 20209(5):442-449. Cited in: PubMed; PMID 32654990.
23. Ahlawat S, Chhabra A, Blakely J. Magnetic resonance neurography of peripheral nerve tumors and tumorlike conditions. Neuroimaging Clin N Am. 2014 Feb;24(1):171-92. Cited in: PubMed; PMID 24210319.
24. Ainsworth KE, Chavhan GB, Gupta AA, et al. Congenital infantile fibrosarcoma: review of imaging features. Pediatr Radiol. 2014 Sep;44(9):1124-9. Cited in: PubMed; PMID 24706181.
25. Ajmal S, Keating M, Wilhelm M. Multifocal Soft Tissue Cryptococcosis in a Renal Transplant Recipient: The Importance of Suspecting Atypical Pathogens in the Immunocompromised Host. Exp Clin Transplant. 2021 Jun;19(6):609-612. Cited in: PubMed; PMID 29957160.
26. Akahoshi K, Oya M, Koga T, et al. Clinical usefulness of endoscopic ultrasound-guided fine needle aspiration for gastric subepithelial lesions smaller than 2 cm. J Gastrointestin Liver Dis. 2014 Dec;23(4):405-12. Cited in: PubMed; PMID 25531999.
27. Akasbi Y, Arifi S, El Idrissi M, et al. Soft-tissue metastasis revealing a pancreatic adenocarcinoma: one case report and a review of literature. Pan Afr Med J. 201211:32. Cited in: PubMed; PMID 22514766.
28. Akbulut M, Gunhan-Bilgen I, Zekioglu O, et al. Fine needle aspiration cytology of inflammatory myofibroblastic tumour (inflammatory pseudotumour) of the breast: a case report and review of the literature. Cytopathology. 2007 Dec;18(6):384-7. Cited in: PubMed; PMID 17944956.
29. Akerman M. Fine-needle aspiration cytology of soft tissue sarcoma: benefits and limitations. Sarcoma. 19982(3-4):155-61. Cited in: PubMed; PMID 18521248.
30. Akerman M, Domanski HA. The complex cytological features of synovial sarcoma in fine needle aspirates, an analysis of four illustrative cases. Cytopathology. 2007 Aug;18(4):234-40. Cited in: PubMed; PMID 17559565.
31. Akerman M, Domanski HA. The cytology of soft tissue tumours. Monogr Clin Cytol. 200316:IX-X, 1-112. Cited in: PubMed; PMID 14518076.
32. Akerman M, Ryd W, Skytting B, et al. Fine-needle aspiration of synovial sarcoma: criteria for diagnosis: retrospective reexamination of 37 cases, including ancillary diagnostics. A Scandinavian Sarcoma Group study. Diagn Cytopathol. 2003 May;28(5):232-8. Cited in: PubMed; PMID 12722117.
33. Akerman M, Rydholm A, Persson BM. Aspiration cytology of soft-tissue tumors. The 10-year experience at an orthopedic oncology center. Acta Orthop Scand. 1985 Oct;56(5):407-12. Cited in: PubMed; PMID 4072661.
34. Akhtar K, Zaheer S, Ahmad S, et al. Sister Mary Joseph's nodule: a rare cytologic presentation. Clin Pract. 2011 Mar;1(1):e6. Cited in: PubMed; PMID 24765279.
35. Akhtar M, Ali MA, Bakry M, et al. Fine-needle aspiration biopsy diagnosis of rhabdomyosarcoma: cytologic, histologic, and ultrastructural correlations. Diagn Cytopathol. 19928(5):465-74. Cited in: PubMed; PMID 1396025.
36. Akhtar M, Ali MA, Sabbah R, et al. Small round cell tumor with divergent differentiation: cytologic, histologic, and ultrastructural findings. Diagn Cytopathol. 199411(2):159-64. Cited in: PubMed; PMID 7813364.
37. Akhtar M, Iqbal MA, Mourad W, et al. Fine-needle aspiration biopsy diagnosis of small round cell tumors of childhood: A comprehensive approach. Diagn Cytopathol. 1999 Aug;21(2):81-91. Cited in: PubMed; PMID 10425044.
38. Akomea-Agyin C, Dussek JE, Anderson DR, et al. Pulmonary artery sarcoma mimicking pulmonary embolism: successful surgical intervention. Ann Thorac Surg. 1996 May;61(5):1536-8. Cited in: PubMed; PMID 8633981.
39. Al Dandan O, Hassan A, Al Muhaish M, et al. Concomitant bilateral elastofibroma in the infrascapular and gluteal regions: a report of a rare case. BMC Musculoskelet Disord. 2020 Jan;21(1):16. Cited in: PubMed; PMID 31914985.
40. Al Kindi HN, Ibrahim AM, Roshdy M, et al. Clinical, cellular, and molecular characterisation of cardiac rhabdomyoma in tuberous sclerosis. Cardiol Young. 2021 Aug;31(8):1297-1305. Cited in: PubMed; PMID 33602381.
42. Alaggio R, Coffin CM, Weiss SW, et al. Liposarcomas in young patients: a study of 82 cases occurring in patients younger than 22 years of age. Am J Surg Pathol. 2009 May;33(5):645-58. Cited in: PubMed; PMID 19194281.
43. Alaggio R, Ninfo V, Rosolen A, et al. Primitive myxoid mesenchymal tumor of infancy: a clinicopathologic report of 6 cases. Am J Surg Pathol. 2006 Mar;30(3):388-94. Cited in: PubMed; PMID 16538060.
44. Alaggio R, Zhang L, Sung YS, et al. A Molecular Study of Pediatric Spindle and Sclerosing Rhabdomyosarcoma: Identification of Novel and Recurrent VGLL2-related Fusions in Infantile Cases. Am J Surg Pathol. 2016 Feb;40(2):224-35. Cited in: PubMed; PMID 26501226.
45. AlAwaji AI, Alsaadi MJ, Bauones S. Prevalence of elastofibroma dorsi found incidentally upon chest computed tomography scan: A tertiary care center experience. Saudi Med J. 2022 Feb;43(2):156-160. Cited in: PubMed; PMID 35110340.
46. Al Hmada Y, Schaefer IM, Fletcher CDM. Hibernoma Mimicking Atypical Lipomatous Tumor: 64 Cases of a Morphologically Distinct Subset. Am J Surg Pathol. 2018 Jul;42(7):951-957. Cited in: PubMed; PMID 29629919.
47. Ali SZ, Hoon V, Hoda S, et al. Solitary fibrous tumor. A cytologic-histologic study with clinical, radiologic, and immunohistochemical correlations. Cancer. 1997 Apr;81(2):116-21. Cited in: PubMed; PMID 9126139.
48. Al-Ibraheemi A, Ahrens WA, Fritchie K, et al. Malignant Tenosynovial Giant Cell Tumor: The True "Synovial Sarcoma?" A Clinicopathologic, Immunohistochemical, and Molecular Cytogenetic Study of 10 Cases, Supporting Origin from Synoviocytes. Mod Pathol. 2019 Feb;32(2):242-251. Cited in: PubMed; PMID 30206409.
49. Al-Ibraheemi A, Broehm C, Tanas MR, et al. Desmoplastic Small Round Cell Tumors With Atypical Presentations: A Report of 34 Cases. Int J Surg Pathol. 2019 May;27(3):236-243. Cited in: PubMed; PMID 30522375.
50. Allison DB, Simner PJ, Ali SZ. Identification of infectious organisms in cytopathology: A review of ancillary diagnostic techniques. Cancer Cytopathol. 2018 Aug;126 Suppl 8:643-653. Cited in: PubMed; PMID 30156776.
51. Allison DB, VandenBussche CJ, Rooper LM, et al. Nodular fasciitis of the parotid gland: A challenging diagnosis on FNA. Cancer Cytopathol. 2018 Oct;126(10):872-880. Cited in: PubMed; PMID 30311731.
52. Allison DB, Wakely PE, Siddiqui MT, et al. Nodular fasciitis: A frequent diagnostic pitfall on fine-needle aspiration. Cancer Cytopathol. 2017 Jan;125(1):20-29. Cited in: PubMed; PMID 27525591.
53. Almeida MM, Nunes AM, Frable WJ. Malignant melanoma of soft tissue. A report of three cases with diagnosis by fine needle aspiration cytology. Acta Cytol. 199438(2):241-6. Cited in: PubMed; PMID 8147218.
54. Alston ELJ, Thangaiah JJ, Rowsey R, et al. Pediatric-type Myoid Neoplasms of Somatic Soft Tissue: A Clinicopathological and Molecular Genetic Study of 78 Tumors, Highlighting Indolent Clinical Behavior and Frequent SRF

Gene Rearrangements. Mod Pathol. 2025 Jan;38(5):100722. Cited in: PubMed; PMID 39864664.
55. Altmayer S, Verma N, Dicks EA, et al. Imaging musculoskeletal soft tissue infections. Semin Ultrasound CT MR. 2020 Feb;41(1):85-98. Cited in: PubMed; PMID 31964497.
56. Álvarez-Rodriguez F, Gimeno-Aranguez M, López-Varela C, et al. Fine-needle aspiration cytology of mammary myofibroblastoma: a report of six cases. Acta Cytol. 201256(5):501-5. Cited in: PubMed; PMID 23075890.
57. Amary F, Perez-Casanova L, Ye H, et al. Synovial chondromatosis and soft tissue chondroma: extraosseous cartilaginous tumor defined by FN1 gene rearrangement. Mod Pathol. 2019 Dec;32(12):1762-1771. Cited in: PubMed; PMID 31273315.
58. Amary MF, Berisha F, Bernardi Fdel C, et al. Detection of SS18-SSX fusion transcripts in formalin-fixed paraffin-embedded neoplasms: analysis of conventional RT-PCR, qRT-PCR and dual color FISH as diagnostic tools for synovial sarcoma. Mod Pathol. 2007 Apr;20(4):482-96. Cited in: PubMed; PMID 17334349.
59. Amer HZ, Hameed M. Intraosseous benign notochordal cell tumor. Arch Pathol Lab Med. 2010 Feb;134(2):283-8. Cited in: PubMed; PMID 20121620.
60. Amita K, Govind AM, Pechiat T, et al. Candida Albicans Infection Masquerading as a Soft Tissue Tumour Diagnosed by Fine Needle Aspiration Cytology. J Clin Diagn Res. 2017 Jul;11(7):ED18-ED20. Cited in: PubMed; PMID 28892913.
62. Anderson T, Zhang L, Hameed M, et al. Thoracic epithelioid malignant vascular tumors: a clinicopathologic study of 52 cases with emphasis on pathologic grading and molecular studies of WWTR1-CAMTA1 fusions. Am J Surg Pathol. 2015 Jan;39(1):132-9. Cited in: PubMed; PMID 25353289.
63. Angelico G, Broggi G, Spadola S, et al. PET/CT-Detected myofibroblastoma of the breast with bizarre cells: A potential diagnostic pitfall of malignancy. Breast J. 2021 Sep;27(9):726-730. Cited in: PubMed; PMID 34196064.
64. Angervall L, Dahl I, Kindblom LG, et al. Spindle cell lipoma. Acta Pathol Microbiol Scand A. 1976 Nov;84(6):477-87. Cited in: PubMed; PMID 998247.
65. Antonescu C. Round cell sarcomas beyond Ewing: emerging entities. Histopathology. 2014 Jan;64(1):26-37. Cited in: PubMed; PMID 24215322.
66. Antonescu CR. Emerging soft tissue tumors with kinase fusions: An overview of the recent literature with an emphasis on diagnostic criteria. Genes Chromosomes Cancer. 2020 Aug;59(8):437-444. Cited in: PubMed; PMID 32243019.
67. Antonescu CR, Dal Cin P, Nafa K, et al. EWSR1-CREB1 is the predominant gene fusion in angiomatoid fibrous histiocytoma. Genes Chromosomes Cancer. 2007 Dec;46(12):1051-60. Cited in: PubMed; PMID 17724745.
68. Antonescu CR, Dickson BC, Sung YS, et al. Recurrent YAP1 and MAML2 Gene Rearrangements in Retiform and Composite Hemangioendothelioma. Am J Surg Pathol. 2020 Dec;44(12):1677-1684. Cited in: PubMed; PMID 32991341.
69. Antonescu CR, Elahi A, Healey JH, et al. Monoclonality of multifocal myxoid liposarcoma: confirmation by analysis of TLS-CHOP or EWS-CHOP rearrangements. Clin Cancer Res. 2000 Jul;6(7):2788-93. Cited in: PubMed; PMID 10914725.
70. Antonescu CR, Le Loarer F, Mosquera JM, et al. Novel YAP1-TFE3 fusion defines a distinct subset of epithelioid hemangioendothelioma. Genes Chromosomes Cancer. 2013 Aug;52(8):775-84. Cited in: PubMed; PMID 23737213.
71. Antonescu CR, Owosho AA, Zhang L, et al. Sarcomas With CIC-rearrangements Are a Distinct Pathologic Entity With Aggressive Outcome: A Clinicopathologic and Molecular Study of 115 Cases. Am J Surg Pathol. 2017 Jul;41(7):941-949. Cited in: PubMed; PMID 28346326.
72. Antonescu CR, Tschernyavsky SJ, Decuseara R, et al. Prognostic impact of P53 status, TLS-CHOP fusion transcript structure, and histological grade in myxoid liposarcoma: a molecular and clinicopathologic study of 82 cases. Clin Cancer Res. 2001 Dec;7(12):3977-87. Cited in: PubMed; PMID 11751490.
73. Antonescu CR, Zhang L, Chang NE, et al. EWSR1-POU5F1 fusion in soft tissue myoepithelial tumors. A molecular analysis of sixty-six cases, including soft tissue, bone, and visceral lesions, showing common involvement of the EWSR1 gene. Genes Chromosomes Cancer. 2010 Dec;49(12):1114-24. Cited in: PubMed; PMID 20815032.
74. Antonescu CR, Zhang L, Nielsen GP, et al. Consistent t(1;10) with rearrangements of TGFBR3 and MGEA5 in both myxoinflammatory fibroblastic sarcoma and hemosiderotic fibrolipomatous tumor. Genes Chromosomes Cancer. 2011 Oct;50(10):757-64. Cited in: PubMed; PMID 21717526.
75. Antonescu CR, Zhang L, Shao SY, et al. Frequent PLAG1 gene rearrangements in skin and soft tissue myoepithelioma with ductal differentiation. Genes Chromosomes Cancer. 2013 Jul;52(7):675-82. Cited in: PubMed; PMID 23630011.
76. Aoyama T, Fukumoto A, Shigita K, et al. Successful Endoscopic Sclerotherapy Using Polidocanol for Small Bowel Hemangioma. Intern Med. 2020 Jul;59(14):1727-1730. Cited in: PubMed; PMID 32238724.
77. Arbajian E, Puls F, Magnusson L, et al. Recurrent EWSR1-CREB3L1 gene fusions in sclerosing epithelioid fibrosarcoma. Am J Surg Pathol. 2014 Jun;38(6):801-8. Cited in: PubMed; PMID 24441665.
78. Argani P, Antonescu CR, Illei PB, et al. Primary renal neoplasms with the ASPL-TFE3 gene fusion of alveolar soft part sarcoma: a distinctive tumor entity previously included among renal cell carcinomas of children and adolescents. Am J Pathol. 2001 Jul;159(1):179-92. Cited in: PubMed; PMID 11438465.
79. Argani P, Lal P, Hutchinson B, et al. Aberrant nuclear immunoreactivity for TFE3 in neoplasms with TFE3 gene fusions: a sensitive and specific immunohistochemical assay. Am J Surg Pathol. 2003 Jun;27(6):750-61. Cited in: PubMed; PMID 12766578.
80. Ariizumi T, Kawashima H, Yamagishi T, et al. Diagnostic accuracy of fine needle aspiration cytology and core needle biopsy in bone and soft tissue tumor: A comparative study of the image-guided and blindly performed procedure. Ann Diagn Pathol. 2022 Aug;59:151936. Cited in: PubMed; PMID 35427924.
81. Armstrong SM, Demicco EG. What's new in fibroblastic tumors? Virchows Arch. 2020 Jan;476(1):41-55. Cited in: PubMed; PMID 31828431.
82. Arndt CA, Hammond S, Rodeberg D, et al. Significance of persistent mature rhabdomyoblasts in bladder/prostate rhabdomyosarcoma: Results from IRS IV. J Pediatr Hematol Oncol. 2006 Sep;28(9):563-7. Cited in: PubMed; PMID 17006261.
83. Arnold MA, Anderson JR, Gastier-Foster JM, et al. Histology, Fusion Status, and Outcome in Alveolar Rhabdomyosarcoma With Low-Risk Clinical Features: A Report From the Children's Oncology Group. Pediatr Blood Cancer. 2016 Apr;63(4):634-9. Cited in: PubMed; PMID 26756883.
84. Aronow ME, Wiley HE, Gaudric A, et al. VON HIPPEL-LINDAU DISEASE: Update on Pathogenesis and Systemic Aspects. Retina. 2019 Dec;39(12):2243-2253. Cited in: PubMed; PMID 31095066.
85. Asahina M, Saito T, Arakawa A, et al. A case of primary spindle cell variant of embryonal rhabdomyosarcoma of the prostate. Int J Clin Exp Pathol. 20147(8):5181-5. Cited in: PubMed; PMID 25197394.
86. Asano Y, Miwa S, Yamamoto N, et al. A scoring system combining clinical, radiological, and histopathological examinations for differential diagnosis between lipoma and atypical lipomatous tumor/well-differentiated liposarcoma. Sci Rep. 2022 Jan;12(1):237. Cited in: PubMed; PMID 34997060.
87. Atahan S, Aksu O, Ekinci C. Cytologic diagnosis and subtyping of rhabdomyosarcoma. Cytopathology. 1998 Dec;9(6):389-97. Cited in: PubMed; PMID 9861531.
88. Ataş E, Koç O, Artık HA. Clinical features and treatment results in children with hemangioma. Turk J Pediatr. 201759(3):254-260. Cited in: PubMed; PMID 29376569.
89. Baffour FI, Wenger DE, Broski SM. 18F-FDG PET/CT imaging features of lipomatous tumors. Am J Nucl Med Mol Imaging. 202010(1):74-82. Cited in: PubMed; PMID 32211221.
90. Bague S, Folpe AL. Dermatofibrosarcoma protuberans presenting as a subcutaneous mass: a clinicopathological study of 15 cases with exclusive or near-exclusive subcutaneous involvement. Am J Dermatopathol. 2008 Aug;30(4):327-32. Cited in: PubMed; PMID 18645303.
91. Baheti AD, Tirumani SH, Rosenthal MH, et al. Myxoid soft-tissue neoplasms: comprehensive update of the taxonomy and MRI features. AJR Am J Roentgenol. 2015 Feb;204(2):374-85. Cited in: PubMed; PMID 25615761.
92. Bahrami A, Dalton JD, Krane JF, et al. A subset of cutaneous and soft tissue mixed tumors are genetically linked to their salivary gland counterpart. Genes Chromosomes Cancer. 2012 Feb;51(2):140-8. Cited in: PubMed; PMID 22038920.
93. Bahrami A, Folpe AL. Adult-type fibrosarcoma: A reevaluation of 163 putative cases diagnosed at a single institution over a 48-year period. Am J Surg Pathol. 2010 Oct;34(10):1504-13. Cited in: PubMed; PMID 20829680.
94. Bahrami A, Gown AM, Baird GS, et al. Aberrant expression of epithelial and neuroendocrine markers in alveolar rhabdomyosarcoma: a potentially serious diagnostic pitfall. Mod Pathol. 2008 Jul;21(7):795-806. Cited in: PubMed; PMID 18487991.
95. Bajpai M, Pardhe N. Cytopathological Diagnosis and Differential Diagnoses of Facial Spindle Cell Lipoma. J Cytol. 201835(1):66-67. Cited in: PubMed; PMID 29403177.
96. Bakiratharajan D, Rekhi B. Ossifying Fibromyxoid Tumor: An Update. Arch Pathol Lab Med. 2016 Apr;140(4):371-5. Cited in: PubMed; PMID 27028395.
97. Bala N, Gupta N, Sachdeva M, et al. A Diagnostic Dilemma in Fine-Needle Aspiration Cytology: Spindle Cell/Pleomorphic Lipoma. Cureus. 2022 Jan;14(1):e20919. Cited in: PubMed; PMID 35154916.
98. Bale TA, Oviedo A, Kozakewich H, et al. Intracranial myxoid mesenchymal tumors with EWSR1-CREB family gene fusions: myxoid variant of angiomatoid fibrous histiocytoma or novel entity? Brain Pathol. 2018 Mar;28(2):183-191. Cited in: PubMed; PMID 28281318.
99. Balestreire E, Haught JM, English JC. Multiple subcutaneous lipomas induced by HAART in the absence of protease inhibitors. Arch Dermatol. 2007 Dec;143(12):1596-7. Cited in: PubMed; PMID 18087023.
100. Banach BS, Antic T, Bridge JA, et al. Fine-needle aspiration of dermatofibrosarcoma protuberans metastasizing to hemithorax with superior vena cava compression: Case report and literature review. Diagn Cytopathol. 2019 Aug;47(8):797-802. Cited in: PubMed; PMID 30919592.
101. Bane BL, Evans HL, Ro JY, et al. Extraskeletal osteosarcoma. A clinicopathologic review of 26 cases. Cancer. 1990 Jun;65(12):2762-70. Cited in: PubMed; PMID 2160317.
102. Baranov E, Black MA, Fletcher CDM, et al. Nuclear expression of DDIT3 distinguishes high-grade myxoid liposarcoma from other round cell sarcomas. Mod Pathol. 2021 Jul;34(7):1367-1372. Cited in: PubMed; PMID 33731886.
103. Baranov E, Hornick JL. Soft Tissue Special Issue: Fibroblastic and Myofibroblastic Neoplasms of the Head and Neck. Head Neck Pathol. 2020 Mar;14(1):43-58. Cited in: PubMed; PMID 31950474.
104. Baranov E, McBride MJ, Bellizzi AM, et al. A Novel SS18-SSX Fusion-specific Antibody for the Diagnosis of Synovial Sarcoma. Am J Surg Pathol. 2020 Jul;44(7):922-933. Cited in: PubMed; PMID 32141887.
105. Barbazza R, Chiarelli S, Quintarelli GF, et al. Role of fine-needle aspiration cytology in the preoperative evaluation of smooth muscle tumors. Diagn Cytopathol. 1997 Apr;16(4):326-30. Cited in: PubMed; PMID 9143825.
106. Barnoud R, Sabourin JC, Pasquier D, et al. Immunohistochemical expression of WT1 by desmoplastic small round cell tumor: a comparative study with other small round cell tumors. Am J Surg Pathol. 2000 Jun;24(6):830-6. Cited in: PubMed; PMID 10843285.
107. Barr FG, Chatten J, D'Cruz CM, et al. Molecular assays for chromosomal translocations in the diagnosis of pediatric soft tissue sarcomas. JAMA. 1995 Feb;273(7):553-7. Cited in: PubMed; PMID 7530783.
108. Barr ML, Jilaveanu LB, Camp RL, et al. PAX-8 expression in renal tumours and distant sites: a useful marker of primary and metastatic renal cell carcinoma? J Clin Pathol. 2015 Jan;68(1):12-7. Cited in: PubMed; PMID 25315900.
109. Barrena S, Almeida J, Del Carmen García-Macias M, et al. Flow cytometry immunophenotyping of fine-needle aspiration specimens: utility in the diagnosis and classification of non-Hodgkin lymphomas. Histopathology. 2011 May;58(6):906-18. Cited in: PubMed; PMID 21438908.
110. Barretina J, Taylor BS, Banerji S, et al. Subtype-specific genomic alterations define new targets for soft-tissue sarcoma therapy. Nat Genet. 2010 Aug;42(8):715-21. Cited in: PubMed; PMID 20601955.
111. Barroca H, Bom-Sucesso M. Fine needle biopsy with cytology in paediatrics: the importance of a multidisciplinary approach and the role of ancillary techniques. Cytopathology. 2014 Feb;25(1):6-20. Cited in: PubMed; PMID 24138725.
112. Bartoš V, Hamarová K. Cutaneous and Subcutaneous Metastases of Adenocarcinoma as a Dominant Clinical Manifestation of Malignancy of Unknown Origin - a Case Report. Klin Onkol. 201831(2):143-147. Cited in: PubMed; PMID 29708358.
113. Bartuma H, Nord KH, Macchia G, et al. Gene expression and single nucleotide polymorphism array analyses of spindle cell lipomas and conventional lipomas with 13q14 deletion. Genes Chromosomes Cancer. 2011 Aug;50(8):619-32. Cited in: PubMed; PMID 21563233.

114. Barwad A, Banik T, Gorsi U, et al. Fine needle aspiration cytology of myositis ossificans. Diagn Cytopathol. 2011 Jun;39(6):432-4. Cited in: PubMed; PMID 20954272.
115. Battaglia M, Vanel D, Pollastri P, et al. Imaging patterns in elastofibroma dorsi. Eur J Radiol. 2009 Oct;72(1):16-21. Cited in: PubMed; PMID 19539441.
117. Beals C, Rogers A, Wakely P, et al. Hibernomas: a single-institution experience and review of literature. Med Oncol. 2014 Jan;31(1):769. Cited in: PubMed; PMID 24248814.
118. Bekers EM, Eijkelenboom A, Grünberg K, et al. Myositis ossificans - Another condition with USP6 rearrangement, providing evidence of a relationship with nodular fasciitis and aneurysmal bone cyst. Ann Diagn Pathol. 2018 Jun;34:56-59. Cited in: PubMed; PMID 29661729.
119. Bellevicine C, Malapelle U, Vigliar E, et al. How to prepare cytological samples for molecular testing. J Clin Pathol. 2017 Oct;70(10):819-826. Cited in: PubMed; PMID 28739858.
120. Bennert KW, Abdul-Karim FW. Fine needle aspiration cytology vs. needle core biopsy of soft tissue tumors. A comparison. Acta Cytol. 199438(3):381-4. Cited in: PubMed; PMID 8191828.
121. Bennett JA, Braga AC, Pinto A, et al. Uterine PEComas: A Morphologic, Immunohistochemical, and Molecular Analysis of 32 Tumors. Am J Surg Pathol. 2018 Oct;42(10):1370-1383. Cited in: PubMed; PMID 30001237.
122. Bera G, Das RN, Bisht J, et al. Cytological diagnosis of mesoblastic nephroma: A report of three cases with summary of prior published cases. Diagn Cytopathol. 2016 Oct;44(10):823-7. Cited in: PubMed; PMID 27324404.
123. Berardo MD, Powers CN, Wakely PE, et al. Fine-needle aspiration cytopathology of malignant fibrous histiocytoma. Cancer. 1997 Aug;81(4):228-37. Cited in: PubMed; PMID 9292738.
124. Berg JC, Scheithauer BW, Spinner RJ, et al. Plexiform schwannoma: a clinicopathologic overview with emphasis on the head and neck region. Hum Pathol. 2008 May;39(5):633-40. Cited in: PubMed; PMID 18439936.
125. Berger-Richardson D, Swallow CJ. Needle tract seeding after percutaneous biopsy of sarcoma: Risk/benefit considerations. Cancer. 2017 Feb;123(4):560-567. Cited in: PubMed; PMID 27859013.
126. Berlin O, Stener B, Kindblom LG, et al. Leiomyosarcomas of venous origin in the extremities. A correlated clinical, roentgenologic, and morphologic study with diagnostic and surgical implications. Cancer. 1984 Nov;54(10):2147-59. Cited in: PubMed; PMID 6488138.
127. Bernstein KE, Lattes R. Nodular (pseudosarcomatous) fasciitis, a nonrecurrent lesion: clinicopathologic study of 134 cases. Cancer. 1982 Apr;49(8):1668-78. Cited in: PubMed; PMID 6279273.
128. Berry AB, Jaffee I, Greenberg M, et al. Nodular Fasciitis: Definitive Diagnosis by Fine Needle Aspiration. Acta Cytol. 201660(1):19-24. Cited in: PubMed; PMID 26981858.
129. Betz BL, Dixon CA, Weigelin HC, et al. The use of stained cytologic direct smears for ALK gene rearrangement analysis of lung adenocarcinoma. Cancer Cytopathol. 2013 Sep;121(9):489-99. Cited in: PubMed; PMID 23536384.
130. Bhagavan BS, Dorfman HD, Murthy MS, et al. Intravascular bronchiolo-alveolar tumor (IVBAT): A low-grade sclerosing epithelioid angiosarcoma of lung. Am J Surg Pathol. 1982 Jan;6(1):41-52. Cited in: PubMed; PMID 6282146.
131. Bhardwaj N, Rohilla M, Trehan A, et al. MYCN amplification and International Neuroblastoma Risk Group stratification on fine-needle aspiration biopsy and their correlation to survival in neuroblastoma. J Clin Pathol. 2022 Apr. Cited in: PubMed; PMID 35414524.
132. Bhattacharya B, Dilworth HP, Iacobuzio-Donahue C, et al. Nuclear beta-catenin expression distinguishes deep fibromatosis from other benign and malignant fibroblastic and myofibroblastic lesions. Am J Surg Pathol. 2005 May;29(5):653-9. Cited in: PubMed; PMID 15832090.
133. Bian Y, Jordan AG, Rupp M, et al. Effusion cytology of desmoplastic small round cell tumor of the pleura. A case report. Acta Cytol. 199337(1):77-82. Cited in: PubMed; PMID 7679537.
134. Bianchi G, Charoenlap C, Cocchi S, et al. Clear cell sarcoma of soft tissue: a retrospective review and analysis of 31 cases treated at Istituto Ortopedico Rizzoli. Eur J Surg Oncol. 2014 May;40(5):505-510. Cited in: PubMed; PMID 24560887.
135. Billings SD, Folpe AL. Diagnostically challenging spindle cell lipomas: a report of 34 "low-fat" and "fat-free" variants. Am J Dermatopathol. 2007 Oct;29(5):437-42. Cited in: PubMed; PMID 17890910.
136. Billings SD, Folpe AL, Weiss SW. Do leiomyomas of deep soft tissue exist? An analysis of highly differentiated smooth muscle tumors of deep soft tissue supporting two distinct subtypes. Am J Surg Pathol. 2001 Sep;25(9):1134-42. Cited in: PubMed; PMID 11688572.
137. Billings SD, Giblen G, Fanburg-Smith JC. Superficial low-grade fibromyxoid sarcoma (Evans tumor): a clinicopathologic analysis of 19 cases with a unique observation in the pediatric population. Am J Surg Pathol. 2005 Feb;29(2):204-10. Cited in: PubMed; PMID 15644777.
138. Binh MB, Guillou L, Hostein I, et al. Dedifferentiated liposarcomas with divergent myosarcomatous differentiation developed in the internal trunk: a study of 27 cases and comparison to conventional dedifferentiated liposarcomas and leiomyosarcomas. Am J Surg Pathol. 2007 Oct;31(10):1557-66. Cited in: PubMed; PMID 17895758.
139. Binh MB, Sastre-Garau X, Guillou L, et al. MDM2 and CDK4 immunostainings are useful adjuncts in diagnosing well-differentiated and dedifferentiated liposarcoma subtypes: a comparative analysis of 559 soft tissue neoplasms with genetic data. Am J Surg Pathol. 2005 Oct;29(10):1340-7. Cited in: PubMed; PMID 16160477.
140. Bixby SD, Hettmer S, Taylor GA, et al. Synovial sarcoma in children: imaging features and common benign mimics. AJR Am J Roentgenol. 2010 Oct;195(4):1026-32. Cited in: PubMed; PMID 20858835.
141. Blacksin MF, White LM, Hameed M, et al. Granular cell tumor of the extremity: magnetic resonance imaging characteristics with pathologic correlation. Skeletal Radiol. 2005 Oct;34(10):625-31. Cited in: PubMed; PMID 16003548.
142. Bledsoe JR, Della-Torre E, Rovati L, et al. IgG4-related disease: review of the histopathologic features, differential diagnosis, and therapeutic approach. APMIS. 2018 Jun;126(6):459-476. Cited in: PubMed; PMID 29924455.
143. Bode-Lesniewska B, Zhao J, Speel EJ, et al. Gains of 12q13-14 and overexpression of mdm2 are frequent findings in intimal sarcomas of the pulmonary artery. Virchows Arch. 2001 Jan;438(1):57-65. Cited in: PubMed; PMID 11213836.
144. Boikos SA, Pappo AS, Killian JK, et al. Molecular Subtypes of KIT/PDGFRA Wild-Type Gastrointestinal Stromal Tumors: A Report From the National Institutes of Health Gastrointestinal Stromal Tumor Clinic. JAMA Oncol. 2016 Jul;2(7):922-8. Cited in: PubMed; PMID 27011036.
145. Boland JM, Colby TV, Folpe AL. Intrathoracic peripheral nerve sheath tumors-a clinicopathological study of 75 cases. Hum Pathol. 2015 Mar;46(3):419-25. Cited in: PubMed; PMID 25595633.
146. Boman F, Chastagner P, Floquet J, et al. [Histological and immunohistochemical diagnosis of bone marrow metastases of neuroblastomas]. Bull Cancer. 199178(10):943-51. Cited in: PubMed; PMID 1768940.
147. Bonifaz A, Tirado-Sánchez A, Calderón L, et al. Mycetoma: experience of 482 cases in a single center in Mexico. PLoS Negl Trop Dis. 2014 Aug;8(8):e3102. Cited in: PubMed; PMID 25144462.
148. Boucher LD, Swanson PE, Stanley MW, et al. Cytology of angiosarcoma. Findings in fourteen fine-needle aspiration biopsy specimens and one pleural fluid specimen. Am J Clin Pathol. 2000 Aug;114(2):210-9. Cited in: PubMed; PMID 10941336.
149. Boudabbous S, Hamard M, Saiji E, et al. What morphological MRI features enable differentiation of low-grade from high-grade soft tissue sarcoma? BJR Open. 20224(1):20210081. Cited in: PubMed; PMID 36105415.
150. Boudjemaa S, Petit A, Dainese L, et al. Congenital Disseminated Extrarenal Malignant Rhabdoid Tumor. Pediatr Dev Pathol. 201518(5):401-4. Cited in: PubMed; PMID 25751458.
151. Bourdeaut F, Lequin D, Brugières L, et al. Frequent hSNF5/INI1 germline mutations in patients with rhabdoid tumor. Clin Cancer Res. 2011 Jan;17(1):31-8. Cited in: PubMed; PMID 21208904.
152. Bourgeau M, Martinez A, Deeb KK, et al. Cytologic features of hepatic YAP1-TFE3 rearranged epithelioid hemangioendothelioma. Diagn Cytopathol. 2021 Dec;49(12):E447-E452. Cited in: PubMed; PMID 34411462.
153. Bouvier C, Le Loarer F, Macagno N, et al. Recurrent novel THBS1-ADGRF5 gene fusion in a new tumor subtype "Acral FibroChondroMyxoid Tumors". Mod Pathol. 2020 Jul;33(7):1360-1368. Cited in: PubMed; PMID 32047233.
154. Brady EJ, Hameed M, Tap WD, et al. Imaging features and clinical course of undifferentiated round cell sarcomas with CIC-DUX4 and BCOR-CCNB3 translocations. Skeletal Radiol. 2021 Mar;50(3):521-529. Cited in: PubMed; PMID 32840647.
155. Brandser EA, Goree JC, El-Khoury GY. Elastofibroma dorsi: prevalence in an elderly patient population as revealed by CT. AJR Am J Roentgenol. 1998 Oct;171(4):977-80. Cited in: PubMed; PMID 9762978.
156. Braun V, Prey S, Gurioli C, et al. Congenital haemangiomas: a single-centre retrospective review. BMJ Paediatr Open. 20204(1):e000816. Cited in: PubMed; PMID 33324762.
157. Bridge JA, Sreekantaiah C, Neff JR, et al. Cytogenetic findings in clear cell sarcoma of tendons and aponeuroses. Malignant melanoma of soft parts. Cancer Genet Cytogenet. 1991 Mar;52(1):101-6. Cited in: PubMed; PMID 2009504.
158. Brisse H, Orbach D, Klijanienko J, et al. Imaging and diagnostic strategy of soft tissue tumors in children. Eur Radiol. 2006 May;16(5):1147-64. Cited in: PubMed; PMID 16411083.
159. Brisse HJ, Orbach D, Klijanienko J. Soft tissue tumours: imaging strategy. Pediatr Radiol. 2010 Jun;40(6):1019-28. Cited in: PubMed; PMID 20432021.
160. Brodeur GM, Pritchard J, Berthold F, et al. Revisions of the international criteria for neuroblastoma diagnosis, staging, and response to treatment. J Clin Oncol. 1993 Aug;11(8):1466-77. Cited in: PubMed; PMID 8336186.
161. Brooks JK, Scheper MA, Kramer RE, et al. Intraoral proliferative myositis: case report and literature review. Head Neck. 2007 Apr;29(4):416-20. Cited in: PubMed; PMID 17111425.
162. Bruehl FK, Cooper KL, Kilpatrick SE, et al. Intramammary Angiomatoid Fibrous Histiocytoma, a Rare EWSR1 Rearranged Mesenchymal Neoplasm in a Previously Unreported Anatomic Location with Review of the Cleveland Clinic Experience. Case Rep Pathol. 20192019:9012878. Cited in: PubMed; PMID 31236300.
163. Buitendijk S, van de Ven CP, Dumans TG, et al. Pediatric aggressive fibromatosis: a retrospective analysis of 13 patients and review of literature. Cancer. 2005 Sep;104(5):1090-9. Cited in: PubMed; PMID 16015632.
164. Burk DL, Brunberg JA, Kanal E, et al. Spinal and paraspinal neurofibromatosis: surface coil MR imaging at 1.5 T1. Radiology. 1987 Mar;162(3):797-801. Cited in: PubMed; PMID 3101136.
165. Burke AP, Gatto-Weis C, Griego JE, et al. Adult cellular rhabdomyoma of the heart: a report of 3 cases. Hum Pathol. 2002 Nov;33(11):1092-7. Cited in: PubMed; PMID 12454813.
166. Burlingame OO, Kessé KO, Silverman SG, et al. On-site adequacy evaluations performed by cytotechnologists: correlation with final interpretations of 5241 image-guided fine-needle aspiration biopsies. Cancer Cytopathol. 2012 Jun;120(3):177-84. Cited in: PubMed; PMID 21882357.
167. Bystritsky R, Chambers H. Cellulitis and Soft Tissue Infections. Ann Intern Med. 2018 Feb;168(3):ITC17-ITC32. Cited in: PubMed; PMID 29404597.
168. Calonje E, Fletcher CD. Myoid differentiation in dermatofibrosarcoma protuberans and its fibrosarcomatous variant: clinicopathologic analysis of 5 cases. J Cutan Pathol. 1996 Feb;23(1):30-6. Cited in: PubMed; PMID 8720984.
169. Campbell K, Bridge JA, DiMaio D, et al. Dermatofibrosarcoma protuberans with platelet-derived growth factor-D rearrangement; two cases with morphologically distinct presentations. J Cutan Pathol. 2022 Mar;49(3):274-277. Cited in: PubMed; PMID 34628665.
170. Campione S, Cozzolino I, Mainenti P, et al. Hepatic epithelioid hemangioendothelioma: Pitfalls in the diagnosis on fine needle cytology and "small biopsy" and review of the literature. Pathol Res Pract. 2015 Sep;211(9):702-5. Cited in: PubMed; PMID 26187370.
171. Canacci AM, Nunez C, Getty P, et al. Diagnosis of malignant granular cell tumor metastatic to bone by fine needle aspiration cytology: a case report. Acta Cytol. 201054(2):190-2. Cited in: PubMed; PMID 20391977.
172. Cancer Genome Atlas Research Network. Electronic address: elizabeth.demicco@sinaihealthsystem.ca, Cancer Genome Atlas Research Network. Comprehensive and Integrated Genomic Characterization of Adult Soft Tissue Sarcomas. Cell. 2017 Nov;171(4):950-965.e28. Cited in: PubMed; PMID 29100075.
173. Caraway NP, Fanning CV, Wojcik EM, et al. Cytology of malignant melanoma of soft parts: fine-needle aspirates and exfoliative specimens. Diagn Cytopathol. 1993 Dec;9(6):632-8. Cited in: PubMed; PMID 8143535.
174. Caraway NP, Salina D, Deavers MT, et al. Pulmonary artery intimal sarcoma diagnosed using endobronchial ultrasound-guided transbronchial needle aspiration. Cytojournal. 201512:3. Cited in: PubMed; PMID 25745502.

175. Cardillo M, Zakowski MF, Lin O. Fine-needle aspiration of epithelioid sarcoma: cytology findings in nine cases. Cancer. 2001 Aug;93(4):246-51. Cited in: PubMed; PMID 11507697.

176. Cardoso P, Rosa J, Esteves J, et al. Fine needle aspiration for the diagnosis and treatment of musculoskleletal tumours. Acta Orthop Traumatol Turc. 2017 Jul;51(4):278-283. Cited in: PubMed; PMID 28739192.

177. Carlson JW, Fletcher CD. Immunohistochemistry for beta-catenin in the differential diagnosis of spindle cell lesions: analysis of a series and review of the literature. Histopathology. 2007 Oct;51(4):509-14. Cited in: PubMed; PMID 17711447.

178. Carney JA. Gastric stromal sarcoma, pulmonary chondroma, and extra-adrenal paraganglioma (Carney Triad): natural history, adrenocortical component, and possible familial occurrence. Mayo Clin Proc. 1999 Jun;74(6):543-52. Cited in: PubMed; PMID 10377927.

179. Carney JA. Psammomatous melanotic schwannoma. A distinctive, heritable tumor with special associations, including cardiac myxoma and the Cushing syndrome. Am J Surg Pathol. 1990 Mar;14(3):206-22. Cited in: PubMed; PMID 2305928.

180. Carpenter EL, Mossé YP. Targeting ALK in neuroblastoma--preclinical and clinical advancements. Nat Rev Clin Oncol. 2012 May;9(7):391-9. Cited in: PubMed; PMID 22585002.

181. Carter JM, Weiss SW, Linos K, et al. Superficial CD34-positive fibroblastic tumor: report of 18 cases of a distinctive low-grade mesenchymal neoplasm of intermediate (borderline) malignancy. Mod Pathol. 2014 Feb;27(2):294-302. Cited in: PubMed; PMID 23887307.

182. Carter JM, Wenger DE, Rose PS, et al. Atypical Notochordal Cell Tumors: A Series of Notochordal-derived Tumors That Defy Current Classification Schemes. Am J Surg Pathol. 2017 Jan;41(1):39-48. Cited in: PubMed; PMID 27819871.

183. Carter JM, Wu Y, Blessing MM, et al. Recurrent Genomic Alterations in Soft Tissue Perineuriomas. Am J Surg Pathol. 2018 Dec;42(12):1708-1714. Cited in: PubMed; PMID 30303818.

184. Carvalho SD, Pissaloux D, Crombé A, et al. Pleomorphic Sarcomas: The State of the Art. Surg Pathol Clin. 2019 Mar;12(1):63-105. Cited in: PubMed; PMID 30709449.

185. Cates JM, Rosenberg AE, O'Connell JX, et al. Chondroblastoma-like chondroma of soft tissue: an underrecognized variant and its differential diagnosis. Am J Surg Pathol. 2001 May;25(5):661-6. Cited in: PubMed; PMID 11342780.

186. Cavazzana AO, Schmidt D, Ninfo V, et al. Spindle cell rhabdomyosarcoma. A prognostically favorable variant of rhabdomyosarcoma. Am J Surg Pathol. 1992 Mar;16(3):229-35. Cited in: PubMed; PMID 1599014.

187. Chak A. EUS in submucosal tumors. Gastrointest Endosc. 2002 Oct;56(4 Suppl):S43-8. Cited in: PubMed; PMID 12297748.

188. Chambers M, O'Hern K, Kerr DA. Fine-needle aspiration biopsy for the diagnosis of bone and soft tissue lesions: a systematic review and meta-analysis. J Am Soc Cytopathol. 20209(5):429-441. Cited in: PubMed; PMID 32622858.

189. Chandanwale SS, Buch AC, Chawla KR, et al. Fine needle aspiration cytology of thyroglossal duct cyst: diagnostic pitfalls and a study of 14 cases. Thyroid Res Pract. 2013;10(3):104–7. doi:10.4103/0973-0354.116136.

190. Chang F. Desmoplastic small round cell tumors: cytologic, histologic, and immunohistochemical features. Arch Pathol Lab Med. 2006 May;130(5):728-32. Cited in: PubMed; PMID 16683894.

191. Chang Y, Cesarman E, Pessin MS, et al. Identification of herpesvirus-like DNA sequences in AIDS-associated Kaposi's sarcoma. Science. 1994 Dec;266(5192):1865-9. Cited in: PubMed; PMID 7997879.

192. Charifa A, Azmat CE, Badri T Lipoma Pathology. In: StatPearls. StatPearls Publishing, Treasure Island (FL). 2022. Cited in: PubMed; PMID 29493968.

193. Chase DR, Enzinger FM. Epithelioid sarcoma. Diagnosis, prognostic indicators, and treatment. Am J Surg Pathol. 1985 Apr;9(4):241-63. Cited in: PubMed; PMID 4014539.

194. Chaudet K, Kaimal A, Deshpande V, et al. INI1 negative sarcoma diagnosed as malignant rhabdoid tumor presenting as hydrops fetalis metastatic to the placenta: a case report and review of the literature on congenital sarcomas. J Matern Fetal Neonatal Med. 2021 Nov;34(22):3790-3793. Cited in: PubMed; PMID 31718365.

195. Cheah A, Billings S, Goldblum J, et al. Spindle cell/pleomorphic lipomas of the face: an under-recognized diagnosis. Histopathology. 2015 Feb;66(3):430-7. Cited in: PubMed; PMID 25219904.

196. Cheah AL, Zou Y, Lanigan C, et al. ALK Expression in Angiomatoid Fibrous Histiocytoma: A Potential Diagnostic Pitfall. Am J Surg Pathol. 2019 Jan;43(1):93-101. Cited in: PubMed; PMID 29877921.

197. Chebib I, Hornicek FJ, Nielsen GP, et al. Cytomorphologic features that distinguish schwannoma from other low-grade spindle cell lesions. Cancer Cytopathol. 2015 Mar;123(3):171-9. Cited in: PubMed; PMID 25641870.

198. Chebib I, Jo VY. Application of ancillary studies in soft tissue cytology using a pattern-based approach. Cancer Cytopathol. 2018 Aug;126 Suppl 8:691-710. Cited in: PubMed; PMID 30156774.

199. Chebib I, Jo VY. Round cell sarcoma with CIC-DUX4 gene fusion: Discussion of the distinctive cytomorphologic, immunohistochemical, and molecular features in the differential diagnosis of round cell tumors. Cancer Cytopathol. 2016 May;124(5):350-61. Cited in: PubMed; PMID 26800124.

200. Cheirif-Wolosky O, Novelo-Soto AD, Orozco-Covarrubias L, et al. Infantile hemangioma: an update in the topical and systemic treatments. Bol Med Hosp Infant Mex. 201976(4):167-175. Cited in: PubMed; PMID 31303649.

201. Chelsky ZL, Paulson VA, Chen EY. Molecular analysis of 10 pleomorphic rhabdomyosarcomas reveals potential prognostic markers and druggable targets. Genes Chromosomes Cancer. 2022 Mar;61(3):138-147. Cited in: PubMed; PMID 34773670.

202. Chen AL, Janko E, Pitman MB, et al. Clinical, cytologic, and immunohistochemical features of sarcomas involving body cavity fluids. Cancer Cytopathol. 2019 Dec;127(12):778-784. Cited in: PubMed; PMID 31693303.

203. Chen G, Folpe AL, Colby TV, et al. Angiomatoid fibrous histiocytoma: unusual sites and unusual morphology. Mod Pathol. 2011 Dec;24(12):1560-70. Cited in: PubMed; PMID 21822206.

204. Chen GX, Chen CW, Wen XR, et al. Intravascular Fasciitis of the Jugular Vein Mimicking Thrombosis and Sarcoma: A Case Report. Front Surg. 20218:715249. Cited in: PubMed; PMID 34646860.

205. Chen L, Larsen B, Dermawan JK, et al. Cytomorphology of NUTM1-rearranged sarcoma involving pleural fluid. Diagn Cytopathol. 2022 Sep;50(9):E244-E247. Cited in: PubMed; PMID 35441831.

206. Chen S, Huang H, He S, et al. Spindle cell lipoma: clinicopathologic characterization of 40 cases. Int J Clin Exp Pathol. 201912(7):2613-2621. Cited in: PubMed; PMID 31934089.

207. Chen X, Yu K, Tong GX, et al. Fine needle aspiration of pleomorphic lipoma of the neck: report of two cases. Diagn Cytopathol. 2010 Mar;38(3):184-7. Cited in: PubMed; PMID 19774616.

208. Chen YY, Yen HH, Soon MS. Solitary gastric melanotic schwannoma: sonographic findings. J Clin Ultrasound. 2007 Jan;35(1):52-4. Cited in: PubMed; PMID 17111368.

209. Cheng H, Yang S, Cai S, et al. Clinical and Prognostic Characteristics of 53 Cases of Extracranial Malignant Rhabdoid Tumor in Children. A Single-Institute Experience from 2007 to 2017. Oncologist. 2019 Jul;24(7):e551-e558. Cited in: PubMed; PMID 30914466.

210. Chetty R, Vajpeyi R, Penwick JL. Psammomatous melanotic schwannoma presenting as colonic polyps. Virchows Arch. 2007 Sep;451(3):717-20. Cited in: PubMed; PMID 17622556.

211. Cheung NK, Zhang J, Lu C, et al. Association of age at diagnosis and genetic mutations in patients with neuroblastoma. JAMA. 2012 Mar;307(10):1062-71. Cited in: PubMed; PMID 22416102.

212. Chhieng DC, Cangiarella JF, Symmans WF, et al. Fine-needle aspiration cytology of Hodgkin disease: a study of 89 cases with emphasis on false-negative cases. Cancer. 2001 Feb;93(1):52-9. Cited in: PubMed; PMID 11241266.

213. Chinoy RF, Beotra A, Naresh KN. Fibromatosis of the breast: diagnosis by fine needle aspiration cytology. Acta Cytol. 199842(3):811-2. Cited in: PubMed; PMID 9622714.

214. Chmielecki J, Crago AM, Rosenberg M, et al. Whole-exome sequencing identifies a recurrent NAB2-STAT6 fusion in solitary fibrous tumors. Nat Genet. 2013 Feb;45(2):131-2. Cited in: PubMed; PMID 23313954.

215. Cho HY, Lee M, Takei H, et al. Immunohistochemical comparison of chordoma with chondrosarcoma, myxopapillary ependymoma, and chordoid meningioma. Appl Immunohistochem Mol Morphol. 2009 Mar;17(2):131-8. Cited in: PubMed; PMID 19521276.

216. Cho NH, Lee KG, Jeong MG. Cytologic evaluation of primary malignant vascular tumors of the liver. One case each of angiosarcoma and epithelioid hemangioendothelioma. Acta Cytol. 199741(5):1468-76. Cited in: PubMed; PMID 9305386.

217. Cho YJ, Kim JY. Alveolar soft part sarcoma: clinical presentation, treatment and outcome in a series of 19 patients. Clin Orthop Surg. 2014 Mar;6(1):80-6. Cited in: PubMed; PMID 24605193.

218. Choi JK, van Hoeven K, Brooks JJ, et al. Desmoplastic small round cell tumor presenting in pleural fluid and accompanied by desmin-positive mesothelial cells. Acta Cytol. 199539(2):377-8. Cited in: PubMed; PMID 7887076.

219. Choi LE, Healey JH, Kuk D, et al. Analysis of outcomes in extraskeletal osteosarcoma: a review of fifty-three cases. J Bone Joint Surg Am. 2014 Jan;96(1):e2. Cited in: PubMed; PMID 24382730.

220. Choi YJ, Lee IS, Song YS, et al. Diagnostic performance of diffusion-weighted (DWI) and dynamic contrast-enhanced (DCE) MRI for the differentiation of benign from malignant soft-tissue tumors. J Magn Reson Imaging. 2019 Sep;50(3):798-809. Cited in: PubMed; PMID 30663160.

221. Choudhury M, Jain R, Nangia A, et al. Localized tenosynovial giant cell tumor of tendon sheath. A case report. Acta Cytol. 200044(3):463-6. Cited in: PubMed; PMID 10834013.

222. Chougule A, Taylor MS, Nardi V, et al. Spindle and Round Cell Sarcoma With EWSR1-PATZ1 Gene Fusion: A Sarcoma With Polyphenotypic Differentiation. Am J Surg Pathol. 2019 Feb;43(2):220-228. Cited in: PubMed; PMID 30379650.

223. Chow LT, Chow WH, Lee JC. Fine needle aspiration (FNA) cytology of proliferative fasciitis: report of a case with immunohistochemical study. Cytopathology. 1995 Oct;6(5):349-57. Cited in: PubMed; PMID 8785374.

224. Chrisinger JSA. Update on Lipomatous Tumors with Emphasis on Emerging Entities, Unusual Anatomic Sites, and Variant Histologic Patterns. Surg Pathol Clin. 2019 Mar;12(1):21-33. Cited in: PubMed; PMID 30709444.

225. Chun YS, Wang L, Nascimento AG, et al. Pediatric inflammatory myofibroblastic tumor: anaplastic lymphoma kinase (ALK) expression and prognosis. Pediatr Blood Cancer. 2005 Nov;45(6):796-801. Cited in: PubMed; PMID 15602716.

226. Chung EB, Enzinger FM. Benign lipoblastomatosis. An analysis of 35 cases. Cancer. 1973 Aug;32(2):482-92. Cited in: PubMed; PMID 4353020.

227. Chung EB, Enzinger FM. Chondroma of soft parts. Cancer. 1978 Apr;41(4):1414-24. Cited in: PubMed; PMID 76505.

228. Chung EB, Enzinger FM. Extraskeletal osteosarcoma. Cancer. 1987 Sep;60(5):1132-42. Cited in: PubMed; PMID 3475157.

229. Chung EB, Enzinger FM. Infantile fibrosarcoma. Cancer. 1976 Aug;38(2):729-39. Cited in: PubMed; PMID 974993.

230. Chung EB, Enzinger FM. Malignant melanoma of soft parts. A reassessment of clear cell sarcoma. Am J Surg Pathol. 1983 Jul;7(5):405-13. Cited in: PubMed; PMID 6614306.

231. Chung EB, Enzinger FM. Proliferative fasciitis. Cancer. 1975 Oct;36(4):1450-8. Cited in: PubMed; PMID 1058047.

232. Chung L, Lau SK, Jiang Z, et al. Overlapping features between dedifferentiated liposarcoma and undifferentiated high-grade pleomorphic sarcoma. Am J Surg Pathol. 2009 Nov;33(11):1594-600. Cited in: PubMed; PMID 19574885.

233. Cibas ES, Ducatman BS. Cytology: diagnostic principles and clinical correlates. Philadelphia (PA): Saunders; 2025.

234. Clay MR, Martinez AP, Weiss SW, et al. MDM2 Amplification in Problematic Lipomatous Tumors: Analysis of FISH Testing Criteria. Am J Surg Pathol. 2015 Oct;39(10):1433-9. Cited in: PubMed; PMID 26146760.

235. Clay MR, Martinez AP, Weiss SW, et al. MDM2 and CDK4 Immunohistochemistry: Should It Be Used in Problematic Differentiated Lipomatous Tumors?: A New Perspective. Am J Surg Pathol. 2016 Dec;40(12):1647-1652. Cited in: PubMed; PMID 27508976.

236. Clayton AC, Salomão DR, Keeney GL, et al. Solitary fibrous tumor: a study of cytologic features of six cases diagnosed by fine-needle aspiration. Diagn Cytopathol. 2001 Sep;25(3):172-6. Cited in: PubMed; PMID 11536441.

237. Cloutier JM, Charville GW, Mertens F, et al. "Inflammatory Leiomyosarcoma" and "Histiocyte-rich Rhabdomyoblastic Tumor": a clinicopathological, immunohistochemical and genetic study of 13 cases, with a proposal for reclassification as "Inflammatory Rhabdomyoblastic Tumor". Mod Pathol. 2021 Apr;34(4):758-769. Cited in: PubMed; PMID 33318583.

238. Coffin CM, Alaggio R. Fibroblastic and myofibroblastic tumors in children and

adolescents. Pediatr Dev Pathol. 201215(1 Suppl):127-80. Cited in: PubMed; PMID 22420727.
239. Coffin CM, Hornick JL, Fletcher CD. Inflammatory myofibroblastic tumor: comparison of clinicopathologic, histologic, and immunohistochemical features including ALK expression in atypical and aggressive cases. Am J Surg Pathol. 2007 Apr;31(4):509-20. Cited in: PubMed; PMID 17414097.
240. Coffin CM, Jaszcz W, O'Shea PA, et al. So-called congenital-infantile fibrosarcoma: does it exist and what is it? Pediatr Pathol. 199414(1):133-50. Cited in: PubMed; PMID 8159611.
241. Coffin CM, Lowichik A, Putnam A. Lipoblastoma (LPB): a clinicopathologic and immunohistochemical analysis of 59 cases. Am J Surg Pathol. 2009 Nov;33(11):1705-12. Cited in: PubMed; PMID 19738456.
242. Coffin CM, Patel A, Perkins S, et al. ALK1 and p80 expression and chromosomal rearrangements involving 2p23 in inflammatory myofibroblastic tumor. Mod Pathol. 2001 Jun;14(6):569-76. Cited in: PubMed; PMID 11406658.
243. Coffin CM, Watterson J, Priest JR, et al. Extrapulmonary inflammatory myofibroblastic tumor (inflammatory pseudotumor). A clinicopathologic and immunohistochemical study of 84 cases. Am J Surg Pathol. 1995 Aug;19(8):859-72. Cited in: PubMed; PMID 7611533.
244. Cohen-Gogo S, Cellier C, Coindre JM, et al. Ewing-like sarcomas with BCOR-CCNB3 fusion transcript: a clinical, radiological and pathological retrospective study from the Société Française des Cancers de L'Enfant. Pediatr Blood Cancer. 2014 Dec;61(12):2191-8. Cited in: PubMed; PMID 25176412.
245. Cohn SL, Pearson AD, London WB, et al. The International Neuroblastoma Risk Group (INRG) classification system: an INRG Task Force report. J Clin Oncol. 2009 Jan;27(2):289-97. Cited in: PubMed; PMID 19047291.
246. Coindre JM. Grading of soft tissue sarcomas: review and update. Arch Pathol Lab Med. 2006 Oct;130(10):1448-53. Cited in: PubMed; PMID 17090186.
247. Coindre JM, de Mascarel A, Trojani M, et al. Immunohistochemical study of rhabdomyosarcoma. Unexpected staining with S100 protein and cytokeratin. J Pathol. 1988 Jun;155(2):127-32. Cited in: PubMed; PMID 2455782.
248. Coindre JM, Mariani O, Chibon F, et al. Most malignant fibrous histiocytomas developed in the retroperitoneum are dedifferentiated liposarcomas: a review of 25 cases initially diagnosed as malignant fibrous histiocytoma. Mod Pathol. 2003 Mar;16(3):256-62. Cited in: PubMed; PMID 12640106.
249. Colin P, Lagacé R, Caillaud JM, et al. Fine-needle aspiration in myxofibrosarcoma: experience of Institut Curie. Diagn Cytopathol. 2010 May;38(5):343-6. Cited in: PubMed; PMID 19899126.
250. Collini P, Negri T, Barisella M, et al. High-grade sarcomatous overgrowth in solitary fibrous tumors: a clinicopathologic study of 10 cases. Am J Surg Pathol. 2012 Aug;36(8):1202-15. Cited in: PubMed; PMID 22613995.
251. Collins K, Buckley T, Anderson K, et al. Perivascular Epithelioid Cell Tumor (PEComa) of Pancreas Diagnosed Preoperatively by Endoscopic Ultrasound-Guided Fine-Needle Aspiration: A Case Report and Review of Literature. Diagn Cytopathol. 2017 Jan;45(1):59-65. Cited in: PubMed; PMID 27628738.
252. Collins MH, Chatten J. Lipoblastoma/lipoblastomatosis: a clinicopathologic study of 25 tumors. Am J Surg Pathol. 1997 Oct;21(10):1131-7. Cited in: PubMed; PMID 9331284.
253. Conde E, Suárez-Gauthier A, Benito A, et al. Accurate identification of ALK positive lung carcinoma patients: novel FDA-cleared automated fluorescence in situ hybridization scanning system and ultrasensitive immunohistochemistry. PLoS One. 20149(9):e107200. Cited in: PubMed; PMID 25248157.
254. Conner JR, Hornick JL. SATB2 is a novel marker of osteoblastic differentiation in bone and soft tissue tumours. Histopathology. 2013 Jul;63(1):36-49. Cited in: PubMed; PMID 23701429.
255. Constantin VD, Socea B, Popa F, et al. A histopathological and immunohistochemical approach of surgical emergencies of GIST. An interdisciplinary study. Rom J Morphol Embryol. 201455(2 Suppl):619-27. Cited in: PubMed; PMID 25178335.
256. Copeland H, Makdisi PB, Duncan M, et al. Primary extraskeletal pleural osteosarcoma: a rare pleural identity. Ann Transl Med. 2016 Jun;4(11):220. Cited in: PubMed; PMID 27386494.
257. Corless CL, Fletcher JA, Heinrich MC. Biology of gastrointestinal stromal tumors. J Clin Oncol. 2004 Sep;22(18):3813-25. Cited in: PubMed; PMID 15365079.
258. Costa MJ, Weiss SW. Angiomatoid malignant fibrous histiocytoma. A follow-up study of 108 cases with evaluation of possible histologic predictors of outcome. Am J Surg Pathol. 1990 Dec;14(12):1126-32. Cited in: PubMed; PMID 2174650.
259. Costa S, Byrne M, Pissaloux D, et al. Melanomas Associated With Blue Nevi or Mimicking Cellular Blue Nevi: Clinical, Pathologic, and Molecular Study of 11 Cases Displaying a High Frequency of GNA11 Mutations, BAP1 Expression Loss, and a Predilection for the Scalp. Am J Surg Pathol. 2016 Mar;40(3):368-77. Cited in: PubMed; PMID 26645730.
260. Coyle J, White LM, Dickson B, et al. MRI characteristics of nodular fasciitis of the musculoskeletal system. Skeletal Radiol. 2013 Jul;42(7):975-82. Cited in: PubMed; PMID 23624727.
261. Crago AM, Denton B, Salas S, et al. A prognostic nomogram for prediction of recurrence in desmoid fibromatosis. Ann Surg. 2013 Aug;258(2):347-53. Cited in: PubMed; PMID 23532110.
262. Crapanzano JP. Fine-needle aspiration of renal angiomyolipoma: cytological findings and diagnostic pitfalls in a series of five cases. Diagn Cytopathol. 2005 Jan;32(1):53-7. Cited in: PubMed; PMID 15584043.
263. Crapanzano JP, Cardillo M, Lin O, et al. Cytology of desmoplastic small round cell tumor. Cancer. 2002 Feb;96(1):21-31. Cited in: PubMed; PMID 11836699.
264. Creager AJ, Pitman MB, Geisinger KR. Cytologic features of clear cell sarcoma (malignant melanoma) of soft parts: a study of fine-needle aspirates and exfoliative specimens. Am J Clin Pathol. 2002 Feb;117(2):217-24. Cited in: PubMed; PMID 11863218.
265. Creytens D, Folpe AL, Koelsche C, et al. Myxoid pleomorphic liposarcoma-a clinicopathologic, immunohistochemical, molecular genetic and epigenetic study of 12 cases, suggesting a possible relationship with conventional pleomorphic liposarcoma. Mod Pathol. 2021 Nov;34(11):2043-2049. Cited in: PubMed; PMID 34168281.
266. Creytens D, van Gorp J, Savola S, et al. Atypical spindle cell lipoma: a clinicopathologic, immunohistochemical, and molecular study emphasizing its relationship to classical spindle cell lipoma. Virchows Arch. 2014 Jul;465(1):97-108. Cited in: PubMed; PMID 24659226.
267. Crist J, Hodge JR, Frick M, et al. Magnetic Resonance Imaging Appearance of Schwannomas from Head to Toe: A Pictorial Review. J Clin Imaging Sci. 20177:38. Cited in: PubMed; PMID 29114437.
268. Cronin CT, Keel SB, Grabbe J, et al. Adult rhabdomyoma of the extremity: a case report and review of the literature. Hum Pathol. 2000 Sep;31(9):1074-80. Cited in: PubMed; PMID 11014574.
269. Cummings TJ, Liu K, Jordan LK, et al. Fine-needle aspiration diagnosis of psammomatous melanotic schwannoma. Diagn Cytopathol. 2000 Jul;23(1):55-8. Cited in: PubMed; PMID 10907935.
270. Cuviello A, Goyal A, Zick A, et al. Sporadic Malignant Glomus Tumor of the Brachial Plexus With Response to Targeted Therapy Directed Against Oncogenic BRAF. JCO Precis Oncol. 20182018: Cited in: PubMed; PMID 30556047.
271. da Cunha Santos G, Saieg MA, Troncone G, et al. Cytological preparations for molecular analysis: A review of technical procedures, advantages and limitations for referring samples for testing. Cytopathology. 2018 Apr;29(2):125-132. Cited in: PubMed; PMID 29575423.
272. Dabbs DJ, Abendroth CS, Grenko RT, et al. Immunocytochemistry on the Thinprep processor. Diagn Cytopathol. 1997 Nov;17(5):388-92. Cited in: PubMed; PMID 9360054.
273. Dadone B, Refae S, Lemarié-Delaunay C, et al. Molecular cytogenetics of pediatric adipocytic tumors. Cancer Genet. 2015 Oct;208(10):469-81. Cited in: PubMed; PMID 26319758.
274. Dadone-Montaudié B, Alberti L, Duc A, et al. Alternative PDGFD rearrangements in dermatofibrosarcomas protuberans without PDGFB fusions. Mod Pathol. 2018 Nov;31(11):1683-1693. Cited in: PubMed; PMID 29955147.
275. Dahiya S, Verma K. Malignant melanoma of soft parts a diagnostic pitfall in FNA: a case report. Indian J Pathol Microbiol. 2004 Jan;47(1):54-7. Cited in: PubMed; PMID 15471132.
276. Dahl I, Akerman M. Nodular fasciitis a correlative cytologic and histologic study of 13 cases. Acta Cytol. 198125(3):215-23. Cited in: PubMed; PMID 6942611.
277. Dahl I, Hagmar B, Angervall L. Leiomyosarcoma of the soft tissue. A correlative cytological and histological study of 11 cases. Acta Pathol Microbiol Scand A. 1981 Jul;89(4):285-91. Cited in: PubMed; PMID 7315325.
278. Dahlén A, Debiec-Rychter M, Pedeutour F, et al. Clustering of deletions on chromosome 13 in benign and low-malignant lipomatous tumors. Int J Cancer. 2003 Feb;103(5):616-23. Cited in: PubMed; PMID 12494468.
279. Daigeler A, Vogt PM, Busch K, et al. Elastofibroma dorsi--differential diagnosis in chest wall tumours. World J Surg Oncol. 2007 Feb;5:15. Cited in: PubMed; PMID 17280612.
280. Dal Cin P, Rao U, Jani-Sait S, et al. Chromosomes in the diagnosis of soft tissue tumors. I. Synovial sarcoma. Mod Pathol. 1992 Jul;5(4):357-62. Cited in: PubMed; PMID 1379714.
281. Dal Cin P, Qian X, Cibas ES. The marriage of cytology and cytogenetics. Cancer Cytopathol. 2013 Jun;121(6):279-90. Cited in: PubMed; PMID 23288831.
282. Dalén BP, Meis-Kindblom JM, Sumathi VP, et al. Fine-needle aspiration cytology and core needle biopsy in the preoperative diagnosis of desmoid tumors. Acta Orthop. 2006 Dec;77(6):926-31. Cited in: PubMed; PMID 17260203.
283. Damron TA, Heiner J. Distant soft tissue metastases: a series of 30 new patients and 91 cases from the literature. Ann Surg Oncol. 2000 Aug;7(7):526-34. Cited in: PubMed; PMID 10947022.
284. D'Antonio A, Baldi C, Memoli D, et al. Fine needle aspiration biopsy of intraparotid spindle cell lipoma: a case report. Diagn Cytopathol. 2013 Feb;41(2):171-3. Cited in: PubMed; PMID 22021087.
285. Daroca PJ, Pulitzer DR, LoCicero J. Ossifying fasciitis. Arch Pathol Lab Med. 1982 Dec;106(13):682-5. Cited in: PubMed; PMID 6814399.
286. Das DK. Fine-needle aspiration cytology: its origin, development, and present status with special reference to a developing country, India. Diagn Cytopathol. 2003 Jun;28(6):345-51. Cited in: PubMed; PMID 12768643.
287. Das S, Das RN, Sen A, et al. Cytological and histological correlation of granular cell tumor in a series of three cases. J Cancer Res Ther. 201814(2):459-461. Cited in: PubMed; PMID 29516941.
288. Dashti NK, Wehrs RN, Thomas BC, et al. Spindle cell rhabdomyosarcoma of bone with FUS-TFCP2 fusion: confirmation of a very recently described rhabdomyosarcoma subtype. Histopathology. 2018 Sep;73(3):514-520. Cited in: PubMed; PMID 29758589.
289. Datir A, James SL, Ali K, et al. MRI of soft-tissue masses: the relationship between lesion size, depth, and diagnosis. Clin Radiol. 2008 Apr;63(4):373-8; discussion 379-80. Cited in: PubMed; PMID 18325355.
290. Dave B, Shet T, Chinoy R. Desmoplastic round cell tumor of childhood: can cytology with immunocytochemistry serve as an alternative for tissue diagnosis? Diagn Cytopathol. 2005 Jun;32(6):330-5. Cited in: PubMed; PMID 15880716.
291. Davicioni E, Anderson MJ, Finckenstein FG, et al. Molecular classification of rhabdomyosarcoma--genotypic and phenotypic determinants of diagnosis: a report from the Children's Oncology Group. Am J Pathol. 2009 Feb;174(2):550-64. Cited in: PubMed; PMID 19147825.
292. Davis BH, Dasgupta A, Kussick S, et al. Validation of cell-based fluorescence assays: practice guidelines from the ICSH and ICCS - part II - preanalytical issues. Cytometry B Clin Cytom. 201384(5):286-90. Cited in: PubMed; PMID 24022851.
293. Davis JL, Lockwood CM, Stohr B, et al. Expanding the Spectrum of Pediatric NTRK-rearranged Mesenchymal Tumors. Am J Surg Pathol. 2019 Apr;43(4):435-445. Cited in: PubMed; PMID 30585824.
294. de Almeida M, Stastny JF, Wakely PE, et al. Fine-needle aspiration biopsy of childhood rhabdomyosarcoma: reevaluation of the cytologic criteria for diagnosis. Diagn Cytopathol. 199411(3):231-6. Cited in: PubMed; PMID 7867465.
295. de Almeida MM, Abecassis N, Almeida MO, et al. Fine-needle aspiration cytology of myositis ossificans: a case report. Diagn Cytopathol. 199410(1):41-3. Cited in: PubMed; PMID 8005041.
296. De Beuckeleer LH, De Schepper AM, Vandevenne JE, et al. MR imaging of clear cell sarcoma (malignant melanoma of the soft parts): a multicenter correlative MRI-pathology study of 21 cases and literature review. Skeletal Radiol. 2000 Apr;29(4):187-95. Cited in: PubMed; PMID 10855466.
297. de Jongste AH, Kraan J, van den Broek PD, et al. Use of TransFix™ cerebrospinal fluid storage tubes prevents cellular loss and enhances flow cytometric detection of malignant hematological cells after 18 hours of storage. Cytometry B Clin Cytom. 2014 Jul;86(4):272-9. Cited in: PubMed; PMID 23674509.
298. Debol SM, Stanley MW, Mallery S, et al. Glomus tumor of the stomach: cytologic diagnosis by endoscopic ultrasound-guided fine-needle aspiration. Diagn Cytopathol. 2003 Jun;28(6):316-21. Cited in: PubMed; PMID 12768637.

299. Deenik W, Mooi WJ, Rutgers EJ, et al. Clear cell sarcoma (malignant melanoma) of soft parts: A clinicopathologic study of 30 cases. Cancer. 1999 Sep;86(6):969-75. Cited in: PubMed; PMID 10491522.
300. de Feraudy S, Fletcher CD. Intradermal nodular fasciitis: a rare lesion analyzed in a series of 24 cases. Am J Surg Pathol. 2010 Sep;34(9):1377-81. Cited in: PubMed; PMID 20716998.
301. Degnan AJ, Jelinek JS, Murphey MD. Lipoblastoma: computed tomographic and magnetic resonance imaging features correlate with tumor behavior and pathology. Pediatr Radiol. 2021 Apr;51(4):614-621. Cited in: PubMed; PMID 33151344.
302. DeHart A, Richter G. Hemangioma: Recent Advances. F1000Res. 20198: Cited in: PubMed; PMID 31807282.
303. Delaney D, Diss TC, Presneau N, et al. GNAS1 mutations occur more commonly than previously thought in intramuscular myxoma. Mod Pathol. 2009 May;22(5):718-24. Cited in: PubMed; PMID 19287459.
304. Demaria S, Yee HT, Cangiarella J, et al. Fine needle aspiration of primary pleomorphic liposarcoma of the breast. A case report. Acta Cytol. 199943(6):1131-6. Cited in: PubMed; PMID 10578991.
305. DeMatteo RP, Lewis JJ, Leung D, et al. Two hundred gastrointestinal stromal tumors: recurrence patterns and prognostic factors for survival. Ann Surg. 2000 Jan;231(1):51-8. Cited in: PubMed; PMID 10636102.
306. Demetri GD, von Mehren M, Antonescu CR, et al. NCCN Task Force report: update on the management of patients with gastrointestinal stromal tumors. J Natl Compr Canc Netw. 2010 Apr;8 Suppl 2(0 2):S1-41; quiz S42-4. Cited in: PubMed; PMID 20457867.
307. Demicco EG. Molecular updates in adipocytic neoplasms. Semin Diagn Pathol. 2019 Mar;36(2):85-94. Cited in: PubMed; PMID 30857767.
308. Demicco EG, Harms PW, Patel RM, et al. Extensive survey of STAT6 expression in a large series of mesenchymal tumors. Am J Clin Pathol. 2015 May;143(5):672-82. Cited in: PubMed; PMID 25873501.
309. Demicco EG, Park MS, Araujo DM, et al. Solitary fibrous tumor: a clinicopathological study of 110 cases and proposed risk assessment model. Mod Pathol. 2012 Sep;25(9):1298-306. Cited in: PubMed; PMID 22575866.
310. Demicco EG, Wagner MJ, Maki RG, et al. Risk assessment in solitary fibrous tumors: validation and refinement of a risk stratification model. Mod Pathol. 2017 Oct;30(10):1433-1442. Cited in: PubMed; PMID 28731041.
311. Denda T, Kamoshida S, Kawamura J, et al. Optimal antigen retrieval for ethanol-fixed cytologic smears. Cancer Cytopathol. 2012 Jun;120(3):167-76. Cited in: PubMed; PMID 22434540.
312. Dermawan JK, Azzato EM, Billings SD, et al. YAP1-TFE3-fused hemangioendothelioma: a multi-institutional clinicopathologic study of 24 genetically-confirmed cases. Mod Pathol. 2021 Dec;34(12):2211-2221. Cited in: PubMed; PMID 34381186.
313. Dermawan JK, Azzato EM, Jebastin Thangaiah J, et al. PRRX1-NCOA1-rearranged fibroblastic tumour: a clinicopathological, immunohistochemical and molecular genetic study of six cases of a potentially under-recognised, distinctive mesenchymal tumour. Histopathology. 2021 Dec;79(6):997-1003. Cited in: PubMed; PMID 34272753.
314. de Saint Aubain Somerhausen N, Fletcher CD. Leiomyosarcoma of soft tissue in children: clinicopathologic analysis of 20 cases. Am J Surg Pathol. 1999 Jul;23(7):755-63. Cited in: PubMed; PMID 10403297.
315. de Saint Aubain Somerhausen N, Rubin BP, Fletcher CD. Myxoid solitary fibrous tumor: a study of seven cases with emphasis on differential diagnosis. Mod Pathol. 1999 May;12(5):463-71. Cited in: PubMed; PMID 10349983.
316. Deshpande A, Nelson D, Corless CL, et al. Leiomyoma of the gastrointestinal tract with interstitial cells of Cajal: a mimic of gastrointestinal stromal tumor. Am J Surg Pathol. 2014 Jan;38(1):72-7. Cited in: PubMed; PMID 24145645.
317. Deshpande V, Zen Y, Chan JK, et al. Consensus statement on the pathology of IgG4-related disease. Mod Pathol. 2012 Sep;25(9):1181-92. Cited in: PubMed; PMID 22596100.
318. de Silva MV, Reid R. Myositis ossificans and fibroosseous pseudotumor of digits: a clinicopathological review of 64 cases with emphasis on diagnostic pitfalls. Int J Surg Pathol. 2003 Jul;11(3):187-95. Cited in: PubMed; PMID 12894350.
319. Dewaele B, Floris G, Finalet-Ferreiro J, et al. Coactivated platelet-derived growth factor receptor {alpha} and epidermal growth factor receptor are potential therapeutic targets in intimal sarcoma. Cancer Res. 2010 Sep;70(18):7304-14. Cited in: PubMed; PMID 20685895.
320. Dey P, Mallik MK, Gupta SK, et al. Role of fine needle aspiration cytology in the diagnosis of soft tissue tumours and tumour-like lesions. Cytopathology. 2004 Feb;15(1):32-7. Cited in: PubMed; PMID 14748789.
321. Deyrup AT, Miettinen M, North PE, et al. Angiosarcomas arising in the viscera and soft tissue of children and young adults: a clinicopathologic study of 15 cases. Am J Surg Pathol. 2009 Feb;33(2):264-9. Cited in: PubMed; PMID 18987547.
322. Deyrup AT, Tighiouart M, Montag AG, et al. Epithelioid hemangioendothelioma of soft tissue: a proposal for risk stratification based on 49 cases. Am J Surg Pathol. 2008 Jun;32(6):924-7. Cited in: PubMed; PMID 18551749.
323. Dharmalingam P, MukundaPai M, Nargund A, et al. Doing More with Less: Fine Needle Aspiration Cytology in Pediatric Neoplasms. J Cytol. 202138(3):127-132. Cited in: PubMed; PMID 34703088.
324. Dharmalingam P, Nargund A, MukundaPai M, et al. Primary Ewing sarcoma of the lung diagnosed on cytology: Case report with review of literature. Diagn Cytopathol. 2020 Nov;48(11):1098-1101. Cited in: PubMed; PMID 32369242.
325. Di Vito A, Scali E, Ferraro G, et al. Elastofibroma dorsi: a histochemical and immunohistochemical study. Eur J Histochem. 2015 Feb;59(1):2459. Cited in: PubMed; PMID 25820560.
326. Dias P, Chen B, Dilday B, et al. Strong immunostaining for myogenin in rhabdomyosarcoma is significantly associated with tumors of the alveolar subclass. Am J Pathol. 2000 Feb;156(2):399-408. Cited in: PubMed; PMID 10666368.
327. Dickson BC, Hornick JL, Fletcher CDM, et al. Dermatofibrosarcoma protuberans with a novel COL6A3-PDGFD fusion gene and apparent predilection for breast. Genes Chromosomes Cancer. 2018 Sep;57(9):437-445. Cited in: PubMed; PMID 30014607.
328. Dim DC, Cooley LD, Miranda RN. Clear cell sarcoma of tendons and aponeuroses: a review. Arch Pathol Lab Med. 2007 Jan;131(1):152-6. Cited in: PubMed; PMID 17227118.
329. Dodd LG. Update on liposarcoma: a review for cytopathologists. Diagn Cytopathol. 2012 Dec;40(12):1122-31. Cited in: PubMed; PMID 21932353.
330. Dodd LG, Layfield LJ. Fine-needle aspiration cytology of ganglion cysts. Diagn Cytopathol. 1996 Dec;15(5):377-81. Cited in: PubMed; PMID 8989538.
331. Dodd LG, Major NM. Fine-needle aspiration cytology of articular and periarticular lesions. Cancer. 2002 Jun;96(3):157-65. Cited in: PubMed; PMID 12115304.
332. Dodd LG, Marom EM, Dash RC, et al. Fine-needle aspiration cytology of "ancient" schwannoma. Diagn Cytopathol. 1999 May;20(5):307-11. Cited in: PubMed; PMID 10319234.
333. Dodd LG, Martinez S. Fine-needle aspiration cytology of pseudosarcomatous lesions of soft tissue. Diagn Cytopathol. 2001 Jan;24(1):28-35. Cited in: PubMed; PMID 11135465.
334. Dodd LG, Sara Jiang X, Rao K, et al. Pleomorphic liposarcoma: a cytologic study of five cases. Diagn Cytopathol. 2015 Feb;43(2):138-43. Cited in: PubMed; PMID 24652822.
335. Dodd LG, Ware P, Duncan D, et al. Doing more with less: New markers for sarcoma diagnosis and their applicability to cytology specimens. Diagn Cytopathol. 2016 Apr;44(4):351-60. Cited in: PubMed; PMID 26780171.
336. Dogan S, Becker JC, Rekhtman N, et al. Use of touch imprint cytology as a simple method to enrich tumor cells for molecular analysis. Cancer Cytopathol. 2013 Jul;121(7):354-60. Cited in: PubMed; PMID 23576371.
337. Domanski HA. Elastic fibers in elastofibroma dorsi by fine-needle aspiration. Diagn Cytopathol. 2014 Jul;42(7):609-11. Cited in: PubMed; PMID 23554149.
338. Domanski HA. Fine-needle aspiration cytology of soft tissue lesions: diagnostic challenges. Diagn Cytopathol. 2007 Dec;35(12):768-73. Cited in: PubMed; PMID 18008345.
339. Domanski HA. Fine-needle aspiration smears from lipomatous hemangiopericytoma need not be confused with myxoid liposarcoma. Diagn Cytopathol. 2003 Nov;29(5):287-91. Cited in: PubMed; PMID 14595798.
340. Domanski HA. FNA diagnosis of dermatofibrosarcoma protuberans. Diagn Cytopathol. 2005 May;32(5):299-302. Cited in: PubMed; PMID 15830369.
341. Domanski HA. Low cellularity of fine needle aspirates in the evaluation of spindle cell lipoma. Acta Cytol. 200246(5):1023. Cited in: PubMed; PMID 12365205.
342. Domanski HA. Role of fine needle aspiration cytology in the diagnosis of soft tissue tumours. Cytopathology. 2020 Jul;31(4):271-279. Cited in: PubMed; PMID 32298511.
343. Domanski HA. The Small Round Cell Sarcomas Complexities and Desmoplastic Presentation. Acta Cytol. 202266(4):279-294. Cited in: PubMed; PMID 35417916.
344. Domanski HA, Akerman M, Carlén B, et al. Core-needle biopsy performed by the cytopathologist: a technique to complement fine-needle aspiration of soft tissue and bone lesions. Cancer. 2005 Aug;105(4):229-39. Cited in: PubMed; PMID 15918176.
345. Domanski HA, Akerman M, Engellau J, et al. Fine-needle aspiration of neurilemoma (schwannoma). A clinicocytopathologic study of 116 patients. Diagn Cytopathol. 2006 Jun;34(6):403-12. Cited in: PubMed; PMID 16680779.
346. Domanski HA, Akerman M, Rissler P, et al. Fine-needle aspiration of soft tissue leiomyosarcoma: an analysis of the most common cytologic findings and the value of ancillary techniques. Diagn Cytopathol. 2006 Sep;34(9):597-604. Cited in: PubMed; PMID 16900474.
347. Domanski HA, Carlén B, Jonsson K, et al. Distinct cytologic features of spindle cell lipoma. A cytologic-histologic study with clinical, radiologic, electron microscopic, and cytogenetic correlations. Cancer. 2001 Dec;93(6):381-9. Cited in: PubMed; PMID 11748578.
348. Domanski HA, Carlén B, Sloth M, et al. Elastofibroma dorsi has distinct cytomorphologic features, making diagnostic surgical biopsy unnecessary: cytomorphologic study with clinical, radiologic, and electron microscopic correlations. Diagn Cytopathol. 2003 Dec;29(6):327-33. Cited in: PubMed; PMID 14648789.
349. Domanski HA, Dawiskiba S. Adult rhabdomyoma in fine needle aspirates. A report of two cases. Acta Cytol. 200044(2):223-6. Cited in: PubMed; PMID 10740610.
350. Domanski HA, Gustafson P. Cytologic features of primary, recurrent, and metastatic dermatofibrosarcoma protuberans. Cancer. 2002 Dec;96(6):351-61. Cited in: PubMed; PMID 12478683.
351. Domanski HA, Mertens F, Panagopoulos I, et al. Low-grade fibromyxoid sarcoma is difficult to diagnose by fine needle aspiration cytology: a cytomorphological study of eight cases. Cytopathology. 2009 Oct;20(5):304-14. Cited in: PubMed; PMID 18637810.
352. Domanski HA, Walther CS. FNA cytology of soft tissue and bone tumors. Basel (Switzerland): Karger; 2017. (Monographs in clinical cytology series; vol. 22).
353. Domanski HA. Chapter 3: Sampling procedure, fine needle aspiration (FNA), and core needle biopsy (CNB). In: Klijanienko J, Lagacé R, editors. Soft tissue tumors: a multidisciplinary, decisional diagnostic approach. Hoboken (NJ): Wiley-Blackwell; 2011. pp. 37–59.
354. Dong Q, McKee G, Pitman M, et al. Epithelioid variant of gastrointestinal stromal tumor: Diagnosis by fine-needle aspiration. Diagn Cytopathol. 2003 Aug;29(2):55-60. Cited in: PubMed; PMID 12889040.
355. Downs-Kelly E, Goldblum JR, Patel RM, et al. The utility of fluorescence in situ hybridization (FISH) in the diagnosis of myxoid soft tissue neoplasms. Am J Surg Pathol. 2008 Jan;32(1):8-13. Cited in: PubMed; PMID 18162764.
356. Downs-Kelly E, Shehata BM, López-Terrada D, et al. The utility of FOXO1 fluorescence in situ hybridization (FISH) in formalin-fixed paraffin-embedded specimens in the diagnosis of alveolar rhabdomyosarcoma. Diagn Mol Pathol. 2009 Sep;18(3):138-43. Cited in: PubMed; PMID 19704258.
357. Doyle LA, Fletcher CD, Hornick JL. Nuclear Expression of CAMTA1 Distinguishes Epithelioid Hemangioendothelioma From Histologic Mimics. Am J Surg Pathol. 2016 Jan;40(1):94-102. Cited in: PubMed; PMID 26414223.
358. Doyle LA, Hornick JL, Fletcher CD. PEComa of the gastrointestinal tract: clinicopathologic study of 35 cases with evaluation of prognostic parameters. Am J Surg Pathol. 2013 Dec;37(12):1769-82. Cited in: PubMed; PMID 24061520.
359. Doyle LA, Möller E, Dal Cin P, et al. MUC4 is a highly sensitive and specific marker for low-grade fibromyxoid sarcoma. Am J Surg Pathol. 2011 May;35(5):733-41. Cited in: PubMed; PMID 21415703.
360. Doyle LA, Nelson D, Heinrich MC, et al. Loss of succinate dehydrogenase subunit B (SDHB) expression is limited to a distinctive subset of gastric wild-type gastrointestinal stromal tumours: a comprehensive genotype-phenotype correlation study. Histopathology. 2012 Nov;61(5):801-9. Cited in: PubMed; PMID 22804613.

361. Doyle LA, Vivero M, Fletcher CD, et al. Nuclear expression of STAT6 distinguishes solitary fibrous tumor from histologic mimics. Mod Pathol. 2014 Mar;27(3):390-5. Cited in: PubMed; PMID 24030747.
362. Doyle LA, Wang WL, Dal Cin P, et al. MUC4 is a sensitive and extremely useful marker for sclerosing epithelioid fibrosarcoma: association with FUS gene rearrangement. Am J Surg Pathol. 2012 Oct;36(10):1444-51. Cited in: PubMed; PMID 22982887.
363. Doyle LA, Wong KK, Bueno R, et al. Ewing sarcoma mimicking atypical carcinoid tumor: detection of unexpected genomic alterations demonstrates the use of next generation sequencing as a diagnostic tool. Cancer Genet. 2014207(7-8):335-9. Cited in: PubMed; PMID 25441687.
364. Drachenberg CB, Papadimitriou JC. Alveolar soft part sarcoma. A case report with correlation of fine needle aspiration and ultrastructural cytologic features. Acta Cytol. 199135(6):746-52. Cited in: PubMed; PMID 1950328.
365. Drakos E, Rassidakis GZ, Leventaki V, et al. Nodular lymphocyte predominant Hodgkin lymphoma with clusters of LP Cells, acute inflammation, and fibrosis: a syncytial variant. Am J Surg Pathol. 2009 Nov;33(11):1725-31. Cited in: PubMed; PMID 19730363.
366. Drut R. Malignant rhabdoid tumor of the kidney diagnosed by fine-needle aspiration cytology. Diagn Cytopathol. 19906(2):124-6. Cited in: PubMed; PMID 2159866.
367. Ducatman BS, Scheithauer BW, Piepgras DG, et al. Malignant peripheral nerve sheath tumors. A clinicopathologic study of 120 cases. Cancer. 1986 May;57(10):2006-21. Cited in: PubMed; PMID 3082508.
368. Dupré MP, Courtade-Saidi M. Immunocytochemistry as an adjunct to diagnostic cytology. Ann Pathol. 2012 Dec;32(6):e47-51, 433-7. Cited in: PubMed; PMID 23244485.
369. Dupree WB, Langloss JM, Weiss SW. Pigmented dermatofibrosarcoma protuberans (Bednar tumor). A pathologic, ultrastructural, and immunohistochemical study. Am J Surg Pathol. 1985 Sep;9(9):630-9. Cited in: PubMed; PMID 3901787.
370. Eckardt JJ, Pritchard DJ, Soule EH. Clear cell sarcoma. A clinicopathologic study of 27 cases. Cancer. 1983 Oct;52(8):1482-8. Cited in: PubMed; PMID 6616410.
371. Eddyani M, Fraga AG, Schmitt F, et al. Fine-needle aspiration, an efficient sampling technique for bacteriological diagnosis of nonulcerative Buruli ulcer. J Clin Microbiol. 2009 Jun;47(6):1700-4. Cited in: PubMed; PMID 19386847.
372. Eddyani M, Sopoh GE, Ayelo G, et al. Diagnostic Accuracy of Clinical and Microbiological Signs in Patients With Skin Lesions Resembling Buruli Ulcer in an Endemic Region. Clin Infect Dis. 2018 Aug;67(6):827-834. Cited in: PubMed; PMID 29538642.
373. Eidhof HHM, Gratama JW, Mulder AHL. Comparison of three methods to stabilize bronchoalveolar lavage cells for flowcytometric analysis. Cytometry B Clin Cytom. 2021 May;100(3):377-383. Cited in: PubMed; PMID 32479677.
374. Eigenbrodt ML, Cunningham LF. Fine needle aspiration cytology of a rhabdomyoma of the pharynx. Acta Cytol. 198630(5):528-32. Cited in: PubMed; PMID 3465146.
376. El Zein S, Boccara O, Soupre V, et al. The histopathology of congenital haemangioma and its clinical correlations: a long-term follow-up study of 55 cases. Histopathology. 2020 Aug;77(2):275-283. Cited in: PubMed; PMID 32281140.
377. Elco CP, Mariño-Enríquez A, Abraham JA, et al. Hybrid myxoinflammatory fibroblastic sarcoma/hemosiderotic fibrolipomatous tumor: report of a case providing further evidence for a pathogenetic link. Am J Surg Pathol. 2010 Nov;34(11):1723-7. Cited in: PubMed; PMID 20871391.
378. el-Jabbour JN, Bennett MH, Burke MM, et al. Proliferative myositis. An immunohistochemical and ultrastructural study. Am J Surg Pathol. 1991 Jul;15(7):654-9. Cited in: PubMed; PMID 2058761.
379. El-Rifai W, Sarlomo-Rikala M, Andersson LC, et al. DNA sequence copy number changes in gastrointestinal stromal tumors: tumor progression and prognostic significance. Cancer Res. 2000 Jul;60(14):3899-903. Cited in: PubMed; PMID 10919666.
380. Enzinger FM. Angiomatoid malignant fibrous histiocytoma: a distinct fibrohistiocytic tumor of children and young adults simulating a vascular neoplasm. Cancer. 1979 Dec;44(6):2147-57. Cited in: PubMed; PMID 228836.
381. ENZINGER FM. INTRAMUSCULAR MYXOMA; A REVIEW AND FOLLOW-UP STUDY OF 34 CASES. Am J Clin Pathol. 1965 Feb;43:104-13. Cited in: PubMed; PMID 14253111.
382. Enzinger FM, Dulcey F. Proliferative myositis. Report of thirty-three cases. Cancer. 1967 Dec;20(12):2213-23. Cited in: PubMed; PMID 6073898.
383. Enzinger FM, Harvey DA. Spindle cell lipoma. Cancer. 1975 Nov;36(5):1852-9. Cited in: PubMed; PMID 1192370.
384. Enzinger FM, Shiraki M. Extraskeletal myxoid chondrosarcoma. An analysis of 34 cases. Hum Pathol. 1972 Sep;3(3):421-35. Cited in: PubMed; PMID 4261659.
385. Erickson-Johnson MR, Chou MM, Evers BR, et al. Nodular fasciitis: a novel model of transient neoplasia induced by MYH9-USP6 gene fusion. Lab Invest. 2011 Oct;91(10):1427-33. Cited in: PubMed; PMID 21826056.
386. Errani C, Zhang L, Sung YS, et al. A novel WWTR1-CAMTA1 gene fusion is a consistent abnormality in epithelioid hemangioendothelioma of different anatomic sites. Genes Chromosomes Cancer. 2011 Aug;50(8):644-53. Cited in: PubMed; PMID 21584898.
387. Erwteman AS, Balach T. Clinical evaluation and management of benign soft tissue tumors of the extremities. Cancer Treat Res. 2014162:171-202. Cited in: PubMed; PMID 25070236.
388. Espinosa-Cotton M, Cheung NV. Immunotherapy and Radioimmunotherapy for Desmoplastic Small Round Cell Tumor. Front Oncol. 202111:772862. Cited in: PubMed; PMID 34869013.
389. Esposito S, Bassetti M, Concia E, et al. Diagnosis and management of skin and soft-tissue infections (SSTI). A literature review and consensus statement: an update. J Chemother. 2017 Aug;29(4):197-214. Cited in: PubMed; PMID 28378613.
390. Estrada-Villaseñor E, Cedillo ED, Martínez GR. Scrape cytology of myositis ossificans: report of a case and analysis of the cytologic findings described previously. Diagn Cytopathol. 2008 Jan;36(1):50-3. Cited in: PubMed; PMID 18064693.
391. Evans DG. Neurofibromatosis type 2 (NF2): a clinical and molecular review. Orphanet J Rare Dis. 2009 Jun;4:16. Cited in: PubMed; PMID 19545378.
392. Evans HL. Low-grade fibromyxoid sarcoma: a clinicopathologic study of 33 cases with long-term follow-up. Am J Surg Pathol. 2011 Oct;35(10):1450-62. Cited in: PubMed; PMID 21921785.
393. Ewing CA, Zakowski MF, Lin O. Monophasic synovial sarcoma: a cytologic spectrum. Diagn Cytopathol. 2004 Jan;30(1):19-23. Cited in: PubMed; PMID 14696140.
394. Fabijanić I, Katavić N, Obad Kovačević D. Pleomorphic rhabdomyosarcoma of the submandibular gland: Diagnosis on a cytology sample. Cytopathology. 2020 May;31(3):250-252. Cited in: PubMed; PMID 32159876.
395. Fallen T, Wilson M, Morlan B, et al. Desmoid tumors -- a characterization of patients seen at Mayo Clinic 1976-1999. Fam Cancer. 20065(2):191-4. Cited in: PubMed; PMID 16736290.
396. Falleti J, De Cecio R, Mentone A, et al. Extraskeletal chondroma of the masseter muscle: a case report with review of the literature. Int J Oral Maxillofac Surg. 2009 Aug;38(8):895-9. Cited in: PubMed; PMID 19349148.
397. Fanburg-Smith JC, Devaney KO, Miettinen M, et al. Multiple spindle cell lipomas: a report of 7 familial and 11 nonfamilial cases. Am J Surg Pathol. 1998 Jan;22(1):40-8. Cited in: PubMed; PMID 9422314.
398. Fanburg-Smith JC, Hengge M, Hengge UR, et al. Extrarenal rhabdoid tumors of soft tissue: a clinicopathologic and immunohistochemical study of 18 cases. Ann Diagn Pathol. 1998 Dec;2(6):351-62. Cited in: PubMed; PMID 9930572.
399. Fanburg-Smith JC, Majidi M, Miettinen M. Keratin expression in schwannoma; a study of 115 retroperitoneal and 22 peripheral schwannomas. Mod Pathol. 2006 Jan;19(1):115-21. Cited in: PubMed; PMID 16357842.
400. Fanburg-Smith JC, Meis-Kindblom JM, Fante R, et al. Malignant granular cell tumor of soft tissue: diagnostic criteria and clinicopathologic correlation. Am J Surg Pathol. 1998 Jul;22(7):779-94. Cited in: PubMed; PMID 9669341.
401. Fanburg-Smith JC, Miettinen M. Angiomatoid "malignant" fibrous histiocytoma: a clinicopathologic study of 158 cases and further exploration of the myoid phenotype. Hum Pathol. 1999 Nov;30(11):1336-43. Cited in: PubMed; PMID 10571514.
402. Fanburg-Smith JC, Miettinen M. Liposarcoma with meningothelial-like whorls: a study of 17 cases of a distinctive histological pattern associated with dedifferentiated liposarcoma. Histopathology. 1998 Nov;33(5):414-24. Cited in: PubMed; PMID 9839165.
403. Farshid G, Pradhan M, Goldblum J, et al. Leiomyosarcoma of somatic soft tissues: a tumor of vascular origin with multivariate analysis of outcome in 42 cases. Am J Surg Pathol. 2002 Jan;26(1):14-24. Cited in: PubMed; PMID 11756765.
404. Fassina A, Klijanienko J. Multidisciplinary and multimodal diagnostic approach in paediatric tumours combining fine needle aspiration, core needle biopsy and ancillary techniques. Cytopathology. 2014 Feb;25(1):3-5. Cited in: PubMed; PMID 24411016.
405. Fernandes F, Eloy C, Carimo A, et al. Simultaneous presentation of Kaposi sarcoma and HHV8-associated large B-cell lymphoma in the same lymph node: A rare diagnosis in an HIV-negative patient. Am J Case Rep. 201314:263-6. Cited in: PubMed; PMID 23885287.
406. Ferner RE, Gutmann DH. International consensus statement on malignant peripheral nerve sheath tumors in neurofibromatosis. Cancer Res. 2002 Mar;62(5):1573-7. Cited in: PubMed; PMID 11894862.
407. Ferreira J, Esteves G, Fonseca R, et al. Fine-needle aspiration of lipoblastoma: Cytological, molecular, and clinical features. Cancer Cytopathol. 2017 Dec;125(12):934-939. Cited in: PubMed; PMID 28902468.
408. Ferreiro JA, Nascimento AG. Hyaline-cell rich chondroid syringoma. A tumor mimicking malignancy. Am J Surg Pathol. 1995 Aug;19(8):912-7. Cited in: PubMed; PMID 7541966.
409. Fetsch JF, Miettinen M. Sclerosing perineurioma: a clinicopathologic study of 19 cases of a distinctive soft tissue lesion with a predilection for the fingers and palms of young adults. Am J Surg Pathol. 1997 Dec;21(12):1433-42. Cited in: PubMed; PMID 9414186.
410. Fetsch PA, Simsir A, Brosky K, et al. Comparison of three commonly used cytologic preparations in effusion immunocytochemistry. Diagn Cytopathol. 2002 Jan;26(1):61-6. Cited in: PubMed; PMID 11782091.
411. Field AS, Geddie WR. Role of fine needle aspiration biopsy cytology in the diagnosis of infections. Diagn Cytopathol. 2016 Dec;44(12):1024-1038. Cited in: PubMed; PMID 27555237.
412. Field AS, Pitman M, Cree IA, et al. The rationale for the development and publication of the World Health Organization reporting systems for cytopathology and a brief overview of the first editions of the lung and pancreaticobiliary systems. Cancer Cytopathol. 2023 Dec;131(12):751-761. Cited in: PubMed; PMID 37702127.
413. Field AS, Zarka MA. Practical cytopathology: a diagnostic approach to fine needle aspiration biopsy. St. Louis (MO): Elsevier; 2017.
414. Fielding D, Dalley AJ, Bashirzadeh F, et al. Diff-Quik Cytology Smears from Endobronchial Ultrasound Transbronchial Needle Aspiration Lymph Node Specimens as a Source of DNA for Next-Generation Sequencing Instead of Cell Blocks. Respiration. 201997(6):525-539. Cited in: PubMed; PMID 30731462.
415. Finley JL, Silverman JF, Dabbs DJ, et al. Chordoma: diagnosis by fine-needle aspiration biopsy with histologic, immunocytochemical, and ultrastructural confirmation. Diagn Cytopathol. 1986 Dec;2(4):330-7. Cited in: PubMed; PMID 2431849.
416. Finos L, Righi A, Frisoni T, et al. Primary extraskeletal myxoid chondrosarcoma of bone: Report of three cases and review of the literature. Pathol Res Pract. 2017 May;213(5):461-466. Cited in: PubMed; PMID 28249774.
417. Fiore M, Grosso F, Lo Vullo S, et al. Myxoid/round cell and pleomorphic liposarcomas: prognostic factors and survival in a series of patients treated at a single institution. Cancer. 2007 Jun;109(12):2522-31. Cited in: PubMed; PMID 17510918.
418. Fisher C. Myofibrosarcoma. Virchows Arch. 2004 Sep;445(3):215-23. Cited in: PubMed; PMID 15173943.
419. Fisher C. The diversity of soft tissue tumours with EWSR1 gene rearrangements: a review. Histopathology. 2014 Jan;64(1):134-50. Cited in: PubMed; PMID 24320889.
420. Fleshman R, Mayerson J, Wakely PE. Fine-needle aspiration biopsy of high-grade sarcoma: a report of 107 cases. Cancer. 2007 Dec;111(6):491-8. Cited in: PubMed; PMID 17941014.
421. Fletcher CD, Akerman M, Dal Cin P, et al. Correlation between clinicopathological features and karyotype in lipomatous tumors. A report of 178 cases from the Chromosomes and Morphology (CHAMP) Collaborative Study Group. Am J Pathol. 1996 Feb;148(2):623-30. Cited in: PubMed; PMID 8579124.
422. Fletcher CD, Beham A, Bekir S, et al. Epithelioid angiosarcoma of deep soft tissue: a distinctive tumor readily mistaken for an epithelial neoplasm. Am J Surg Pathol. 1991 Oct;15(10):915-24. Cited in: PubMed; PMID 1718176.
423. Fletcher CD, Martin-Bates E. Spindle cell lipoma: a clinicopathological study with some original observations. Histopathology. 1987 Aug;11(8):803-17. Cited in: PubMed; PMID 3623439.
424. Florentine BD, Cohen AN. Nodular sclerosing classical Hodgkin lymphoma masquerading as acute suppurative-necrotizing

lymphadenitis. Diagn Cytopathol. 2014 Mar;42(3):238-41. Cited in: PubMed; PMID 21965120.
425. Flores-Montero J, de Tute R, Paiva B, et al. Immunophenotype of normal vs. myeloma plasma cells: Toward antibody panel specifications for MRD detection in multiple myeloma. Cytometry B Clin Cytom. 2016 Jan;90(1):61-72. Cited in: PubMed; PMID 26100534.
426. Flucke U, Mentzel T, Verdijk MA, et al. EWSR1-ATF1 chimeric transcript in a myoepithelial tumor of soft tissue: a case report. Hum Pathol. 2012 May;43(5):764-8. Cited in: PubMed; PMID 22154050.
427. Flucke U, Palmedo G, Blankenhorn N, et al. EWSR1 gene rearrangement occurs in a subset of cutaneous myoepithelial tumors: a study of 18 cases. Mod Pathol. 2011 Nov;24(11):1444-50. Cited in: PubMed; PMID 21725291.
428. Flucke U, Tops BB, Verdijk MA, et al. NR4A3 rearrangement reliably distinguishes between the clinicopathologically overlapping entities myoepithelial carcinoma of soft tissue and cellular extraskeletal myxoid chondrosarcoma. Virchows Arch. 2012 Jun;460(6):621-8. Cited in: PubMed; PMID 22569967.
429. Flucke U, Vogels RJ, de Saint Aubain Somerhausen N, et al. Epithelioid Hemangioendothelioma: clinicopathologic, immunhistochemical, and molecular genetic analysis of 39 cases. Diagn Pathol. 2014 Jul;9:131. Cited in: PubMed; PMID 24986479.
430. Foley KM, Woodruff JM, Ellis FT, et al. Radiation-induced malignant and atypical peripheral nerve sheath tumors. Ann Neurol. 1980 Apr;7(4):311-8. Cited in: PubMed; PMID 7377756.
431. Folpe AL, Billings SD, McKenney JK, et al. Expression of claudin-1, a recently described tight junction-associated protein, distinguishes soft tissue perineurioma from potential mimics. Am J Surg Pathol. 2002 Dec;26(12):1620-6. Cited in: PubMed; PMID 12459629.
432. Folpe AL, Chand EM, Goldblum JR, et al. Expression of Fli-1, a nuclear transcription factor, distinguishes vascular neoplasms from potential mimics. Am J Surg Pathol. 2001 Aug;25(8):1061-6. Cited in: PubMed; PMID 11474291.
433. Folpe AL, Devaney K, Weiss SW. Lipomatous hemangiopericytoma: a rare variant of hemangiopericytoma that may be confused with liposarcoma. Am J Surg Pathol. 1999 Oct;23(10):1201-7. Cited in: PubMed; PMID 10524520.
434. Folpe AL, Deyrup AT. Alveolar soft-part sarcoma: a review and update. J Clin Pathol. 2006 Nov;59(11):1127-32. Cited in: PubMed; PMID 17071801.
435. Folpe AL, Fanburg-Smith JC, Miettinen M, et al. Atypical and malignant glomus tumors: analysis of 52 cases, with a proposal for the reclassification of glomus tumors. Am J Surg Pathol. 2001 Jan;25(1):1-12. Cited in: PubMed; PMID 11145243.
436. Folpe AL, Goldblum JR, Rubin BP, et al. Morphologic and immunophenotypic diversity in Ewing family tumors: a study of 66 genetically confirmed cases. Am J Surg Pathol. 2005 Aug;29(8):1025-33. Cited in: PubMed; PMID 16006796.
437. Folpe AL, Lane KL, Paull G, et al. Low-grade fibromyxoid sarcoma and hyalinizing spindle cell tumor with giant rosettes: a clinicopathologic study of 73 cases supporting their identity and assessing the impact of high-grade areas. Am J Surg Pathol. 2000 Oct;24(10):1353-60. Cited in: PubMed; PMID 11023096.
438. Folpe AL, McKenney JK, Bridge JA, et al. Sclerosing rhabdomyosarcoma in adults: report of four cases of a hyalinizing, matrix-rich variant of rhabdomyosarcoma that may be confused with osteosarcoma, chondrosarcoma, or angiosarcoma. Am J Surg Pathol. 2002 Sep;26(9):1175-83. Cited in: PubMed; PMID 12218574.
439. Folpe AL, Mentzel T, Lehr HA, et al. Perivascular epithelioid cell neoplasms of soft tissue and gynecologic origin: a clinicopathologic study of 26 cases and review of the literature. Am J Surg Pathol. 2005 Dec;29(12):1558-75. Cited in: PubMed; PMID 16327428.
440. Folpe AL, Tetzlaff MT, Billings SD, et al. Superficial Neurocristic EWSR1::FLI1 Fusion Tumor: A Distinctive, Clinically Indolent, S100 Protein/SOX10-Positive Neoplasm. Mod Pathol. 2024 Aug;37(8):100537. Cited in: PubMed; PMID 38866368.
441. Foo WC, Cruise MW, Wick MR, et al. Immunohistochemical staining for TLE1 distinguishes synovial sarcoma from histologic mimics. Am J Clin Pathol. 2011 Jun;135(6):839-44. Cited in: PubMed; PMID 21571956.
442. Fowler LJ, Lachar WA. Application of immunohistochemistry to cytology. Arch Pathol Lab Med. 2008 Mar;132(3):373-83. Cited in: PubMed; PMID 18318580.
443. French CA, Mentzel T, Kutzner H, et al. Intradermal spindle cell/pleomorphic lipoma: a distinct subset. Am J Dermatopathol. 2000 Dec;22(6):496-502. Cited in: PubMed; PMID 11190440.
444. Frickmann H, Zautner AE, Moter A, et al. Fluorescence in situ hybridization (FISH) in the microbiological diagnostic routine laboratory: a review. Crit Rev Microbiol. 2017 May;43(3):263-293. Cited in: PubMed; PMID 28129707.
445. Friis RB, Safwat A, Baad-Hansen T, et al. Solitary Fibrous Tumour: A Single Institution Retrospective Study and Further Validation of a Prognostic Risk Assessment System. Clin Oncol (R Coll Radiol). 2018 Dec;30(12):798-804. Cited in: PubMed; PMID 30206022.
446. Fritchie KJ, Goldblum JR, Tubbs RR, et al. The expanded histologic spectrum of myxoid liposarcoma with an emphasis on newly described patterns: implications for diagnosis on small biopsy specimens. Am J Clin Pathol. 2012 Feb;137(2):229-39. Cited in: PubMed; PMID 22261448.
447. Fritzsche FR, Bode PK, Moch H, et al. Determination of the Her-2/neu gene amplification status in cytologic breast cancer specimens using automated silver-enhanced in-situ hybridization (SISH). Am J Surg Pathol. 2010 Aug;34(8):1180-5. Cited in: PubMed; PMID 20661016.
448. Fröstad B, Martinsson T, Tani E, et al. The use of fine-needle aspiration cytology in the molecular characterization of neuroblastoma in children. Cancer. 1999 Apr;87(2):60-8. Cited in: PubMed; PMID 10227595.
449. Fröstad B, Tani E, Kogner P, et al. The clinical use of fine needle aspiration cytology for diagnosis and management of children with neuroblastic tumours. Eur J Cancer. 1998 Mar;34(4):529-36. Cited in: PubMed; PMID 9713304.
450. Fuchs J, Dantonello TM, Blumenstock G, et al. Treatment and outcome of patients suffering from perineal/perianal rhabdomyosarcoma: results from the CWS trials--retrospective clinical study. Ann Surg. 2014 Jun;259(6):1166-72. Cited in: PubMed; PMID 24045440.
451. Fügen A, Elif S, Gülistan G, et al. Fine-needle aspiration cytology of a mammary myofibroblastoma: A case report on the role of immunohistochemistry and cell block preparations and a review of the literature. Diagn Cytopathol. 2016 Dec;44(12):1064-1069. Cited in: PubMed; PMID 27458002.
452. Fukuda Y, Miyake H, Masuda Y, et al. Histogenesis of unique elastinophilic fibers of elastofibroma: ultrastructural and immunohistochemical studies. Hum Pathol. 1987 May;18(5):424-9. Cited in: PubMed; PMID 3552953.
453. Fukunaga M. Expression of D2-40 in lymphatic endothelium of normal tissues and in vascular tumours. Histopathology. 2005 Apr;46(4):396-402. Cited in: PubMed; PMID 15810951.
454. Furlong MA, Fanburg-Smith JC, Miettinen M. The morphologic spectrum of hibernoma: a clinicopathologic study of 170 cases. Am J Surg Pathol. 2001 Jun;25(6):809-14. Cited in: PubMed; PMID 11395560.
455. Furlong MA, Mentzel T, Fanburg-Smith JC. Pleomorphic rhabdomyosarcoma in adults: a clinicopathologic study of 38 cases with emphasis on morphologic variants and recent skeletal muscle-specific markers. Mod Pathol. 2001 Jun;14(6):595-603. Cited in: PubMed; PMID 11406662.
456. Gaballah AH, Jensen CT, Palmquist S, et al. Angiosarcoma: clinical and imaging features from head to toe. Br J Radiol. 2017 Jul;90(1075):20170039. Cited in: PubMed; PMID 28471264.
457. Gaertner EM, Steinberg DM, Huber M, et al. Pulmonary and mediastinal glomus tumors--report of five cases including a pulmonary glomangiosarcoma: a clinicopathologic study with literature review. Am J Surg Pathol. 2000 Aug;24(8):1105-14. Cited in: PubMed; PMID 10935651.
458. Gaetke-Udager K, Yablon CM, Lucas DR, et al. Myxoinflammatory fibroblastic sarcoma: spectrum of disease and imaging presentation. Skeletal Radiol. 2016 Mar;45(3):347-56. Cited in: PubMed; PMID 26563559.
459. Gaffney EF, Dervan PA, Fletcher CD. Pleomorphic rhabdomyosarcoma in adulthood. Analysis of 11 cases with definition of diagnostic criteria. Am J Surg Pathol. 1993 Jun;17(6):601-9. Cited in: PubMed; PMID 8333559.
460. Gajdzis P, Brisse HJ, Klijanienko J. Diagnostic performance of fine-needle aspiration in soft tissue tumors: Application of the World Health Organization System for Reporting Soft Tissue Cytopathology and risk of malignancy assessment. Cancer Cytopathol. 2024 Aug. Cited in: PubMed; PMID 39212584.
461. Gajdzis P, Laé M, Klijanienko J. FNA of epithelioid sarcoma: Curie Institute experience and critical review of the literature. Cancer Cytopathol. 2018 Nov;126(11):934-941. Cited in: PubMed; PMID 30291790.
462. Gajdzis P, Laé M, Pierron G, et al. Fine-Needle Aspiration Features of BCOR-CCNB3 Sarcoma. Am J Clin Pathol. 2020 Feb;153(3):315-321. Cited in: PubMed; PMID 31679010.
463. Gajdzis P, Pierron G, Klijanienko J. Cytology of Undifferentiated Round-Cell Sarcomas of Bone and Soft Tissue: Ewing Sarcoma or Not Ewing Sarcoma, That Is the Question. Acta Cytol. 202266(4):295-306. Cited in: PubMed; PMID 34515032.
464. Galliani CA, Bisceglia M, Del Giudice A, et al. Desmoplastic Small Round Cell Tumor of the Kidney: Report of a Case, Literature Review, and Comprehensive Discussion of the Distinctive Morphologic, Immunohistochemical, and Molecular Features in the Differential Diagnosis of Small Round Cell Tumors Affecting the Kidney. Adv Anat Pathol. 2020 Nov;27(6):408-421. Cited in: PubMed; PMID 32804706.
465. Gambarotti M, Benini S, Gamberi G, et al. CIC-DUX4 fusion-positive round-cell sarcomas of soft tissue and bone: a single-institution morphological and molecular analysis of seven cases. Histopathology. 2016 Oct;69(4):624-34. Cited in: PubMed; PMID 27079694.
466. Gamborino E, Carrilho C, Ferro J, et al. Fine-needle aspiration diagnosis of Kaposi's sarcoma in a developing country. Diagn Cytopathol. 2000 Nov;23(5):322-5. Cited in: PubMed; PMID 11074626.
467. Gandhi A, Mahajan G, Sharma S. Chondroid lipoma mimicking pleomorphic adenoma on cytology. Diagn Cytopathol. 2013 Nov;41(11):1012-3. Cited in: PubMed; PMID 22711496.
468. Ganick DJ, Silverman JF, Holbrook CT, et al. Clinical utility of fine needle aspiration in the diagnosis and management of neuroblastoma. Med Pediatr Oncol. 198816(2):101-6. Cited in: PubMed; PMID 3352532.
469. Gantzer J, Di Marco A, Fabacher T, et al. Conformity to Clinical Practice Guidelines at Initial Management in Adult Soft Tissue and Visceral Tumors since the Implementation of the NetSarc Network in Eastern France. Oncologist. 2019 Aug;24(8):e775-e783. Cited in: PubMed; PMID 31073021.
470. García-Prats MD, Vargas J, De Agustín P. Diagnosis of malignant melanoma of soft parts in a nodal metastasis by fine needle aspiration cytology. Acta Cytol. 199337(5):848-50. Cited in: PubMed; PMID 8362598.
471. Gartner L, Pearce CJ, Saifuddin A. The role of the plain radiograph in the characterisation of soft tissue tumours. Skeletal Radiol. 2009 Jun;38(6):549-58. Cited in: PubMed; PMID 18566812.
472. Gasparotto D, Rossi S, Polano M, et al. Quadruple-Negative GIST Is a Sentinel for Unrecognized Neurofibromatosis Type 1 Syndrome. Clin Cancer Res. 2017 Jan;23(1):273-282. Cited in: PubMed; PMID 27390349.
473. Gaumann A, Petrow P, Mentzel T, et al. Osteopontin expression in primary sarcomas of the pulmonary artery. Virchows Arch. 2001 Nov;439(5):668-74. Cited in: PubMed; PMID 11764388.
474. Gebhard S, Coindre JM, Michels JJ, et al. Pleomorphic liposarcoma: clinicopathologic, immunohistochemical, and follow-up analysis of 63 cases: a study from the French Federation of Cancer Centers Sarcoma Group. Am J Surg Pathol. 2002 May;26(5):601-16. Cited in: PubMed; PMID 11979090.
475. Geller RL, Hookim K, Sullivan HC, et al. Cytologic features of angiosarcoma: A review of 26 cases diagnosed on FNA. Cancer Cytopathol. 2016 Sep;124(9):659-68. Cited in: PubMed; PMID 27088896.
476. Gentles C, Perin J, Berrey H, et al. Soft-tissue chondroma. Orthopedics. 2007 Mar;30(3):180, 241-3. Cited in: PubMed; PMID 17375540.
477. George B, Rivera Rolon MDM, Clement CG. Role of fine-needle aspiration cytology in early diagnosis of fungal infections. Diagn Cytopathol. 2020 Jul;48(7):645-651. Cited in: PubMed; PMID 32352648.
478. Gerleman R, Mortensen MB, Detlefsen S. Desmoid Tumor of the Pancreas: Case Report and Review of a Rare Entity. Int J Surg Pathol. 2015 Oct;23(7):579-84. Cited in: PubMed; PMID 26215223.
479. Ghadimi MP, Liu P, Peng T, et al. Pleomorphic liposarcoma: clinical observations and molecular variables. Cancer. 2011 Dec;117(23):5359-69. Cited in: PubMed; PMID 21598240.
480. Ghanem N, Altehoefer C, Furtwängler A, et al. Computed tomography in gastrointestinal stromal tumors. Eur Radiol. 2003 Jul;13(7):1669-78. Cited in: PubMed; PMID 12835984.
481. Gholami S, Cassidy MR, Kirane A, et al. Size and Location are the Most Important Risk Factors for Malignant Behavior in Resected Solitary Fibrous Tumors. Ann Surg Oncol. 2017 Dec;24(13):3865-3871. Cited in: PubMed; PMID 29039030.
482. Ghosh M, Islam N, Saha H, et al. Cytodiagnosis of inflammatory myofibroblastic tumor: A report of three cases in infants. Diagn

Cytopathol. 2018 Sep;46(9):776-781. Cited in: PubMed; PMID 29673102.
483. Giannikopoulos P, Parham DM. Rhabdomyosarcoma: How Advanced Molecular Methods Are Shaping the Diagnostic and Therapeutic Paradigm. Pediatr Dev Pathol. 202124(5):395-404. Cited in: PubMed; PMID 34107813.
484. Giannini C, Scheithauer BW, Jenkins RB, et al. Soft-tissue perineurioma. Evidence for an abnormality of chromosome 22, criteria for diagnosis, and review of the literature. Am J Surg Pathol. 1997 Feb;21(2):164-73. Cited in: PubMed; PMID 9042282.
485. Gibson TC, Bishop JA, Thompson LD. Parotid Gland Nodular Fasciitis: A Clinicopathologic Series of 12 Cases with a Review of 18 Cases from the Literature. Head Neck Pathol. 2015 Sep;9(3):334-44. Cited in: PubMed; PMID 25472697.
486. Gielen JL, De Schepper AM, Vanhoenacker F, et al. Accuracy of MRI in characterization of soft tissue tumors and tumor-like lesions. A prospective study in 548 patients. Eur Radiol. 2004 Dec;14(12):2320-30. Cited in: PubMed; PMID 15290067.
488. Gisselsson D, Hibbard MK, Dal Cin P, et al. PLAG1 alterations in lipoblastoma: involvement in varied mesenchymal cell types and evidence for alternative oncogenic mechanisms. Am J Pathol. 2001 Sep;159(3):955-62. Cited in: PubMed; PMID 11549588.
489. Gladdy RA, Qin LX, Moraco N, et al. Do radiation-associated soft tissue sarcomas have the same prognosis as sporadic soft tissue sarcomas? J Clin Oncol. 2010 Apr;28(12):2064-9. Cited in: PubMed; PMID 20308666.
490. Gladdy RA, Qin LX, Moraco N, et al. Predictors of survival and recurrence in primary leiomyosarcoma. Ann Surg Oncol. 2013 Jun;20(6):1851-7. Cited in: PubMed; PMID 23354568.
491. Gleason BC, Fletcher CD. Myoepithelial carcinoma of soft tissue in children: an aggressive neoplasm analyzed in a series of 29 cases. Am J Surg Pathol. 2007 Dec;31(12):1813-24. Cited in: PubMed; PMID 18043035.
492. Gleason BC, Hornick JL. Inflammatory myofibroblastic tumours: where are we now? J Clin Pathol. 2008 Apr;61(4):428-37. Cited in: PubMed; PMID 17938159.
493. Gleeson FC, Kipp BR, Kerr SE, et al. Kinase genotype analysis of gastric gastrointestinal stromal tumor cytology samples using targeted next-generation sequencing. Clin Gastroenterol Hepatol. 2015 Jan;13(1):202-6. Cited in: PubMed; PMID 24997326.
494. Gochhait D, Dey P, Rajwanshi A, et al. Spectrum of fungal and parasitic infections on fine needle aspiration cytology. Diagn Cytopathol. 2015 Jun;43(6):450-5. Cited in: PubMed; PMID 25605666.
495. Goetz SP, Robinson RA, Landas SK. Extraskeletal myxoid chondrosarcoma of the pleura. Report of a case clinically simulating mesothelioma. Am J Clin Pathol. 1992 Apr;97(4):498-502. Cited in: PubMed; PMID 1553915.
496. Goldblum JR, Reith JD, Weiss SW. Sarcomas arising in dermatofibrosarcoma protuberans: a reappraisal of biologic behavior in eighteen cases treated by wide local excision with extended clinical follow up. Am J Surg Pathol. 2000 Aug;24(8):1125-30. Cited in: PubMed; PMID 10935653.
497. Goldblum JR, Tuthill RJ. CD34 and factor-XIIIa immunoreactivity in dermatofibrosarcoma protuberans and dermatofibroma. Am J Dermatopathol. 1997 Apr;19(2):147-53. Cited in: PubMed; PMID 9129699.
498. Gomes AL, Bardales RH, Milanezi F, et al. Molecular analysis of c-Kit and PDGFRA in GISTs diagnosed by EUS. Am J Clin Pathol. 2007 Jan;127(1):89-96. Cited in: PubMed; PMID 17145623.
499. González-Cámpora R, Muñoz-Arias G, Otal-Salaverri C, et al. Fine needle aspiration cytology of primary soft tissue tumors. Morphologic analysis of the most frequent types. Acta Cytol. 199236(6):905-17. Cited in: PubMed; PMID 1449029.
500. Gonzalez-Cámpora R, Ríos-Martín JJ, Solórzano-Amoretti A, et al. Fine needle aspiration cytology of an acral myxoinflammatory fibroblastic sarcoma: case report with cytological and cytogenetic findings. Cytopathology. 2008 Apr;19(2):118-23. Cited in: PubMed; PMID 17511780.
501. Gonzalez-Santiago TM, Drage LA. Nontuberculous Mycobacteria: Skin and Soft Tissue Infections. Dermatol Clin. 2015 Jul;33(3):563-77. Cited in: PubMed; PMID 26143432.
502. Goodlad JR, Mentzel T, Fletcher CD. Low grade fibromyxoid sarcoma: clinicopathological analysis of eleven new cases in support of a distinct entity. Histopathology. 1995 Mar;26(3):229-37. Cited in: PubMed; PMID 7797200.
503. Gordon A, McManus A, Anderson J, et al. Chromosomal imbalances in pleomorphic rhabdomyosarcomas and identification of the alveolar rhabdomyosarcoma-associated PAX3-FOXO1A fusion gene in one case. Cancer Genet Cytogenet. 2003 Jan;140(1):73-7. Cited in: PubMed; PMID 12550764.
504. Graadt van Roggen JF, McMenamin ME, Belchis DA, et al. Reticular perineurioma: a distinctive variant of soft tissue perineurioma. Am J Surg Pathol. 2001 Apr;25(4):485-93. Cited in: PubMed; PMID 11257623.
505. Graadt van Roggen JF, Mooi WJ, Hogendoorn PC. Clear cell sarcoma of tendons and aponeuroses (malignant melanoma of soft parts) and cutaneous melanoma: exploring the histogenetic relationship between these two clinicopathological entities. J Pathol. 1998 Sep;186(1):3-7. Cited in: PubMed; PMID 9875133.
506. Granter SR, Weilbaecher KN, Quigley C, et al. Clear cell sarcoma shows immunoreactivity for microphthalmia transcription factor: further evidence for melanocytic differentiation. Mod Pathol. 2001 Jan;14(1):6-9. Cited in: PubMed; PMID 11211309.
507. Grass J, Majenka P, Sedlaczek OL, et al. Granulomatous Reaction to Cosmetic Soft Tissue Filler with Late-onset Inflammatory Response. Acta Derm Venereol. 2020 Aug;100(15):adv00243. Cited in: PubMed; PMID 32725258.
508. Griffiths HJ, Burke J, Bonfiglio TA. Granulomatous pseudotumors in total joint replacement. Skeletal Radiol. 198716(2):146-52. Cited in: PubMed; PMID 3554529.
509. Gronchi A, Miah AB, Dei Tos AP, et al. Soft tissue and visceral sarcomas: ESMO-EURACAN-GENTURIS Clinical Practice Guidelines for diagnosis, treatment and follow-up. Ann Oncol. 2021 Nov;32(11):1348-1365. Cited in: PubMed; PMID 34303806.
510. Gross JM, Perret R, Coindre JM, et al. Lipoblastoma-Like Tumor and Fibrosarcoma-Like Lipomatous Neoplasm Represent the Same Entity: A Clinicopathologic and Molecular Genetic Study of 23 Cases Occurring in Both Men and Women at Diverse Locations. Mod Pathol. 2023 Sep;36(9):100246. Cited in: PubMed; PMID 37307874.
511. Grünewald TGP, Cidre-Aranaz F, Surdez D, et al. Ewing sarcoma. Nat Rev Dis Primers. 2018 Jul;4(1):5. Cited in: PubMed; PMID 29977059.
512. Gu M, Nguyen PT, Cao S, et al. Diagnosis of gastric glomus tumor by endoscopic ultrasound-guided fine needle aspiration biopsy. A case report with cytologic, histologic and immunohistochemical studies. Acta Cytol. 200246(3):560-6. Cited in: PubMed; PMID 12040654.
513. Gui H, Lhospital E, Staddon AP, et al. Combined Sclerosing and Spindle Cell Rhabdomyosarcoma in Previous Craniotomy Site: A Case Report and a Review of the Literature. Int J Surg Pathol. 2019 May;27(3):328-335. Cited in: PubMed; PMID 30270691.
514. Guillou L, Benhattar J, Bonichon F, et al. Histologic grade, but not SYT-SSX fusion type, is an important prognostic factor in patients with synovial sarcoma: a multicenter, retrospective analysis. J Clin Oncol. 2004 Oct;22(20):4040-50. Cited in: PubMed; PMID 15364967.
515. Guillou L, Benhattar J, Gengler C, et al. Translocation-positive low-grade fibromyxoid sarcoma: clinicopathologic and molecular analysis of a series expanding the morphologic spectrum and suggesting potential relationship to sclerosing epithelioid fibrosarcoma: a study from the French Sarcoma Group. Am J Surg Pathol. 2007 Sep;31(9):1387-402. Cited in: PubMed; PMID 17721195.
516. Guillou L, Gebhard S, Coindre JM. Lipomatous hemangiopericytoma: a fat-containing variant of solitary fibrous tumor? Clinicopathologic, immunohistochemical, and ultrastructural analysis of a series in favor of a unifying concept. Hum Pathol. 2000 Sep;31(9):1108-15. Cited in: PubMed; PMID 11014579.
517. Guillou L, Gebhard S, Coindre JM. Orbital and extraorbital giant cell angiofibroma: a giant cell-rich variant of solitary fibrous tumor? Clinicopathologic and immunohistochemical analysis of a series in favor of a unifying concept. Am J Surg Pathol. 2000 Jul;24(7):971-9. Cited in: PubMed; PMID 10895819.
518. Guillou L, Wadden C, Coindre JM, et al. "Proximal-type" epithelioid sarcoma, a distinctive aggressive neoplasm showing rhabdoid features. Clinicopathologic, immunohistochemical, and ultrastructural study of a series. Am J Surg Pathol. 1997 Feb;21(2):130-46. Cited in: PubMed; PMID 9042279.
519. Guiter GE, Gamboni MM, Zakowski MF. The cytology of extraskeletal Ewing sarcoma. Cancer. 1999 Jun;87(3):141-8. Cited in: PubMed; PMID 10385445.
520. Gülhan B, Küpeli S, Yalçin B, et al. An unusual presentation of infantile fibrosarcoma in a male newborn. Am J Perinatol. 2009 May;26(5):331-3. Cited in: PubMed; PMID 19067284.
521. Gunawan B, von Heydebreck A, Sander B, et al. An oncogenetic tree model in gastrointestinal stromal tumours (GISTs) identifies different pathways of cytogenetic evolution with prognostic implications. J Pathol. 2007 Mar;211(4):463-70. Cited in: PubMed; PMID 17226762.
522. Gunaydin SD, Arikan-Akdagli S, Akova M. Fungal infections of the skin and soft tissue. Curr Opin Infect Dis. 2020 Apr;33(2):130-136. Cited in: PubMed; PMID 31990815.
523. Guo T, Zhang L, Chang NE, et al. Consistent MYC and FLT4 gene amplification in radiation-induced angiosarcoma but not in other radiation-associated atypical vascular lesions. Genes Chromosomes Cancer. 2011 Jan;50(1):25-33. Cited in: PubMed; PMID 20949568.
524. Guo Z, Voytovich M, Kurtycz DF, et al. Fine-needle aspiration diagnosis of spindle-cell lipoma: a case report and review of the literature. Diagn Cytopathol. 2000 Nov;23(5):362-5. Cited in: PubMed; PMID 11074636.
525. Gupta K, Dey P, Goldsmith R, et al. Comparison of cytologic features of giant-cell tumor and giant-cell tumor of tendon sheath. Diagn Cytopathol. 2004 Jan;30(1):14-8. Cited in: PubMed; PMID 14696139.
526. Gupta K, Dey P, Vashisht R. Fine-needle aspiration cytology of malignant peripheral nerve sheath tumors. Diagn Cytopathol. 2004 Jul;31(1):1-4. Cited in: PubMed; PMID 15236255.
527. Gupta N, Barwad A, Katamuthu K, et al. Solitary fibrous tumour: a diagnostic challenge for the cytopathologist. Cytopathology. 2012 Aug;23(4):250-5. Cited in: PubMed; PMID 21658137.
528. Gupta N, Rajwanshi A, Mohindra S, et al. Diagnosis of adult rhabdomyoma by fine needle aspiration cytology: a report of 2 cases. Acta Cytol. 201054(5 Suppl):968-72. Cited in: PubMed; PMID 21053579.
529. Gupta R, Mathur SR, Singh P, et al. Cellular mesoblastic nephroma in an infant: report of the cytologic diagnosis of a rare paediatric renal tumor. Diagn Cytopathol. 2009 May;37(5):377-80. Cited in: PubMed; PMID 19217046.
530. Gupta RK, Naran S, Selby RE. Fine needle aspiration cytodiagnosis of subcutaneous fat necrosis of newborn. A case report. Acta Cytol. 199539(4):759-61. Cited in: PubMed; PMID 7631551.
531. Gupta S, Gupta R, Sodhani P. Spindle cell lipoma with predominant nerve sheath tumor-like areas: A potential diagnostic pitfall on aspiration cytology. Diagn Cytopathol. 2015 Dec;43(12):1017-9. Cited in: PubMed; PMID 26457887.
533. Haihua R, Xiaobing W, Jie P, et al. Retrospective analysis of 73 cases of elastofibroma. Ann R Coll Surg Engl. 2020 Feb;102(2):84-93. Cited in: PubMed; PMID 31233334.
534. Hallor KH, Sciot R, Staaf J, et al. Two genetic pathways, t(1;10) and amplification of 3p11-12, in myxoinflammatory fibroblastic sarcoma, haemosiderotic fibrolipomatous tumour, and morphologically similar lesions. J Pathol. 2009 Apr;217(5):716-27. Cited in: PubMed; PMID 19199331.
535. Handa U, Palta A, Mohan H, et al. Aspiration cytology of glomus tumor: a case report. Acta Cytol. 200145(6):1073-6. Cited in: PubMed; PMID 11726106.
536. Haniball J, Sumathi VP, Kindblom LG, et al. Prognostic factors and metastatic patterns in primary myxoid/round-cell liposarcoma. Sarcoma. 20112011:538085. Cited in: PubMed; PMID 22190864.
537. Hanna SA, Tirabosco R, Amin A, et al. Dedifferentiated chordoma: a report of four cases arising 'de novo'. J Bone Joint Surg Br. 2008 May;90(5):652-6. Cited in: PubMed; PMID 18450635.
538. Hanna SL, Kaste S, Jenkins JJ, et al. Epithelioid sarcoma: clinical, MR imaging and pathologic findings. Skeletal Radiol. 2002 Jul;31(7):400-12. Cited in: PubMed; PMID 12107573.
539. Hansen T, Pedersen H, Brauner V, et al. Control specimens for immunocytochemistry in liquid-based cytology. Cytopathology. 2011 Aug;22(4):243-6. Cited in: PubMed; PMID 20482720.
540. Harigopal M, Seshan SV, DeLellis RA, et al. Aspiration cytology of elastofibroma dorsi: case report with ultrastructural and immunohistochemical findings. Diagn Cytopathol. 2002 May;26(5):310-3. Cited in: PubMed; PMID 11992374.
541. Harp E, Caraway NP. FNA of thyroid granular cell tumor. Diagn Cytopathol. 2013 Sep;41(9):825-8. Cited in: PubMed; PMID 22508678.
543. Hart J, Gardner JM, Edgar M, et al. Epithelioid Schwannomas: An Analysis of 58 Cases Including Atypical Variants. Am J Surg Pathol. 2016 May;40(5):704-13. Cited in: PubMed; PMID 26752543.
544. Hasegawa T, Matsuno Y, Shimoda T, et al. Proximal-type epithelioid sarcoma: a clinicopathologic study of 20 cases. Mod Pathol. 2001 Jul;14(7):655-63. Cited in: PubMed; PMID 11454997.
546. Hashimoto H, Tsuneyoshi M, Daimaru Y, et al. Intramuscular myxoma. A clinicopathologic, immunohistochemical, and

electron microscopic study. Cancer. 1986 Aug;58(3):740-7. Cited in: PubMed; PMID 3524794.

547. Hawkins DS, Chi YY, Anderson JR, et al. Addition of Vincristine and Irinotecan to Vincristine, Dactinomycin, and Cyclophosphamide Does Not Improve Outcome for Intermediate-Risk Rhabdomyosarcoma: A Report From the Children's Oncology Group. J Clin Oncol. 2018 Sep;36(27):2770-2777. Cited in: PubMed; PMID 30091945.

548. Hawley IC, Krausz T, Evans DJ, et al. Spindle cell lipoma--a pseudoangiomatous variant. Histopathology. 1994 Jun;24(6):565-9. Cited in: PubMed; PMID 8063285.

550. Hayeri MR, Ziai P, Shehata ML, et al. Soft-Tissue Infections and Their Imaging Mimics: From Cellulitis to Necrotizing Fasciitis. Radiographics. 2016 Oct;36(6):1888-1910. Cited in: PubMed; PMID 27726741.

551. Hayes-Jordan A, LaQuaglia MP, Modak S. Management of desmoplastic small round cell tumor. Semin Pediatr Surg. 2016 Oct;25(5):299-304. Cited in: PubMed; PMID 27955733.

552. Hays DM, Newton W, Soule EH, et al. Mortality among children with rhabdomyosarcomas of the alveolar histologic subtype. J Pediatr Surg. 1983 Aug;18(4):412-7. Cited in: PubMed; PMID 6620082.

553. Heinrich MC, Corless CL, Duensing A, et al. PDGFRA activating mutations in gastrointestinal stromal tumors. Science. 2003 Jan;299(5607):708-10. Cited in: PubMed; PMID 12522257.

554. Henke AC, Salomao DR, Hughes JH. Cellular schwannoma mimics a sarcoma: an example of a potential pitfall in aspiration cytodiagnosis. Diagn Cytopathol. 1999 May;20(5):312-6. Cited in: PubMed; PMID 10319235.

555. Henricks WH, Chu YC, Goldblum JR, et al. Dedifferentiated liposarcoma: a clinicopathological analysis of 155 cases with a proposal for an expanded definition of dedifferentiation. Am J Surg Pathol. 1997 Mar;21(3):271-81. Cited in: PubMed; PMID 9060596.

556. Hernández JL, Rodríguez-Parets JO, Valero JM, et al. High-resolution genome-wide analysis of chromosomal alterations in elastofibroma. Virchows Arch. 2010 Jun;456(6):681-7. Cited in: PubMed; PMID 20422214.

557. Hernández-Ortiz MJ, Valenzuela-Ruiz P, Gonzalez-Estecha A, et al. Fine needle aspiration cytology of primary epithelioid sarcoma of the vulva. A case report. Acta Cytol. 199539(1):100-3. Cited in: PubMed; PMID 7846995.

558. Hewer E, Schmitt AM. Ultrafast Toluidine Blue Staining for Rapid On-Site Evaluation of Cytological Smears. Acta Cytol. 202064(4):375-377. Cited in: PubMed; PMID 31962321.

559. Hibbard MK, Kozakewich HP, Dal Cin P, et al. PLAG1 fusion oncogenes in lipoblastoma. Cancer Res. 2000 Sep;60(17):4869-72. Cited in: PubMed; PMID 10987300.

560. Hibbitts E, Chi YY, Hawkins DS, et al. Refinement of risk stratification for childhood rhabdomyosarcoma using FOXO1 fusion status in addition to established clinical outcome predictors: A report from the Children's Oncology Group. Cancer Med. 2019 Oct;8(14):6437-6448. Cited in: PubMed; PMID 31456361.

561. Hicks J, Dilley A, Patel D, et al. Lipoblastoma and lipoblastomatosis in infancy and childhood: histopathologic, ultrastructural, and cytogenetic features. Ultrastruct Pathol. 200125(4):321-33. Cited in: PubMed; PMID 11577778.

562. Hill DA, Pfeifer JD, Marley EF, et al. WT1 staining reliably differentiates desmoplastic small round cell tumor from Ewing sarcoma/ primitive neuroectodermal tumor. An immunohistochemical and molecular diagnostic study. Am J Clin Pathol. 2000 Sep;114(3):345-53. Cited in: PubMed; PMID 10989634.

563. Hirose T, Scheithauer BW, Sano T. Perineurial malignant peripheral nerve sheath tumor (MPNST): a clinicopathologic, immunohistochemical, and ultrastructural study of seven cases. Am J Surg Pathol. 1998 Nov;22(11):1368-78. Cited in: PubMed; PMID 9808129.

564. Hirota S, Isozaki K, Moriyama Y, et al. Gain-of-function mutations of c-kit in human gastrointestinal stromal tumors. Science. 1998 Jan;279(5350):577-80. Cited in: PubMed; PMID 9438854.

565. Hisaoka M, Ishida T, Kuo TT, et al. Clear cell sarcoma of soft tissue: a clinicopathologic, immunohistochemical, and molecular analysis of 33 cases. Am J Surg Pathol. 2008 Mar;32(3):452-60. Cited in: PubMed; PMID 18300804.

566. Hodge JC, Pearce KE, Wang X, et al. Molecular cytogenetic analysis for TFE3 rearrangement in Xp11.2 renal cell carcinoma and alveolar soft part sarcoma: validation and clinical experience with 75 cases. Mod Pathol. 2014 Jan;27(1):113-27. Cited in: PubMed; PMID 23828314.

567. Hoekstra HJ, Haas RLM, Verhoef C, et al. Adherence to Guidelines for Adult (Non-GIST) Soft Tissue Sarcoma in the Netherlands: A Plea for Dedicated Sarcoma Centers. Ann Surg Oncol. 2017 Oct;24(11):3279-3288. Cited in: PubMed; PMID 28748443.

568. Hofvander J, Jo VY, Ghanei I, et al. Comprehensive genetic analysis of a paediatric pleomorphic myxoid liposarcoma reveals near-haploidization and loss of the RB1 gene. Histopathology. 2016 Jul;69(1):141-147. Cited in: PubMed; PMID 26647907.

569. Holck S, Bredesen JL. Solid glomus tumor presenting as an axillary mass: report of a case with morphologic study, including cytologic characteristics. Acta Cytol. 199640(3):555-62. Cited in: PubMed; PMID 8669195.

570. Hombal SM. Fine needle aspiration cytology of malignant melanoma of soft parts: a case report and literature review. Cytopathology. 2000 Feb;11(1):61-6. Cited in: PubMed; PMID 10714378.

571. Hondar Wu HT, Chen W, Lee O, et al. Imaging and pathological correlation of soft-tissue chondroma: a serial five-case study and literature review. Clin Imaging. 200630(1):32-6. Cited in: PubMed; PMID 16377482.

572. Hoot AC, Russo P, Judkins AR, et al. Immunohistochemical analysis of hSNF5/ INI1 distinguishes renal and extra-renal malignant rhabdoid tumors from other pediatric soft tissue tumors. Am J Surg Pathol. 2004 Nov;28(11):1485-91. Cited in: PubMed; PMID 15489652.

573. Hornick JL. Limited biopsies of soft tissue tumors: the contemporary role of immunohistochemistry and molecular diagnostics. Mod Pathol. 2019 Jan;32(Suppl 1):27-37. Cited in: PubMed; PMID 30600320.

574. Hornick JL. Subclassification of pleomorphic sarcomas: How and why should we care? Ann Diagn Pathol. 2018 Dec;37:118-124. Cited in: PubMed; PMID 30340082.

575. Hornick JL, Bosenberg MW, Mentzel T, et al. Pleomorphic liposarcoma: clinicopathologic analysis of 57 cases. Am J Surg Pathol. 2004 Oct;28(10):1257-67. Cited in: PubMed; PMID 15371941.

576. Hornick JL, Dal Cin P, Fletcher CD. Loss of INI1 expression is characteristic of both conventional and proximal-type epithelioid sarcoma. Am J Surg Pathol. 2009 Apr;33(4):542-50. Cited in: PubMed; PMID 19033866.

577. Hornick JL, Fletcher CD. Cutaneous myoepithelioma: a clinicopathologic and immunohistochemical study of 14 cases. Hum Pathol. 2004 Jan;35(1):14-24. Cited in: PubMed; PMID 14745720.

578. Hornick JL, Fletcher CD. Intraarticular nodular fasciitis--a rare lesion: clinicopathologic analysis of a series. Am J Surg Pathol. 2006 Feb;30(2):237-41. Cited in: PubMed; PMID 16434899.

579. Hornick JL, Fletcher CD. Myoepithelial tumors of soft tissue: a clinicopathologic and immunohistochemical study of 101 cases with evaluation of prognostic parameters. Am J Surg Pathol. 2003 Sep;27(9):1183-96. Cited in: PubMed; PMID 12960802.

580. Hornick JL, Fletcher CD. PEComa: what do we know so far? Histopathology. 2006 Jan;48(1):75-82. Cited in: PubMed; PMID 16359539.

581. Hornick JL, Fletcher CD. Soft tissue perineurioma: clinicopathologic analysis of 81 cases including those with atypical histologic features. Am J Surg Pathol. 2005 Jul;29(7):845-58. Cited in: PubMed; PMID 15958848.

582. Hornick JL, Nielsen GP. Beyond "Triton": Malignant Peripheral Nerve Sheath Tumors With Complete Heterologous Rhabdomyoblastic Differentiation Mimicking Spindle Cell Rhabdomyosarcoma. Am J Surg Pathol. 2019 Oct;43(10):1323-1330. Cited in: PubMed; PMID 31107719.

583. Hoshi M, Oebisu N, Iwai T, et al. Review of the referral documents of patients with malignant soft tissue tumors. Sci Rep. 2022 Nov;12(1):19527. Cited in: PubMed; PMID 36376458.

584. Hosler GA, Steinberg DM, Sheth S, et al. Inflammatory pseudotumor: a diagnostic dilemma in cytopathology. Diagn Cytopathol. 2004 Oct;31(4):267-70. Cited in: PubMed; PMID 15452903.

585. Hostein I, Andraud-Fregeville M, Guillou L, et al. Rhabdomyosarcoma: value of myogenin expression analysis and molecular testing in diagnosing the alveolar subtype: an analysis of 109 paraffin-embedded specimens. Cancer. 2004 Dec;101(12):2817-24. Cited in: PubMed; PMID 15536621.

586. Hottenrott G, Mentzel T, Peters A, et al. Intravascular ("intimal") epithelioid angiosarcoma: clinicopathological and immunohistochemical analysis of three cases. Virchows Arch. 1999 Nov;435(5):473-8. Cited in: PubMed; PMID 10592050.

587. Hourani R, Taslakian B, Shabb NS, et al. Fibroblastic and myofibroblastic tumors of the head and neck: comprehensive imaging-based review with pathologic correlation. Eur J Radiol. 2015 Feb;84(2):250-60. Cited in: PubMed; PMID 25467227.

588. Housini I, Dabbs DJ. Fine needle aspiration cytology of perineurioma. Report of a case with histologic, immunohistochemical and ultrastructural studies. Acta Cytol. 199034(3):420-4. Cited in: PubMed; PMID 2160770.

589. Howitt BE, Fletcher CD. Mammary-type Myofibroblastoma: Clinicopathologic Characterization in a Series of 143 Cases. Am J Surg Pathol. 2016 Mar;40(3):361-7. Cited in: PubMed; PMID 26523539.

590. Hu J, Tipps AMP, Hasteh F, et al. Intranodal palisaded myofibroblastoma of para-esophageal lymph node: Case report with cytologic and histologic findings. Diagn Cytopathol. 2019 Dec;47(12):1306-1309. Cited in: PubMed; PMID 31400261.

591. Huang EC, Ghazikhanian V, Qian X. Giant cell-rich osteosarcoma of the parotid gland: An exceptionally rare entity at an unusual site. Diagn Cytopathol. 2016 Dec;44(12):1107-1111. Cited in: PubMed; PMID 27561385.

592. Huang HY, Antonescu CR. Sinonasal smooth muscle cell tumors: a clinicopathologic and immunohistochemical analysis of 12 cases with emphasis on the low-grade end of the spectrum. Arch Pathol Lab Med. 2003 Mar;127(3):297-304. Cited in: PubMed; PMID 12653572.

593. Huang HY, Brennan MF, Singer S, et al. Distant metastasis in retroperitoneal dedifferentiated liposarcoma is rare and rapidly fatal: a clinicopathological study with emphasis on the low-grade myxofibrosarcoma-like pattern as an early sign of dedifferentiation. Mod Pathol. 2005 Jul;18(7):976-84. Cited in: PubMed; PMID 15832195.

594. Huang HY, Lal P, Qin J, et al. Low-grade myxofibrosarcoma: a clinicopathologic analysis of 49 cases treated at a single institution with simultaneous assessment of the efficacy of 3-tier and 4-tier grading systems. Hum Pathol. 2004 May;35(5):612-21. Cited in: PubMed; PMID 15138937.

595. Huang SC, Chen HW, Zhang L, et al. Novel FUS-KLF17 and EWSR1-KLF17 fusions in myoepithelial tumors. Genes Chromosomes Cancer. 2015 May;54(5):267-75. Cited in: PubMed; PMID 25706482.

596. Huang YH, Lu YC, Huang HY, et al. Fine-needle aspiration cytology of melanotic schwannoma in the submandibular gland. Diagn Cytopathol. 2021 Jan;49(1):142-145. Cited in: PubMed; PMID 32583622.

597. Hummel P, Cangiarella JF, Cohen JM, et al. Transthoracic fine-needle aspiration biopsy of pulmonary spindle cell and mesenchymal lesions: a study of 61 cases. Cancer. 2001 Jun;93(3):187-98. Cited in: PubMed; PMID 11391606.

598. Humphreys S, Pambakian H, McKee PH, et al. Soft tissue chondroma--a study of 15 tumours. Histopathology. 1986 Feb;10(2):147-59. Cited in: PubMed; PMID 3957252.

599. Hung JH, Hsueh C, Liao CY, et al. Pulmonary Hilar Tumor: An Unusual Presentation of Sclerosing Hemangioma. Case Rep Med. 20162016:8919012. Cited in: PubMed; PMID 27761142.

600. Hung YP, Fletcher CD, Hornick JL. Evaluation of NKX2-2 expression in round cell sarcomas and other tumors with EWSR1 rearrangement: imperfect specificity for Ewing sarcoma. Mod Pathol. 2016 Apr;29(4):370-80. Cited in: PubMed; PMID 26847175.

601. Hung YP, Lovitch SB, Qian X. Histiocytic sarcoma: New insights into FNA cytomorphology and molecular characteristics. Cancer Cytopathol. 2017 Aug;125(8):604-614. Cited in: PubMed; PMID 28805986.

602. Husain M, Nguyen GK. Malignant melanoma of soft parts diagnosed by needle aspiration cytology and electron microscopy. Diagn Cytopathol. 1995 Jul;13(1):89-92. Cited in: PubMed; PMID 7587885.

603. Huwait H, Meneghetti A, Nielsen TO. Kaposi sarcoma of the adrenal gland resembling epithelioid angiosarcoma: a case report. Sarcoma. 20112011:898257. Cited in: PubMed; PMID 21845069.

604. Hwang DG, Qian X, Hornick JL. DOG1 antibody is a highly sensitive and specific marker for gastrointestinal stromal tumors in cytology cell blocks. Am J Clin Pathol. 2011 Mar;135(3):448-53. Cited in: PubMed; PMID 21350101.

605. Hwang S, Kelliher E, Hameed M. Imaging features of low-grade fibromyxoid sarcoma (Evans tumor). Skeletal Radiol. 2012 Sep;41(10):1263-72. Cited in: PubMed; PMID 22576969.

606. Ibrahim RM, Steenstrup Jensen S, Juel J. Clear cell sarcoma-A review. J Orthop. 2018 Dec;15(4):963-966. Cited in: PubMed; PMID 30210202.

607. Ikeda K, Tate G, Suzuki T, et al. Comparison of immunocytochemical sensitivity between formalin-fixed and alcohol-fixed specimens reveals the diagnostic value of alcohol-fixed cytocentrifuged preparations in malignant effusion

cytology. Am J Clin Pathol. 2011 Dec;136(6):934-42. Cited in: PubMed; PMID 22095380.
608. Ikeda K, Tate G, Suzuki T, et al. Fine needle aspiration cytology of primary proximal-type epithelioid sarcoma of the perineum: a case report. Acta Cytol. 200549(3):314-8. Cited in: PubMed; PMID 15966295.
609. Ilaslan H, Joyce M, Bauer T, et al. Decubital ischemic fasciitis: clinical, pathologic, and MRI features of pseudosarcoma. AJR Am J Roentgenol. 2006 Nov;187(5):1338-41. Cited in: PubMed; PMID 17056926.
610. Indave Ruiz BI, Armon S, Watanabe R, et al. Clonality, Mutation and Kaposi Sarcoma: A Systematic Review. Cancers (Basel). 2022 Feb;14(5): Cited in: PubMed; PMID 35267506.
611. International Academy of Cytology – International Agency for Research on Cancer – World Health Organization Joint Editorial Board. WHO Reporting System for Lung Cytopathology. Lyon (France): International Agency for Research on Cancer; 2022. (IAC-IARC-WHO cytopathology reporting systems series, 1st ed.; vol. 1). https://publications.iarc.fr/620.
612. International Academy of Cytology – International Agency for Research on Cancer – World Health Organization Joint Editorial Board. WHO Reporting System for Lymph Node, Spleen, and Thymus Cytopathology. Lyon (France): International Agency for Research on Cancer; 2024. (IAC-IARC-WHO cytopathology reporting systems series, 1st ed.; vol. 3). https://publications.iarc.who.int/644.
613. International Academy of Cytology – International Agency for Research on Cancer – World Health Organization Joint Editorial Board. WHO Reporting System for Pancreaticobiliary Cytopathology. Lyon (France): International Agency for Research on Cancer; 2022. (IAC-IARC-WHO cytopathology reporting systems series, 1st ed.; vol. 2). https://publications.iarc.fr/621.
614. International Society for the Study of Vascular Anomalies. ISSVA Classification of Vascular Anomalies, 2018 Classification (approved at the May 2018 General Assembly in Amsterdam, the Netherlands); 2018. Available from: https://www.issva.org/classification.
615. Iqbal CW, St Peter S, Ishitani MB. Pediatric dermatofibrosarcoma protuberans: multi-institutional outcomes. J Surg Res. 2011 Sep;170(1):69-72. Cited in: PubMed; PMID 21429521.
616. Ireland DC, Soule EH, Ivins JC. Myxoma of somatic soft tissues. A report of 58 patients, 3 with multiple tumors and fibrous dysplasia of bone. Mayo Clin Proc. 1973 Jun;48(6):401-10. Cited in: PubMed; PMID 4709710.
617. Irwin MS, Park JR. Neuroblastoma: paradigm for precision medicine. Pediatr Clin North Am. 2015 Feb;62(1):225-56. Cited in: PubMed; PMID 25435121.
618. Ishak KG, Sesterhenn IA, Goodman ZD, et al. Epithelioid hemangioendothelioma of the liver: a clinicopathologic and follow-up study of 32 cases. Hum Pathol. 1984 Sep;15(9):839-52. Cited in: PubMed; PMID 6088383.
619. Ishi K, Suzuki F, Saito A, et al. Cytodiagnosis of malignant melanoma of soft tissue: report of a case with diagnosis by intraoperative cytology. Acta Cytol. 199842(5):1177-80. Cited in: PubMed; PMID 9755678.
620. Italiano A, Sung YS, Zhang L, et al. High prevalence of CIC fusion with double-homeobox (DUX4) transcription factors in EWSR1-negative undifferentiated small blue round cell sarcomas. Genes Chromosomes Cancer. 2012 Mar;51(3):207-18. Cited in: PubMed; PMID 22072439.
621. Ito K, Kubota K, Morooka M, et al. Diagnostic usefulness of 18F-FDG PET/CT in the differentiation of pulmonary artery sarcoma and pulmonary embolism. Ann Nucl Med. 2009 Sep;23(7):671-6. Cited in: PubMed; PMID 19680740.
622. Iyer RS, Schaunaman G, Pruthi S, et al. Imaging of pediatric desmoplastic small-round-cell tumor with pathologic correlation. Curr Probl Diagn Radiol. 201342(1):26-32. Cited in: PubMed; PMID 23146167.
623. Iyer VK, Kapila K, Verma K. Fine-needle aspiration cytology of giant cell tumor of tendon sheath. Diagn Cytopathol. 2003 Aug;29(2):105-10. Cited in: PubMed; PMID 12889051.
624. Jahanseir K, Xing D, Greipp PT, et al. PDGFB Rearrangements in Dermatofibrosarcoma Protuberans of the Vulva: A Study of 11 Cases Including Myxoid and Fibrosarcomatous Variants. Int J Gynecol Pathol. 2018 Nov;37(6):537-546. Cited in: PubMed; PMID 29140881.
625. Jain D, Mathur SR, Iyer VK. Cell blocks in cytopathology: a review of preparative methods, utility in diagnosis and role in ancillary studies. Cytopathology. 2014 Dec;25(6):356-71. Cited in: PubMed; PMID 25113785.
626. Jain D, Roy-Chowdhuri S. Molecular Pathology of Lung Cancer Cytology Specimens: A Concise Review. Arch Pathol Lab Med. 2018 Sep;142(9):1127-1133. Cited in: PubMed; PMID 29547001.
627. Jaiprakash P, Radhakrishnan B, Kudva R, et al. Nodular Fasciitis - Fine Needle Aspiration Cytology Diagnosis and Its Pitfalls, with Review of Literature. Iran J Pathol. 201914(1):76-82. Cited in: PubMed; PMID 31531104.
628. Jakowski JD, Wakely PE. Cytopathology of extraskeletal myxoid chondrosarcoma: report of 8 cases. Cancer. 2007 Oct;111(5):298-305. Cited in: PubMed; PMID 17676582.
629. Jansen-Landheer ML, Krijnen P, Oostindiër MJ, et al. Improved diagnosis and treatment of soft tissue sarcoma patients after implementation of national guidelines: a population-based study. Eur J Surg Oncol. 2009 Dec;35(12):1326-32. Cited in: PubMed; PMID 19525085.
630. Järvi OH, Länsimies PH. Subclinical elastofibromas in the scapular region in an autopsy series. Acta Pathol Microbiol Scand A. 1975 Jan;83(1):87-108. Cited in: PubMed; PMID 1124654.
631. Jebastin Thangaiah J, Hanley K, Nomani L, et al. Cytologic features and immunohistochemical findings of epithelioid hemangioendothelioma (EHE) in effusion: A case series. Diagn Cytopathol. 2021 Jan;49(1):E24-E30. Cited in: PubMed; PMID 32797671.
632. Jelinek JS, Wu A, Wallace M, et al. Imaging of spindle cell lipoma. Clin Radiol. 2020 May;75(5):396.e15-396.e21. Cited in: PubMed; PMID 31932047.
633. Jennings LJ, Arcila ME, Corless C, et al. Guidelines for Validation of Next-Generation Sequencing-Based Oncology Panels: A Joint Consensus Recommendation of the Association for Molecular Pathology and College of American Pathologists. J Mol Diagn. 2017 May;19(3):341-365. Cited in: PubMed; PMID 28341590.
634. Jennings TA, Peterson L, Axiotis CA, et al. Angiosarcoma associated with foreign body material. A report of three cases. Cancer. 1988 Dec;62(11):2436-44. Cited in: PubMed; PMID 3052791.
635. Jha P, Moosavi C, Fanburg-Smith JC. Giant cell fibroblastoma: an update and addition of 86 new cases from the Armed Forces Institute of Pathology, in honor of Dr. Franz M. Enzinger. Ann Diagn Pathol. 2007 Apr;11(2):81-8. Cited in: PubMed; PMID 17349565.
636. Jilong Y, Jian W, Xiaoyan Z, et al. Analysis of APC/beta-catenin genes mutations and Wnt signalling pathway in desmoid-type fibromatosis. Pathology. 2007 Jun;39(3):319-25. Cited in: PubMed; PMID 17558858.
637. Jiménez-Heffernan JA, Rodríguez-García AM, Cima L, et al. A comprehensive review of the "tigroid" background cytological concept: what, when, where and why? Pathologica. 2022 Apr;114(2):121-127. Cited in: PubMed; PMID 35481562.
638. Jin B, Saleh H. Pitfalls in the diagnosis of adult rhabdomyoma by fine needle aspiration: report of a case and a brief literature review. Diagn Cytopathol. 2009 Jul;37(7):483-6. Cited in: PubMed; PMID 19217050.
639. Jin M, Chowsilpa S, Ali SZ, et al. Mesenchymal neoplasms of the tubular gut and adjacent structures: experience with EUS-guided fine-needle aspiration cytopathology. J Am Soc Cytopathol. 20209(6):528-539. Cited in: PubMed; PMID 32622859.
640. Jin M, Wakely PE. Lymph node cytopathology: Essential ancillary studies as applied to lymphoproliferative neoplasms. Cancer Cytopathol. 2018 Aug;126 Suppl 8:615-626. Cited in: PubMed; PMID 30156771.
641. Jing X, Li QK, Bedrossian U, et al. Morphologic and immunocytochemical performances of effusion cell blocks prepared using 3 different methods. Am J Clin Pathol. 2013 Feb;139(2):177-82. Cited in: PubMed; PMID 23355202.
642. Jiwani S, Gokden M, Lindberg M, et al. Fine-needle aspiration cytology of epithelioid malignant peripheral nerve sheath tumor: A case report and review of the literature. Diagn Cytopathol. 2016 Mar;44(3):226-31. Cited in: PubMed; PMID 26646298.
643. Jo VY. Applications of Ancillary Testing in the Cytologic Diagnosis of Soft Tissue Neoplasms. Surg Pathol Clin. 2018 Sep;11(3):633-656. Cited in: PubMed; PMID 30190145.
644. Jo VY. EWSR1 fusions: Ewing sarcoma and beyond. Cancer Cytopathol. 2020 Apr;128(4):229-231. Cited in: PubMed; PMID 31995669.
645. Jo VY, and Qian X. Chapter 18: Molecular diagnostics in bone and soft tissue tumors. In: Roy-Chowdhuri S, VanderLaan PA, Stewart JM, et al., editors. Molecular diagnostics in cytopathology: a practical handbook for the practicing pathologist. London (UK): Springer; 2019. pp. 425–89.
646. Jo VY, Antonescu CR, Dickson BC, et al. Cutaneous Syncytial Myoepithelioma Is Characterized by Recurrent EWSR1-PBX3 Fusions. Am J Surg Pathol. 2019 Oct;43(10):1349-1354. Cited in: PubMed; PMID 31135487.
647. Jo VY, Antonescu CR, Zhang L, et al. Cutaneous syncytial myoepithelioma: clinicopathologic characterization in a series of 38 cases. Am J Surg Pathol. 2013 May;37(5):710-8. Cited in: PubMed; PMID 23588365.
648. Jo VY, Fletcher CD. Epithelioid malignant peripheral nerve sheath tumor: clinicopathologic analysis of 63 cases. Am J Surg Pathol. 2015 May;39(5):673-82. Cited in: PubMed; PMID 25602794.
649. Jo VY, Fletcher CD. p63 immunohistochemical staining is limited in soft tissue tumors. Am J Clin Pathol. 2011 Nov;136(5):762-6. Cited in: PubMed; PMID 22031315.
650. Jo VY, Fletcher CDM. SMARCB1/INI1 Loss in Epithelioid Schwannoma: A Clinicopathologic and Immunohistochemical Study of 65 Cases. Am J Surg Pathol. 2017 Aug;41(8):1013-1022. Cited in: PubMed; PMID 28368924.
651. Jo VY, Hornick JL, Qian X. Utility of brachyury in distinction of chordoma from cytomorphologic mimics in fine-needle aspiration and core needle biopsy. Diagn Cytopathol. 2014 Aug;42(8):647-52. Cited in: PubMed; PMID 24554551.
652. Joensuu H. Risk stratification of patients diagnosed with gastrointestinal stromal tumor. Hum Pathol. 2008 Oct;39(10):1411-9. Cited in: PubMed; PMID 18774375.
653. Joensuu H, Martin-Broto J, Nishida T, et al. Follow-up strategies for patients with gastrointestinal stromal tumour treated with or without adjuvant imatinib after surgery. Eur J Cancer. 2015 Aug;51(12):1611-7. Cited in: PubMed; PMID 26022432.
654. John A, Lee N, Lim A, et al. Triceps mass - A rare presentation of renal cell carcinoma. Urol Case Rep. 2022 Jul;43:102079. Cited in: PubMed; PMID 35520031.
655. Jones C, Liu K, Hirschowitz S, et al. Concordance of histopathologic and cytologic grading in musculoskeletal sarcomas: can grades obtained from analysis of the fine-needle aspirates serve as the basis for therapeutic decisions? Cancer. 2002 Apr;96(2):83-91. Cited in: PubMed; PMID 11954025.
657. Joshi VV, Cantor AB, Altshuler G, et al. Conventional versus modified morphologic criteria for ganglioneuroblastoma. A review of cases from the Pediatric Oncology Group. Arch Pathol Lab Med. 1996 Sep;120(9):859-65. Cited in: PubMed; PMID 9140292.
658. Joshi VV, Silverman JF. Pathology of neuroblastic tumors. Semin Diagn Pathol. 1994 May;11(2):107-17. Cited in: PubMed; PMID 7809504.
659. Jóźwiak S, Kawalec W, Dłuzewska J, et al. Cardiac tumours in tuberous sclerosis: their incidence and course. Eur J Pediatr. 1994 Mar;153(3):155-7. Cited in: PubMed; PMID 8181495.
660. Jun DW, Lee OY, Park CK, et al. Cutaneous metastases of pancreatic carcinoma as a first clinical manifestation. Korean J Intern Med. 2005 Sep;20(3):260-3. Cited in: PubMed; PMID 16295788.
661. Jurcić V, Zidar A, Montiel MD, et al. Myxoinflammatory fibroblastic sarcoma: a tumor not restricted to acral sites. Ann Diagn Pathol. 2002 Oct;6(5):272-80. Cited in: PubMed; PMID 12376919.
662. Jurczyk M, Zhu B, Laskin W, et al. Pitfalls in the diagnosis of hepatic epithelioid hemangioendothelioma by FNA and needle core biopsy. Diagn Cytopathol. 2014 Jun;42(6):516-20. Cited in: PubMed; PMID 23288560.
663. Kaffenberger BH, Wakely PE, Mayerson JL. Local recurrence rate of fine-needle aspiration biopsy in primary high-grade sarcomas. J Surg Oncol. 2010 Jun;101(7):618-21. Cited in: PubMed; PMID 20461770.
664. Kai K, Kusano K, Sakai M, et al. Active neovascularization and possible vascular-centric development of gastric and periscapular elastofibromas. Virchows Arch. 2009 Feb;454(2):181-8. Cited in: PubMed; PMID 19132384.
665. Kajtár B, Tornóczky T, Kálmán E, et al. CD99-positive undifferentiated round cell sarcoma diagnosed on fine needle aspiration cytology, later found to harbour a CIC-DUX4 translocation: a recently described entity. Cytopathology. 2014 Apr;25(2):129-32. Cited in: PubMed; PMID 23834194.
666. Kandemir NO, Yurdakan G, Bektas S, et al. Classic Kaposi sarcoma with sarcoid-like granulomas: a case report and literature review. Exp Mol Pathol. 2009 Oct;87(2):89-93. Cited in: PubMed; PMID 19679122.
668. Kang Y, Pekmezci M, Folpe AL, et al. Diagnostic utility of SOX10 to distinguish malignant peripheral nerve sheath tumor from synovial sarcoma, including intraneural synovial sarcoma. Mod Pathol. 2014 Jan;27(1):55-61. Cited in: PubMed; PMID 23929265.
669. Kannan S, Chong HH, Chew B, et al. Leiomyosarcoma in the extremities and trunk wall: systematic review and meta-analysis of the oncological outcomes. World J Surg Oncol. 2022 Apr;20(1):124. Cited in: PubMed; PMID 35436892.

670. Kao EY, Ardic F, Fadra N, et al. Chondroid Synoviocytic Neoplasm: A Clinicopathologic, Immunohistochemical, and Molecular Genetic Study of a Distinctive Tumor of Synoviocytes. Mod Pathol. 2024 Nov;37(11):100598. Cited in: PubMed; PMID 39181450.
671. Kao SC. Overview of the clinical and imaging features of the most common non-rhabdomyosarcoma soft-tissue sarcomas. Pediatr Radiol. 2019 Oct;49(11):1524-1533. Cited in: PubMed; PMID 31620852.
672. Kao YC, Owosho AA, Sung YS, et al. BCOR-CCNB3 Fusion Positive Sarcomas: A Clinicopathologic and Molecular Analysis of 36 Cases With Comparison to Morphologic Spectrum and Clinical Behavior of Other Round Cell Sarcomas. Am J Surg Pathol. 2018 May;42(5):604-615. Cited in: PubMed; PMID 29300189.
673. Kao YC, Sung YS, Chen CL, et al. ETV transcriptional upregulation is more reliable than RNA sequencing algorithms and FISH in diagnosing round cell sarcomas with CIC gene rearrangements. Genes Chromosomes Cancer. 2017 Jun;56(6):501-510. Cited in: PubMed; PMID 28233365.
674. Kao YC, Sung YS, Zhang L, et al. Recurrent BCOR Internal Tandem Duplication and YWHAE-NUTM2B Fusions in Soft Tissue Undifferentiated Round Cell Sarcoma of Infancy: Overlapping Genetic Features With Clear Cell Sarcoma of Kidney. Am J Surg Pathol. 2016 Aug;40(8):1009-20. Cited in: PubMed; PMID 26945340.
675. Kapila K, Ghosal N, Gill SS, et al. Cytomorphology of lipomatous tumors of soft tissue. Acta Cytol. 200347(4):555-62. Cited in: PubMed; PMID 12920746.
676. Kapoor N, Shinagare AB, Jagannathan JP, et al. Clinical and radiologic features of extraskeletal myxoid chondrosarcoma including initial presentation, local recurrence, and metastases. Radiol Oncol. 2014 Sep;48(3):235-42. Cited in: PubMed; PMID 25177237.
677. Karamchandani JR, Nielsen TO, van de Rijn M, et al. Sox10 and S100 in the diagnosis of soft-tissue neoplasms. Appl Immunohistochem Mol Morphol. 2012 Oct;20(5):445-50. Cited in: PubMed; PMID 22495377.
678. Karamzadeh Dashti N, Bahrami A, Lee SJ, et al. BRAF V600E Mutations Occur in a Subset of Glomus Tumors, and Are Associated With Malignant Histologic Characteristics. Am J Surg Pathol. 2017 Nov;41(11):1532-1541. Cited in: PubMed; PMID 28834810.
679. Karnak I, Senocak ME, Ciftci AO, et al. Inflammatory myofibroblastic tumor in children: diagnosis and treatment. J Pediatr Surg. 2001 Jun;36(6):908-12. Cited in: PubMed; PMID 11381424.
680. Kasper B, Lecointe-Artzner E, Wait S, et al. Working to improve the management of sarcoma patients across Europe: a policy checklist. BMC Cancer. 2018 Apr;18(1):424. Cited in: PubMed; PMID 29661168.
681. Kasraeian S, Allison DC, Ahlmann ER, et al. A comparison of fine-needle aspiration, core biopsy, and surgical biopsy in the diagnosis of extremity soft tissue masses. Clin Orthop Relat Res. 2010 Nov;468(11):2992-3002. Cited in: PubMed; PMID 20512437.
682. Kato S, Kikuchi K, Chinen K, et al. Diagnostic utility of endoscopic ultrasound-guided fine-needle aspiration biopsy for glomus tumor of the stomach. World J Gastroenterol. 2015 Jun;21(22):7052-8. Cited in: PubMed; PMID 26078584.
683. Kaur I, Handa U, Kundu R, et al. Role of fine-needle aspiration cytology and core needle biopsy in diagnosing musculoskeletal neoplasms. J Cytol. 201633(1):7-12. Cited in: PubMed; PMID 27011434.
684. Kaur M, Chatterjee D, Kundu R, et al. Spindle cell lipoma mimicking pleomorphic adenoma: A diagnostic challenge on cytology. Diagn Cytopathol. 2019 Apr;47(4):341-344. Cited in: PubMed; PMID 30468314.
685. Kay PA, Nascimento AG, Unni KK, et al. Chordoma. Cytomorphologic findings in 14 cases diagnosed by fine needle aspiration. Acta Cytol. 200347(2):202-8. Cited in: PubMed; PMID 12685190.
686. Kelly KM, Womer RB, Sorensen PH, et al. Common and variant gene fusions predict distinct clinical phenotypes in rhabdomyosarcoma. J Clin Oncol. 1997 May;15(5):1831-6. Cited in: PubMed; PMID 9164192.
687. Kembhavi SA, Shah S, Rangarajan V, et al. Imaging in neuroblastoma: An update. Indian J Radiol Imaging. 201525(2):129-36. Cited in: PubMed; PMID 25969636.
688. Kendall BS, Liang CY, Lancaster KJ, et al. Ischemic fasciitis. Report of a case with fine needle aspiration findings. Acta Cytol. 199741(2):598-602. Cited in: PubMed; PMID 9100807.
689. Keppens C, Tack V, Hart N', et al. A stitch in time saves nine: external quality assessment rounds demonstrate improved quality of biomarker analysis in lung cancer. Oncotarget. 2018 Apr;9(29):20524-20538. Cited in: PubMed; PMID 29755669.
690. Kerbrat A, Beaufrere A, Neiva-Vaz C, et al. Rhabdomyosarcoma and rhabdomyoma associated with nevoid basal cell carcinoma syndrome: Local treatment strategy. Pediatr Dermatol. 2018 Jul;35(4):e245-e247. Cited in: PubMed; PMID 29799139.
691. Kerimaa P, Marttila A, Hyvönen P, et al. MRI-guided biopsy and fine needle aspiration biopsy (FNAB) in the diagnosis of musculoskeletal lesions. Eur J Radiol. 2013 Dec;82(12):2328-33. Cited in: PubMed; PMID 24099641.
692. Kerl K, Nowacki M, Leuschner I, et al. Infantile fibrosarcoma - an important differential diagnosis of congenital vascular tumors. Pediatr Hematol Oncol. 2012 Sep;29(6):545-8. Cited in: PubMed; PMID 22812410.
693. KERN WH. Proliferative myositis; a pseudosarcomatous reaction to injury: a report of seven cases. Arch Pathol. 1960 Feb;69:209-16. Cited in: PubMed; PMID 14408614.
694. Kerr DA, Thompson LDR, Tafe LJ, et al. Clinicopathologic and Genomic Characterization of Inflammatory Myofibroblastic Tumors of the Head and Neck: Highlighting a Novel Fusion and Potential Diagnostic Pitfall. Am J Surg Pathol. 2021 Dec;45(12):1707-1719. Cited in: PubMed; PMID 34001695.
695. Kerridge WD, Kryvenko ON, Thompson A, et al. Fat Necrosis of the Breast: A Pictorial Review of the Mammographic, Ultrasound, CT, and MRI Findings with Histopathologic Correlation. Radiol Res Pract. 20152015:613139. Cited in: PubMed; PMID 25861475.
696. Khalbuss WE, Teot LA, Monaco SE. Diagnostic accuracy and limitations of fine-needle aspiration cytology of bone and soft tissue lesions: a review of 1114 cases with cytological-histological correlation. Cancer Cytopathol. 2010 Feb;118(1):24-32. Cited in: PubMed; PMID 20091838.
697. Khamaysi I, Naroditsky I, Malkin L. Primary synovial sarcoma of the mediastinum: a rare tumor diagnosed by endoscopic ultrasound-fine needle biopsy (EUS-FNB)-Cytomorphologic, immunohistochemical, and molecular analysis. Clin J Gastroenterol. 2021 Aug;14(4):961-964. Cited in: PubMed; PMID 33792887.
698. Khandakar B, Chen H. Ultrasound-guided fine needle aspiration cytology of angiosarcoma of head and neck: a review of cytomorphologic features and discussion of diagnostic pitfall of aspiration cytology of vascular lesions. Diagn Cytopathol. 2021 Jul;49(7):902-906. Cited in: PubMed; PMID 33964187.
699. Khandeparkar SG, Joshi A, Khande T, et al. A rare case of giant soft tissue chondroma of the wrist: A cytopathological study with review of the literature. J Cytol. 2014 Jan;31(1):40-3. Cited in: PubMed; PMID 25190983.
700. Khashper A, Zheng J, Nahal A, et al. Imaging characteristics of spindle cell lipoma and its variants. Skeletal Radiol. 2014 May;43(5):591-7. Cited in: PubMed; PMID 24554024.
701. Khatib Y, Khade AL, Shah VB, et al. Cytohistological Features of Spindle Cell Lipoma- A Case Report with Differential Diagnosis. J Clin Diagn Res. 2017 Feb;11(2):ED10-ED11. Cited in: PubMed; PMID 28384874.
702. Khong PL, Goh WH, Wong VC, et al. MR imaging of spinal tumors in children with neurofibromatosis 1. AJR Am J Roentgenol. 2003 Feb;180(2):413-7. Cited in: PubMed; PMID 12540444.
703. Khoo M, Pressney I, Hargunani R, et al. Melanotic schwannoma: an 11-year case series. Skeletal Radiol. 2016 Jan;45(1):29-34. Cited in: PubMed; PMID 26386847.
704. Kilpatrick SE, Bergman S, Pettenati MJ, et al. The usefulness of cytogenetic analysis in fine needle aspirates for the histologic subtyping of sarcomas. Mod Pathol. 2006 Jun;19(6):815-9. Cited in: PubMed; PMID 16557276.
705. Kilpatrick SE, Cappellari JO, Bos GD, et al. Is fine-needle aspiration biopsy a practical alternative to open biopsy for the primary diagnosis of sarcoma? Experience with 140 patients. Am J Clin Pathol. 2001 Jan;115(1):59-68. Cited in: PubMed; PMID 11190808.
706. Kilpatrick SE, Doyon J, Choong PF, et al. The clinicopathologic spectrum of myxoid and round cell liposarcoma. A study of 95 cases. Cancer. 1996 Apr;77(8):1450-8. Cited in: PubMed; PMID 8608528.
707. Kilpatrick SE, Hitchcock MG, Kraus MD, et al. Mixed tumors and myoepitheliomas of soft tissue: a clinicopathologic study of 19 cases with a unifying concept. Am J Surg Pathol. 1997 Jan;21(1):13-22. Cited in: PubMed; PMID 8990137.
708. Kilpatrick SE, Inwards CY, Fletcher CD, et al. Myxoid chondrosarcoma (chordoid sarcoma) of bone: a report of two cases and review of the literature. Cancer. 1997 May;79(10):1903-10. Cited in: PubMed; PMID 9149016.
709. Kilpatrick SE, Teot LA, Stanley MW, et al. Fine-needle aspiration biopsy of synovial sarcoma. A cytomorphologic analysis of primary, recurrent, and metastatic tumors. Am J Clin Pathol. 1996 Dec;106(6):769-75. Cited in: PubMed; PMID 8980353.
710. Kilpatrick SE, Ward WG. Myxofibrosarcoma of soft tissues: cytomorphologic analysis of a series. Diagn Cytopathol. 1999 Jan;20(1):6-9. Cited in: PubMed; PMID 9884819.
711. Kilpatrick SE, Ward WG, Bos GD. The value of fine-needle aspiration biopsy in the differential diagnosis of adult myxoid sarcoma. Cancer. 2000 Jun;90(3):167-77. Cited in: PubMed; PMID 10896330.
712. Kilpatrick SE, Ward WG, Cappellari JO, et al. Fine-needle aspiration biopsy of soft tissue sarcomas. A cytomorphologic analysis with emphasis on histologic subtyping, grading, and therapeutic significance. Am J Clin Pathol. 1999 Aug;112(2):179-88. Cited in: PubMed; PMID 10439797.
713. Kim DW, Shin JH, Lee HJ, et al. Spindle cell rhabdomyosacoma of uterus: a case study. Korean J Pathol. 2013 Aug;47(4):388-91. Cited in: PubMed; PMID 24009636.
714. Kim JH, Jung IY, Song JE, et al. Profiles of Extrapulmonary Nontuberculous Mycobacteria Infections and Predictors for Species: A Multicenter Retrospective Study. Pathogens. 2020 Nov;9(11): Cited in: PubMed; PMID 33202553.
715. Kim L, Park IS, Han JY, et al. Aspiration cytology of fibrosarcomatous variant of dermatofibrosarcoma protuberans with osteoclast-like giant cells in the chest wall: a case report. Acta Cytol. 200549(6):644-9. Cited in: PubMed; PMID 16450905.
716. Kim Y, Moses M, Zegarelli DJ, et al. Cartilage choristoma (soft tissue chondroma): a rare presentation in the lower lip. J Clin Pediatr Dent. 200933(3):253-4. Cited in: PubMed; PMID 19476101.
717. Kirshtein B, Meirovitz M, Okon E, et al. Sister Mary Joseph's nodule as the first presenting sign of primary fallopian tube adenocarcinoma. J Minim Invasive Gynecol. 200613(3):234-6. Cited in: PubMed; PMID 16698532.
718. Kirwadi A, Abdul-Halim R, Fernando M, et al. MR imaging features of spindle cell lipoma. Skeletal Radiol. 2014 Feb;43(2):191-6. Cited in: PubMed; PMID 24240205.
719. Kishore B, Khare P, Gupta RJ, et al. A rare case of paratesticular pleomorphic rhabdomyosarcoma diagnosed by fine needle aspiration: a case report. Diagn Cytopathol. 2010 Feb;38(2):121-6. Cited in: PubMed; PMID 19790247.
720. Kitagawa Y, Tsunoda R, Nanno M, et al. Combined Use of Magnetic Resonance Imaging and Fine-Needle Aspiration Cytology for Diagnosis of Soft-Tissue Tumors. J Nippon Med Sch. 2020 May;87(2):54-59. Cited in: PubMed; PMID 31611506.
721. Klapsinou E, Despoina P, Dimitra D. Cytologic findings and potential pitfalls in proliferative myositis and myositis ossificans diagnosed by fine needle aspiration cytology: report of four cases and review of the literature. Diagn Cytopathol. 2012 Mar;40(3):239-44. Cited in: PubMed; PMID 20890998.
722. Kleer CG, Unni KK, McLeod RA. Epithelioid hemangioendothelioma of bone. Am J Surg Pathol. 1996 Nov;20(11):1301-11. Cited in: PubMed; PMID 8898834.
723. Klevos G, Jose J, Pretell-Mazzini J, et al. Hibernoma. Am J Orthop (Belle Mead NJ). 2015 Jun;44(6):284-7. Cited in: PubMed; PMID 26046999.
724. Klijanienko J, Caillaud JM, Lagacé R. Cytohistologic correlations in schwannomas (neurilemmomas), including "ancient," cellular, and epithelioid variants. Diagn Cytopathol. 2006 Aug;34(8):517-22. Cited in: PubMed; PMID 16850489.
725. Klijanienko J, Caillaud JM, Lagacé R. Fine-needle aspiration in liposarcoma: cytohistologic correlative study including well-differentiated, myxoid, and pleomorphic variants. Diagn Cytopathol. 2004 May;30(5):307-12. Cited in: PubMed; PMID 15108227.
726. Klijanienko J, Caillaud JM, Lagacé R. Fine-needle aspiration of primary and recurrent benign fibrous histiocytoma: classic, aneurysmal, and myxoid variants. Diagn Cytopathol. 2004 Dec;31(6):387-91. Cited in: PubMed; PMID 15540171.
727. Klijanienko J, Caillaud JM, Lagacé R. Fine-needle aspiration of primary and recurrent dermatofibrosarcoma protuberans. Diagn Cytopathol. 2004 Apr;30(4):261-5. Cited in: PubMed; PMID 15048962.
728. Klijanienko J, Caillaud JM, Lagacé R, et al. Comparative fine-needle aspiration and pathologic study of malignant fibrous histiocytoma: cytodiagnostic features of 95 tumors in 71 patients. Diagn Cytopathol. 2003 Dec;29(6):320-6. Cited in: PubMed; PMID 14648788.
729. Klijanienko J, Caillaud JM, Lagacé R, et al. Cytohistologic correlations in 56 synovial sarcomas in 36 patients: the Institut Curie experience.

Diagn Cytopathol. 2002 Aug;27(2):96-102. Cited in: PubMed; PMID 12203876.
730. Klijanienko J, Caillaud JM, Lagacé R, et al. Cytohistologic correlations in angiosarcoma including classic and epithelioid variants: Institut Curie's experience. Diagn Cytopathol. 2003 Sep;29(3):140-5. Cited in: PubMed; PMID 12951681.
731. Klijanienko J, Caillaud JM, Lagacé R, et al. Cytohistologic correlations of 24 malignant peripheral nerve sheath tumor (MPNST) in 17 patients: the Institut Curie experience. Diagn Cytopathol. 2002 Aug;27(2):103-8. Cited in: PubMed; PMID 12203877.
732. Klijanienko J, Caillaud JM, Lagacé R, et al. Fine-needle aspiration of leiomyosarcoma: a correlative cytohistopathological study of 96 tumors in 68 patients. Diagn Cytopathol. 2003 Mar;28(3):119-25. Cited in: PubMed; PMID 12619091.
733. Klijanienko J, Caillaud JM, Orbach D, et al. Cyto-histological correlations in primary, recurrent and metastatic rhabdomyosarcoma: the institut Curie's experience. Diagn Cytopathol. 2007 Aug;35(8):482-7. Cited in: PubMed; PMID 17636492.
734. Klijanienko J, Caillaud JM, Orbach D, et al. Cyto-histological correlations in primary, recurrent, and metastatic bone and soft tissue osteosarcoma. Institut Curie's experience. Diagn Cytopathol. 2007 May;35(5):270-5. Cited in: PubMed; PMID 17427216.
735. Klijanienko J, Cohen-Gogo S, Choucair ML, et al. Chapter 1: General considerations. In: Klijanienko J, Pohar Marinšek Ž, Domanski HA, editors. Small volume biopsy in pediatric tumors: an atlas for diagnostic pathology. Cham (Switzerland): Springer; 2018. pp. 1–59.
736. Klijanienko J, Colin P, Couturier J, et al. Fine-needle aspiration in desmoplastic small round cell tumor: a report of 10 new tumors in 8 patients with clinicopathological and molecular correlations with review of the literature. Cancer Cytopathol. 2014 May;122(5):386-93. Cited in: PubMed; PMID 24639098.
737. Klijanienko J, Couturier J, Bourdeaut F, et al. Fine-needle aspiration as a diagnostic technique in 50 cases of primary Ewing sarcoma/peripheral neuroectodermal tumor. Institut Curie's experience. Diagn Cytopathol. 2012 Jan;40(1):19-25. Cited in: PubMed; PMID 22180234.
738. Klijanienko J, Couturier J, Brisse H, et al. Diagnostic and prognostic information obtained on fine-needle aspirates of primary neuroblastic tumors: Proposal for a cytology prognostic score. Cancer Cytopathol. 2011 Dec;119(6):411-23. Cited in: PubMed; PMID 21774092.
739. Klijanienko J, Lagacé R, editors. Soft tissue tumors: a multidisciplinary, decisional diagnostic approach. Hoboken (NJ): Wiley-Blackwell; 2011.
740. Klijanienko J, Pierron G, Sastre-Garau X, et al. Value of combined cytology and molecular information in the diagnosis of soft tissue tumors. Cancer Cytopathol. 2015 Mar;123(3):141-51. Cited in: PubMed; PMID 25487166.
741. Kloboves-Prevodnik VV, Us-Krasovec M, Gale N, et al. Cytological features of lipoblastoma: a report of three cases. Diagn Cytopathol. 2005 Sep;33(3):195-200. Cited in: PubMed; PMID 16078242.
742. Knebel C, Neumann J, Schwaiger BJ, et al. Differentiating atypical lipomatous tumors from lipomas with magnetic resonance imaging: a comparison with MDM2 gene amplification status. BMC Cancer. 2019 Apr;19(1):309. Cited in: PubMed; PMID 30943944.
743. Kocjan G, Sams V, Davidson T. Dermatofibrosarcoma protuberans as a diagnostic pitfall in fine-needle aspiration diagnosis of angiosarcoma of the breast. Diagn Cytopathol. 1996 Feb;14(1):94-5. Cited in: PubMed; PMID 8834087.
744. Koelsche C, Benhamida JK, Kommoss FKF, et al. Intimal sarcomas and undifferentiated cardiac sarcomas carry mutually exclusive MDM2, MDM4, and CDK6 amplifications and share a common DNA methylation signature. Mod Pathol. 2021 Dec;34(12):2122-2129. Cited in: PubMed; PMID 34312479.
746. Koelsche C, Schweizer L, Renner M, et al. Nuclear relocation of STAT6 reliably predicts NAB2-STAT6 fusion for the diagnosis of solitary fibrous tumour. Histopathology. 2014 Nov;65(5):613-22. Cited in: PubMed; PMID 24702701.
747. Kohashi K, Izumi T, Oda Y, et al. Infrequent SMARCB1/INI1 gene alteration in epithelioid sarcoma: a useful tool in distinguishing epithelioid sarcoma from malignant rhabdoid tumor. Hum Pathol. 2009 Mar;40(3):349-55. Cited in: PubMed; PMID 18973917.
748. Kohashi K, Yamada Y, Hotokebuchi Y, et al. ERG and SALL4 expressions in SMARCB1/INI1-deficient tumors: a useful tool for distinguishing epithelioid sarcoma from malignant rhabdoid tumor. Hum Pathol. 2015 Feb;46(2):225-30. Cited in: PubMed; PMID 25479928.
749. Kollur SM, El Hag IA. Fine-needle aspiration cytology of metastatic nasopharyngeal carcinoma in cervical lymph nodes: comparison with metastatic squamous-cell carcinoma, and Hodgkin's and non-Hodgkin's lymphoma. Diagn Cytopathol. 2003 Jan;28(1):18-22. Cited in: PubMed; PMID 12508177.
750. Kong CS, Cha I. Nodular fasciitis: diagnosis by fine needle aspiration biopsy. Acta Cytol. 200448(4):473-7. Cited in: PubMed; PMID 15296335.
751. Kosemehmetoglu K, Vrana JA, Folpe AL. TLE1 expression is not specific for synovial sarcoma: a whole section study of 163 soft tissue and bone neoplasms. Mod Pathol. 2009 Jul;22(7):872-8. Cited in: PubMed; PMID 19363472.
752. Koshy A, Jain R, Srinivasan R, et al. Cytopathological spectrum of peripheral neuroblastic tumours in fine needle aspiration cytology and categorisation as per International Neuroblastoma Pathology Classification. Cytopathology. 2019 Nov;30(6):634-643. Cited in: PubMed; PMID 31231909.
753. Köster J, Ghanei I, Domanski HA. Comparative cytological and histological assessment of 828 primary soft tissue and bone lesions, and proposal for a system for reporting soft tissue cytopathology. Cytopathology. 2021 Jan;32(1):7-19. Cited in: PubMed; PMID 32926591.
754. Kottu R, Prayaga AK. Synovial sarcoma with relevant immunocytochemistry and special emphasis on the monophasic fibrous variant. J Cytol. 2010 Apr;27(2):47-50. Cited in: PubMed; PMID 21157548.
755. Kovach SJ, Fischer AC, Katzman PJ, et al. Inflammatory myofibroblastic tumors. J Surg Oncol. 2006 Oct;94(5):385-91. Cited in: PubMed; PMID 16967468.
756. Kraan J, Sleijfer S, Strijbos MH, et al. External quality assurance of circulating tumor cell enumeration using the CellSearch(®) system: a feasibility study. Cytometry B Clin Cytom. 2011 Mar;80(2):112-8. Cited in: PubMed; PMID 21337491.
757. Kransdorf MJ. Malignant soft-tissue tumors in a large referral population: distribution of diagnoses by age, sex, and location. AJR Am J Roentgenol. 1995 Jan;164(1):129-34. Cited in: PubMed; PMID 7998525.
758. Krogerus L, Kholová I. Cell Block in Cytological Diagnostics: Review of Preparatory Techniques. Acta Cytol. 201862(4):237-243. Cited in: PubMed; PMID 29909418.
759. Kubota F, Matsuyama A, Shibuya R, et al. Desmin-positivity in spindle cells: under-recognized immunophenotype of lipoblastoma. Pathol Int. 2013 Jul;63(7):353-7. Cited in: PubMed; PMID 23865573.
760. Kulkarni MP, Gosavi AV, Anvikar AR, et al. Cytodiagnosis of congenital mesoblastic nephroma: a case report. Diagn Cytopathol. 2013 Mar;41(3):234-8. Cited in: PubMed; PMID 23417966.
761. Kumar N, Das PM, Jain S, et al. Melanoma of the soft parts: diagnosis of metastatic and recurrent tumors by aspiration cytology. Diagn Cytopathol. 2003 Jun;28(6):295-300. Cited in: PubMed; PMID 12768633.
762. Kumar R, Rekhi B, Shirazi N, et al. Spectrum of cytomorphological features, including literature review, of an extraskeletal myxoid chondrosarcoma with t(9;22)(q22;q12) (TEC/EWS) results in one case. Diagn Cytopathol. 2008 Dec;36(12):868-75. Cited in: PubMed; PMID 18925568.
763. Kumar S, Chowdhury N. Accuracy, limitations and pitfalls in the diagnosis of soft tissue tumors by fine needle aspiration cytology. Indian J Pathol Microbiol. 2007 Jan;50(1):42-5. Cited in: PubMed; PMID 17474257.
764. Kumaran A, Puthenparambath S. Fine-needle aspiration diagnosis of nodular fasciitis: A case report. J Cytol. 201633(3):172-174. Cited in: PubMed; PMID 27756994.
765. Kumaratilake JS, Krishnan R, Lomax-Smith J, et al. Elastofibroma: disturbed elastic fibrillogenesis by periosteal-derived cells? An immunoelectron microscopic and in situ hybridization study. Hum Pathol. 1991 Oct;22(10):1017-29. Cited in: PubMed; PMID 1842374.
766. Kura MM, Aliporewala VM, Jorwekar SP, et al. Epithelioid sarcoma: A rare neoplasm presenting in a sporotrichoid pattern. Indian J Dermatol Venereol Leprol. 202187(5):690-692. Cited in: PubMed; PMID 34379944.
767. Kurata K, Anan K, Ishikawa N, et al. A case of primary extraskeletal osteosarcoma of the breast. Surg Case Rep. 2018 Sep;4(1):121. Cited in: PubMed; PMID 30232644.
768. Kurzawa P, Kattapuram S, Hornicek FJ, et al. Primary myoepithelioma of bone: a report of 8 cases. Am J Surg Pathol. 2013 Jul;37(7):960-8. Cited in: PubMed; PMID 23681076.
769. Küsters-Vandevelde HV, Klaasen A, Küsters B, et al. Activating mutations of the GNAQ gene: a frequent event in primary melanocytic neoplasms of the central nervous system. Acta Neuropathol. 2010 Mar;119(3):317-23. Cited in: PubMed; PMID 19936769.
771. Ladanyi M, Antonescu CR, Drobnjak M, et al. The precrystalline cytoplasmic granules of alveolar soft part sarcoma contain monocarboxylate transporter 1 and CD147. Am J Pathol. 2002 Apr;160(4):1215-21. Cited in: PubMed; PMID 11943706.
772. Ladanyi M, Antonescu CR, Leung DH, et al. Impact of SYT-SSX fusion type on the clinical behavior of synovial sarcoma: a multi-institutional retrospective study of 243 patients. Cancer Res. 2002 Jan;62(1):135-40. Cited in: PubMed; PMID 11782370.
773. Lae ME, Roche PC, Jin L, et al. Desmoplastic small round cell tumor: a clinicopathologic, immunohistochemical, and molecular study of 32 tumors. Am J Surg Pathol. 2002 Jul;26(7):823-35. Cited in: PubMed; PMID 12131150.
774. Lai C, Long JR, Larsen BT, et al. Percutaneous biopsy of musculoskeletal tumors and the potential for needle tract seeding: technical considerations, current controversies, and outcomes. Skeletal Radiol. 2023 Mar;52(3):505-516. Cited in: PubMed; PMID 36255472.
775. Lane KL, Shannon RJ, Weiss SW. Hyalinizing spindle cell tumor with giant rosettes: a distinctive tumor closely resembling low-grade fibromyxoid sarcoma. Am J Surg Pathol. 1997 Dec;21(12):1481-8. Cited in: PubMed; PMID 9414192.
776. Laskin WB, Fetsch JF, Miettinen M. Myxoinflammatory fibroblastic sarcoma: a clinicopathologic analysis of 104 cases, with emphasis on predictors of outcome. Am J Surg Pathol. 2014 Jan;38(1):1-12. Cited in: PubMed; PMID 24121178.
777. Laskin WB, Silverman TA, Enzinger FM. Postradiation soft tissue sarcomas. An analysis of 53 cases. Cancer. 1988 Dec;62(11):2330-40. Cited in: PubMed; PMID 3179948.
778. Lasota J, Fetsch JF, Wozniak A, et al. The neurofibromatosis type 2 gene is mutated in perineurial cell tumors: a molecular genetic study of eight cases. Am J Pathol. 2001 Apr;158(4):1223-9. Cited in: PubMed; PMID 11290539.
779. Latz S, Ellinger J, Goltz D, et al. Spindle cell rhabdomyosarcoma of the prostate. Int J Urol. 2013 Sep;20(9):935-7. Cited in: PubMed; PMID 23320845.
780. Lau K, Massad M, Pollak C, et al. Clinical patterns and outcome in epithelioid hemangioendothelioma with or without pulmonary involvement: insights from an internet registry in the study of a rare cancer. Chest. 2011 Nov;140(5):1312-1318. Cited in: PubMed; PMID 21546438.
781. Lauer DH, Enzinger FM. Cranial fasciitis of childhood. Cancer. 1980 Jan;45(2):401-6. Cited in: PubMed; PMID 7351023.
782. Laurini JA, Zhang L, Goldblum JR, et al. Low-grade fibromyxoid sarcoma of the small intestine: report of 4 cases with molecular cytogenetic confirmation. Am J Surg Pathol. 2011 Jul;35(7):1069-73. Cited in: PubMed; PMID 21677541.
783. Layfield LJ. Soft tissue tumor diagnosis: A three prong approach utilizing pattern analysis, immunocytochemistry, and molecular diagnostics. Diagn Cytopathol. 2020 Mar;48(3):265-284. Cited in: PubMed; PMID 31868988.
784. Layfield LJ, Anders KH, Glasgow BJ, et al. Fine-needle aspiration of primary soft-tissue lesions. Arch Pathol Lab Med. 1986 May;110(5):420-4. Cited in: PubMed; PMID 3754426.
785. Layfield LJ, Dodd L, Klijanienko J. Myxoid neoplasms of bone and soft tissue: a pattern-based approach. J Am Soc Cytopathol. 202110(3):278-292. Cited in: PubMed; PMID 33168472.
787. Layfield LJ, Mooney EE, Dodd LG. Not by blood alone: diagnosis of hemangiomas by fine-needle aspiration. Diagn Cytopathol. 1998 Oct;19(4):250-4. Cited in: PubMed; PMID 9784986.
788. Layfield LJ, Stegelmeier P, Wang L, et al. Core needle biopsy for the diagnosis of primary soft tissue lesions: Accuracy and diagnostic challenges. Diagn Cytopathol. 2022 Sep;50(9):442-450. Cited in: PubMed; PMID 35791462.
789. Layfield LJ, Wallander ML. Diagnosis of gastrointestinal stromal tumors from minute specimens: cytomorphology, immunohistochemistry, and molecular diagnostic findings. Diagn Cytopathol. 2012 Jun;40(6):484-90. Cited in: PubMed; PMID 22351482.
790. Le BH, Boyer PJ, Lewis JE, et al. Granular cell tumor: immunohistochemical assessment of inhibin-alpha, protein gene product 9.5, S100 protein, CD68, and Ki-67 proliferative index with clinical correlation. Arch Pathol Lab Med. 2004 Jul;128(7):771-5. Cited in: PubMed; PMID 15214825.

791. Le Guellec S, Chibon F, Ouali M, et al. Are peripheral purely undifferentiated pleomorphic sarcomas with MDM2 amplification dedifferentiated liposarcomas? Am J Surg Pathol. 2014 Mar;38(3):293-304. Cited in: PubMed; PMID 24525499.
792. Le Guellec S, Decouvelaere AV, Filleron T, et al. Malignant Peripheral Nerve Sheath Tumor Is a Challenging Diagnosis: A Systematic Pathology Review, Immunohistochemistry, and Molecular Analysis in 160 Patients From the French Sarcoma Group Database. Am J Surg Pathol. 2016 Jul;40(7):896-908. Cited in: PubMed; PMID 27158754.
793. Le Guellec S, Velasco V, Pérot G, et al. ETV4 is a useful marker for the diagnosis of CIC-rearranged undifferentiated round-cell sarcomas: a study of 127 cases including mimicking lesions. Mod Pathol. 2016 Dec;29(12):1523-1531. Cited in: PubMed; PMID 27562494.
794. Le HB, Lee ST, Munk PL. Image-guided musculoskeletal biopsies. Semin Intervent Radiol. 2010 Jun;27(2):191-8. Cited in: PubMed; PMID 21629408.
795. Le Loarer F, Cleven AHG, Bouvier C, et al. A subset of epithelioid and spindle cell rhabdomyosarcomas is associated with TFCP2 fusions and common ALK upregulation. Mod Pathol. 2020 Mar;33(3):404-419. Cited in: PubMed; PMID 31383960.
796. Le Loarer F, Pissaloux D, Watson S, et al. Clinicopathologic Features of CIC-NUTM1 Sarcomas, a New Molecular Variant of the Family of CIC-Fused Sarcomas. Am J Surg Pathol. 2019 Feb;43(2):268-276. Cited in: PubMed; PMID 30407212.
797. Le Loarer F, Zhang L, Fletcher CD, et al. Consistent SMARCB1 homozygous deletions in epithelioid sarcoma and in a subset of myoepithelial carcinomas can be reliably detected by FISH in archival material. Genes Chromosomes Cancer. 2014 Jun;53(6):475-86. Cited in: PubMed; PMID 24585572.
798. Lecoutere E, Creytens D. Atypical spindle cell/pleomorphic lipomatous tumor. Histol Histopathol. 2020 Aug;35(8):769-778. Cited in: PubMed; PMID 32068239.
799. Lee AY, Agaram NP, Qin LX, et al. Optimal Percent Myxoid Component to Predict Outcome in High-Grade Myxofibrosarcoma and Undifferentiated Pleomorphic Sarcoma. Ann Surg Oncol. 2016 Mar;23(3):818-25. Cited in: PubMed; PMID 26759307.
800. Lee JC, Chou HC, Wang CH, et al. Myoepithelioma-like Hyalinizing Epithelioid Tumors of the Hand With Novel OGT-FOXO3 Fusions. Am J Surg Pathol. 2020 Mar;44(3):387-395. Cited in: PubMed; PMID 31567281.
801. Lee JC, Thomas JM, Phillips S, et al. Aggressive fibromatosis: MRI features with pathologic correlation. AJR Am J Roentgenol. 2006 Jan;186(1):247-54. Cited in: PubMed; PMID 16357411.
802. Lee JC, Wu JM, Liau JY, et al. Cytopathologic features of epithelioid inflammatory myofibroblastic sarcoma with correlation of histopathology, immunohistochemistry, and molecular cytogenetic analysis. Cancer Cytopathol. 2015 Aug;123(8):495-504. Cited in: PubMed; PMID 26139079.
803. Lee JS, Fetsch JF, Wasdhal DA, et al. A review of 40 patients with extraskeletal osteosarcoma. Cancer. 1995 Dec;76(11):2253-9. Cited in: PubMed; PMID 8635029.
804. Lee LH, Bos GD, Marsh WL, et al. Fine-needle aspiration cytology of sclerosing perineurioma. Ann Diagn Pathol. 2004 Apr;8(2):80-6. Cited in: PubMed; PMID 15060885.
805. Lee TK, Miyamoto H, Osunkoya AO, et al. Smooth muscle neoplasms of the urinary bladder: a clinicopathologic study of 51 cases. Am J Surg Pathol. 2010 Apr;34(4):502-9. Cited in: PubMed; PMID 20154594.
806. Leelatian N, Doxie DB, Greenplate AR, et al. Preparing Viable Single Cells from Human Tissue and Tumors for Cytomic Analysis. Curr Protoc Mol Biol. 2017 Apr;118:25C.1.1-25C.1.23. Cited in: PubMed; PMID 28369679.
807. Lefebvre G, Le Corroller T. Ultrasound and MR imaging of peripheral nerve tumors: the state of the art. Skeletal Radiol. 2022 Jun. Cited in: PubMed; PMID 35713690.
808. Lehmer LM, Moore JB, Ragsdale BD. Ischemic fasciitis: enhanced diagnostic resolution through clinical, histopathologic and radiologic correlation in 17 cases. J Cutan Pathol. 2016 Sep;43(9):740-8. Cited in: PubMed; PMID 27161342.
810. Lemeur M, Mattei JC, Souteyrand P, et al. Prognostic factors for the recurrence of myxoid liposarcoma: 20 cases with up to 8 years follow-up. Orthop Traumatol Surg Res. 2015 Feb;101(1):103-7. Cited in: PubMed; PMID 25583234.
811. Lemos MM, Karlen J, Tani E. Fine-needle aspiration cytology of angiomatoid malignant fibrous histiocytoma. Diagn Cytopathol. 2005 Aug;33(2):116-21. Cited in: PubMed; PMID 16007669.
812. Lemos MM, Kindblom LG, Meis-Kindblom JM, et al. Fine-needle aspiration characteristics of hibernoma. Cancer. 2001 Jun;93(3):206-10. Cited in: PubMed; PMID 11391608.
813. Leung LY, Shu SJ, Chan AC, et al. Nodular fasciitis: MRI appearance and literature review. Skeletal Radiol. 2002 Jan;31(1):9-13. Cited in: PubMed; PMID 11807586.
814. Leung SW, Bédard YC. Immunocytochemical staining on ThinPrep processed smears. Mod Pathol. 1996 Mar;9(3):304-6. Cited in: PubMed; PMID 8685232.
815. Leuschner I, Newton WA, Schmidt D, et al. Spindle cell variants of embryonal rhabdomyosarcoma in the paratesticular region. A report of the Intergroup Rhabdomyosarcoma Study. Am J Surg Pathol. 1993 Mar;17(3):221-30. Cited in: PubMed; PMID 8434703.
816. Lew WY. Spindle cell lipoma of the breast: a case report and literature review. Diagn Cytopathol. 1993 Aug;9(4):434-7. Cited in: PubMed; PMID 8261850.
817. Li G, Ogose A, Kawashima H, et al. Cytogenetic and real-time quantitative reverse-transcriptase polymerase chain reaction analyses in pleomorphic rhabdomyosarcoma. Cancer Genet Cytogenet. 2009 Jul;192(1):1-9. Cited in: PubMed; PMID 19480930.
818. Li J, Yin WH, Takeuchi K, et al. Inflammatory myofibroblastic tumor with RANBP2 and ALK gene rearrangement: a report of two cases and literature review. Diagn Pathol. 2013 Sep;8:147. Cited in: PubMed; PMID 24034896.
819. Li WS, Liao IC, Wen MC, et al. BCOR-CCNB3-positive soft tissue sarcoma with round-cell and spindle-cell histology: a series of four cases highlighting the pitfall of mimicking poorly differentiated synovial sarcoma. Histopathology. 2016 Nov;69(5):792-801. Cited in: PubMed; PMID 27228320.
820. Libbrecht S, Van Dorpe J, Creytens D. The Rapidly Expanding Group of RB1-Deleted Soft Tissue Tumors: An Updated Review. Diagnostics (Basel). 2021 Mar;11(3): Cited in: PubMed; PMID 33802620.
821. Lidang Jensen M, Schumacher B, Myhre Jensen O, et al. Extraskeletal osteosarcomas: a clinicopathologic study of 25 cases. Am J Surg Pathol. 1998 May;22(5):588-94. Cited in: PubMed; PMID 9591729.
822. Liegl B, Bennett MW, Fletcher CD. Microcystic/reticular schwannoma: a distinct variant with predilection for visceral locations. Am J Surg Pathol. 2008 Jul;32(7):1080-7. Cited in: PubMed; PMID 18520439.
823. Liegl B, Fletcher CD. Ischemic fasciitis: analysis of 44 cases indicating an inconsistent association with immobility or debilitation. Am J Surg Pathol. 2008 Oct;32(10):1546-52. Cited in: PubMed; PMID 18724246.
824. Lim GS, Oliva E. The morphologic spectrum of uterine PEC-cell associated tumors in a patient with tuberous sclerosis. Int J Gynecol Pathol. 2011 Mar;30(2):121-8. Cited in: PubMed; PMID 21293289.
825. Lim SM, Chang H, Cha YJ, et al. Validation of ALK/ROS1 Dual Break Apart FISH Probe probe in non-small-cell lung cancer. Lung Cancer. 2017 Sep;111:79-83. Cited in: PubMed; PMID 28838404.
826. Lindberg GM, Maitra A, Gokaslan ST, et al. Low grade fibromyxoid sarcoma: fine-needle aspiration cytology with histologic, cytogenetic, immunohistochemical, and ultrastructural correlation. Cancer. 1999 Apr;87(2):75-82. Cited in: PubMed; PMID 10227597.
827. Lindeman NI, Cagle PT, Aisner DL, et al. Updated Molecular Testing Guideline for the Selection of Lung Cancer Patients for Treatment With Targeted Tyrosine Kinase Inhibitors: Guideline From the College of American Pathologists, the International Association for the Study of Lung Cancer, and the Association for Molecular Pathology. J Thorac Oncol. 2018 Mar;13(3):323-358. Cited in: PubMed; PMID 29396253.
828. Lintusaari J, Vesaniemi E, Kalfert D, et al. IgG4-positive plasma cells in Hashimoto thyroiditis: IgG4-related disease or inflammation-related IgG4-positivity? APMIS. 2020 Sep;128(9):531-538. Cited in: PubMed; PMID 32578252.
829. Lips DJ, Barker N, Clevers H, et al. The role of APC and beta-catenin in the aetiology of aggressive fibromatosis (desmoid tumors). Eur J Surg Oncol. 2009 Jan;35(1):3-10. Cited in: PubMed; PMID 18722078.
830. Liu D, Quinonez G, Latosinsky S. Dedifferentiated liposarcoma with a paraganglioma-like histologic pattern: a case report and review of the literature. Arch Pathol Lab Med. 2004 Jul;128(7):788-91. Cited in: PubMed; PMID 15214821.
831. Liu H, Sukov WR, Ro JY. The t(1;10)(p22;q24) TGFBR3/MGEA5 Translocation in Pleomorphic Hyalinizing Angiectatic Tumor, Myxoinflammatory Fibroblastic Sarcoma, and Hemosiderotic Fibrolipomatous Tumor. Arch Pathol Lab Med. 2019 Feb;143(2):212-221. Cited in: PubMed; PMID 29979612.
832. Liu K, Layfield LJ, Coogan AC, et al. Diagnostic accuracy in fine-needle aspiration of soft tissue and bone lesions. Influence of clinical history and experience. Am J Clin Pathol. 1999 May;111(5):632-40. Cited in: PubMed; PMID 10230353.
833. Liu W, Bui MM, Cheong D, et al. Hibernoma: comparing imaging appearance with more commonly encountered benign or low-grade lipomatous neoplasms. Skeletal Radiol. 2013 Aug;42(8):1073-8. Cited in: PubMed; PMID 23385517.
834. Liu Y, Zheng Q, Wang C, et al. Granular cell tumors overexpress TFE3 without gene rearrangement: Evaluation of immunohistochemistry and break-apart FISH in 45 cases. Oncol Lett. 2019 Dec;18(6):6355-6360. Cited in: PubMed; PMID 31788112.
835. Liu Z, Mira JL, Vu H. Diagnosis of malignant granular cell tumor by fine needle aspiration cytology: Acta Cytol. 200145(6):1011-21. Cited in: PubMed; PMID 11726096.
836. Llombart-Bosch A, Machado I, Navarro S, et al. Histological heterogeneity of Ewing's sarcoma/PNET: an immunohistochemical analysis of 415 genetically confirmed cases with clinical support. Virchows Arch. 2009 Nov;455(5):397-411. Cited in: PubMed; PMID 19841938.
837. Logan PM, Connell DG, O'Connell JX, et al. Image-guided percutaneous biopsy of musculoskeletal tumors: an algorithm for selection of specific biopsy techniques. AJR Am J Roentgenol. 1996 Jan;166(1):137-41. Cited in: PubMed; PMID 8571862.
838. Longhi A, Bielack SS, Grimer R, et al. Extraskeletal osteosarcoma: A European Musculoskeletal Oncology Society study on 266 patients. Eur J Cancer. 2017 Mar;74:9-16. Cited in: PubMed; PMID 28167373.
839. Lopez J, Rayhrer CS. Ischemic fasciitis conversion to myxofibrosarcoma: A case report. Int J Surg Case Rep. 2021 Dec;89:106664. Cited in: PubMed; PMID 34896963.
840. López-Ferrer P, Jiménez-Heffernan JA, Vicandi B, et al. Cytologic features of alveolar soft part sarcoma: report of three cases. Diagn Cytopathol. 2002 Aug;27(2):115-9. Cited in: PubMed; PMID 12203880.
841. Lopez-Nunez O, Alaggio R, Ranganathan S, et al. New molecular insights into the pathogenesis of lipoblastomas: clinicopathologic, immunohistochemical, and molecular analysis in pediatric cases. Hum Pathol. 2020 Oct;104:30-41. Cited in: PubMed; PMID 32692992.
842. López-Ríos F, Alberti N, Pérez-Barrios A, et al. Aspiration biopsy of pleomorphic lipoma of the breast. A case report. Acta Cytol. 200044(2):255-8. Cited in: PubMed; PMID 10740617.
843. Lorigan JG, O'Keeffe FN, Evans HL, et al. The radiologic manifestations of alveolar soft-part sarcoma. AJR Am J Roentgenol. 1989 Aug;153(2):335-9. Cited in: PubMed; PMID 2750619.
844. Louis CU, Shohet JM. Neuroblastoma: molecular pathogenesis and therapy. Annu Rev Med. 201566:49-63. Cited in: PubMed; PMID 25386934.
845. Lozano MD, Echeveste JI, Abengozar M, et al. Cytology Smears in the Era of Molecular Biomarkers in Non-Small Cell Lung Cancer: Doing More With Less. Arch Pathol Lab Med. 2018 Mar;142(3):291-298. Cited in: PubMed; PMID 29494220.
846. Lu HC, Eulo V, Apicelli AJ, et al. Aberrant ATRX protein expression is associated with poor overall survival in NF1-MPNST. Oncotarget. 2018 May;9(33):23018-23028. Cited in: PubMed; PMID 29796169.
847. Lu L, Lao IW, Liu X, et al. Nodular fasciitis: a retrospective study of 272 cases from China with clinicopathologic and radiologic correlation. Ann Diagn Pathol. 2015 Jun;19(3):180-5. Cited in: PubMed; PMID 25890487.
848. Lucas DR. Myxoinflammatory Fibroblastic Sarcoma: Review and Update. Arch Pathol Lab Med. 2017 Nov;141(11):1503-1507. Cited in: PubMed; PMID 29072951.
849. Lucas DR, Fletcher CD, Adsay NV, et al. High-grade extraskeletal myxoid chondrosarcoma: a high-grade epithelioid malignancy. Histopathology. 1999 Sep;35(3):201-8. Cited in: PubMed; PMID 10469211.
850. Ludwig K, Alaggio R, Zin A, et al. BCOR-CCNB3 Undifferentiated Sarcoma-Does Immunohistochemistry Help in the Identification? Pediatr Dev Pathol. 201720(4):321-329. Cited in: PubMed; PMID 28420319.
851. Lund JJ, Xia L, Kerr S, et al. The utility of a touch preparation in the diagnosis of fluctuant subcutaneous fat necrosis of the newborn. Pediatr Dermatol. 200926(2):241-3. Cited in: PubMed; PMID 19419492.
852. Lundgren L, Kindblom LG, Willems J, et al. Proliferative myositis and fasciitis. A light and electron microscopic, cytologic,

DNA-cytometric and immunohistochemical study. APMIS. 1992 May;100(5):437-48. Cited in: PubMed; PMID 1586481.
854. Luzar B, Martin B, Fisher C, et al. Cutaneous malignant glomus tumours: applicability of currently established malignancy criteria for tumours occurring in the skin. Pathology. 2018 Dec;50(7):711-717. Cited in: PubMed; PMID 30314644.
855. Lynskey SJ, Pianta MJ. MRI and thallium features of pigmented villonodular synovitis and giant cell tumours of tendon sheaths: a retrospective single centre study of imaging and literature review. Br J Radiol. 201588(1056):20150528. Cited in: PubMed; PMID 26440548.
856. Ma Y, Feng J, Zhao J, et al. PHOX2B as a Reliable Marker for Neuroblastoma in Tissue and Cytology Specimens. J Neuropathol Exp Neurol. 2021 Dec;80(12):1108-1116. Cited in: PubMed; PMID 34965292.
857. Machado I, López-Soto MV, Rubio L, et al. Soft tissue myoepithelial carcinoma with rhabdoid-like features and EWSR1 rearrangement: Fine needle aspiration cytology with histologic correlation. Diagn Cytopathol. 2015 May;43(5):421-6. Cited in: PubMed; PMID 25693574.
858. Machado I, Navarro S, López-Guerrero JA, et al. Neuroendocrine differentiation in a large series of genetically-confirmed Ewing's sarcoma family tumor: Does it provide any diagnostic or prognostic information? Pathol Res Pract. 2021 Mar;219:153362. Cited in: PubMed; PMID 33610950.
859. Machado I, Yoshida A, Morales MGN, et al. Review with novel markers facilitates precise categorization of 41 cases of diagnostically challenging, "undifferentiated small round cell tumors". A clinicopathologic, immunophenotypic and molecular analysis. Ann Diagn Pathol. 2018 Jun;34:1-12. Cited in: PubMed; PMID 29661713.
860. Maire G, Forus A, Foa C, et al. 11q13 alterations in two cases of hibernoma: large heterozygous deletions and rearrangement breakpoints near GARP in 11q13.5. Genes Chromosomes Cancer. 2003 Aug;37(4):389-95. Cited in: PubMed; PMID 12800150.
861. Majoor BCJ, van de Sande MAJ, Appelman-Dijkstra NM, et al. Prevalence and Clinical Features of Mazabraud Syndrome: A Multicenter European Study. J Bone Joint Surg Am. 2019 Jan;101(2):160-168. Cited in: PubMed; PMID 30653046.
862. Makhlouf HR, Ishak KG, Goodman ZD. Epithelioid hemangioendothelioma of the liver: a clinicopathologic study of 137 cases. Cancer. 1999 Feb;85(3):562-82. Cited in: PubMed; PMID 10091730.
863. Makise N, Sekimizu M, Kubo T, et al. Clarifying the Distinction Between Malignant Peripheral Nerve Sheath Tumor and Dedifferentiated Liposarcoma: A Critical Reappraisal of the Diagnostic Utility of MDM2 and H3K27me3 Status. Am J Surg Pathol. 2018 May;42(5):656-664. Cited in: PubMed; PMID 29309298.
864. Malami SA, Ochicha O. A review of the utilization of fine needle aspiration in clinical practice and research in Nigeria. Cytojournal. 20118:12. Cited in: PubMed; PMID 21760830.
865. Malapelle U, Mayo-de-Las-Casas C, Molina-Vila MA, et al. Consistency and reproducibility of next-generation sequencing and other multigene mutational assays: A worldwide ring trial study on quantitative cytological molecular reference specimens. Cancer Cytopathol. 2017 Aug;125(8):615-626. Cited in: PubMed; PMID 28475299.
866. Maleki S, Cajigas A, Moss J, et al. Fine-needle aspiration biopsy of prostate synovial sarcoma: A case report and review of the literature. Diagn Cytopathol. 2017 Feb;45(2):168-172. Cited in: PubMed; PMID 27774755.
867. Malempati S, Hawkins DS. Rhabdomyosarcoma: review of the Children's Oncology Group (COG) Soft-Tissue Sarcoma Committee experience and rationale for current COG studies. Pediatr Blood Cancer. 2012 Jul;59(1):5-10. Cited in: PubMed; PMID 22378628.
868. Mallik MK, Dey P, Gupta SK, et al. Grading of soft tissue sarcomas on fine-needle aspiration cytology smear. Diagn Cytopathol. 2010 Feb;38(2):109-12. Cited in: PubMed; PMID 19688763.
869. Mandelia A, Agarwala S, Sharma A, et al. Assessment of fine needle aspiration cytology samples for molecular genetic analysis in neuroblastoma. Pediatr Surg Int. 2013 Nov;29(11):1131-8. Cited in: PubMed; PMID 23979398.
870. Manner J, Radlwimmer B, Hohenberger P, et al. MYC high level gene amplification is a distinctive feature of angiosarcomas after irradiation or chronic lymphedema. Am J Pathol. 2010 Jan;176(1):34-9. Cited in: PubMed; PMID 20008140.
871. Manucha V, Sun CC. Cytologic findings and differential diagnosis in hepatic Epithelioid hemangioendothelioma: a case report. Acta Cytol. 200852(6):713-7. Cited in: PubMed; PMID 19068677.
872. Marchetti A, Barberis M, Papotti M, et al. ALK rearrangement testing by FISH analysis in non-small-cell lung cancer patients: results of the first italian external quality assurance scheme. J Thorac Oncol. 2014 Oct;9(10):1470-6. Cited in: PubMed; PMID 25170637.
873. Marchetti A, Felicioni L, Buttitta F. Assessing EGFR mutations. N Engl J Med. 2006 Feb;354(5):526-8; author reply 526-8. Cited in: PubMed; PMID 16452569.
874. Marco V, Sirvent J, Alvarez Moro J, et al. Malignant melanotic schwannoma fine-needle aspiration biopsy findings. Diagn Cytopathol. 1998 Apr;18(4):284-6. Cited in: PubMed; PMID 9557264.
875. Mardekian SK, Solomides CC, Gong JZ, et al. Comparison of Chromogenic In Situ Hybridization and Fluorescence In Situ Hybridization for the Evaluation of MDM2 Amplification in Adipocytic Tumors. J Clin Lab Anal. 2015 Nov;29(6):462-8. Cited in: PubMed; PMID 25132285.
876. Mariño-Enríquez A, Fletcher CD, Dal Cin P, et al. Dedifferentiated liposarcoma with "homologous" lipoblastic (pleomorphic liposarcoma-like) differentiation: clinicopathologic and molecular analysis of a series suggesting revised diagnostic criteria. Am J Surg Pathol. 2010 Aug;34(8):1122-31. Cited in: PubMed; PMID 20588177.
877. Mariño-Enríquez A, Hornick JL, Dal Cin P, et al. Dedifferentiated liposarcoma and pleomorphic liposarcoma: a comparative study of cytomorphology and MDM2/CDK4 expression on fine-needle aspiration. Cancer Cytopathol. 2014 Feb;122(2):128-37. Cited in: PubMed; PMID 24227706.
878. Mariño-Enriquez A, Nascimento AF, Ligon AH, et al. Atypical Spindle Cell Lipomatous Tumor: Clinicopathologic Characterization of 232 Cases Demonstrating a Morphologic Spectrum. Am J Surg Pathol. 2017 Feb;41(2):234-244. Cited in: PubMed; PMID 27879515.
879. Mariño-Enríquez A, Wang WL, Roy A, et al. Epithelioid inflammatory myofibroblastic sarcoma: An aggressive intra-abdominal variant of inflammatory myofibroblastic tumor with nuclear membrane or perinuclear ALK. Am J Surg Pathol. 2011 Jan;35(1):135-44. Cited in: PubMed; PMID 21164297.
880. Martignoni G, Gobbo S, Camparo P, et al. Differential expression of cathepsin K in neoplasms harboring TFE3 gene fusions. Mod Pathol. 2011 Oct;24(10):1313-9. Cited in: PubMed; PMID 21602817.
881. Martin L, Combemale P, Dupin M, et al. The atrophic variant of dermatofibrosarcoma protuberans in childhood: a report of six cases. Br J Dermatol. 1998 Oct;139(4):719-25. Cited in: PubMed; PMID 10025975.
882. Martín Broto J. Advancing towards Better Cooperation for Better Sarcoma Prognoses. Oncology. 201895 Suppl 1:5-10. Cited in: PubMed; PMID 30554196.
883. Martinez SJ, Moreno CC, Vinson EN, et al. Angiomatoid fibrous histiocytoma: novel MR imaging findings. Skeletal Radiol. 2016 May;45(5):661-70. Cited in: PubMed; PMID 26919861.
884. Martínez Trufero J, Pajares Bernad I, Torres Ramón I, et al. Desmoid-Type Fibromatosis: Who, When, and How to Treat. Curr Treat Options Oncol. 2017 May;18(5):29. Cited in: PubMed; PMID 28439797.
885. Martínez-Onsurbe P, Jiménez-Heffernan JA, Guadalix-Hidalgo G. Fine needle aspiration cytology of intranodal myofibroblastoma. A case report. Acta Cytol. 200246(6):1143-7. Cited in: PubMed; PMID 12462097.
886. Maruyama R, Nakano M, Yamashita S, et al. Fine needle aspiration cytology of clear cell sarcoma. Report of a case with immunocytochemical, immunohistochemical and ultrastructural studies. Acta Cytol. 199236(6):937-42. Cited in: PubMed; PMID 1449032.
887. Masson-Lecomte A, Rocher L, Ferlicot S, et al. High-flow priapism due to a malignant glomus tumor (glomangiosarcoma) of the corpus cavernosum. J Sex Med. 2011 Dec;8(12):3518-22. Cited in: PubMed; PMID 19912496.
888. Matevossian E, Brücher BL, Nährig J, et al. Glomus tumor of the stomach simulating a gastrointestinal stromal tumor: a case report and review of literature. Case Rep Gastroenterol. 2008 Jan;2(1):1-5. Cited in: PubMed; PMID 21490829.
889. Mathur S, Kapila K, Verma K. Accuracy of cytological grading of spindle-cell sarcomas. Diagn Cytopathol. 2003 Aug;29(2):79-83. Cited in: PubMed; PMID 12889044.
890. Matsuyama A, Hisaoka M, Hashimoto H. PLAG1 expression in mesenchymal tumors: an immunohistochemical study with special emphasis on the pathogenetical distinction between soft tissue myoepithelioma and pleomorphic adenoma of the salivary gland. Pathol Int. 2012 Jan;62(1):1-7. Cited in: PubMed; PMID 22192798.
891. Matsuyama A, Shiba E, Umekita Y, et al. Clinicopathologic Diversity of Undifferentiated Sarcoma With BCOR-CCNB3 Fusion: Analysis of 11 Cases With a Reappraisal of the Utility of Immunohistochemistry for BCOR and CCNB3. Am J Surg Pathol. 2017 Dec;41(12):1713-1721. Cited in: PubMed; PMID 28877060.
892. Matter MS, Chijioke O, Savic S, et al. Narrative review of molecular pathways of kinase fusions and diagnostic approaches for their detection in non-small cell lung carcinomas. Transl Lung Cancer Res. 2020 Dec;9(6):2645-2655. Cited in: PubMed; PMID 33489824.
894. Matusik J, Wiberg A, Sloboda J, et al. Fine needle aspiration in nodular fasciitis of the face. Cytopathology. 2002 Apr;13(2):128-32. Cited in: PubMed; PMID 11952752.
895. Matyakhina L, Bei TA, McWhinney SR, et al. Genetics of carney triad: recurrent losses at chromosome 1 but lack of germline mutations in genes associated with paragangliomas and gastrointestinal stromal tumors. J Clin Endocrinol Metab. 2007 Aug;92(8):2938-43. Cited in: PubMed; PMID 17535989.
896. Mavrogenis AF, Coll-Mesa L, Drago G, et al. Hibernomas: clinicopathological features, diagnosis, and treatment of 17 cases. Orthopedics. 2011 Nov;34(11):e755-9. Cited in: PubMed; PMID 22049958.
897. Mayr-Kanhäuser S, Behmel A, Aberer W. Multiple glomus tumors of the skin with male-to-male transmission over four generations. J Invest Dermatol. 2001 Mar;116(3):475-6. Cited in: PubMed; PMID 11231328.
898. McCarter MD, Lewis JJ, Antonescu CR, et al. Extraskeletal osteosarcoma: analysis of outcome of a rare neoplasm. Sarcoma. 20004(3):119-23. Cited in: PubMed; PMID 18521290.
899. McCarthy AJ, Chetty R. Tumours composed of fat are no longer a simple diagnosis: an overview of fatty tumours with a spindle cell component. J Clin Pathol. 2018 Jun;71(6):483-492. Cited in: PubMed; PMID 29358476.
900. McCarville MB, Muzzafar S, Kao SC, et al. Imaging features of alveolar soft-part sarcoma: a report from Children's Oncology Group Study ARST0332. AJR Am J Roentgenol. 2014 Dec;203(6):1345-52. Cited in: PubMed; PMID 25415714.
901. McCluggage WG, Lioe TF, McClelland HR, et al. Rhabdomyosarcoma of the uterus: report of two cases, including one of the spindle cell variant. Int J Gynecol Cancer. 200212(1):128-32. Cited in: PubMed; PMID 11860548.
902. McCuaig CC. Update on classification and diagnosis of vascular malformations. Curr Opin Pediatr. 2017 Aug;29(4):448-454. Cited in: PubMed; PMID 28654575.
903. McCuiston A, Bishop JA. Usefulness of NKX2.2 Immunohistochemistry for Distinguishing Ewing Sarcoma from Other Sinonasal Small Round Blue Cell Tumors. Head Neck Pathol. 2018 Mar;12(1):89-94. Cited in: PubMed; PMID 28616785.
904. McCullough AL, Scotland TR, Dundas SR, et al. The impact of a managed clinical network on referral patterns of sarcoma patients in Grampian. Scott Med J. 2014 May;59(2):108-13. Cited in: PubMed; PMID 24692232.
905. McGregor DK, Krishnan B, Green L. Fine-needle aspiration of adult rhabdomyoma: a case report with review of the literature. Diagn Cytopathol. 2003 Feb;28(2):92-5. Cited in: PubMed; PMID 12561029.
906. McKee PH, Fletcher CD. Dermatofibrosarcoma protuberans presenting in infancy and childhood. J Cutan Pathol. 1991 Aug;18(4):241-6. Cited in: PubMed; PMID 1939782.
907. McMaster ML, Goldstein AM, Bromley CM, et al. Chordoma: incidence and survival patterns in the United States, 1973-1995. Cancer Causes Control. 2001 Jan;12(1):1-11. Cited in: PubMed; PMID 11227920.
908. McMenamin ME, Fletcher CD. Expanding the spectrum of malignant change in schwannomas: epithelioid malignant change, epithelioid malignant peripheral nerve sheath tumor, and epithelioid angiosarcoma: a study of 17 cases. Am J Surg Pathol. 2001 Jan;25(1):13-25. Cited in: PubMed; PMID 11145248.
909. McMenamin ME, Fletcher CD. Mammary-type myofibroblastoma of soft tissue: a tumor closely related to spindle cell lipoma. Am J Surg Pathol. 2001 Aug;25(8):1022-9. Cited in: PubMed; PMID 11474286.
910. Meazza C, Bisogno G, Gronchi A, et al. Aggressive fibromatosis in children and adolescents: the Italian experience. Cancer. 2010 Jan;116(1):233-40. Cited in: PubMed; PMID 19950127.
911. Megahed M. Histopathological variants of neurofibroma. A study of 114 lesions. Am J Dermatopathol. 1994 Oct;16(5):486-95. Cited in: PubMed; PMID 7528474.

912. Meis JM, Enzinger FM. Proliferative fasciitis and myositis of childhood. Am J Surg Pathol. 1992 Apr;16(4):364-72. Cited in: PubMed; PMID 1566969.
913. Meis-Kindblom JM, Bergh P, Gunterberg B, et al. Extraskeletal myxoid chondrosarcoma: a reappraisal of its morphologic spectrum and prognostic factors based on 117 cases. Am J Surg Pathol. 1999 Jun;23(6):636-50. Cited in: PubMed; PMID 10366145.
914. Meis-Kindblom JM, Kindblom LG. Acral myxoinflammatory fibroblastic sarcoma: a low-grade tumor of the hands and feet. Am J Surg Pathol. 1998 Aug;22(8):911-24. Cited in: PubMed; PMID 9706971.
915. Meis-Kindblom JM, Kindblom LG. Angiosarcoma of soft tissue: a study of 80 cases. Am J Surg Pathol. 1998 Jun;22(6):683-97. Cited in: PubMed; PMID 9630175.
916. Meister P, Bückmann FW, Konrad E. Extent and level of fascial involvement in 100 cases with nodular fasciitis. Virchows Arch A Pathol Anat Histol. 1978 Oct;380(2):177-85. Cited in: PubMed; PMID 153036.
917. Mello CA, Campos FAB, Santos TG, et al. Desmoplastic Small Round Cell Tumor: A Review of Main Molecular Abnormalities and Emerging Therapy. Cancers (Basel). 2021 Jan;13(3): Cited in: PubMed; PMID 33525546.
918. Menge F, Jakob J, Kasper B, et al. Clinical Presentation of Gastrointestinal Stromal Tumors. Visc Med. 2018 Oct;34(5):335-340. Cited in: PubMed; PMID 30498699.
919. Mentzel T, Beham A, Calonje E, et al. Epithelioid hemangioendothelioma of skin and soft tissues: clinicopathologic and immunohistochemical study of 30 cases. Am J Surg Pathol. 1997 Apr;21(4):363-74. Cited in: PubMed; PMID 9130982.
920. Mentzel T, Beham A, Katenkamp D, et al. Fibrosarcomatous ("high-grade") dermatofibrosarcoma protuberans: clinicopathologic and immunohistochemical study of a series of 41 cases with emphasis on prognostic significance. Am J Surg Pathol. 1998 May;22(5):576-87. Cited in: PubMed; PMID 9591728.
921. Mentzel T, Calonje E, Wadden C, et al. Myxofibrosarcoma. Clinicopathologic analysis of 75 cases with emphasis on the low-grade variant. Am J Surg Pathol. 1996 Apr;20(4):391-405. Cited in: PubMed; PMID 8604805.
922. Mentzel T, Dry S, Katenkamp D, et al. Low-grade myofibroblastic sarcoma: analysis of 18 cases in the spectrum of myofibroblastic tumors. Am J Surg Pathol. 1998 Oct;22(10):1228-38. Cited in: PubMed; PMID 9777985.
923. Mentzel T, Katenkamp D. Intraneural angiosarcoma and angiosarcoma arising in benign and malignant peripheral nerve sheath tumours: clinicopathological and immunohistochemical analysis of four cases. Histopathology. 1999 Aug;35(2):114-20. Cited in: PubMed; PMID 10460655.
924. Mentzel T, Katenkamp D. Sclerosing, pseudovascular rhabdomyosarcoma in adults. Clinicopathological and immunohistochemical analysis of three cases. Virchows Arch. 2000 Apr;436(4):305-11. Cited in: PubMed; PMID 10834531.
925. Mentzel T, Kutzner H. Reticular and plexiform perineurioma: clinicopathological and immunohistochemical analysis of two cases and review of perineurial neoplasms of skin and soft tissues. Virchows Arch. 2005 Oct;447(4):677-82. Cited in: PubMed; PMID 16133356.
926. Mentzel T, Palmedo G, Kuhnen C. Well-differentiated spindle cell liposarcoma ('atypical spindle cell lipomatous tumor') does not belong to the spectrum of atypical lipomatous tumor but has a close relationship to spindle cell lipoma: clinicopathologic, immunohistochemical, and molecular analysis of six cases. Mod Pathol. 2010 May;23(5):729-36. Cited in: PubMed; PMID 20228779.
927. Mentzel T, Schärer L, Kazakov DV, et al. Myxoid dermatofibrosarcoma protuberans: clinicopathologic, immunohistochemical, and molecular analysis of eight cases. Am J Dermatopathol. 2007 Oct;29(5):443-8. Cited in: PubMed; PMID 17890911.
928. Merck C, Hagmar B. Myxofibrosarcoma: a correlative cytologic and histologic study of 13 cases examined by fine needle aspiration cytology. Acta Cytol. 198024(2):137-44. Cited in: PubMed; PMID 6154396.
929. Merkel DE, Dressler LG, McGuire WL. Flow cytometry, cellular DNA content, and prognosis in human malignancy. J Clin Oncol. 1987 Oct;5(10):1690-703. Cited in: PubMed; PMID 3309200.
930. Meyer A, Szajnbok P, Koszka AJM, et al. A rare sporadic pancreatic desmoid fibromatosis with splenic vein invasion diagnosed by CT scan-guided core needle biopsy: a case report with possible differential diagnosis from metastatic colorectal or renal cancer. J Surg Case Rep. 2021 Jun;2021(6):rjab257. Cited in: PubMed; PMID 34194727.
931. Meyerson J, Pan YL, Spaeth M, et al. Pediatric Ganglion Cysts: A Retrospective Review. Hand (N Y). 2019 Jul;14(4):445-448. Cited in: PubMed; PMID 29310457.
932. Michael CW, Bedrossian CC. The implementation of liquid-based cytology for lung and pleural-based diseases. Acta Cytol. 201458(6):563-73. Cited in: PubMed; PMID 25427721.
933. Michal M. Inflammatory myxoid tumor of the soft parts with bizarre giant cells. Pathol Res Pract. 1998194(8):529-33. Cited in: PubMed; PMID 9779486.
934. Michal M, Berry RS, Rubin BP, et al. EWSR1-SMAD3-rearranged Fibroblastic Tumor: An Emerging Entity in an Increasingly More Complex Group of Fibroblastic/Myofibroblastic Neoplasms. Am J Surg Pathol. 2018 Oct;42(10):1325-1333. Cited in: PubMed; PMID 29957732.
935. Michal M, Miettinen M. Myoepitheliomas of the skin and soft tissues. Report of 12 cases. Virchows Arch. 1999 May;434(5):393-400. Cited in: PubMed; PMID 10389622.
936. Michelow P, Field AS. Spindle Cell Lesions of the Breast on Fine-Needle Aspiration Biopsy: A Miscellany of Masses. Acta Cytol. 201963(4):328-339. Cited in: PubMed; PMID 31117069.
937. Michelow P, Omar T, Field A, et al. The cytopathology of mycobacterial infection. Diagn Cytopathol. 2016 Mar;44(3):255-62. Cited in: PubMed; PMID 26800030.
938. Miettinen M. Smooth muscle tumors of soft tissue and non-uterine viscera: biology and prognosis. Mod Pathol. 2014 Jan;27 Suppl 1(Suppl 1):S17-29. Cited in: PubMed; PMID 24384850.
939. Miettinen M, Enzinger FM. Epithelioid variant of pleomorphic liposarcoma: a study of 12 cases of a distinctive variant of high-grade liposarcoma. Mod Pathol. 1999 Jul;12(7):722-8. Cited in: PubMed; PMID 10430277.
940. Miettinen M, Fanburg-Smith JC, Virolainen M, et al. Epithelioid sarcoma: an immunohistochemical analysis of 112 classical and variant cases and a discussion of the differential diagnosis. Hum Pathol. 1999 Aug;30(8):934-42. Cited in: PubMed; PMID 10452506.
941. Miettinen M, Fetsch JF. Distribution of keratins in normal endothelial cells and a spectrum of vascular tumors: implications in tumor diagnosis. Hum Pathol. 2000 Sep;31(9):1062-7. Cited in: PubMed; PMID 11014572.
942. Miettinen M, Furlong M, Sarlomo-Rikala M, et al. Gastrointestinal stromal tumors, intramural leiomyomas, and leiomyosarcomas in the rectum and anus: a clinicopathologic, immunohistochemical, and molecular genetic study of 144 cases. Am J Surg Pathol. 2001 Sep;25(9):1121-33. Cited in: PubMed; PMID 11688571.
943. Miettinen M, Höckerstedt K, Reitamo J, et al. Intramuscular myxoma--a clinicopathological study of twenty-three cases. Am J Clin Pathol. 1985 Sep;84(3):265-72. Cited in: PubMed; PMID 4036856.
944. Miettinen M, Lasota J. Gastrointestinal stromal tumors: pathology and prognosis at different sites. Semin Diagn Pathol. 2006 May;23(2):70-83. Cited in: PubMed; PMID 17193820.
945. Miettinen M, McCue PA, Sarlomo-Rikala M, et al. Sox10--a marker for not only schwannian and melanocytic neoplasms but also myoepithelial cell tumors of soft tissue: a systematic analysis of 5134 tumors. Am J Surg Pathol. 2015 Jun;39(6):826-35. Cited in: PubMed; PMID 25724000.
946. Miettinen M, Paal E, Lasota J, et al. Gastrointestinal glomus tumors: a clinicopathologic, immunohistochemical, and molecular genetic study of 32 cases. Am J Surg Pathol. 2002 Mar;26(3):301-11. Cited in: PubMed; PMID 11859201.
947. Miettinen M, Sarlomo-Rikala M, Sobin LH, et al. Esophageal stromal tumors: a clinicopathologic, immunohistochemical, and molecular genetic study of 17 cases and comparison with esophageal leiomyomas and leiomyosarcomas. Am J Surg Pathol. 2000 Feb;24(2):211-22. Cited in: PubMed; PMID 10680889.
948. Miettinen M, Sobin LH. Gastrointestinal stromal tumors in the appendix: a clinicopathologic and immunohistochemical study of four cases. Am J Surg Pathol. 2001 Nov;25(11):1433-7. Cited in: PubMed; PMID 11684962.
949. Miettinen M, Wang Z, Lasota J, et al. Nuclear Brachyury Expression Is Consistent in Chordoma, Common in Germ Cell Tumors and Small Cell Carcinomas, and Rare in Other Carcinomas and Sarcomas: An Immunohistochemical Study of 5229 Cases. Am J Surg Pathol. 2015 Oct;39(10):1305-12. Cited in: PubMed; PMID 26099010.
950. Miettinen M, Wang Z, McCue PA, et al. SALL4 expression in germ cell and non-germ cell tumors: a systematic immunohistochemical study of 3215 cases. Am J Surg Pathol. 2014 Mar;38(3):410-20. Cited in: PubMed; PMID 24525512.
951. Miettinen M, Wang Z, Sarlomo-Rikala M, et al. ERG expression in epithelioid sarcoma: a diagnostic pitfall. Am J Surg Pathol. 2013 Oct;37(10):1580-5. Cited in: PubMed; PMID 23774169.
952. Miettinen M, Wang ZF, Lasota J. DOG1 antibody in the differential diagnosis of gastrointestinal stromal tumors: a study of 1840 cases. Am J Surg Pathol. 2009 Sep;33(9):1401-8. Cited in: PubMed; PMID 19606013.
953. Miettinen M, Wang ZF, Paetau A, et al. ERG transcription factor as an immunohistochemical marker for vascular endothelial tumors and prostatic carcinoma. Am J Surg Pathol. 2011 Mar;35(3):432-41. Cited in: PubMed; PMID 21317715.
954. Miettinen M, Wang ZF, Sarlomo-Rikala M, et al. Succinate dehydrogenase-deficient GISTs: a clinicopathologic, immunohistochemical, and molecular genetic study of 66 gastric GISTs with predilection to young age. Am J Surg Pathol. 2011 Nov;35(11):1712-21. Cited in: PubMed; PMID 21997692.
955. Minoda Y, Akahoshi K, Oya M, et al. Gastric glomus tumor diagnosed by endoscopic ultrasound-guided fine-needle aspiration biopsy: report of a case. Fukuoka Igaku Zasshi. 2014 Apr;105(4):105-9. Cited in: PubMed; PMID 25076782.
956. Minoletti F, Miozzo M, Pedeutour F, et al. Involvement of chromosomes 17 and 22 in dermatofibrosarcoma protuberans. Genes Chromosomes Cancer. 1995 May;13(1):62-5. Cited in: PubMed; PMID 7541645.
957. Mito JK, Qian X, Doyle LA, et al. Role of Histone H3K27 Trimethylation Loss as a Marker for Malignant Peripheral Nerve Sheath Tumor in Fine-Needle Aspiration and Small Biopsy Specimens. Am J Clin Pathol. 2017 Aug;148(2):179-189. Cited in: PubMed; PMID 28898989.
958. Miura Y, Keira Y, Ogino J, et al. Detection of specific genetic abnormalities by fluorescence in situ hybridization in soft tissue tumors. Pathol Int. 2012 Jan;62(1):16-27. Cited in: PubMed; PMID 22192800.
959. Mizuguchi K, Minato H, Onishi H, et al. Cytopathological findings of primary pulmonary Ewing family of tumors with EWSR1 translocation: A case report. Thorac Cancer. 2016 Sep;7(5):602-606. Cited in: PubMed; PMID 27766786.
960. Mobarki M, Dumollard JM, Dal Col P, et al. Granular cell tumor a study of 42 cases and systemic review of the literature. Pathol Res Pract. 2020 Apr;216(4):152865. Cited in: PubMed; PMID 32089415.
961. Mobley BC, McKenney JK, Bangs CD, et al. Loss of SMARCB1/INI1 expression in poorly differentiated chordomas. Acta Neuropathol. 2010 Dec;120(6):745-53. Cited in: PubMed; PMID 21057957.
962. Moffarah AS, Al Mohajer M, Hurwitz BL, et al. Skin and Soft Tissue Infections. Microbiol Spectr. 2016 Aug;4(4): Cited in: PubMed; PMID 27726817.
963. Mohajeri A, Tayebwa J, Collin A, et al. Comprehensive genetic analysis identifies a pathognomonic NAB2/STAT6 fusion gene, nonrandom secondary genomic imbalances, and a characteristic gene expression profile in solitary fibrous tumor. Genes Chromosomes Cancer. 2013 Oct;52(10):873-86. Cited in: PubMed; PMID 23761323.
964. Mohanty SK, Pradhan D, Stavropoulos S, et al. Diagnosis of gastric glomus tumour by endoscopic ultrasound-guided fine needle aspiration cytology: a case report. Cytopathology. 2014 Jun;25(3):205-7. Cited in: PubMed; PMID 23635014.
965. Moholkar S, Sebire NJ, Roebuck DJ. Radiological-pathological correlation in lipoblastoma and lipoblastomatosis. Pediatr Radiol. 2006 Aug;36(8):851-6. Cited in: PubMed; PMID 16775739.
966. Moisini I, Amin K, Mallery S, et al. Efficacy of endoscopic-guided fine-needle aspiration in the diagnosis of gastrointestinal spindle cell tumors. Diagn Cytopathol. 2018 Aug;46(8):663-669. Cited in: PubMed; PMID 31012545.
967. Mojica WD, Kuntzman T. Elastofibroma dorsi: elaboration of cytologic features and review of its pathogenesis. Diagn Cytopathol. 2000 Dec;23(6):393-6. Cited in: PubMed; PMID 11074644.
968. Mokhtari M, Kumar PV, Rezazadeh S. Confusing cytological findings in myositis ossificans. Acta Cytol. 201256(5):565-70. Cited in: PubMed; PMID 23075901.
969. Molina-Ruiz AM, Cerroni L, Kutzner H, et al. Immunohistochemistry in the diagnosis of cutaneous bacterial infections. Am J Dermatopathol. 2015 Mar;37(3):179-93; quiz 194-6. Cited in: PubMed; PMID 25699977.
970. Möller E, Hornick JL, Magnusson L, et al. FUS-CREB3L2/L1-positive sarcomas show a specific gene expression profile with upregulation of CD24 and FOXL1. Clin Cancer Res. 2011 May;17(9):2646-56. Cited in: PubMed; PMID 21536545.
971. Möller E, Mandahl N, Mertens F, et al. Molecular identification of COL6A3-CSF1

fusion transcripts in tenosynovial giant cell tumors. Genes Chromosomes Cancer. 2008 Jan;47(1):21-5. Cited in: PubMed; PMID 17918257.
972. Momosaka D, Togao O, Hiwatashi A, et al. Spindle cell/sclerosing rhabdomyosarcoma with intracranial invasion without destroying the bone of the skull base: a case report and literature review. Acta Radiol Open. 2017 Aug;6(8):2058460117727316. Cited in: PubMed; PMID 28839951.
973. Montgomery EA, Devaney KO, Giordano TJ, et al. Inflammatory myxohyaline tumor of distal extremities with virocyte or Reed-Sternberg-like cells: a distinctive lesion with features simulating inflammatory conditions, Hodgkin's disease, and various sarcomas. Mod Pathol. 1998 Apr;11(4):384-91. Cited in: PubMed; PMID 9578090.
974. Montgomery EA, Meis JM. Nodular fasciitis. Its morphologic spectrum and immunohistochemical profile. Am J Surg Pathol. 1991 Oct;15(10):942-8. Cited in: PubMed; PMID 1928550.
975. Montgomery EA, Meis JM, Mitchell MS, et al. Atypical decubital fibroplasia. A distinctive fibroblastic pseudotumor occurring in debilitated patients. Am J Surg Pathol. 1992 Jul;16(7):708-15. Cited in: PubMed; PMID 1530110.
976. Moreau LC, Turcotte R, Ferguson P, et al. Myxoid\round cell liposarcoma (MRCLS) revisited: an analysis of 418 primarily managed cases. Ann Surg Oncol. 2012 Apr;19(4):1081-8. Cited in: PubMed; PMID 22052112.
977. Morotti RA, Nicol KK, Parham DM, et al. An immunohistochemical algorithm to facilitate diagnosis and subtyping of rhabdomyosarcoma: the Children's Oncology Group experience. Am J Surg Pathol. 2006 Aug;30(8):962-8. Cited in: PubMed; PMID 16861966.
979. Moskowitz C, Edelstein C, Oh M, et al. Retinal capillary hemangioma in von Hippel-Lindau disease. Can J Ophthalmol. 2005 Apr;40(2):192-4. Cited in: PubMed; PMID 16049535.
980. Mosquera JM, Fletcher CD. Expanding the spectrum of malignant progression in solitary fibrous tumors: a study of 8 cases with a discrete anaplastic component--is this dedifferentiated SFT? Am J Surg Pathol. 2009 Sep;33(9):1314-21. Cited in: PubMed; PMID 19718788.
981. Mosquera JM, Sboner A, Zhang L, et al. Novel MIR143-NOTCH fusions in benign and malignant glomus tumors. Genes Chromosomes Cancer. 2013 Nov;52(11):1075-87. Cited in: PubMed; PMID 23999936.
982. Mossé YP. Anaplastic Lymphoma Kinase as a Cancer Target in Pediatric Malignancies. Clin Cancer Res. 2016 Feb;22(3):546-52. Cited in: PubMed; PMID 26503946.
983. Mosunjac MB, Johnston EI, Mosunjac MI. Fine-needle aspiration cytologic diagnosis of metastatic melanotic schwannoma: familial case of a mother and daughter with Carney's complex and literature review. Diagn Cytopathol. 2007 Feb;35(2):130-4. Cited in: PubMed; PMID 17230569.
984. Moten AS, Zhao H, Wu H, et al. Malignant granular cell tumor: Clinical features and long-term survival. J Surg Oncol. 2018 Nov;118(6):891-897. Cited in: PubMed; PMID 30196562.
985. Mou Y, Jiao Q, Wang Y, et al. Musculoskeletal actinomycosis in children: a case report. BMC Infect Dis. 2021 Dec;21(1):1220. Cited in: PubMed; PMID 34876043.
986. Mravic M, LaChaud G, Nguyen A, et al. Clinical and histopathological diagnosis of glomus tumor: an institutional experience of 138 cases. Int J Surg Pathol. 2015 May;23(3):181-8. Cited in: PubMed; PMID 25614464.
987. Mukherjee D, Chaichana KL, Gokaslan ZL, et al. Survival of patients with malignant primary osseous spinal neoplasms: results from the Surveillance, Epidemiology, and End Results (SEER) database from 1973 to 2003. J Neurosurg Spine. 2011 Feb;14(2):143-50. Cited in: PubMed; PMID 21184634.
988. Mukherjee S, Bandyopadhyay G, Saha S, et al. Cytodiagnosis of glomus tumor. J Cytol. 2010 Jul;27(3):104-5. Cited in: PubMed; PMID 21187877.
989. Muñoz Arias G, González-Cámpora R, Ríos Martin JJ, et al. Elastofibroma: cytologic findings using fine needle aspiration. Acta Cytol. 200751(3):497-9. Cited in: PubMed; PMID 17536569.
990. Murakami S, Isozaki H, Shou T, et al. Primary osteosarcoma of the breast. Pathol Int. 2009 Feb;59(2):111-5. Cited in: PubMed; PMID 19154266.
991. Murali R, Doubrovsky A, Watson GF, et al. Diagnosis of metastatic melanoma by fine-needle biopsy: analysis of 2,204 cases. Am J Clin Pathol. 2007 Mar;127(3):385-97. Cited in: PubMed; PMID 17276948.
992. Murali R, Zarka MA, Ocal IT, et al. Cytologic features of epithelioid hemangioendothelioma. Am J Clin Pathol. 2011 Nov;136(5):739-46. Cited in: PubMed; PMID 22031312.
993. Muratori F, Bettini L, Frenos F, et al. Myxoid Liposarcoma: Prognostic Factors and Metastatic Pattern in a Series of 148 Patients Treated at a Single Institution. Int J Surg Oncol. 20182018:8928706. Cited in: PubMed; PMID 29977616.
994. Murphey MD, Smith WS, Smith SE, et al. From the archives of the AFIP. Imaging of musculoskeletal neurogenic tumors: radiologic-pathologic correlation. Radiographics. 199919(5):1253-80. Cited in: PubMed; PMID 10489179.
995. Murugan P, Basu D, Kumar S, et al. Clear cell sarcoma of the soft parts arising in the rectus abdominis in a child - aspiration cytology of a rare case. Cytojournal. 2007 Jul;4:15. Cited in: PubMed; PMID 17631685.
996. Muyanja D, Kalyesubula R, Namukwaya E, et al. Diagnostic accuracy of fine needle aspiration cytology in providing a diagnosis of cervical lymphadenopathy among HIV-infected patients. Afr Health Sci. 2015 Mar;15(1):107-16. Cited in: PubMed; PMID 25834538.
997. Naeem R, Lux ML, Huang SF, et al. Ring chromosomes in dermatofibrosarcoma protuberans are composed of interspersed sequences from chromosomes 17 and 22. Am J Pathol. 1995 Dec;147(6):1553-8. Cited in: PubMed; PMID 7495279.
998. Nagamine N, Nohara Y, Ito E. Elastofibroma in Okinawa. A clinicopathologic study of 170 cases. Cancer. 1982 Nov;50(9):1794-805. Cited in: PubMed; PMID 7116305.
999. Nagano S, Yahiro Y, Yokouchi M, et al. Doppler ultrasound for diagnosis of soft tissue sarcoma: efficacy of ultrasound-based screening score. Radiol Oncol. 2015 Jun;49(2):135-40. Cited in: PubMed; PMID 26029024.
1000. Nagao K, Ito H, Yoshida H. Chromosomal translocation t(X;18) in human synovial sarcomas analyzed by fluorescence in situ hybridization using paraffin-embedded tissue. Am J Pathol. 1996 Feb;148(2):601-9. Cited in: PubMed; PMID 8579122.
1001. Nagira K, Yamamoto T, Akisue T, et al. Reliability of fine-needle aspiration biopsy in the initial diagnosis of soft-tissue lesions. Diagn Cytopathol. 2002 Dec;27(6):354-61. Cited in: PubMed; PMID 12451566.
1002. Nagira K, Yamamoto T, Akisue T, et al. Scrape and fine-needle aspiration cytology of elastofibroma. Anticancer Res. 200222(6B):3561-7. Cited in: PubMed; PMID 12552956.
1003. Nagira K, Yamamoto T, Akisue T, et al. Scrape and fine-needle aspiration cytology of extraskeletal osteosarcoma. Diagn Cytopathol. 2002 Sep;27(3):177-80. Cited in: PubMed; PMID 12203867.
1004. Nakamura Y, Ohta Y, Itoh S, et al. Elastofibroma dorsi. Cytologic, histologic, immunohistochemical and ultrastructural studies. Acta Cytol. 199236(4):559-62. Cited in: PubMed; PMID 1636353.
1005. Nambirajan A, Jain D. Cell blocks in cytopathology: An update. Cytopathology. 2018 Dec;29(6):505-524. Cited in: PubMed; PMID 30153355.
1006. Nambirajan A, Jain D, Malik P, et al. Metastatic alveolar soft part sarcoma of the lung: Metastatic alveolar soft part sarcoma of the lung-a morphologic pitfall on cytology and aberrant CD10 expression on histology. Diagn Cytopathol. 2016 Mar;44(3):250-4. Cited in: PubMed; PMID 26693959.
1007. Narendra S, Valente A, Tull J, et al. DDIT3 gene break-apart as a molecular marker for diagnosis of myxoid liposarcoma--assay validation and clinical experience. Diagn Mol Pathol. 2011 Dec;20(4):218-24. Cited in: PubMed; PMID 22089349.
1008. Narváez JA, Martinez S, Dodd LG, et al. Acral myxoinflammatory fibroblastic sarcomas: MRI findings in four cases. AJR Am J Roentgenol. 2007 May;188(5):1302-5. Cited in: PubMed; PMID 17449774.
1009. Nascimento AF, Bertoni F, Fletcher CD. Epithelioid variant of myxofibrosarcoma: expanding the clinicomorphologic spectrum of myxofibrosarcoma in a series of 17 cases. Am J Surg Pathol. 2007 Jan;31(1):99-105. Cited in: PubMed; PMID 17197925.
1010. Nascimento AF, Fletcher CD. Spindle cell rhabdomyosarcoma in adults. Am J Surg Pathol. 2005 Aug;29(8):1106-13. Cited in: PubMed; PMID 16006807.
1011. Nascimento AG, Unii KK, Pritchard DJ, et al. A clinicopathologic study of 20 cases of large-cell (atypical) Ewing's sarcoma of bone. Am J Surg Pathol. 1980 Feb;4(1):29-36. Cited in: PubMed; PMID 7361993.
1012. Navarro OM. Pearls and Pitfalls in the Imaging of Soft-Tissue Masses in Children. Semin Ultrasound CT MR. 2020 Oct;41(5):498-512. Cited in: PubMed; PMID 32980096.
1013. Nemanqani D, Mourad WA. Cytomorphologic features of fine-needle aspiration of liposarcoma. Diagn Cytopathol. 1999 Feb;20(2):67-9. Cited in: PubMed; PMID 9951599.
1014. Nese N, Martignoni G, Fletcher CD, et al. Pure epithelioid PEComas (so-called epithelioid angiomyolipoma) of the kidney: A clinicopathologic study of 41 cases: detailed assessment of morphology and risk stratification. Am J Surg Pathol. 2011 Feb;35(2):161-76. Cited in: PubMed; PMID 21263237.
1015. Neuville A, Collin F, Bruneval P, et al. Intimal sarcoma is the most frequent primary cardiac sarcoma: clinicopathologic and molecular retrospective analysis of 100 primary cardiac sarcomas. Am J Surg Pathol. 2014 Apr;38(4):461-9. Cited in: PubMed; PMID 24625414.
1016. Ng E, Tandon AA, Ho BC, et al. Characterising benign fibrous soft-tissue tumours in adults: why is it so difficult and what do we need to know? Clin Radiol. 2015 Jul;70(7):684-97. Cited in: PubMed; PMID 25782339.
1017. Ng VY, Thomas K, Crist M, et al. Fine needle aspiration for clinical triage of extremity soft tissue masses. Clin Orthop Relat Res. 2010 Apr;468(4):1120-8. Cited in: PubMed; PMID 19763717.
1018. Nguyen T, Eltorky MA. Intranodal palisaded myofibroblastoma. Arch Pathol Lab Med. 2007 Feb;131(2):306-10. Cited in: PubMed; PMID 17284119.
1019. Nicol KK, Ward WG, Savage PD, et al. Fine-needle aspiration biopsy of skeletal versus extraskeletal osteosarcoma. Cancer. 1998 Jun;84(3):176-85. Cited in: PubMed; PMID 9678733.
1020. Nielsen GP, Dickersin GR, Provenzal JM, et al. Lipomatous hemangiopericytoma. A histologic, ultrastructural and immunohistochemical study of a unique variant of hemangiopericytoma. Am J Surg Pathol. 1995 Jul;19(7):748-56. Cited in: PubMed; PMID 7793472.
1021. Nielsen GP, O'Connell JX, Rosenberg AE. Intramuscular myxoma: a clinicopathologic study of 51 cases with emphasis on hypercellular and hypervascular variants. Am J Surg Pathol. 1998 Oct;22(10):1222-7. Cited in: PubMed; PMID 9777984.
1022. Niemann TH, Bottles K. Cytologic diagnosis of metastatic epithelioid sarcoma. A cytologic mimic of squamous cell carcinoma. Am J Clin Pathol. 1993 Aug;100(2):171-3. Cited in: PubMed; PMID 8356950.
1023. Nieuwenhuis MH, Casparie M, Mathus-Vliegen LM, et al. A nation-wide study comparing sporadic and familial adenomatous polyposis-related desmoid-type fibromatoses. Int J Cancer. 2011 Jul;129(1):256-61. Cited in: PubMed; PMID 20830713.
1024. Nilsson B, Bümming P, Meis-Kindblom JM, et al. Gastrointestinal stromal tumors: the incidence, prevalence, clinical course, and prognostication in the preimatinib mesylate era--a population-based study in western Sweden. Cancer. 2005 Feb;103(4):821-9. Cited in: PubMed; PMID 15648083.
1025. Nishi SP, Brey NV, Sanchez RL. Dermal nodular fasciitis: three case reports of the head and neck and literature review. J Cutan Pathol. 2006 May;33(5):378-82. Cited in: PubMed; PMID 16640547.
1026. Nishijima Y, Hirato J, Fukuda T. Pleomorphic rhabdomyosarcoma arising in the anterior mediastinum: A case report with cytological features of imprint and liquid-based cytology specimens. Diagn Cytopathol. 2017 Apr;45(4):333-338. Cited in: PubMed; PMID 28024111.
1027. Nishio J, Nakayama S, Nabeshima K, et al. Biology and Management of Dedifferentiated Liposarcoma: State of the Art and Perspectives. J Clin Med. 2021 Jul;10(15): Cited in: PubMed; PMID 34362013.
1028. Nishio J, Nakayama S, Nabeshima K, et al. Current Update on the Diagnosis, Management and Pathogenesis of Elastofibroma Dorsi. Anticancer Res. 2021 May;41(5):2211-2215. Cited in: PubMed; PMID 33952447.
1029. Nishio JN, Iwasaki H, Ohjimi Y, et al. Gain of Xq detected by comparative genomic hybridization in elastofibroma. Int J Mol Med. 2002 Sep;10(3):277-80. Cited in: PubMed; PMID 12165800.
1030. Nonaka D, Chiriboga L, Rubin BP. Sox10: a pan-schwannian and melanocytic marker. Am J Surg Pathol. 2008 Sep;32(9):1291-8. Cited in: PubMed; PMID 18636017.
1031. Nord KH, Magnusson L, Isaksson M, et al. Concomitant deletions of tumor suppressor genes MEN1 and AIP are essential for the pathogenesis of the brown fat tumor hibernoma. Proc Natl Acad Sci U S A. 2010 Dec;107(49):21122-7. Cited in: PubMed; PMID 21078971.
1032. North PE. Pediatric Vascular Tumors and Malformations. Surg Pathol Clin. 2010 Sep;3(3):455-94. Cited in: PubMed; PMID 26839221.
1033. North PE, Waner M, Buckmiller L, et al. Vascular tumors of infancy and childhood: beyond capillary hemangioma. Cardiovasc Pathol. 200615(6):303-17. Cited in: PubMed; PMID 17113009.

1034. Noujaim J, Thway K, Jones RL, et al. Adult Pleomorphic Rhabdomyosarcoma: A Multicentre Retrospective Study. Anticancer Res. 2015 Nov;35(11):6213-7. Cited in: PubMed; PMID 26504053.

1035. Nystrom LM, Reimer NB, Reith JD, et al. Multidisciplinary management of soft tissue sarcoma. ScientificWorldJournal. 20132013:852462. Cited in: PubMed; PMID 23983648.

1036. Oberlin O, Rey A, Lyden E, et al. Prognostic factors in metastatic rhabdomyosarcomas: results of a pooled analysis from United States and European cooperative groups. J Clin Oncol. 2008 May;26(14):2384-9. Cited in: PubMed; PMID 18467730.

1037. O'Connell JX, Wehrli BM, Nielsen GP, et al. Giant cell tumors of soft tissue: a clinicopathologic study of 18 benign and malignant tumors. Am J Surg Pathol. 2000 Mar;24(3):386-95. Cited in: PubMed; PMID 10716152.

1038. Oda Y, Miyajima K, Kawaguchi K, et al. Pleomorphic leiomyosarcoma: clinicopathologic and immunohistochemical study with special emphasis on its distinction from ordinary leiomyosarcoma and malignant fibrous histiocytoma. Am J Surg Pathol. 2001 Aug;25(8):1030-8. Cited in: PubMed; PMID 11474287.

1039. Oda Y, Tsuneyoshi M. Extrarenal rhabdoid tumors of soft tissue: clinicopathological and molecular genetic review and distinction from other soft-tissue sarcomas with rhabdoid features. Pathol Int. 2006 Jun;56(6):287-95. Cited in: PubMed; PMID 16704491.

1040. Odashiro AN, Odashiro Miiji LN, Odashiro DN, et al. Mammary myofibroblastoma: report of two cases with fine-needle aspiration cytology and review of the cytology literature. Diagn Cytopathol. 2004 Jun;30(6):406-10. Cited in: PubMed; PMID 15176028.

1041. Ogun GO. Fine needle Aspiration Biopsy (FNAB) in the initial evaluation and diagnosis of palpable soft tissue lesions and with histologic correlation. Pan Afr Med J. 201520:44. Cited in: PubMed; PMID 26090002.

1043. Okamatsu C, London WB, Naranjo A, et al. Clinicopathological characteristics of ganglioneuroma and ganglioneuroblastoma: a report from the CCG and COG. Pediatr Blood Cancer. 2009 Oct;53(4):563-9. Cited in: PubMed; PMID 19530234.

1044. Okamoto S, Hisaoka M, Ishida T, et al. Extraskeletal myxoid chondrosarcoma: a clinicopathologic, immunohistochemical, and molecular analysis of 18 cases. Hum Pathol. 2001 Oct;32(10):1116-24. Cited in: PubMed; PMID 11679947.

1045. Okamoto S, Hisaoka M, Meis-Kindblom JM, et al. Juxta-articular myxoma and intramuscular myxoma are two distinct entities. Activating Gs alpha mutation at Arg 201 codon does not occur in juxta-articular myxoma. Virchows Arch. 2002 Jan;440(1):12-5. Cited in: PubMed; PMID 11942570.

1046. Olaleye O, Fu B, Moorthy R, et al. Left supraclavicular spindle cell lipoma. Int J Otolaryngol. 20102010:942152. Cited in: PubMed; PMID 20508829.

1047. Oliva MS, Smimmo A, Vitiello R, et al. Elastofibroma dorsi: What's new? Orthop Rev (Pavia). 2020 Jun;12(Suppl 1):8708. Cited in: PubMed; PMID 32913617.

1048. Oliveira AM, Chou MM. USP6-induced neoplasms: the biologic spectrum of aneurysmal bone cyst and nodular fasciitis. Hum Pathol. 2014 Jan;45(1):1-11. Cited in: PubMed; PMID 23769422.

1049. Oliveira AM, Dei Tos AP, Fletcher CD, et al. Primary giant cell tumor of soft tissues: a study of 22 cases. Am J Surg Pathol. 2000 Feb;24(2):248-56. Cited in: PubMed; PMID 10680893.

1050. Olson MT, Ali SZ. Myxofibrosarcoma: cytomorphologic findings and differential diagnosis on fine needle aspiration. Acta Cytol. 201256(1):15-24. Cited in: PubMed; PMID 22236741.

1051. Orbach D, Rey A, Cecchetto G, et al. Infantile fibrosarcoma: management based on the European experience. J Clin Oncol. 2010 Jan;28(2):318-23. Cited in: PubMed; PMID 19917847.

1052. Ordi J, Riverola A, Solé M, et al. Fine needle aspiration of myofibroblastoma of the breast in a man. A report of two cases. Acta Cytol. 199236(2):194-8. Cited in: PubMed; PMID 1543005.

1053. O'Regan KN, Jagannathan J, Krajewski K, et al. Imaging of liposarcoma: classification, patterns of tumor recurrence, and response to treatment. AJR Am J Roentgenol. 2011 Jul;197(1):W37-43. Cited in: PubMed; PMID 21700993.

1054. Orell SR. Pitfalls in fine needle aspiration cytology. Cytopathology. 2003 Aug;14(4):173-82. Cited in: PubMed; PMID 12873307.

1055. O'Sullivan PJ, Harris AC, Munk PL. Radiological imaging features of non-uterine leiomyosarcoma. Br J Radiol. 2008 Jan;81(961):73-81. Cited in: PubMed; PMID 17681989.

1056. Otsuka H, Kohashi K, Yoshimoto M, et al. Immunohistochemical evaluation of H3K27 trimethylation in malignant peripheral nerve sheath tumors. Pathol Res Pract. 2018 Mar;214(3):417-425. Cited in: PubMed; PMID 29482987.

1057. Oumarou Hama H, Aboudharam G, Barbieri R, et al. Immunohistochemical diagnosis of human infectious diseases: a review. Diagn Pathol. 2022 Jan;17(1):17. Cited in: PubMed; PMID 35094696.

1058. Owens CL, Sharma R, Ali SZ. Deep fibromatosis (desmoid tumor): cytopathologic characteristics, clinicoradiologic features, and immunohistochemical findings on fine-needle aspiration. Cancer. 2007 Jun;111(3):166-72. Cited in: PubMed; PMID 17477374.

1059. Ozaki S, Kasashima S, Kawashima A, et al. Fine needle aspiration cytology findings of myxoinflammatory fibroblastic sarcoma: A case report. Diagn Cytopathol. 2018 Sep;46(9):739-743. Cited in: PubMed; PMID 28544823.

1060. Paal E, Miettinen M. Retroperitoneal leiomyomas: a clinicopathologic and immunohistochemical study of 56 cases with a comparison to retroperitoneal leiomyosarcomas. Am J Surg Pathol. 2001 Nov;25(11):1355-63. Cited in: PubMed; PMID 11684951.

1061. PACK GT, TABAH EJ. Dermato-fibrosarcoma protuberans. A report of 39 cases. AMA Arch Surg. 1951 Mar;62(3):391-411. Cited in: PubMed; PMID 14799050.

1062. Pagliuca F, Ronchi A, Cozzolino I, et al. Mesenchymal neoplasms: Is it time for cytology? New perspectives for the pre-operative diagnosis of soft tissue tumors in the molecular era. Pathol Res Pract. 2020 Jun;216(6):152923. Cited in: PubMed; PMID 32303388.

1063. Pai T, Nair N, Pantvaidya G, et al. Metastatic nasopharyngeal carcinoma presenting as an isolated breast mass: A diagnostic pitfall and a review of literature. Indian J Pathol Microbiol. 201760(1):119-121. Cited in: PubMed; PMID 28195109.

1064. Pal S, Nautiyal N, Kaira K, et al. Cytological Features of Cutaneous Granular Cell Tumor: A Brief Report. J Cytol. 201936(4):217-218. Cited in: PubMed; PMID 31741584.

1065. Palicelli A, Ramponi A, Valente G, et al. S-100 Immunohistochemical Positivity in Rhabdomyoma: An Underestimated Potential Diagnostic Pitfall in Routine Practice. Diagnostics (Basel). 2022 Apr;12(4): Cited in: PubMed; PMID 35453940.

1066. Palmer HE, Mukunyadzi P, Culbreth W, et al. Subgrouping and grading of soft-tissue sarcomas by fine-needle aspiration cytology: a histopathologic correlation study. Diagn Cytopathol. 2001 May;24(5):307-16. Cited in: PubMed; PMID 11335959.

1067. Panagopoulos I, Mertens F, Dêbiec-Rychter M, et al. Molecular genetic characterization of the EWS/ATF1 fusion gene in clear cell sarcoma of tendons and aponeuroses. Int J Cancer. 2002 Jun;99(4):560-7. Cited in: PubMed; PMID 11992546.

1068. Pandey G, Jalaly F. Fine needle aspiration cytology of soft tissue lesion: our institutional experience. IOSR J Dent Med Sci. 2021;20(4):1–4. doi:10.9790/0853-2004020104.

1069. Pang LJ, Chang B, Zou H, et al. Alveolar soft part sarcoma: a bimarker diagnostic strategy using TFE3 immunoassay and ASPL-TFE3 fusion transcripts in paraffin-embedded tumor tissues. Diagn Mol Pathol. 2008 Dec;17(4):245-52. Cited in: PubMed; PMID 18382356.

1070. Pang Y, Xie F, Cao H, et al. Mutational inactivation of mTORC1 repressor gene DEPDC5 in human gastrointestinal stromal tumors. Proc Natl Acad Sci U S A. 2019 Nov;116(45):22746-22753. Cited in: PubMed; PMID 31636198.

1071. Pantanowitz L, Dezube BJ. Kaposi sarcoma in unusual locations. BMC Cancer. 2008 Jul;8:190. Cited in: PubMed; PMID 18605999.

1072. Papillard-Maréchal S, Brisse HJ, Pannier S, et al. [Pseudotumoral soft tissue masses in children and adolescents]. Arch Pediatr. 2015 Jan;22(1):14-23. Cited in: PubMed; PMID 25435271.

1073. Papke DJ, Jo VY. Practical Application of Cytology and Core Biopsy in the Diagnosis of Mesenchymal Tumors. Surg Pathol Clin. 2019 Mar;12(1):227-248. Cited in: PubMed; PMID 30709446.

1074. Parham DM. Pathologic classification of rhabdomyosarcomas and correlations with molecular studies. Mod Pathol. 2001 May;14(5):506-14. Cited in: PubMed; PMID 11353062.

1075. Parham DM, Barr FG. Classification of rhabdomyosarcoma and its molecular basis. Adv Anat Pathol. 2013 Nov;20(6):387-97. Cited in: PubMed; PMID 24113309.

1076. Parham DM, Weeks DA, Beckwith JB. The clinicopathologic spectrum of putative extrarenal rhabdoid tumors. An analysis of 42 cases studied with immunohistochemistry or electron microscopy. Am J Surg Pathol. 1994 Oct;18(10):1010-29. Cited in: PubMed; PMID 8092393.

1077. Parish JM, Rosenow EC, Swensen SJ, et al. Pulmonary artery sarcoma. Clinical features. Chest. 1996 Dec;110(6):1480-8. Cited in: PubMed; PMID 8989065.

1078. Park SJ, Park CJ, Kim S, et al. Detection of bone marrow metastases of neuroblastoma with immunohistochemical staining of CD56, chromogranin A, and synaptophysin. Appl Immunohistochem Mol Morphol. 2010 Jul;18(4):348-52. Cited in: PubMed; PMID 20216406.

1079. Parmar V, Peters RT, Cheesman E, et al. Congenital infantile fibrosarcoma of the colon: a case series and literature review. Pediatr Surg Int. 2014 Oct;30(10):1079-85. Cited in: PubMed; PMID 25150723.

1080. Partridge JC, Cipriani N, Faquin WC, et al. Periarticular Cysts of the Temporomandibular Joint Are More Frequently Synovial Than Ganglion. J Oral Maxillofac Surg. 2016 Jul;74(7):1396-402. Cited in: PubMed; PMID 26902711.

1081. Pasini B, McWhinney SR, Bei T, et al. Clinical and molecular genetics of patients with the Carney-Stratakis syndrome and germline mutations of the genes coding for the succinate dehydrogenase subunits SDHB, SDHC, and SDHD. Eur J Hum Genet. 2008 Jan;16(1):79-88. Cited in: PubMed; PMID 17667967.

1082. Pasmant E, Parfait B, Luscan A, et al. Neurofibromatosis type 1 molecular diagnosis: what can NGS do for you when you have a large gene with loss of function mutations? Eur J Hum Genet. 2015 May;23(5):596-601. Cited in: PubMed; PMID 25074460.

1083. Pasquali S, Gronchi A, Strauss D, et al. Resectable extra-pleural and extra-meningeal solitary fibrous tumours: A multi-centre prognostic study. Eur J Surg Oncol. 2016 Jul;42(7):1064-70. Cited in: PubMed; PMID 26924782.

1084. Patchefsky AS, Enzinger FM. Intravascular fasciitis: a report of 17 cases. Am J Surg Pathol. 1981 Jan;5(1):29-36. Cited in: PubMed; PMID 7246849.

1085. Patel KU, Szabo SS, Hernandez VS, et al. Dermatofibrosarcoma protuberans COL1A1-PDGFB fusion is identified in virtually all dermatofibrosarcoma protuberans cases when investigated by newly developed multiplex reverse transcription polymerase chain reaction and fluorescence in situ hybridization assays. Hum Pathol. 2008 Feb;39(2):184-93. Cited in: PubMed; PMID 17950782.

1086. Patel NR, Chrisinger JSA, Demicco EG, et al. USP6 activation in nodular fasciitis by promoter-swapping gene fusions. Mod Pathol. 2017 Nov;30(11):1577-1588. Cited in: PubMed; PMID 28752842.

1087. Pedeutour F, Coindre JM, Sozzi G, et al. Supernumerary ring chromosomes containing chromosome 17 sequences. A specific feature of dermatofibrosarcoma protuberans? Cancer Genet Cytogenet. 1994 Aug;76(1):1-9. Cited in: PubMed; PMID 8076341.

1088. Pedeutour F, Lacour JP, Perrin C, et al. Another case of t(17;22)(q22;q13) in an infantile dermatofibrosarcoma protuberans. Cancer Genet Cytogenet. 1996 Jul;89(2):175-6. Cited in: PubMed; PMID 8697429.

1089. Pedeutour F, Simon MP, Minoletti F, et al. Ring 22 chromosomes in dermatofibrosarcoma protuberans are low-level amplifiers of chromosome 17 and 22 sequences. Cancer Res. 1995 Jun;55(11):2400-3. Cited in: PubMed; PMID 7757993.

1090. Pedeutour F, Simon MP, Minoletti F, et al. Translocation, t(17;22)(q22;q13), in dermatofibrosarcoma protuberans: a new tumor-associated chromosome rearrangement. Cytogenet Cell Genet. 199672(2-3):171-4. Cited in: PubMed; PMID 8978765.

1091. Pekmezci M, Cuevas-Ocampo AK, Perry A, et al. Significance of H3K27me3 loss in the diagnosis of malignant peripheral nerve sheath tumors. Mod Pathol. 2017 Dec;30(12):1710-1719. Cited in: PubMed; PMID 28776579.

1092. Pekmezci M, Reuss DE, Hirbe AC, et al. Morphologic and immunohistochemical features of malignant peripheral nerve sheath tumors and cellular schwannomas. Mod Pathol. 2015 Feb;28(2):187-200. Cited in: PubMed; PMID 25189642.

1093. Pelletier J, Gottlieb M, Long B, et al. Necrotizing Soft Tissue Infections (NSTI): Pearls and Pitfalls for the Emergency Clinician. J Emerg Med. 2022 Apr;62(4):480-491. Cited in: PubMed; PMID 35115188.

1094. Pellín A, Monteagudo C, López-Ginés C, et al. New type of chimeric fusion product between the EWS and ATFI genes in clear cell sarcoma (malignant melanoma of soft parts). Genes Chromosomes Cancer. 1998 Dec;23(4):358-60. Cited in: PubMed; PMID 9824209.

1095. Pendse AA, Dodd LG. Fine-needle-aspiration cytology of a proximal type epithelioid sarcoma: A case report. Diagn Cytopathol. 2015 Oct;43(10):859-62. Cited in: PubMed;

PMID 26138930.
1096. Peng WX, Kudo M, Yamamoto T, et al. Nodular fasciitis in the parotid gland: a case report and review of the literature. Diagn Cytopathol. 2013 Sep;41(9):829-33. Cited in: PubMed; PMID 23749727.
1097. Perlman S. Von Hippel-Lindau disease and Sturge-Weber syndrome. Handb Clin Neurol. 2018148:823-826. Cited in: PubMed; PMID 29478617.
1098. Perosio PM, Weiss SW. Ischemic fasciitis: a juxta-skeletal fibroblastic proliferation with a predilection for elderly patients. Mod Pathol. 1993 Jan;6(1):69-72. Cited in: PubMed; PMID 8426859.
1099. Perret R, Tallegas M, Velasco V, et al. Recurrent YAP1::MAML2 fusions in "nodular necrotizing" variants of myxoinflammatory fibroblastic sarcoma: a comprehensive study of 7 cases. Mod Pathol. 2022 Oct;35(10):1398-1404. Cited in: PubMed; PMID 35546636.
1100. Perry MD, Furlong JW, Johnston WW. Fine needle aspiration cytology of metastatic dermatofibrosarcoma protuberans. A case report. Acta Cytol. 198630(5):507-12. Cited in: PubMed; PMID 3465142.
1101. Perry MD, Gore M, Seigler HF, et al. Fine needle aspiration biopsy of metastatic melanoma. A morphologic analysis of 174 cases. Acta Cytol. 198630(4):385-96. Cited in: PubMed; PMID 3461649.
1102. Peters TL, Kumar V, Polikepahad S, et al. BCOR-CCNB3 fusions are frequent in undifferentiated sarcomas of male children. Mod Pathol. 2015 Apr;28(4):575-86. Cited in: PubMed; PMID 25360585.
1103. Petscavage-Thomas JM, Walker EA, Logie CI, et al. Soft-tissue myxomatous lesions: review of salient imaging features with pathologic comparison. Radiographics. 201434(4):964-80. Cited in: PubMed; PMID 25019435.
1104. Pettinato G, Insabato L, De Chiara A, et al. Epithelioid hemangioendothelioma of soft tissue. Fine needle aspiration cytology, histology, electron microscopy and immunohistochemistry of a case. Acta Cytol. 198630(2):194-200. Cited in: PubMed; PMID 3515816.
1105. Pettinato G, Manivel JC, De Rosa G, et al. Angiomatoid malignant fibrous histiocytoma: cytologic, immunohistochemical, ultrastructural, and flow cytometric study of 20 cases. Mod Pathol. 1990 Jul;3(4):479-87. Cited in: PubMed; PMID 2170972.
1106. Pettinato G, Manivel JC, Petrella G, et al. Fine needle aspiration cytology, immunocytochemistry and electron microscopy of fibromatosis of the breast. Report of two cases. Acta Cytol. 199135(4):403-8. Cited in: PubMed; PMID 1927173.
1107. Pierron G, Tirode F, Lucchesi C, et al. A new subtype of bone sarcoma defined by BCOR-CCNB3 gene fusion. Nat Genet. 2012 Mar;44(4):461-6. Cited in: PubMed; PMID 22387997.
1108. Pileri SA, Ascani S, Cox MC, et al. Myeloid sarcoma: clinico-pathologic, phenotypic and cytogenetic analysis of 92 adult patients. Leukemia. 2007 Feb;21(2):340-50. Cited in: PubMed; PMID 17170724.
1109. Pires CAA, Noronha MAN, Monteiro JCMS, et al. Kaposi's sarcoma in persons living with HIV/AIDS: a case series in a tertiary referral hospital. An Bras Dermatol. 201893(4):524-528. Cited in: PubMed; PMID 30066758.
1110. Pisapia P, Bellevicine C, Malapelle U, et al. Bird's eye view of modern cytopathology: Report from the seventh international Molecular Cytopathology Meeting in Naples, Italy, 2018. Cancer Cytopathol. 2019 Jun;127(6):350-357. Cited in: PubMed; PMID 31135103.
1111. Pisapia P, Lozano MD, Vigliar E, et al. ALK and ROS1 testing on lung cancer cytologic samples: Perspectives. Cancer Cytopathol. 2017 Nov;125(11):817-830. Cited in: PubMed; PMID 28743163.
1112. Pisapia P, Pepe F, Sgariglia R, et al. Next generation sequencing in cytology. Cytopathology. 2021 Sep;32(5):588-595. Cited in: PubMed; PMID 33792981.
1113. Pisharodi LR, Cary D, Bernacki EG. Elastofibroma dorsi: diagnostic problems and pitfalls. Diagn Cytopathol. 199410(3):242-4. Cited in: PubMed; PMID 8050332.
1114. Plaza JA, Ballestín C, Pérez-Barrios A, et al. Cytologic, cytochemical, immunocytochemical and ultrastructural diagnosis of a sacrococcygeal chordoma in a fine needle aspiration biopsy specimen. Acta Cytol. 198933(1):89-92. Cited in: PubMed; PMID 2644745.
1115. Plaza JA, Mayerson J, Wakely PE. Nodular fasciitis of the hand: a potential diagnostic pitfall in fine-needle aspiration cytopathology. Am J Clin Pathol. 2005 Mar;123(3):388-93. Cited in: PubMed; PMID 15716235.
1116. Plaza JA, Perez-Montiel D, Mayerson J, et al. Metastases to soft tissue: a review of 118 cases over a 30-year period. Cancer. 2008 Jan;112(1):193-203. Cited in: PubMed; PMID 18040999.
1117. Pohar-Marinsek Z, Bracko M. Rhabdomyosarcoma. Cytomorphology, subtyping and differential diagnostic dilemmas. Acta Cytol. 200044(4):524-32. Cited in: PubMed; PMID 10934943.
1118. Pohar-Marinsek Z, Flezar M, Lamovec J. Acral myxoinflammatory fibroblastic sarcoma in FNAB samples: can we distinguish it from other myxoid lesions? Cytopathology. 2003 Apr;14(2):73-8. Cited in: PubMed; PMID 12713479.
1119. Pohar-Marinsek Z, Zidar A. Epithelioid sarcoma in FNAB smears. Diagn Cytopathol. 1994 Dec;11(4):367-72. Cited in: PubMed; PMID 7534682.
1120. Popok SM, Naib ZM. Fine needle aspiration cytology of myositis ossificans. Diagn Cytopathol. 19851(3):236-40. Cited in: PubMed; PMID 3836091.
1121. Porteus C, Gan Q, Gong Y, et al. Sclerosing epithelioid fibrosarcoma: cytologic characterization with histologic, immunohistologic, molecular, and clinical correlation of 8 cases. J Am Soc Cytopathol. 20209(6):513-519. Cited in: PubMed; PMID 32624384.
1122. Portugal R, Barroca H. Clear cell sarcoma, cellular mesoblastic nephroma and metanephric adenoma: cytological features and differential diagnosis with Wilms tumour. Cytopathology. 2008 Apr;19(2):80-5. Cited in: PubMed; PMID 17681013.
1123. Powers CN. Diagnosis of infectious diseases: a cytopathologist's perspective. Clin Microbiol Rev. 1998 Apr;11(2):341-65. Cited in: PubMed; PMID 9564567.
1124. Powers CN, Berardo MD, Frable WJ. Fine-needle aspiration biopsy: pitfalls in the diagnosis of spindle-cell lesions. Diagn Cytopathol. 199410(3):232-40; discussion 241. Cited in: PubMed; PMID 8050331.
1125. Powers CN, Hurt MA, Frable WJ. Fine-needle aspiration biopsy: dermatofibrosarcoma protuberans. Diagn Cytopathol. 19939(2):145-50. Cited in: PubMed; PMID 8513707.
1126. Presneau N, Shalaby A, Ye H, et al. Role of the transcription factor T (brachyury) in the pathogenesis of sporadic chordoma: a genetic and functional-based study. J Pathol. 2011 Feb;223(3):327-35. Cited in: PubMed; PMID 21171078.
1128. Price SK, Kahn LB, Saxe N. Dermal and intravascular fasciitis. Unusual variants of nodular fasciitis. Am J Dermatopathol. 1993 Dec;15(6):539-43. Cited in: PubMed; PMID 8311183.
1129. Prieto-Granada C, Zhang L, Chen HW, et al. A genetic dichotomy between pure sclerosing epithelioid fibrosarcoma (SEF) and hybrid SEF/low-grade fibromyxoid sarcoma: a pathologic and molecular study of 18 cases. Genes Chromosomes Cancer. 2015 Jan;54(1):28-38. Cited in: PubMed; PMID 25231134.
1130. Prieto-Granada CN, Wiesner T, Messina JL, et al. Loss of H3K27me3 Expression Is a Highly Sensitive Marker for Sporadic and Radiation-induced MPNST. Am J Surg Pathol. 2016 Apr;40(4):479-89. Cited in: PubMed; PMID 26645727.
1131. Prieto-Rodríguez M, Camañas-Sanz A, Bas T, et al. Psammomatous melanotic schwannoma localized in the mediastinum: diagnosis by fine-needle aspiration cytology. Diagn Cytopathol. 1998 Oct;19(4):298-302. Cited in: PubMed; PMID 9784997.
1132. Proietti A, Alì G, Pelliccioni S, et al. Anaplastic lymphoma kinase gene rearrangements in cytological samples of non-small cell lung cancer: comparison with histological assessment. Cancer Cytopathol. 2014 Jun;122(6):445-53. Cited in: PubMed; PMID 24648382.
1133. Pulitzer DR, Martin PC, Reed RJ. Epithelioid glomus tumor. Hum Pathol. 1995 Sep;26(9):1022-7. Cited in: PubMed; PMID 7672784.
1134. Puls F, Niblett A, Marland G, et al. BCOR-CCNB3 (Ewing-like) sarcoma: a clinicopathologic analysis of 10 cases, in comparison with conventional Ewing sarcoma. Am J Surg Pathol. 2014 Oct;38(10):1307-18. Cited in: PubMed; PMID 24805859.
1135. Purandare NC, Shah S, Agrawal A, et al. Spectrum of Flurodeoxyglucose Positron Emission Tomography/Computerized Tomography Findings in Tumors and Tumor-Like Conditions of the Musculoskeletal System. Indian J Nucl Med. 202136(3):327-339. Cited in: PubMed; PMID 34658562.
1136. Purgina B, Jaffe R, Monaco SE, et al. Cytomorphology of Erdheim-Chester disease presenting as a retroperitoneal soft tissue lesion. Cytojournal. 20118:22. Cited in: PubMed; PMID 22279491.
1137. Pusztaszeri M, Triponez F, Pache JC, et al. Riedel's thyroiditis with increased IgG4 plasma cells: evidence for an underlying IgG4-related sclerosing disease? Thyroid. 2012 Sep;22(9):964-8. Cited in: PubMed; PMID 22827716.
1138. Qian X, Hornick JL, Cibas ES, et al. Angiomatoid fibrous histiocytoma a series of five cytologic cases with literature review and emphasis on diagnostic pitfalls. Diagn Cytopathol. 2012 Aug;40 Suppl 2:E86-93. Cited in: PubMed; PMID 22045622.
1139. Qualman S, Lynch J, Bridge J, et al. Prevalence and clinical impact of anaplasia in childhood rhabdomyosarcoma : a report from the Soft Tissue Sarcoma Committee of the Children's Oncology Group. Cancer. 2008 Dec;113(11):3242-7. Cited in: PubMed; PMID 18985676.
1140. Quante M, Patel NK, Hill S, et al. Epithelioid hemangioendothelioma presenting in the skin: a clinicopathologic study of eight cases. Am J Dermatopathol. 1998 Dec;20(6):541-6. Cited in: PubMed; PMID 9855348.
1141. Raab SS, Silverman JF, McLeod DL, et al. Fine needle aspiration biopsy of fibromatoses. Acta Cytol. 199337(3):323-8. Cited in: PubMed; PMID 8498134.
1142. Radu O, Pantanowitz L. Kaposi sarcoma. Arch Pathol Lab Med. 2013 Feb;137(2):289-94. Cited in: PubMed; PMID 23368874.
1143. Rakheja D, Cunningham JC, Mitui M, et al. A subset of cranial fasciitis is associated with dysregulation of the Wnt/beta-catenin pathway. Mod Pathol. 2008 Nov;21(11):1330-6. Cited in: PubMed; PMID 18587328.
1144. Ramani NS, Chen H, Broaddus RR, et al. Utilization of cytology smears improves success rates of RNA-based next-generation sequencing gene fusion assays for clinically relevant predictive biomarkers. Cancer Cytopathol. 2021 May;129(5):374-382. Cited in: PubMed; PMID 33119213.
1145. Raney RB, Meza J, Anderson JR, et al. Treatment of children and adolescents with localized parameningeal sarcoma: experience of the Intergroup Rhabdomyosarcoma Study Group protocols IRS-II through -IV, 1978-1997. Med Pediatr Oncol. 2002 Jan;38(1):22-32. Cited in: PubMed; PMID 11835233.
1146. Rani D, Gupta A. Cytological Diagnosis and Misdiagnosis of Nodular Fasciitis. J Cytol. 201936(4):196-199. Cited in: PubMed; PMID 31741577.
1147. Rankine AJ, Filion PR, Platten MA, et al. Perineurioma: a clinicopathological study of eight cases. Pathology. 2004 Aug;36(4):309-15. Cited in: PubMed; PMID 15370128.
1148. Rao IS, Singh MK, Gupta SD, et al. Utility of fine-needle aspiration cytology in the classification of leprosy. Diagn Cytopathol. 2001 May;24(5):317-21. Cited in: PubMed; PMID 11335960.
1149. Rao U, Cheng A, Didolkar MS. Extraosseous osteogenic sarcoma: clinicopathological study of eight cases and review of literature. Cancer. 1978 Apr;41(4):1488-96. Cited in: PubMed; PMID 346199.
1150. Rao UN, Hanan SH, Lotze MT, et al. Distant skin and soft tissue metastases from sarcomas. J Surg Oncol. 1998 Oct;69(2):94-8. Cited in: PubMed; PMID 9808512.
1151. Rao V, Rekhi B. Cytomorphological spectrum, including immunohistochemical results of 16 cases of clear cell sarcoma of soft tissue, along with positive EWSR1 gene rearrangement result in two cases. Cytopathology. 2020 Jul;31(4):280-287. Cited in: PubMed; PMID 32356379.
1152. Rau AR, Kini H, Verghese R. Tigroid background in fine-needle aspiration cytology of clear cell sarcoma. Diagn Cytopathol. 2006 May;34(5):355-7. Cited in: PubMed; PMID 16604557.
1153. Ravi S, Gochhait D, Stephen N, et al. Giant cell tumour-like features of myositis ossificans in cytology-a case report. Cytopathology. 2020 Sep;31(5):471-474. Cited in: PubMed; PMID 31991033.
1154. Reeves BR, Fletcher CD, Gusterson BA. Translocation t(12;22)(q13;q13) is a nonrandom rearrangement in clear cell sarcoma. Cancer Genet Cytogenet. 1992 Dec;64(2):101-3. Cited in: PubMed; PMID 1486556.
1155. Reimann JD, Fletcher CD. Myxoid dermatofibrosarcoma protuberans: a rare variant analyzed in a series of 23 cases. Am J Surg Pathol. 2007 Sep;31(9):1371-7. Cited in: PubMed; PMID 17721193.
1156. Reiseter T, Nordshus T, Borthne A, et al. Lipoblastoma: MRI appearances of a rare paediatric soft tissue tumour. Pediatr Radiol. 1999 Jul;29(7):542-5. Cited in: PubMed; PMID 10398794.
1157. Reitamo JJ, Häyry P, Nykyri E, et al. The desmoid tumor. I. Incidence, sex-, age- and anatomical distribution in the Finnish population. Am J Clin Pathol. 1982 Jun;77(6):665-73. Cited in: PubMed; PMID 7091046.
1158. Reith JD, Goldblum JR, Lyles RH, et al. Extragastrointestinal (soft tissue) stromal tumors: an analysis of 48 cases with emphasis on histologic predictors of outcome. Mod Pathol. 2000 May;13(5):577-85. Cited in: PubMed; PMID 10824931.

1159. Rekhi B. Core Needle Biopsy versus Fine Needle Aspiration Cytology in Bone and Soft Tissue Tumors. J Cytol. 201936(2):118-123. Cited in: PubMed; PMID 30992649.
1160. Rekhi B. Fine needle aspiration cytology of a superficial CD34-positive fibroblastic tumour, including differential diagnoses and recent updates. Cytopathology. 2023 Jan;34(1):66-71. Cited in: PubMed; PMID 36151940.
1161. Rekhi B, Adamane S, Ghodke K, et al. Angiomatoid fibrous histiocytoma: Clinicopathological spectrum of five cases, including EWSR1-CREB1 positive result in a single case. Indian J Pathol Microbiol. 201659(2):148-52. Cited in: PubMed; PMID 27166030.
1162. Rekhi B, Baheti AD, Patkar S. Dedifferentiated liposarcoma with heterologous spindle cell rhabdomyoblastic de-differentiation: An unusual pattern expanding the morphological spectrum. Indian J Pathol Microbiol. 202063(4):630-633. Cited in: PubMed; PMID 33154322.
1163. Rekhi B, Dermawan JK, Fritchie KJ, et al. EWSR1::ATF1 fusions characterize a group of extra-abdominal epithelioid and round cell mesenchymal neoplasms, phenotypically overlapping with sclerosing epithelioid fibrosarcomas, and intra-abdominal FET::CREB fusion neoplasms. Virchows Arch. 2024 Dec;485(6):995-1005. Cited in: PubMed; PMID 39031200.
1164. Rekhi B, Desai S, Jambhekar NA. Epithelioid variant of a pleomorphic liposarcoma displaying arborizing vascular arrangements on cytology smears: a case report of an interesting cytomorphologic pattern in an uncommon tumor. Acta Cytol. 201054(5 Suppl):963-7. Cited in: PubMed; PMID 21053578.
1165. Rekhi B, Deshmukh M, Jambhekar NA. Low-grade fibromyxoid sarcoma: a clinicopathologic study of 18 cases, including histopathologic relationship with sclerosing epithelioid fibrosarcoma in a subset of cases. Ann Diagn Pathol. 2011 Oct;15(5):303-11. Cited in: PubMed; PMID 21550274.
1166. Rekhi B, Dodd L, Dharavath B, et al. Cytomorphology of spindle cell/sclerosing rhabdomyosarcoma, including MYOD1 (LI22R) mutation result. Diagn Cytopathol. 2022 Dec;50(12):E367-E372. Cited in: PubMed; PMID 35929754.
1167. Rekhi B, Gorad BD, Chinoy RF. Clinicopathological features with outcomes of a series of conventional and proximal-type epithelioid sarcomas, diagnosed over a period of 10 years at a tertiary cancer hospital in India. Virchows Arch. 2008 Aug;453(2):141-53. Cited in: PubMed; PMID 18607629.
1168. Rekhi B, Gorad BD, Chinoy RF. Proximal-type epithelioid sarcoma--a rare, aggressive subtype of epithelioid sarcoma presenting as a recurrent perineal mass in a middle-aged male. World J Surg Oncol. 2007 Mar;5:28. Cited in: PubMed; PMID 17341294.
1169. Rekhi B, Gorad BD, Kakade AC, et al. Scope of FNAC in the diagnosis of soft tissue tumors--a study from a tertiary cancer referral center in India. Cytojournal. 2007 Oct;4:20. Cited in: PubMed; PMID 17973999.
1170. Rekhi B, Gupta C, Chinnaswamy G, et al. Clinicopathologic features of 300 rhabdomyosarcomas with emphasis upon differential expression of skeletal muscle specific markers in the various subtypes: A single institutional experience. Ann Diagn Pathol. 2018 Oct;36:50-60. Cited in: PubMed; PMID 30098515.
1171. Rekhi B, Ingle A, Agarwal M, et al. Alveolar soft part sarcoma 'revisited': clinicopathological review of 47 cases from a tertiary cancer referral centre, including immunohistochemical expression of TFE3 in 22 cases and 21 other tumours. Pathology. 2012 Jan;44(1):11-7. Cited in: PubMed; PMID 22173238.
1172. Rekhi B, Jambhekar NA. Immunohistochemical validation of INI1/SMARCB1 in a spectrum of musculoskeletal tumors: an experience at a Tertiary Cancer Referral Centre. Pathol Res Pract. 2013 Dec;209(12):758-66. Cited in: PubMed; PMID 24075062.
1173. Rekhi B, Karmarkar S. Clinicocytopathological spectrum, including uncommon forms, of nine cases of chordomas with immunohistochemical results, including brachyury immunostaining: A single institutional experience. Cytopathology. 2019 Mar;30(2):229-235. Cited in: PubMed; PMID 30218622.
1174. Rekhi B, Kembhavi P, Mishra SN. Cytomorphological features and literature review of CIC-DUX4-positive sarcoma, confirmed by reverse transcription polymerase chain reaction in a paediatric patient. Cytopathology. 2021 Jan;32(1):120-126. Cited in: PubMed; PMID 33399252.
1175. Rekhi B, Kosemehmetoglu K, Tezel GG, et al. Clinicopathologic features and immunohistochemical spectrum of 11 cases of epithelioid malignant peripheral nerve sheath tumors, including INI1/SMARCB1 results and BRAF V600E analysis. APMIS. 2017 Aug;125(8):679-689. Cited in: PubMed; PMID 28452074.
1176. Rekhi B, Rao V, Ramadwar M. Revisiting cytomorphology, including unusual features and clinical scenarios of 8 cases of alveolar soft part sarcoma with TFE3 immunohistochemical staining in 7 cases. Cytopathology. 2021 Jan;32(1):20-28. Cited in: PubMed; PMID 32853443.
1177. Rekhi B, Shetty O, Ramadwar M, et al. Role of fine needle aspiration cytology in the diagnosis of a rare case of a poorly differentiated synovial sarcoma with "Rhabdoid" features, including treatment implications. Diagn Cytopathol. 2017 Jul;45(7):662-667. Cited in: PubMed; PMID 28345284.
1178. Rekhi B, Singh N. Spectrum of cytopathologic features of epithelioid sarcoma in a series of 7 uncommon cases with immunohistochemical results, including loss of INI1/SMARCB1 in two test cases. Diagn Cytopathol. 2016 Jul;44(7):636-42. Cited in: PubMed; PMID 27145123.
1179. Rekhi B, Sridhar E, Viswanathan S, et al. ALK+ anaplastic large cell lymphoma with cohesive, perivascular arrangements on cytology, mimicking a soft tissue sarcoma: a report of 2 cases. Acta Cytol. 201054(1):75-8. Cited in: PubMed; PMID 20306994.
1180. Rekhi B, Upadhyay P, Ramteke MP, et al. MYOD1 (L122R) mutations are associated with spindle cell and sclerosing rhabdomyosarcomas with aggressive clinical outcomes. Mod Pathol. 2016 Dec;29(12):1532-1540. Cited in: PubMed; PMID 27562493.
1181. Rekhtman N, Kazi S, Yao J, et al. Depletion of Core Needle Biopsy Cellularity and DNA Content as a Result of Vigorous Touch Preparations. Arch Pathol Lab Med. 2015 Jul;139(7):907-12. Cited in: PubMed; PMID 25521802.
1182. Renn A, Adejolu M, Messiou C, et al. Overview of malignant soft-tissue sarcomas of the limbs. Clin Radiol. 2021 Dec;76(12):940. e1-940.e16. Cited in: PubMed; PMID 34607656.
1183. Renshaw AA, Perez-Atayde AR, Fletcher JA, et al. Cytology of typical and atypical Ewing's sarcoma/PNET. Am J Clin Pathol. 1996 Nov;106(5):620-4. Cited in: PubMed; PMID 8929472.
1184. Resnick JM, Fanning CV, Caraway NP, et al. Percutaneous needle biopsy diagnosis of benign neurogenic neoplasms. Diagn Cytopathol. 1997 Jan;16(1):17-25. Cited in: PubMed; PMID 9034731.
1185. Richardson SO, Huibers MMH, de Weger RA, et al. One-fits-all pretreatment protocol facilitating Fluorescence In Situ Hybridization on formalin-fixed paraffin-embedded, fresh frozen and cytological slides. Mol Cytogenet. 201912:27. Cited in: PubMed; PMID 31236139.
1186. Ritchie DA, Aniq H, Davies AM, et al. Hibernoma--correlation of histopathology and magnetic-resonance-imaging features in 10 cases. Skeletal Radiol. 2006 Aug;35(8):579-89. Cited in: PubMed; PMID 16642344.
1187. Rizer M, Singer AD, Edgar M, et al. The histological variants of liposarcoma: predictive MRI findings with prognostic implications, management, follow-up, and differential diagnosis. Skeletal Radiol. 2016 Sep;45(9):1193-204. Cited in: PubMed; PMID 27209201.
1188. Roake CM, Artandi SE. DNA repair: Telomere-lengthening mechanism revealed. Nature. 2016 Nov;539(7627):35-36. Cited in: PubMed; PMID 27760112.
1189. Robinson DR, Wu YM, Kalyana-Sundaram S, et al. Identification of recurrent NAB2-STAT6 gene fusions in solitary fibrous tumor by integrative sequencing. Nat Genet. 2013 Feb;45(2):180-5. Cited in: PubMed; PMID 23313952.
1190. Robson AM, Calonje E. Cutaneous perineurioma: a poorly recognized tumour often misdiagnosed as epithelioid histiocytoma. Histopathology. 2000 Oct;37(4):332-9. Cited in: PubMed; PMID 11012740.
1191. Rodriguez FJ, Graham MK, Brosnan-Cashman JA, et al. Telomere alterations in neurofibromatosis type 1-associated solid tumors. Acta Neuropathol Commun. 2019 Aug;7(1):139. Cited in: PubMed; PMID 31462295.
1192. Roh MH. The utilization of cytologic and small biopsy samples for ancillary molecular testing. Mod Pathol. 2019 Jan;32(Suppl 1):77-85. Cited in: PubMed; PMID 30600323.
1193. Romero-Guadarrama MB, Jiménez-Becerra S, Durán-Padilla MA, et al. Mediastinal pleomorphic liposarcoma diagnosed by fine needle aspiration biopsy: a case report. Acta Cytol. 200751(3):440-2. Cited in: PubMed; PMID 17536551.
1195. Ronchi A, Panarese I, Aquino G, et al. Synovial sarcoma diagnosis on fine needle cytology sample confirmed by fluorescence in situ hybridisation. Cytopathology. 2019 May;30(3):314-317. Cited in: PubMed; PMID 30417957.
1196. Rööser B, Herrlin K, Rydholm A, et al. Pseudomalignant myositis ossificans. Clinical, radiologic, and cytologic diagnosis in 5 cases. Acta Orthop Scand. 1989 Aug;60(4):457-60. Cited in: PubMed; PMID 2816324.
1197. Rosai J. Soft Tissues. In: Goldblum JR, Lamps LW, McKenney JK. Rosai and Ackerman's surgical pathology. 11th ed. Philadelphia, PA: Elsevier; 2017.
1199. Rosenberg AE. Pseudosarcomas of soft tissue. Arch Pathol Lab Med. 2008 Apr;132(4):579-86. Cited in: PubMed; PMID 18384209.
1201. Rossi S, Fletcher CD. Angiosarcoma arising in hemangioma/vascular malformation: report of four cases and review of the literature. Am J Surg Pathol. 2002 Oct;26(10):1319-29. Cited in: PubMed; PMID 12360047.
1202. Rossi S, Miceli R, Messerini L, et al. Natural history of imatinib-naive GISTs: a retrospective analysis of 929 cases with long-term follow-up and development of a survival nomogram based on mitotic index and size as continuous variables. Am J Surg Pathol. 2011 Nov;35(11):1646-56. Cited in: PubMed; PMID 21997685.
1203. Rossi S, Orvieto E, Furlanetto A, et al. Utility of the immunohistochemical detection of FLI-1 expression in round cell and vascular neoplasm using a monoclonal antibody. Mod Pathol. 2004 May;17(5):547-52. Cited in: PubMed; PMID 15001993.
1204. Rossi S, Szuhai K, Ijszenga M, et al. EWSR1-CREB1 and EWSR1-ATF1 fusion genes in angiomatoid fibrous histiocytoma. Clin Cancer Res. 2007 Dec;13(24):7322-8. Cited in: PubMed; PMID 18094413.
1205. Roy-Chowdhuri S, Dacic S, Ghofrani M, et al. Collection and Handling of Thoracic Small Biopsy and Cytology Specimens for Ancillary Studies: Guideline From the College of American Pathologists in Collaboration With the American College of Chest Physicians, Association for Molecular Pathology, American Society of Cytopathology, American Thoracic Society, Pulmonary Pathology Society, Papanicolaou Society of Cytopathology, Society of Interventional Radiology, and Society of Thoracic Radiology. Arch Pathol Lab Med. 2020 May. Cited in: PubMed; PMID 32401054.
1206. Roy-Chowdhuri S, Pisapia P, Salto-Tellez M, et al. Invited review-next-generation sequencing: a modern tool in cytopathology. Virchows Arch. 2019 Jul;475(1):3-11. Cited in: PubMed; PMID 30877381.
1207. Roy-Chowdhuri S, Stewart J. Preanalytic Variables in Cytology: Lessons Learned From Next-Generation Sequencing-The MD Anderson Experience. Arch Pathol Lab Med. 2016 Nov;140(11):1191-1199. Cited in: PubMed; PMID 27333361.
1208. Rubens DJ, Fultz PJ, Gottlieb RH, et al. Effective ultrasonographically guided intervention for diagnosis of musculoskeletal lesions. J Ultrasound Med. 1997 Dec;16(12):831-42. Cited in: PubMed; PMID 9401998.
1209. Rubin BP, Goldblum JR. Pathology of soft tissue sarcoma. J Natl Compr Canc Netw. 2007 Apr;5(4):411-8. Cited in: PubMed; PMID 17442232.
1210. Rudzinski ER, Anderson JR, Chi YY, et al. Histology, fusion status, and outcome in metastatic rhabdomyosarcoma: A report from the Children's Oncology Group. Pediatr Blood Cancer. 2017 Dec;64(12): Cited in: PubMed; PMID 28521080.
1211. Rudzinski ER, Anderson JR, Hawkins DS, et al. The World Health Organization Classification of Skeletal Muscle Tumors in Pediatric Rhabdomyosarcoma: A Report From the Children's Oncology Group. Arch Pathol Lab Med. 2015 Oct;139(10):1281-7. Cited in: PubMed; PMID 25989287.
1212. Rudzinski ER, Teot LA, Anderson JR, et al. Dense pattern of embryonal rhabdomyosarcoma, a lesion easily confused with alveolar rhabdomyosarcoma: a report from the Soft Tissue Sarcoma Committee of the Children's Oncology Group. Am J Clin Pathol. 2013 Jul;140(1):82-90. Cited in: PubMed; PMID 23765537.
1213. Rydholm A. Management of patients with soft-tissue tumors. Strategy developed at a regional oncology center. Acta Orthop Scand Suppl. 1983203:13-77. Cited in: PubMed; PMID 6581679.
1214. Rydholm A, Berg NO. Size, site and clinical incidence of lipoma. Factors in the differential diagnosis of lipoma and sarcoma. Acta Orthop Scand. 1983 Dec;54(6):929-34. Cited in: PubMed; PMID 6670522.
1215. Ryu HS, Lee SS, Choi HS, et al. A case of pulmonary malignant epithelioid hemangioendothelioma misdiagnosed as adenocarcinoma by fine needle aspiration cytology. Diagn Cytopathol. 2011 Nov;39(11):801-7. Cited in: PubMed; PMID 21994192.
1216. Saad A, Azzopardi C, Patel A, et al. Myositis ossificans revisited - The largest

reported case series. J Clin Orthop Trauma. 2021 Jun;17:123-127. Cited in: PubMed; PMID 33816108.
1217. Saad RS, Takei H, Lipscomb J, et al. Nodular fasciitis of parotid region: a pitfall in the diagnosis of pleomorphic adenomas on fine-needle aspiration cytology. Diagn Cytopathol. 2005 Sep;33(3):191-4. Cited in: PubMed; PMID 16078254.
1218. Sachdeva MP, Goldblum JR, Rubin BP, et al. Low-fat and fat-free pleomorphic lipomas: a diagnostic challenge. Am J Dermatopathol. 2009 Jul;31(5):423-6. Cited in: PubMed; PMID 19542913.
1220. Saito T. Glomus tumor of the penis. Int J Urol. 2000 Mar;7(3):115-7. Cited in: PubMed; PMID 10750892.
1221. Saito Y, Miyajima C, Nakao K, et al. Highly malignant submandibular extraskeletal osteosarcoma in a young patient. Auris Nasus Larynx. 2008 Dec;35(4):576-8. Cited in: PubMed; PMID 18242029.
1222. Sakhadeo U, Mundhe R, DeSouza MA, et al. Pleomorphic lipoma: A gentle giant of pathology. J Cytol. 201532(3):201-3. Cited in: PubMed; PMID 26729985.
1223. Sakuma T, Matsuo K, Koike S, et al. Fine needle aspiration cytology of nodular fasciitis of the breast. Diagn Cytopathol. 2015 Mar;43(3):222-9. Cited in: PubMed; PMID 24862506.
1224. Salas S, Dufresne A, Bui B, et al. Prognostic factors influencing progression-free survival determined from a series of sporadic desmoid tumors: a wait-and-see policy according to tumor presentation. J Clin Oncol. 2011 Sep;29(26):3553-8. Cited in: PubMed; PMID 21844500.
1225. Salas S, Resseguier N, Blay JY, et al. Prediction of local and metastatic recurrence in solitary fibrous tumor: construction of a risk calculator in a multicenter cohort from the French Sarcoma Group (FSG) database. Ann Oncol. 2017 Aug;28(8):1979-1987. Cited in: PubMed; PMID 28838212.
1226. Salem Shabb N, Boulos F, Tawil A, et al. Clear cell sarcoma (malignant melanoma of soft parts): fine-needle aspiration cytology of a highly pigmented tumor. Diagn Cytopathol. 2003 Jun;28(6):313-5. Cited in: PubMed; PMID 12768636.
1227. Sanfilippo R, Miceli R, Grosso F, et al. Myxofibrosarcoma: prognostic factors and survival in a series of patients treated at a single institution. Ann Surg Oncol. 2011 Mar;18(3):720-5. Cited in: PubMed; PMID 20878245.
1228. Sangiorgio V, Daniele L, Gallo T, et al. Ultrasound-guided fine needle aspiration cytology in the diagnosis of hepatic and pancreatic perivascular epithelioid cell tumors: A case series. Diagn Cytopathol. 2019 Apr;47(4):315-319. Cited in: PubMed; PMID 30417984.
1229. Santiago T, Clay MR, Allen SJ, et al. Recurrent BCOR internal tandem duplication and BCOR or BCL6 expression distinguish primitive myxoid mesenchymal tumor of infancy from congenital infantile fibrosarcoma. Mod Pathol. 2018 Feb;31(2):374. Cited in: PubMed; PMID 29430000.
1230. Santos F, Martins C, Lemos MM. Fine-needle aspiration features of extraskeletal myxoid chondrosarcoma: A study of cytological and molecular features. Diagn Cytopathol. 2018 Nov;46(11):950-957. Cited in: PubMed; PMID 30353688.
1231. Saoud C, Schowinsky J, Ali SZ. Myxoid Soft Tissue Tumors: A 20-Year Experience on Fine Needle Aspiration with Application of the Proposed WHO Reporting System for Soft Tissue Cytopathology. Acta Cytol. 202367(5):468-481. Cited in: PubMed; PMID 37231794.
1232. Sápi Z, Antal I, Pápai Z, et al. Diagnosis of soft tissue tumors by fine-needle aspiration with combined cytopathology and ancillary techniques. Diagn Cytopathol. 2002 Apr;26(4):232-42. Cited in: PubMed; PMID 11933269.
1233. Sápi Z, Lippai Z, Papp G, et al. Nodular fasciitis: a comprehensive, time-correlated investigation of 17 cases. Mod Pathol. 2021 Dec;34(12):2192-2199. Cited in: PubMed; PMID 34381187.
1234. Saqi A, Nisbet L, Gagneja P, et al. Primary pleural epithelioid hemangioendothelioma with rhabdoid phenotype: report and review of the literature. Diagn Cytopathol. 2007 Apr;35(4):203-8. Cited in: PubMed; PMID 17351942.
1235. Saqi A, Yu GH, Marshall MB. Fine-needle aspiration of hibernoma. Diagn Cytopathol. 2003 Jul;29(1):44-5. Cited in: PubMed; PMID 12827716.
1236. Sargar K, Kao SC, Spunt SL, et al. MRI and CT of Low-Grade Fibromyxoid Sarcoma in Children: A Report From Children's Oncology Group Study ARST0332. AJR Am J Roentgenol. 2015 Aug;205(2):414-20. Cited in: PubMed; PMID 26204295.
1237. Sarkar D, Ray S, Saha M, et al. Alveolar rhabdomyosarcoma with multiple distal metastases. A case report and review of literature. BMJ Case Rep. 2012 Sep;2012: Cited in: PubMed; PMID 22948994.
1238. Sartelli M, Guirao X, Hardcastle TC, et al. 2018 WSES/SIS-E consensus conference: recommendations for the management of skin and soft-tissue infections. World J Emerg Surg. 201813:58. Cited in: PubMed; PMID 30564282.
1239. Satish S, Shivalingaiah SC, Ravishankar S, et al. Fine needle aspiration cytology of pseudosarcomatous reactive lesions of soft tissues: A report of two cases. J Cytol. 2012 Oct;29(4):264-6. Cited in: PubMed; PMID 23326034.
1240. Satturwar S, Rekhtman N, Lin O, et al. An update on touch preparations of small biopsies. J Am Soc Cytopathol. 20209(5):322-331. Cited in: PubMed; PMID 32417160.
1241. Satturwar S, Wakely PE, Pantanowitz L. Approach to FNA of Myxoid Soft Tissue Tumors. Adv Anat Pathol. 2022 Nov;29(6):380-388. Cited in: PubMed; PMID 35878421.
1242. Satturwar SP, Khader SN, Quiroga-Garza GM. Fluorescent in-situ hybridization test performed on cell blocks is useful for establishing germ cell origin of metastatic tumors with unusual clinical presentation. Diagn Cytopathol. 2022 Sep;50(9):E267-E274. Cited in: PubMed; PMID 35612406.
1243. Sauter JL, Grogg KL, Vrana JA, et al. Young investigator challenge: Validation and optimization of immunohistochemistry protocols for use on cellient cell block specimens. Cancer Cytopathol. 2016 Feb;124(2):89-100. Cited in: PubMed; PMID 26882197.
1244. Savic S, Bode B, Diebold J, et al. Detection of ALK-positive non-small-cell lung cancers on cytological specimens: high accuracy of immunocytochemistry with the 5A4 clone. J Thorac Oncol. 2013 Aug;8(8):1004-11. Cited in: PubMed; PMID 23689429.
1245. Savic S, Bubendorf L. Common Fluorescence In Situ Hybridization Applications in Cytology. Arch Pathol Lab Med. 2016 Dec;140(12):1323-1330. Cited in: PubMed; PMID 27479335.
1246. Savic S, Bubendorf L. Role of fluorescence in situ hybridization in lung cancer cytology. Acta Cytol. 201256(6):611-21. Cited in: PubMed; PMID 23207439.
1247. Savic S, Glatz K, Schoenegg R, et al. Multitarget fluorescence in situ hybridization elucidates equivocal lung cytology. Chest. 2006 Jun;129(6):1629-35. Cited in: PubMed; PMID 16778285.
1248. Sbaraglia M, Righi A, Gambarotti M, et al. Ewing sarcoma and Ewing-like tumors. Virchows Arch. 2020 Jan;476(1):109-119. Cited in: PubMed; PMID 31802230.
1249. Scapa JV, Cloutier JM, Raghavan SS, et al. DDIT3 Immunohistochemistry Is a Useful Tool for the Diagnosis of Myxoid Liposarcoma. Am J Surg Pathol. 2021 Feb;45(2):230-239. Cited in: PubMed; PMID 32815829.
1250. Schaefer IM, Al-Ibraheemi A, Qian X. Cytomorphologic Spectrum of SMARCB1-Deficient Soft Tissue Neoplasms. Am J Clin Pathol. 2021 Jul;156(2):229-245. Cited in: PubMed; PMID 33608696.
1251. Schaefer IM, Dong F, Garcia EP, et al. Recurrent SMARCB1 Inactivation in Epithelioid Malignant Peripheral Nerve Sheath Tumors. Am J Surg Pathol. 2019 Jun;43(6):835-843. Cited in: PubMed; PMID 30864974.
1252. Schaefer IM, Fletcher CD. Myxoid variant of so-called angiomatoid "malignant fibrous histiocytoma": clinicopathologic characterization in a series of 21 cases. Am J Surg Pathol. 2014 Jun;38(6):816-23. Cited in: PubMed; PMID 24503754.
1253. Schaefer IM, Fletcher CD, Hornick JL. Loss of H3K27 trimethylation distinguishes malignant peripheral nerve sheath tumors from histologic mimics. Mod Pathol. 2016 Jan;29(1):4-13. Cited in: PubMed; PMID 26585554.
1254. Schaefer IM, Fletcher JA, Nielsen GP, et al. Immunohistochemistry for histone H3G34W and H3K36M is highly specific for giant cell tumor of bone and chondroblastoma, respectively, in FNA and core needle biopsy. Cancer Cytopathol. 2018 Aug;126(8):552-566. Cited in: PubMed; PMID 29757500.
1255. Schaefer IM, Hornick JL. SWI/SNF complex-deficient soft tissue neoplasms: An update. Semin Diagn Pathol. 2021 May;38(3):222-231. Cited in: PubMed; PMID 32646614.
1256. Schaefer IM, Wang Y, Liang CW, et al. MAX inactivation is an early event in GIST development that regulates p16 and cell proliferation. Nat Commun. 2017 Mar;8:14674. Cited in: PubMed; PMID 28270683.
1257. Scherübl H, Faiss S, Knoefel WT, et al. Management of early asymptomatic gastrointestinal stromal tumors of the stomach. World J Gastrointest Endosc. 2014 Jul;6(7):266-71. Cited in: PubMed; PMID 25031785.
1258. Schleiermacher G, Mosseri V, London WB, et al. Segmental chromosomal alterations have prognostic impact in neuroblastoma: a report from the INRG project. Br J Cancer. 2012 Oct;107(8):1418-22. Cited in: PubMed; PMID 22976801.
1259. Schmidt RL, Witt BL, Lopez-Calderon LE, et al. The influence of rapid onsite evaluation on the adequacy rate of fine-needle aspiration cytology: a systematic review and meta-analysis. Am J Clin Pathol. 2013 Mar;139(3):300-8. Cited in: PubMed; PMID 23429365.
1260. Schmitt FC, AC Mera A. Fine needle aspiration cytology presentation of a cellular variant of breast myofibroblastoma. Report of a case with immunohistochemical studies. Acta Cytol. 199842(3):721-4. Cited in: PubMed; PMID 9622694.
1262. Schneider V, Smyczek B. Sister Mary Joseph's nodule. Diagnosis of umbilical metastases by fine needle aspiration. Acta Cytol. 199034(4):555-8. Cited in: PubMed; PMID 2375224.
1263. Schneider-Stock R, Walter H, Radig K, et al. MDM2 amplification and loss of heterozygosity at Rb and p53 genes: no simultaneous alterations in the oncogenesis of liposarcomas. J Cancer Res Clin Oncol. 1998124(10):532-40. Cited in: PubMed; PMID 9829856.
1264. Schoolmeester JK, Howitt BE, Hirsch MS, et al. Perivascular epithelioid cell neoplasm (PEComa) of the gynecologic tract: clinicopathologic and immunohistochemical characterization of 16 cases. Am J Surg Pathol. 2014 Feb;38(2):176-88. Cited in: PubMed; PMID 24418852.
1265. Schrijver WA, van der Groep P, Hoefnagel LD, et al. Influence of decalcification procedures on immunohistochemistry and molecular pathology in breast cancer. Mod Pathol. 2016 Dec;29(12):1460-1470. Cited in: PubMed; PMID 27562496.
1266. Schubert PT, Razack R, Vermaak A, et al. Fine-needle aspiration cytology of subcutaneous fat necrosis of the newborn: the cytology spectrum with review of the literature. Diagn Cytopathol. 2012 Mar;40(3):245-7. Cited in: PubMed; PMID 22334526.
1267. Schulz B, Altendorf-Hofmann A, Kirchner T, et al. Loss of CD34 and high IGF2 are associated with malignant transformation in solitary fibrous tumors. Pathol Res Pract. 2014 Feb;210(2):92-7. Cited in: PubMed; PMID 24360568.
1268. Schwartz JG, Zollars PR. Fine needle aspiration cytology of malignant melanoma of soft parts. Report of two cases. Acta Cytol. 199034(3):397-400. Cited in: PubMed; PMID 2343698.
1269. Sciot R, Bekaert J. Spindle cell lipoma with extramedullary haematopoiesis. Histopathology. 2001 Aug;39(2):215-6. Cited in: PubMed; PMID 11493343.
1270. Sciot R, Rosai J, Dal Cin P, et al. Analysis of 35 cases of localized and diffuse tenosynovial giant cell tumor: a report from the Chromosomes and Morphology (CHAMP) study group. Mod Pathol. 1999 Jun;12(6):576-9. Cited in: PubMed; PMID 10392632.
1272. SĘdek Ł, Kulis J, SŁota Ł, et al. The influence of fixation of biological samples on cell count and marker expression stability in flow cytometric analyses. Cent Eur J Immunol. 202045(2):206-213. Cited in: PubMed; PMID 33456333.
1273. Sehgal IS, Gupta N, Dhooria S, et al. Processing and Reporting of Cytology Specimens from Mediastinal Lymph Nodes Collected using Endobronchial Ultrasound-Guided Transbronchial Needle Aspiration: A State-of-the-Art Review. J Cytol. 202037(2):72-81. Cited in: PubMed; PMID 32606494.
1274. Seidal T, Walaas L, Kindblom LG, et al. Cytology of embryonal rhabdomyosarcoma: a cytologic, light microscopic, electron microscopic, and immunohistochemical study of seven cases. Diagn Cytopathol. 19884(4):292-9. Cited in: PubMed; PMID 3076110.
1275. Selby DM, Stocker JT, Ishak KG. Angiosarcoma of the liver in childhood: a clinicopathologic and follow-up study of 10 cases. Pediatr Pathol. 199212(4):485-98. Cited in: PubMed; PMID 1409148.
1276. Sengupta S, Mondal SK, Mallick MG, et al. Role of cytology in diagnosis of soft tissue sarcomas with special reference to false positive cases. J Cytol. 2009 Jan;26(1):15-9. Cited in: PubMed; PMID 21938143.
1277. Sepe PS, Moparty B, Pitman MB, et al. EUS-guided FNA for the diagnosis of GI stromal cell tumors: sensitivity and cytologic yield. Gastrointest Endosc. 2009 Aug;70(2):254-61. Cited in: PubMed; PMID 19482280.
1278. Shabb N, Sneige N, Fanning CV, et al. Fine-needle aspiration cytology of alveolar soft-part sarcoma. Diagn Cytopathol. 19917(3):293-8. Cited in: PubMed; PMID 1879268.
1279. Shah KK, McHugh JB, Folpe AL, et al. Dermatofibrosarcoma Protuberans of Distal Extremities and Acral Sites: A Clinicopathologic Analysis of 27 Cases. Am J Surg Pathol. 2018 Mar;42(3):413-419. Cited in: PubMed; PMID 29240584.

1280. Shahabi A, Israel AK, Sullivan CB, et al. Fine needle aspiration biopsy of epithelioid-mesenchymal neoplasm with PTCH1-GLI1 fusion: A case report. Diagn Cytopathol. 2022 Aug;50(8):E223-E229. Cited in: PubMed; PMID 35514197.
1282. Shan Y, Cai J, Han Y, et al. An analysis of the diagnosis, clinical characteristics, treatment, and survival outcomes of 36 extracranial malignant rhabdoid tumor patients. Transl Pediatr. 2021 Jun;10(6):1598-1609. Cited in: PubMed; PMID 34295774.
1283. Sharma A, Thangaiah JJ, Shetty S, et al. Bone and soft tissue sarcomas in cerebrospinal fluid and effusion: A 20-year review at our institution. Cancer Cytopathol. 2021 Oct;129(10):776-787. Cited in: PubMed; PMID 34233079.
1284. Sharma K, Yadav SK, Valluru B, et al. Significance of MRI in the diagnosis and differentiation of clear cell sarcoma of tendon and aponeurosis (CCSTA): A case report. Medicine (Baltimore). 2018 Aug;97(31):e11012. Cited in: PubMed; PMID 30075493.
1285. Sharma S, Gupta N, Rajwanshi A, et al. Inflammatory myofibroblastic tumour: a diagnostic challenge on fine needle aspiration cytology. Cytopathology. 2016 Dec;27(6):512-516. Cited in: PubMed; PMID 27087029.
1286. Sheng W, Lu L, Wang J. Cellular angiolipoma: a clinicopathological and immunohistochemical study of 12 cases. Am J Dermatopathol. 2013 Apr;35(2):220-5. Cited in: PubMed; PMID 22935891.
1287. Shiba S, Imaoka H, Shioji K, et al. Clinical characteristics of Japanese patients with epithelioid hemangioendothelioma: a multicenter retrospective study. BMC Cancer. 2018 Oct;18(1):993. Cited in: PubMed; PMID 30340559.
1288. Shibayama T, Okamoto T, Nakashima Y, et al. Screening of BCOR-CCNB3 sarcoma using immunohistochemistry for CCNB3: A clinicopathological report of three pediatric cases. Pathol Int. 2015 Aug;65(8):410-4. Cited in: PubMed; PMID 26037154.
1289. Shidham VB. CellBlockistry: Chemistry and art of cell-block making - A detailed review of various historical options with recent advances. Cytojournal. 201916:12. Cited in: PubMed; PMID 31367220.
1290. Shield PW, Cosier J, Ellerby G, et al. Rapid on-site evaluation of fine needle aspiration specimens by cytology scientists: a review of 3032 specimens. Cytopathology. 2014 Oct;25(5):322-9. Cited in: PubMed; PMID 24844295.
1291. Shih AR, Chebib I, Deshpande V, et al. Molecular characteristics of poorly differentiated chordoma. Genes Chromosomes Cancer. 2019 Nov;58(11):804-808. Cited in: PubMed; PMID 31135077.
1292. Shih AR, Cote GM, Chebib I, et al. Clinicopathologic characteristics of poorly differentiated chordoma. Mod Pathol. 2018 Aug;31(8):1237-1245. Cited in: PubMed; PMID 29483606.
1293. Shim HS, Choi YD, Cho NH. Malignant glomus tumor of the urinary bladder. Arch Pathol Lab Med. 2005 Jul;129(7):940-2. Cited in: PubMed; PMID 15974822.
1294. Shimada H, Ambros IM, Dehner LP, et al. Terminology and morphologic criteria of neuroblastic tumors: recommendations by the International Neuroblastoma Pathology Committee. Cancer. 1999 Jul;86(2):349-63. Cited in: PubMed; PMID 10421272.
1295. Shimada H, Ambros IM, Dehner LP, et al. The International Neuroblastoma Pathology Classification (the Shimada system). Cancer. 1999 Jul;86(2):364-72. Cited in: PubMed; PMID 10421273.
1296. Shimada S, Ishizawa T, Ishizawa K, et al. Dedifferentiated liposarcoma with rhabdomyoblastic differentiation. Virchows Arch. 2005 Nov;447(5):835-41. Cited in: PubMed; PMID 16012847.
1297. Shimizu S, Hashimoto H, Enjoji M. Nodular fasciitis: an analysis of 250 patients. Pathology. 1984 Apr;16(2):161-6. Cited in: PubMed; PMID 6462780.
1298. Shin C, Low I, Ng D, et al. USP6 gene rearrangement in nodular fasciitis and histological mimics. Histopathology. 2016 Nov;69(5):784-791. Cited in: PubMed; PMID 27271298.
1299. Shinagare AB, Ramaiya NH, Jagannathan JP, et al. A to Z of desmoid tumors. AJR Am J Roentgenol. 2011 Dec;197(6):W1008-14. Cited in: PubMed; PMID 22109314.
1300. Shirley MD, Tang H, Gallione CJ, et al. Sturge-Weber syndrome and port-wine stains caused by somatic mutation in GNAQ. N Engl J Med. 2013 May;368(21):1971-9. Cited in: PubMed; PMID 23656586.
1301. Shmookler BM, Enzinger FM. Pleomorphic lipoma: a benign tumor simulating liposarcoma. A clinicopathologic analysis of 48 cases. Cancer. 1981 Jan;47(1):126-33. Cited in: PubMed; PMID 7459800.
1302. Shu H, Ma Q, Li A, et al. Diagnostic Performance of US and MRI in Predicting Malignancy of Soft Tissue Masses: Using a Scoring System. Front Oncol. 202212:853232. Cited in: PubMed; PMID 35574339.
1303. SHUGART RR, SOULE EH, JOHNSON EW. GLOMUS TUMOR. Surg Gynecol Obstet. 1963 Sep;117:334-40. Cited in: PubMed; PMID 14080348.
1304. Siddiqa A, Haider A, Mehmood M, et al. A 58-Year-Old Man with a Painful Gluteal Mass as the First Presentation of Metastatic Adenocarcinoma of the Lung. Am J Case Rep. 2021 Mar;22:e928122. Cited in: PubMed; PMID 33664218.
1305. Siegel GW, Biermann JS, Chugh R, et al. The multidisciplinary management of bone and soft tissue sarcoma: an essential organizational framework. J Multidiscip Healthc. 20158:109-15. Cited in: PubMed; PMID 25733913.
1306. Silverman JF, Landreneau RJ, Sturgis CD, et al. Small-cell variant of synovial sarcoma: fine-needle aspiration with ancillary features and potential diagnostic pitfalls. Diagn Cytopathol. 2000 Aug;23(2):118-23. Cited in: PubMed; PMID 10888758.
1307. Silverman JF, Olson PR, Dabbs DJ, et al. Fine-needle aspiration cytology of a mediastinal seminoma associated with multilocular thymic cyst. Diagn Cytopathol. 1999 Apr;20(4):224-8. Cited in: PubMed; PMID 10204106.
1309. Simon MP, Pedeutour F, Sirvent N, et al. Deregulation of the platelet-derived growth factor B-chain gene via fusion with collagen gene COL1A1 in dermatofibrosarcoma protuberans and giant-cell fibroblastoma. Nat Genet. 1997 Jan;15(1):95-8. Cited in: PubMed; PMID 8988177.
1310. Simpson KW, Albores-Saavedra J. HMB-45 reactivity in conventional uterine leiomyosarcomas. Am J Surg Pathol. 2007 Jan;31(1):95-8. Cited in: PubMed; PMID 17197924.
1311. Singh HK, Kilpatrick SE, Silverman JF. Fine needle aspiration biopsy of soft tissue sarcomas: utility and diagnostic challenges. Adv Anat Pathol. 2004 Jan;11(1):24-37. Cited in: PubMed; PMID 14676638.
1312. Singh S, Paul S, Dhall K, et al. Nodular fasciitis: a diagnostic challenge. Indian J Pathol Microbiol. 201356(3):288-90. Cited in: PubMed; PMID 24152513.
1314. Sinovic J, Bridge JA. Translocation (2;17) in recurrent dermatofibrosarcoma protuberans. Cancer Genet Cytogenet. 1994 Jul;75(2):156-7. Cited in: PubMed; PMID 8055483.
1315. Sio TT, Vu CC, Sohawon S, et al. Extraskeletal Osteosarcoma: An International Rare Cancer Network Study. Am J Clin Oncol. 2016 Feb;39(1):32-6. Cited in: PubMed; PMID 24401667.
1316. Sioletic S, Dal Cin P, Fletcher CD, et al. Well-differentiated and dedifferentiated liposarcomas with prominent myxoid stroma: analysis of 56 cases. Histopathology. 2013 Jan;62(2):287-93. Cited in: PubMed; PMID 23020289.
1317. Sirohi D, Smith SC, Epstein JI, et al. Pericytic tumors of the kidney-a clinicopathologic analysis of 17 cases. Hum Pathol. 2017 Jun;64:106-117. Cited in: PubMed; PMID 28438616.
1318. Skapek SX, Ferrari A, Gupta AA, et al. Rhabdomyosarcoma. Nat Rev Dis Primers. 2019 Jan;5(1):1. Cited in: PubMed; PMID 30617281.
1319. Skoog L, Tani E. Immunocytochemistry: an indispensable technique in routine cytology. Cytopathology. 2011 Aug;22(4):215-29. Cited in: PubMed; PMID 21771092.
1320. Slater DN, Cotton DW, Azzopardi JG. Oncocytic glomus tumour: a new variant. Histopathology. 1987 May;11(5):523-31. Cited in: PubMed; PMID 3038728.
1321. Sloan EA, Chiang J, Villanueva-Meyer JE, et al. Intracranial mesenchymal tumor with FET-CREB fusion-A unifying diagnosis for the spectrum of intracranial myxoid mesenchymal tumors and angiomatoid fibrous histiocytoma-like neoplasms. Brain Pathol. 2021 Jul;31(4):e12918. Cited in: PubMed; PMID 33141488.
1322. Slotkin EK, Bowman AS, Levine MF, et al. Comprehensive Molecular Profiling of Desmoplastic Small Round Cell Tumor. Mol Cancer Res. 2021 Jul;19(7):1146-1155. Cited in: PubMed; PMID 33753552.
1323. Smith SC, Gooding WE, Elkins M, et al. Solitary Fibrous Tumors of the Head and Neck: A Multi-Institutional Clinicopathologic Study. Am J Surg Pathol. 2017 Dec;41(12):1642-1656. Cited in: PubMed; PMID 28877055.
1324. Smith TA, Easley KA, Goldblum JR. Myxoid/round cell liposarcoma of the extremities. A clinicopathologic study of 29 cases with particular attention to extent of round cell liposarcoma. Am J Surg Pathol. 1996 Feb;20(2):171-80. Cited in: PubMed; PMID 8554106.
1325. Sola Pérez J, Pérez-Guillermo M, Bas Bernal A, et al. Malignant rhabdoid tumor of soft tissues: a cytopathological and immunohistochemical study. Diagn Cytopathol. 19928(4):369-73. Cited in: PubMed; PMID 1322263.
1326. Sola-Pérez J, Pérez-Guillermo M, Bas-Bernal A, et al. Melanocytic schwannoma: the cytologic aspect in fine-needle aspiration cytology (FNAC): report of a case located in the spinal cord. Diagn Cytopathol. 199411(3):291-6. Cited in: PubMed; PMID 7867475.
1327. Somerhausen NS, Fletcher CD. Diffuse-type giant cell tumor: clinicopathologic and immunohistochemical analysis of 50 cases with extraarticular disease. Am J Surg Pathol. 2000 Apr;24(4):479-92. Cited in: PubMed; PMID 10757395.
1329. Song W, van Hemel BM, Suurmeijer AJH. Suitability of the CellientTM cell block method for diagnosing soft tissue and bone tumors. Diagn Cytopathol. 2018 Apr;46(4):299-305. Cited in: PubMed; PMID 29318761.
1330. Soni PB, Verma AK, Chandoke RK, et al. A prospective study of soft tissue tumors histocytopathology correlation. Patholog Res Int. 20142014:678628. Cited in: PubMed; PMID 24876987.
1331. Sonobe H, Furihata M, Iwata J, et al. Dermatofibrosarcoma protuberans harboring t(9;22)(q32;q12.2). Cancer Genet Cytogenet. 1999 Apr;110(1):14-8. Cited in: PubMed; PMID 10198616.
1332. Sood N, Rewri S, Nigam JS. Small cell extraskeletal osteosarcoma: a rare case report. Rare Tumors. 2014 Jan;6(1):5029. Cited in: PubMed; PMID 24711902.
1333. Sordillo PP, Hajdu SI, Magill GB, et al. Extraosseous osteogenic sarcoma. A review of 48 patients. Cancer. 1983 Feb;51(4):727-34. Cited in: PubMed; PMID 6571801.
1334. Sorensen PH, Lynch JC, Qualman SJ, et al. PAX3-FKHR and PAX7-FKHR gene fusions are prognostic indicators in alveolar rhabdomyosarcoma: a report from the children's oncology group. J Clin Oncol. 2002 Jun;20(11):2672-9. Cited in: PubMed; PMID 12039929.
1335. Soslow RA, Yin P, Steinberg CR, et al. Cytopathologic features of hepatic epithelioid hemangioendothelioma. Diagn Cytopathol. 1997 Jul;17(1):50-3. Cited in: PubMed; PMID 9218904.
1336. Specht K, Sung YS, Zhang L, et al. Distinct transcriptional signature and immunoprofile of CIC-DUX4 fusion-positive round cell tumors compared to EWSR1-rearranged Ewing sarcomas: further evidence toward distinct pathologic entities. Genes Chromosomes Cancer. 2014 Jul;53(7):622-33. Cited in: PubMed; PMID 24723486.
1337. Specht K, Zhang L, Sung YS, et al. Novel BCOR-MAML3 and ZC3H7B-BCOR Gene Fusions in Undifferentiated Small Blue Round Cell Sarcomas. Am J Surg Pathol. 2016 Apr;40(4):433-42. Cited in: PubMed; PMID 26752546.
1338. Sperandeo M, Trovato FM, Melillo N, et al. The role of ultrasound-guided fine needle aspiration biopsy in musculoskeletal diseases. Eur J Radiol. 2017 May;90:234-244. Cited in: PubMed; PMID 28583640.
1339. Sredni ST, Tomita T. Rhabdoid tumor predisposition syndrome. Pediatr Dev Pathol. 201518(1):49-58. Cited in: PubMed; PMID 25494491.
1340. Sridhar S, Al-Moallem B, Kamal H, et al. New insights into the genetics of neuroblastoma. Mol Diagn Ther. 2013 Apr;17(2):63-9. Cited in: PubMed; PMID 23329364.
1341. Srinivasan R, Gautam U, Gupta R, et al. Synovial sarcoma: diagnosis on fine-needle aspiration by morphology and molecular analysis. Cancer. 2009 Apr;117(2):128-36. Cited in: PubMed; PMID 19267417.
1342. Stacchini A, Demurtas A, Aliberti S. Extranodal Lymphoproliferative Processes and Flow Cytometry. Acta Cytol. 201660(4):315-325. Cited in: PubMed; PMID 27537785.
1343. Stanley MW, Skoog L, Tani EM, et al. Nodular fasciitis: spontaneous resolution following diagnosis by fine-needle aspiration. Diagn Cytopathol. 19939(3):322-4. Cited in: PubMed; PMID 8519200.
1344. Stegmaier S, Poremba C, Schaefer KL, et al. Prognostic value of PAX-FKHR fusion status in alveolar rhabdomyosarcoma: a report from the cooperative soft tissue sarcoma study group (CWS). Pediatr Blood Cancer. 2011 Sep;57(3):406-14. Cited in: PubMed; PMID 21254373.
1345. Stelow EB, Murad FM, Debol SM, et al. A limited immunocytochemical panel for the distinction of subepithelial gastrointestinal mesenchymal neoplasms sampled by endoscopic ultrasound-guided fine-needle aspiration. Am J Clin Pathol. 2008 Feb;129(2):219-25. Cited in: PubMed; PMID 18208801.
1346. Stelow EB, Stanley MW, Mallery S, et al. Endoscopic ultrasound-guided fine-needle aspiration findings of gastrointestinal leiomyomas and gastrointestinal stromal tumors. Am J Clin Pathol. 2003 May;119(5):703-8. Cited in: PubMed; PMID 12760289.

1347. Stenman G, Kindblom LG, Angervall L. Reciprocal translocation t(12;22)(q13;q13) in clear-cell sarcoma of tendons and aponeuroses. Genes Chromosomes Cancer. 1992 Mar;4(2):122-7. Cited in: PubMed; PMID 1373311.
1348. Stevens DL, Bryant AE, Goldstein EJ. Necrotizing Soft Tissue Infections. Infect Dis Clin North Am. 2021 Mar;35(1):135-155. Cited in: PubMed; PMID 33303335.
1349. Stewart B, Manglik N, Zhao B, et al. Aortic intimal sarcoma: report of two cases with immunohistochemical analysis for pathogenesis. Cardiovasc Pathol. 201322(5):351-6. Cited in: PubMed; PMID 23628153.
1350. Stewart BD, Nascimento AF. Palmar and plantar fibromatosis: a review. J Pathol Transl Med. 2021 Jul;55(4):265-270. Cited in: PubMed; PMID 34225446.
1351. Stewart DR, Sloan JL, Yao L, et al. Diagnosis, management, and complications of glomus tumours of the digits in neurofibromatosis type 1. J Med Genet. 2010 Aug;47(8):525-32. Cited in: PubMed; PMID 20530151.
1352. Stoll LM, Li QK. Cytology of fine-needle aspiration of inflammatory myofibroblastic tumor. Diagn Cytopathol. 2011 Sep;39(9):663-72. Cited in: PubMed; PMID 20730898.
1353. Stone AB, Mallery JS, Stewart J, et al. A rare sporadic pancreatic desmoid fibromatosis diagnosed by endoscopic ultrasound-guided fine-needle aspiration: Case report and literature review. Diagn Cytopathol. 2021 Feb;49(2):E49-E54. Cited in: PubMed; PMID 32857922.
1354. Stratakis CA, Carney JA. The triad of paragangliomas, gastric stromal tumours and pulmonary chondromas (Carney triad), and the dyad of paragangliomas and gastric stromal sarcomas (Carney-Stratakis syndrome): molecular genetics and clinical implications. J Intern Med. 2009 Jul;266(1):43-52. Cited in: PubMed; PMID 19522824.
1355. Strauss DC, Qureshi YA, Hayes AJ, et al. The role of core needle biopsy in the diagnosis of suspected soft tissue tumours. J Surg Oncol. 2010 Oct;102(5):523-9. Cited in: PubMed; PMID 20872955.
1356. Styring E, Billing V, Hartman L, et al. Simple guidelines for efficient referral of soft-tissue sarcomas: a population-based evaluation of adherence to guidelines and referral patterns. J Bone Joint Surg Am. 2012 Jul;94(14):1291-6. Cited in: PubMed; PMID 22810399.
1357. Sugiura Y, Nagaishi M, Takano I, et al. Convexity dural chondroma: a case report with pathological and molecular analysis. Clin Neuropathol. 201534(1):13-8. Cited in: PubMed; PMID 25250651.
1358. Sukov WR, Franco MF, Erickson-Johnson M, et al. Frequency of USP6 rearrangements in myositis ossificans, brown tumor, and cherubism: molecular cytogenetic evidence that a subset of "myositis ossificans-like lesions" are the early phases in the formation of soft-tissue aneurysmal bone cyst. Skeletal Radiol. 2008 Apr;37(4):321-7. Cited in: PubMed; PMID 18265974.
1359. Sullivan LM, Folpe AL, Pawel BR, et al. Epithelioid sarcoma is associated with a high percentage of SMARCB1 deletions. Mod Pathol. 2013 Mar;26(3):385-92. Cited in: PubMed; PMID 23060122.
1360. Sultan I, Rodriguez-Galindo C, Saab R, et al. Comparing children and adults with synovial sarcoma in the Surveillance, Epidemiology, and End Results program, 1983 to 2005: an analysis of 1268 patients. Cancer. 2009 Aug;115(15):3537-47. Cited in: PubMed; PMID 19514087.
1361. Sun J, Zhang Z, Xiao Y, et al. Skeletal Muscle Metastasis From Renal Cell Carcinoma: A Case Series and Literature Review. Front Surg. 20229:762540. Cited in: PubMed; PMID 35310441.
1362. Sunitsch S, Gilg MM, Kashofer K, et al. Detection of GNAS mutations in intramuscular / cellular myxomas as diagnostic tool in the classification of myxoid soft tissue tumors. Diagn Pathol. 2018 Aug;13(1):52. Cited in: PubMed; PMID 30111377.
1363. Surabhi VR, Chua S, Patel RP, et al. Inflammatory Myofibroblastic Tumors: Current Update. Radiol Clin North Am. 2016 May;54(3):553-63. Cited in: PubMed; PMID 27153788.
1364. Surace C, Panagopoulos I, Pålsson E, et al. A novel FISH assay for SS18-SSX fusion type in synovial sarcoma. Lab Invest. 2004 Sep;84(9):1185-92. Cited in: PubMed; PMID 15208645.
1366. Suster D, Michal M, Huang H, et al. Myxoinflammatory fibroblastic sarcoma: an immunohistochemical and molecular genetic study of 73 cases. Mod Pathol. 2020 Dec;33(12):2520-2533. Cited in: PubMed; PMID 32514165.
1367. Suster S, Moran CA, Koss MN. Epithelioid hemangioendothelioma of the anterior mediastinum. Clinicopathologic, immunohistochemical, and ultrastructural analysis of 12 cases. Am J Surg Pathol. 1994 Sep;18(9):871-81. Cited in: PubMed; PMID 8067508.
1368. Suster S, Rosai J. Intranodal hemorrhagic spindle-cell tumor with "amianthoid" fibers. Report of six cases of a distinctive mesenchymal neoplasm of the inguinal region that simulates Kaposi's sarcoma. Am J Surg Pathol. 1989 May;13(5):347-57. Cited in: PubMed; PMID 2712187.
1369. Suthipintawong C, Leong AS, Vinyuvat S. Immunostaining of cell preparations: a comparative evaluation of common fixatives and protocols. Diagn Cytopathol. 1996 Aug;15(2):167-74. Cited in: PubMed; PMID 8872443.
1370. Suurmeijer AJH, Dickson BC, Swanson D, et al. A morphologic and molecular reappraisal of myoepithelial tumors of soft tissue, bone, and viscera with EWSR1 and FUS gene rearrangements. Genes Chromosomes Cancer. 2020 Jun;59(6):348-356. Cited in: PubMed; PMID 31994243.
1371. Svarvar C, Böhling T, Berlin O, et al. Clinical course of nonvisceral soft tissue leiomyosarcoma in 225 patients from the Scandinavian Sarcoma Group. Cancer. 2007 Jan;109(2):282-91. Cited in: PubMed; PMID 17154171.
1372. Taefi A, Matsukuma K, Chak E. Massive Epithelioid Hemangioendothelioma Causing Noncirrhotic Portal Hypertension. Clin Gastroenterol Hepatol. 2019 Jun;17(7):A19. Cited in: PubMed; PMID 29609064.
1373. Tamborini E, Casieri P, Miselli F, et al. Analysis of potential receptor tyrosine kinase targets in intimal and mural sarcomas. J Pathol. 2007 Jun;212(2):227-35. Cited in: PubMed; PMID 17471466.
1374. Tamiolakis D, Mygdakos N, Tsamis I, et al. Aspiration and Brushing Cytology in tumors and tumor-like conditions of the tongue: A Study of 27 Cases. Stomatologija. 201517(2):67-72. Cited in: PubMed; PMID 26879271.
1375. Tan H, Wang B, Xiao H, et al. Radiologic and Clinicopathologic Findings of Inflammatory Myofibroblastic Tumor. J Comput Assist Tomogr. 2017 Jan;41(1):90-97. Cited in: PubMed; PMID 27224222.
1376. Tan PH, Lai LM, Carrington EV, et al. Fat necrosis of the breast--a review. Breast. 2006 Jun;15(3):313-8. Cited in: PubMed; PMID 16198567.
1377. Tanas MR, Goldblum JR. Fluorescence in situ hybridization in the diagnosis of soft tissue neoplasms: a review. Adv Anat Pathol. 2009 Nov;16(6):383-91. Cited in: PubMed; PMID 19851129.
1378. Tanas MR, Rubin BP, Montgomery EA, et al. Utility of FISH in the diagnosis of angiomatoid fibrous histiocytoma: a series of 18 cases. Mod Pathol. 2010 Jan;23(1):93-7. Cited in: PubMed; PMID 19801966.
1379. Tang S, Dodd LG. CIC-DUX4 sarcoma diagnosed by fine-needle aspiration cytology: A case report. Diagn Cytopathol. 2018 Nov;46(11):958-963. Cited in: PubMed; PMID 30353686.
1380. Tani E, Wejde J, Åström K, et al. FNA cytology of solitary fibrous tumors and the diagnostic value of STAT6 immunocytochemistry. Cancer Cytopathol. 2018 Jan;126(1):36-43. Cited in: PubMed; PMID 28914981.
1381. Tani EM, Stanley MW, Skoog L. Fine needle aspiration cytology presentation of bilateral mammary fibromatosis. Report of a case. Acta Cytol. 198832(4):555-8. Cited in: PubMed; PMID 3400396.
1382. Tanwar P, Gupta N, Vasishta RK, et al. Fine needle aspiration cytology in fibromatosis. J Cytol. 2012 Jan;29(1):66-8. Cited in: PubMed; PMID 22438623.
1383. Tao LC, Davidson DD. Aspiration biopsy cytology of smooth muscle tumors. A cytologic approach to the differentiation between leiomyosarcoma and leiomyoma. Acta Cytol. 199337(3):300-8. Cited in: PubMed; PMID 8498132.
1384. Tasli F, Vardar E, Argon A, et al. Histochemical and immunohistochemical characteristics of elastofibromas. Pol J Pathol. 2014 Jun;65(2):120-4. Cited in: PubMed; PMID 25119171.
1385. Tateishi U, Hasegawa T, Kusumoto M, et al. Radiologic manifestations of proximal-type epithelioid sarcoma of the soft tissues. AJR Am J Roentgenol. 2002 Oct;179(4):973-7. Cited in: PubMed; PMID 12239049.
1386. Taweevisit M, Thorner PS. Distinctive features of low-grade myofibroblastic sarcoma on aspiration cytology: A case report. Cytopathology. 2018 Dec;29(6):578-581. Cited in: PubMed; PMID 30079453.
1387. TAYLOR HB, HELWIG EB. Dermatofibrosarcoma protuberans. A study of 115 cases. Cancer. 196215:717-25. Cited in: PubMed; PMID 13919964.
1388. Teefey SA, Dahiya N, Middleton WD, et al. Ganglia of the hand and wrist: a sonographic analysis. AJR Am J Roentgenol. 2008 Sep;191(3):716-20. Cited in: PubMed; PMID 18716098.
1389. Tepe M, Polat MA, Calisir C, et al. Prevalence of elastofibroma dorsi on CT: Is it really an uncommon entity? Acta Orthop Traumatol Turc. 2019 May;53(3):195-198. Cited in: PubMed; PMID 31031128.
1390. Terrier-Lacombe MJ, Guillou L, Maire G, et al. Dermatofibrosarcoma protuberans, giant cell fibroblastoma, and hybrid lesions in children: clinicopathologic comparative analysis of 28 cases with molecular data--a study from the French Federation of Cancer Centers Sarcoma Group. Am J Surg Pathol. 2003 Jan;27(1):27-39. Cited in: PubMed; PMID 12502925.
1391. Terry J, Saito T, Subramanian S, et al. TLE1 as a diagnostic immunohistochemical marker for synovial sarcoma emerging from gene expression profiling studies. Am J Surg Pathol. 2007 Feb;31(2):240-6. Cited in: PubMed; PMID 17255769.
1392. Thakkar SD, Feigen U, Mautner VF. Spinal tumours in neurofibromatosis type 1: an MRI study of frequency, multiplicity and variety. Neuroradiology. 1999 Sep;41(9):625-9. Cited in: PubMed; PMID 10525761.
1393. Thampi S, Matthay KK, Boscardin WJ, et al. Clinical Features and Outcomes Differ between Skeletal and Extraskeletal Osteosarcoma. Sarcoma. 20142014:902620. Cited in: PubMed; PMID 25294959.
1394. Thejasvi K, Niveditha SR, Suguna BV, et al. Cytomorphology of hibernoma: a report of 2 cases. Acta Cytol. 201054(5 Suppl):875-8. Cited in: PubMed; PMID 21053560.
1395. Thiesse P, Hany MA, Combaret V, et al. Assessment of percutaneous fine needle aspiration cytology as a technique to provide diagnostic and prognostic information in neuroblastoma. Eur J Cancer. 2000 Aug;36(12):1544-51. Cited in: PubMed; PMID 10930802.
1396. Thirumala S, Desai M, Kannan V. Diagnostic pitfalls in fine needle aspiration cytology of pleomorphic lipoma. A case report. Acta Cytol. 200044(4):653-6. Cited in: PubMed; PMID 10934961.
1397. Thomas J, Adeyi AO, Olu-Eddo AO, et al. Fine needle aspiration cytology in the management of childhood palpable masses: Ibadan experience. J Trop Pediatr. 1999 Dec;45(6):378. Cited in: PubMed; PMID 10667013.
1398. Thomson TA, Horsman D, Bainbridge TC. Cytogenetic and cytologic features of chondroid lipoma of soft tissue. Mod Pathol. 1999 Jan;12(1):88-91. Cited in: PubMed; PMID 9950168.
1399. Thool AA, Raut WK, Lele VR, et al. Fine needle aspiration cytology of soft tissue chondroma. A case report. Acta Cytol. 200145(1):86-8. Cited in: PubMed; PMID 11213511.
1400. Thunnissen FB, Arends JW, Buchholtz RT, et al. Fine needle aspiration cytology of inflammatory pseudotumor of the lung (plasma cell granuloma). Report of four cases. Acta Cytol. 198933(6):917-21. Cited in: PubMed; PMID 2588924.
1401. Thway K. Well-differentiated liposarcoma and dedifferentiated liposarcoma: An updated review. Semin Diagn Pathol. 2019 Mar;36(2):112-121. Cited in: PubMed; PMID 30852045.
1402. Thway K. What's new in adipocytic neoplasia? Histopathology. 2022 Jan;80(1):76-97. Cited in: PubMed; PMID 34958506.
1403. Thway K, Fisher C. Angiomatoid fibrous histiocytoma: the current status of pathology and genetics. Arch Pathol Lab Med. 2015 May;139(5):674-82. Cited in: PubMed; PMID 25927151.
1404. Thway K, Fisher C. Tumors with EWSR1-CREB1 and EWSR1-ATF1 fusions: the current status. Am J Surg Pathol. 2012 Jul;36(7):e1-e11. Cited in: PubMed; PMID 22510762.
1405. Thway K, Fisher C. Undifferentiated and dedifferentiated soft tissue neoplasms: Immunohistochemical surrogates for differential diagnosis. Semin Diagn Pathol. 2021 Nov;38(6):170-186. Cited in: PubMed; PMID 34602314.
1406. Thway K, Flora R, Shah C, et al. Diagnostic utility of p16, CDK4, and MDM2 as an immunohistochemical panel in distinguishing well-differentiated and dedifferentiated liposarcomas from other adipocytic tumors. Am J Surg Pathol. 2012 Mar;36(3):462-9. Cited in: PubMed; PMID 22301498.
1407. Thway K, Flora RS, Fisher C. Chondroid lipoma: an update and review. Ann Diagn Pathol. 2012 Jun;16(3):230-4. Cited in: PubMed; PMID 22607659.
1408. Thway K, Noujaim J, Zaidi S, et al. Desmoplastic Small Round Cell Tumor: Pathology, Genetics, and Potential Therapeutic Strategies. Int J Surg Pathol. 2016 Dec;24(8):672-684. Cited in: PubMed; PMID 27621277.
1409. Thway K, Robertson D, Thway Y, et al. Dedifferentiated liposarcoma with meningothelial-like whorls, metaplastic bone formation, and CDK4, MDM2, and p16 expression: a morphologic and immunohistochemical study. Am J Surg Pathol. 2011 Mar;35(3):356-63. Cited in: PubMed; PMID 21317707.

1410. Thway K, Wang J, Swansbury J, et al. Fluorescence In Situ Hybridization for MDM2 Amplification as a Routine Ancillary Diagnostic Tool for Suspected Well-Differentiated and Dedifferentiated Liposarcomas: Experience at a Tertiary Center. Sarcoma. 20152015:812089. Cited in: PubMed; PMID 25810689.
1411. Tirabosco R, Mangham DC, Rosenberg AE, et al. Brachyury expression in extra-axial skeletal and soft tissue chordomas: a marker that distinguishes chordoma from mixed tumor/myoepithelioma/parachordoma in soft tissue. Am J Surg Pathol. 2008 Apr;32(4):572-80. Cited in: PubMed; PMID 18301055.
1412. Todorović-Raković N. Chromogenic In Situ Hybridization (CISH) as a Method for Detection of C-Myc Amplification in Formalin-Fixed Paraffin-Embedded Tumor Tissue: An Update. Methods Mol Biol. 20212318:313-320. Cited in: PubMed; PMID 34019299.
1413. Toi PCh, Siddaraju N, Basu D. Fine-needle aspiration cytology of granular cell tumor: A report of two cases. J Cytol. 2013 Jul;30(3):195-7. Cited in: PubMed; PMID 24130413.
1414. Toll AD, Wakely PE, Ali SZ. Acral myxoinflammatory fibroblastic sarcoma: cytopathologic findings on fine-needle aspiration. Acta Cytol. 201357(2):134-8. Cited in: PubMed; PMID 23406831.
1415. Tong GX, Hamele-Bena D, Borczuk A, et al. Fine needle aspiration biopsy of epithelioid hemangioendothelioma of the oral cavity: report of one case and review of literature. Diagn Cytopathol. 2006 Mar;34(3):218-23. Cited in: PubMed; PMID 16470861.
1416. Tong TR, Chow TC, Chan OW, et al. Clear-cell sarcoma diagnosis by fine-needle aspiration: cytologic, histologic, and ultrastructural features; potential pitfalls; and literature review. Diagn Cytopathol. 2002 Mar;26(3):174-80. Cited in: PubMed; PMID 11892024.
1417. Torres-Mora J, Dry S, Li X, et al. Malignant melanotic schwannian tumor: a clinicopathologic, immunohistochemical, and gene expression profiling study of 40 cases, with a proposal for the reclassification of "melanotic schwannoma". Am J Surg Pathol. 2014 Jan;38(1):94-105. Cited in: PubMed; PMID 24145644.
1418. Traina F, Errani C, Toscano A, et al. Current concepts in the biopsy of musculoskeletal tumors: AAOS exhibit selection. J Bone Joint Surg Am. 2015 Jan;97(2):e7. Cited in: PubMed; PMID 25609446.
1419. Travis JA, Bridge JA. Significance of both numerical and structural chromosomal abnormalities in clear cell sarcoma. Cancer Genet Cytogenet. 1992 Dec;64(2):104-6. Cited in: PubMed; PMID 1486557.
1420. Travis WD, Wold LE. Immunoperoxidase staining of fine needle aspiration specimens previously stained by the Papanicolaou technique. Acta Cytol. 198731(4):517-20. Cited in: PubMed; PMID 2440215.
1421. Trihia HJ, Novkovic N, Provatas I, et al. Primary Alveolar Rhabdomyosarcoma of the Breast in an Adult: An Extremely Rare Case. Case Rep Pathol. 20192019:6098747. Cited in: PubMed; PMID 31032134.
1422. Tripathy S, Parida GK, Naswa N, et al. Elastofibroma Dorsi: Findings on 18F-Fluorodeoxyglucose Positron Emission Tomography-Computed Tomography. Indian J Nucl Med. 201934(3):258-259. Cited in: PubMed; PMID 31293317.
1423. Trovik CS, Bauer HC, Brosjö O, et al. Fine needle aspiration (FNA) cytology in the diagnosis of recurrent soft tissue sarcoma. Cytopathology. 1998 Oct;9(5):320-8. Cited in: PubMed; PMID 9800130.
1424. Tsai HK, Hornick JL, Vivero M. INSM1 expression in a subset of thoracic malignancies and small round cell tumors: rare potential pitfalls for small cell carcinoma. Mod Pathol. 2020 Aug;33(8):1571-1580. Cited in: PubMed; PMID 32203089.
1425. Tsang AK, Wong FC, Ng PW, et al. Fine needle aspiration cytology of dermatofibrosarcoma protuberans in the breast: a case report. Pathology. 2005 Feb;37(1):84-6. Cited in: PubMed; PMID 15875741.
1426. Tsubakimoto M, Yamashiro T, Tsuchiya N, et al. MRI findings and demographics of elastofibroma dorsi: assessment of diffusion-weighted imaging and contrast enhancement patterns. Acta Radiol. 2018 Jun;59(6):709-715. Cited in: PubMed; PMID 28920444.
1427. Tsuda Y, Matsuyama A, Makihara K, et al. Nuclear expression of MDM2 in hibernoma: a potential diagnostic pitfall. Virchows Arch. 2021 Mar;478(3):527-534. Cited in: PubMed; PMID 32815035.
1428. Tsuneyoshi M, Dorfman HD, Bauer TW. Epithelioid hemangioendothelioma of bone. A clinicopathologic, ultrastructural, and immunohistochemical study. Am J Surg Pathol. 1986 Nov;10(11):754-64. Cited in: PubMed; PMID 2430475.
1429. Turcotte RE. Giant cell tumor of bone. Orthop Clin North Am. 2006 Jan;37(1):35-51. Cited in: PubMed; PMID 16311110.
1430. Turner JH, Richmon JD. Head and neck rhabdomyosarcoma: a critical analysis of population-based incidence and survival data. Otolaryngol Head Neck Surg. 2011 Dec;145(6):967-73. Cited in: PubMed; PMID 21873599.
1431. Ud Din N, Ahmad Z, Zreik R, et al. Abdominopelvic and Retroperitoneal Low-Grade Fibromyxoid Sarcoma: A Clinicopathologic Study of 13 Cases. Am J Clin Pathol. 2018 Jan;149(2):128-134. Cited in: PubMed; PMID 29385413.
1432. Ud Din N, Zhang P, Sukov WR, et al. Spindle Cell Lipomas Arising at Atypical Locations. Am J Clin Pathol. 2016 Oct;146(4):487-95. Cited in: PubMed; PMID 27686175.
1433. Ulrich JD, Specht K, Schlitter AM, et al. A rare case of perivascular epithelioid cell tumor (PEComa) of the pancreas diagnosed by endoscopic ultrasound. Endosc Int Open. 2020 Jan;8(1):E25-E28. Cited in: PubMed; PMID 31921981.
1434. Ushijima M, Hashimoto H, Tsuneyoshi M, et al. Giant cell tumor of the tendon sheath (nodular tenosynovitis). A study of 207 cases to compare the large joint group with the common digit group. Cancer. 1986 Feb;57(4):875-84. Cited in: PubMed; PMID 3943019.
1435. Val-Bernal JF, Martino M, Terán A, et al. Endoscopic ultrasound-guided fine-needle aspiration cytology in the diagnosis of leiomyomas of the gastrointestinal tract. Rev Esp Patol. 201952(3):154-162. Cited in: PubMed; PMID 31213256.
1436. Vallat-Decouvelaere AV, Wassef M, Lot G, et al. Spinal melanotic schwannoma: a tumour with poor prognosis. Histopathology. 1999 Dec;35(6):558-66. Cited in: PubMed; PMID 10583580.
1438. Van Geertruyden J, Lorea P, Goldschmidt D, et al. Glomus tumours of the hand. A retrospective study of 51 cases. J Hand Surg Br. 1996 Apr;21(2):257-60. Cited in: PubMed; PMID 8732413.
1440. VandenBussche CJ, Adams CL, McDonald OG, et al. The fine needle aspiration of translocation sarcomas. Cytopathology. 2017 Oct;28(5):356-363. Cited in: PubMed; PMID 28718513.
1441. VandenBussche CJ, Wakely PE, Siddiqui MT, et al. Cytopathologic characteristics of epithelioid vascular malignancies. Acta Cytol. 201458(4):356-66. Cited in: PubMed; PMID 25195738.
1442. van der Zwan SM, DeMatteo RP. Gastrointestinal stromal tumor: 5 years later. Cancer. 2005 Nov;104(9):1781-8. Cited in: PubMed; PMID 16136600.
1443. van Roggen JF, McMenamin ME, Fletcher CD. Cellular myxoma of soft tissue: a clinicopathological study of 38 cases confirming indolent clinical behaviour. Histopathology. 2001 Sep;39(3):287-97. Cited in: PubMed; PMID 11532040.
1444. Van Treeck BJ, Fritchie KJ. Updates in spindle cell/pleomorphic lipomas. Semin Diagn Pathol. 2019 Mar;36(2):105-111. Cited in: PubMed; PMID 30850230.
1445. Vargas AC, Selinger C, Satgunaseelan L, et al. FISH analysis of selected soft tissue tumors: Diagnostic experience in a tertiary center. Asia Pac J Clin Oncol. 2019 Feb;15(1):38-47. Cited in: PubMed; PMID 29806089.
1446. Vasei N, Shishegar A, Ghalkhani F, et al. Fat necrosis in the Breast: A systematic review of clinical. Lipids Health Dis. 2019 Jun;18(1):139. Cited in: PubMed; PMID 31185981.
1447. Ventura RA, Martin-Subero JI, Jones M, et al. FISH analysis for the detection of lymphoma-associated chromosomal abnormalities in routine paraffin-embedded tissue. J Mol Diagn. 2006 May;8(2):141-51. Cited in: PubMed; PMID 16645199.
1448. Vera-Alvarez J, García-Prats MD, Marigil-Gómez M, et al. Elastofibroma dorsi diagnosed by fine needle aspiration cytology. Acta Cytol. 200852(2):264-6. Cited in: PubMed; PMID 18500010.
1449. Vibhakar AM, Cassels JA, Botchu R, et al. Imaging update on soft tissue sarcoma. J Clin Orthop Trauma. 2021 Nov;22:101568. Cited in: PubMed; PMID 34567971.
1450. Vidyavathi K, Udayakumar M, Prasad CB, et al. Glomus tumor mimicking eccrine spiradenoma on fine needle aspiration. J Cytol. 2009 Jan;26(1):46-8. Cited in: PubMed; PMID 21938152.
1451. Vigliar E, Malapelle U, de Luca C, et al. Challenges and opportunities of next-generation sequencing: a cytopathologist's perspective. Cytopathology. 2015 Oct;26(5):271-83. Cited in: PubMed; PMID 26399861.
1452. Viguer JM, Jiménez-Heffernan JA, Vicandi B, et al. Cytologic features of synovial sarcoma with emphasis on the monophasic fibrous variant: a morphologic and immunocytochemical analysis of bcl-2 protein expression. Cancer. 1998 Feb;84(1):50-6. Cited in: PubMed; PMID 9500652.
1453. Vincent J, Maleki Z. Elastofibroma: cytomorphologic, histologic, and radiologic findings in five cases. Diagn Cytopathol. 2012 Aug;40 Suppl 2:E99-E103. Cited in: PubMed; PMID 21630483.
1454. Vinette-Leduc D, Yazdi HM. Fine-needle aspiration biopsy of a glomus tumor of the stomach. Diagn Cytopathol. 2001 May;24(5):340-2. Cited in: PubMed; PMID 11335965.
1455. Virayavanich W, Ringler MD, Chin CT, et al. CT-guided biopsy of bone and soft-tissue lesions: role of on-site immediate cytologic evaluation. J Vasc Interv Radiol. 2011 Jul;22(7):1024-30. Cited in: PubMed; PMID 21570872.
1456. Vistica DT, Krosky PM, Kenney S, et al. Immunohistochemical discrimination between the ASPL-TFE3 fusion proteins of alveolar soft part sarcoma. J Pediatr Hematol Oncol. 2008 Jan;30(1):46-52. Cited in: PubMed; PMID 18176180.
1457. Voltaggio L, Murray R, Lasota J, et al. Gastric schwannoma: a clinicopathologic study of 51 cases and critical review of the literature. Hum Pathol. 2012 May;43(5):650-9. Cited in: PubMed; PMID 22137423.
1458. Voskuil RT, Mayerson JL, Scharschmidt TJ. The utility of fine-needle aspiration: how FNA has affected our musculoskeletal oncology practice. J Am Soc Cytopathol. 20209(6):596-601. Cited in: PubMed; PMID 32773338.
1459. Vujovic S, Henderson S, Presneau N, et al. Brachyury, a crucial regulator of notochordal development, is a novel biomarker for chordomas. J Pathol. 2006 Jun;209(2):157-65. Cited in: PubMed; PMID 16538613.
1460. Wagner RD, Wang EK, Lloyd MS, et al. Cranial Fasciitis: A Systematic Review and Diagnostic Approach to a Pediatric Scalp Mass. J Craniofac Surg. 2016 Jan;27(1):e65-71. Cited in: PubMed; PMID 26703041.
1461. Wake LM, VandenBussche CJ, Ali SZ, et al. Flow cytometric analysis of fine needle aspirates is affected by tumor subtype, but not by anatomic location nor technique. Diagn Cytopathol. 2020 Jun;48(6):538-546. Cited in: PubMed; PMID 32212260.
1462. Wakely PE. Atypical spindle cell/pleomorphic lipomatous tumour (ASPLT): A report of three FNA cases and comparison with spindle cell/pleomorphic lipoma cytopathology. Cytopathology. 2023 Jul;34(4):346-352. Cited in: PubMed; PMID 36856555.
1463. Wakely PE. Cytopathology of myxofibrosarcoma: a study of 66 cases and literature review. J Am Soc Cytopathol. 202110(3):300-309. Cited in: PubMed; PMID 33041221.
1464. Wakely PE. Extraskeletal myxoid chondrosarcoma: combining cytopathology with molecular testing to achieve diagnostic accuracy. J Am Soc Cytopathol. 202110(3):293-299. Cited in: PubMed; PMID 32828707.
1465. Wakely PE. Myxomatous soft tissue tumors: correlation of cytopathology and histopathology. Ann Diagn Pathol. 1999 Aug;3(4):227-42. Cited in: PubMed; PMID 10459049.
1466. Wakely PE, Ali SZ, Bishop JA. The cytopathology of malignant peripheral nerve sheath tumor: a report of 55 fine-needle aspiration cases. Cancer Cytopathol. 2012 Oct;120(5):334-41. Cited in: PubMed; PMID 22434579.
1467. Wakely PE, Almeida M, Frable WJ. Fine-needle aspiration biopsy cytology of myositis ossificans. Mod Pathol. 1994 Jan;7(1):23-5. Cited in: PubMed; PMID 8159649.
1468. Wakely PE, Giacomantonio M. Fine needle aspiration cytology of metastatic malignant rhabdoid tumor. Acta Cytol. 198630(5):533-7. Cited in: PubMed; PMID 3465147.
1469. Wakely PE, Jin M. Myxoid liposarcoma: Fine-needle aspiration cytopathology in the molecular era. A report of 24 cases. J Am Soc Cytopathol. 20165(3):162-169. Cited in: PubMed; PMID 31042519.
1470. Wakely PE, Kneisl JS. Soft tissue aspiration cytopathology. Cancer. 2000 Oct;90(5):292-8. Cited in: PubMed; PMID 11038426.
1471. Wakely PE, McDermott JE, Ali SZ. Cytopathology of alveolar soft part sarcoma: a report of 10 cases. Cancer. 2009 Dec;117(6):500-7. Cited in: PubMed; PMID 19787801.
1472. Wakely PE, Rekhi B. Cytopathology of solitary fibrous tumor: a series of 34 cases. J Am Soc Cytopathol. 202110(4):382-390. Cited in: PubMed; PMID 34049841.
1473. Wakely PE, Siddiqui MT. Fine-needle aspiration cytopathology of soft tissue myoepithelioma: an analysis of seven cases. J Am Soc Cytopathol. 202211(1):31-39. Cited in: PubMed; PMID 34649776.
1474. Walaas L, Angervall L, Hagmar B, et al. A correlative cytologic and histologic study of malignant fibrous histiocytoma: an analysis of 40 cases examined by fine-needle aspiration cytology. Diagn Cytopathol. 19862(1):46-54. Cited in: PubMed; PMID 2424689.
1475. Walaas L, Kindblom LG. Fine-needle aspiration biopsy in the preoperative diagnosis

of chordoma: a study of 17 cases with application of electron microscopic, histochemical, and immunocytochemical examination. Hum Pathol. 1991 Jan;22(1):22-8. Cited in: PubMed; PMID 1702083.
1476. Walaas L, Kindblom LG. Lipomatous tumors: a correlative cytologic and histologic study of 27 tumors examined by fine needle aspiration cytology. Hum Pathol. 1985 Jan;16(1):6-18. Cited in: PubMed; PMID 2579013.
1477. Walterhouse DO, Pappo AS, Meza JL, et al. Shorter-duration therapy using vincristine, dactinomycin, and lower-dose cyclophosphamide with or without radiotherapy for patients with newly diagnosed low-risk rhabdomyosarcoma: a report from the Soft Tissue Sarcoma Committee of the Children's Oncology Group. J Clin Oncol. 2014 Nov;32(31):3547-52. Cited in: PubMed; PMID 25267746.
1478. Walther C, Domanski HA, von Steyern FV, et al. Chromosome banding analysis of cells from fine-needle aspiration biopsy samples from soft tissue and bone tumors: is it clinically meaningful? Cancer Genet. 2011 Apr;204(4):203-6. Cited in: PubMed; PMID 21536238.
1479. Wang G, Jacobson JA, Feng FY, et al. Sonography of wrist ganglion cysts: variable and noncystic appearances. J Ultrasound Med. 2007 Oct;26(10):1323-8; quiz 1330-1. Cited in: PubMed; PMID 17901135.
1480. Wang G, Tucker T, Ng TL, et al. Fine-needle aspiration of soft tissue myoepithelioma. Diagn Cytopathol. 2016 Feb;44(2):152-5. Cited in: PubMed; PMID 26644362.
1481. Wang H, Jacobson A, Harmon DC, et al. Prognostic factors in alveolar soft part sarcoma: A SEER analysis. J Surg Oncol. 2016 Apr;113(5):581-6. Cited in: PubMed; PMID 26804150.
1482. Wang JC, Li WS, Kao YC, et al. Clinicopathological and molecular characterisation of USP6-rearranged soft tissue neoplasms: the evidence of genetic relatedness indicates an expanding family with variable bone-forming capacity. Histopathology. 2021 Apr;78(5):676-689. Cited in: PubMed; PMID 33000481.
1483. Wang L, Zehir A, Sadowska J, et al. Consistent copy number changes and recurrent PRKAR1A mutations distinguish Melanotic Schwannomas from Melanomas: SNP-array and next generation sequencing analysis. Genes Chromosomes Cancer. 2015 Aug;54(8):463-471. Cited in: PubMed; PMID 26031761.
1484. Wang MX, Devine C, Segaran N, et al. Current update on molecular cytogenetics, diagnosis and management of gastrointestinal stromal tumors. World J Gastroenterol. 2021 Nov;27(41):7125-7133. Cited in: PubMed; PMID 34887632.
1485. Wang Y, Marino-Enriquez A, Bennett RR, et al. Dystrophin is a tumor suppressor in human cancers with myogenic programs. Nat Genet. 2014 Jun;46(6):601-6. Cited in: PubMed; PMID 24793134.
1486. Wangsiricharoen S, Ali SZ, Wakely PE. Cytopathology of myxoinflammatory fibroblastic sarcoma: a series of eight cases and review of the literature. J Am Soc Cytopathol. 202110(3):310-320. Cited in: PubMed; PMID 33431307.
1487. Wangsiricharoen S, Larman TC, Wakely PE, et al. Cytopathology of extra-renal perivascular epithelioid cell tumor (PEComa): a series of 7 cases and review of the literature. J Am Soc Cytopathol. 202110(2):175-186. Cited in: PubMed; PMID 33162379.
1488. Wargotz ES, Weiss SW, Norris HJ. Myofibroblastoma of the breast. Sixteen cases of a distinctive benign mesenchymal tumor. Am J Surg Pathol. 1987 Jul;11(7):493-502. Cited in: PubMed; PMID 3037930.
1489. Warpe BM. Kaposi Sarcoma as Initial Presentation of HIV Infection. N Am J Med Sci. 2014 Dec;6(12):650-2. Cited in: PubMed; PMID 25599055.
1490. Watabe S, Kikuchi Y, Mukaiyama J, et al. Cytological features of BCOR-CCNB3 sarcoma: Comparison with Ewing sarcoma and synovial sarcoma. Cytopathology. 2021 Nov;32(6):771-778. Cited in: PubMed; PMID 34265123.
1491. Waters BL, Panagopoulos I, Allen EF. Genetic characterization of angiomatoid fibrous histiocytoma identifies fusion of the FUS and ATF-1 genes induced by a chromosomal translocation involving bands 12q13 and 16p11. Cancer Genet Cytogenet. 2000 Sep;121(2):109-16. Cited in: PubMed; PMID 11063792.
1492. Watson S, Perrin V, Guillemot D, et al. Transcriptomic definition of molecular subgroups of small round cell sarcomas. J Pathol. 2018 May;245(1):29-40. Cited in: PubMed; PMID 29431183.
1493. Weber MH, Kilpatrick SE, Bergman S. The cytologic diagnosis of epithelioid myxofibrosarcoma: a case report. Diagn Cytopathol. 2012 Aug;40 Suppl 2:E140-3. Cited in: PubMed; PMID 22927294.
1494. Webster P, Wujanto L, Fisher C, et al. Malignancies confined to disused arteriovenous fistulae in renal transplant patients: an important differential diagnosis. Am J Nephrol. 201134(1):42-8. Cited in: PubMed; PMID 21659738.
1495. Weinreb I, Rubin BP, Goldblum JR. Pleomorphic angiomatoid fibrous histiocytoma: a case confirmed by fluorescence in situ hybridization analysis for EWSR1 rearrangement. J Cutan Pathol. 2008 Sep;35(9):855-60. Cited in: PubMed; PMID 18422688.
1496. Weir MM, Rosenberg AE, Bell DA. Grading of spindle cell sarcomas in fine-needle aspiration biopsy specimens. Am J Clin Pathol. 1999 Dec;112(6):784-90. Cited in: PubMed; PMID 10587701.
1497. Weiss SW, Enzinger FM. Epithelioid hemangioendothelioma: a vascular tumor often mistaken for a carcinoma. Cancer. 1982 Sep;50(5):970-81. Cited in: PubMed; PMID 7093931.
1498. Weiss SW, Gnepp DR, Bratthauer GL. Palisaded myofibroblastoma. A benign mesenchymal tumor of lymph node. Am J Surg Pathol. 1989 May;13(5):341-6. Cited in: PubMed; PMID 2712186.
1499. Weiss SW, Ishak KG, Dail DH, et al. Epithelioid hemangioendothelioma and related lesions. Semin Diagn Pathol. 1986 Nov;3(4):259-87. Cited in: PubMed; PMID 3303234.
1500. Wenger DE, Wold LE. Benign vascular lesions of bone: radiologic and pathologic features. Skeletal Radiol. 2000 Feb;29(2):63-74. Cited in: PubMed; PMID 10741493.
1501. West RB, Corless CL, Chen X, et al. The novel marker, DOG1, is expressed ubiquitously in gastrointestinal stromal tumors irrespective of KIT or PDGFRA mutation status. Am J Pathol. 2004 Jul;165(1):107-13. Cited in: PubMed; PMID 15215166.
1502. WHO Classification of Tumours Editorial Board. Haematolymphoid tumours. Lyon (France): International Agency for Research on Cancer; 2024. (WHO classification of tumours series, 5th ed.; vol. 11). https://publications.iarc.who.int/637.
1503. WHO Classification of Tumours Editorial Board. Soft tissue and bone tumours. Lyon (France): International Agency for Research on Cancer; 2020. (WHO classification of tumours series, 5th ed.; vol. 3). https://publications.iarc.who.int/588.
1504. Wickham MQ, Youens KE, Dodd LG. Acral myxoinflammatory fibroblastic sarcoma fine needle aspiration: a case report. Diagn Cytopathol. 2012 Aug;40 Suppl 2:E144-8. Cited in: PubMed; PMID 21548124.
1505. Wieczorek TJ, Krane JF, Domanski HA, et al. Cytologic findings in granular cell tumors, with emphasis on the diagnosis of malignant granular cell tumor by fine-needle aspiration biopsy. Cancer. 2001 Dec;93(6):398-408. Cited in: PubMed; PMID 11748580.
1506. Wile AG, Evans HL, Romsdahl MM. Leiomyosarcoma of soft tissue: a clinicopathologic study. Cancer. 1981 Aug;48(4):1022-32. Cited in: PubMed; PMID 7272926.
1507. Wilkerson BW, Crim JR, Hung M, et al. Characterization of synovial sarcoma calcification. AJR Am J Roentgenol. 2012 Dec;199(6):W730-4. Cited in: PubMed; PMID 23169746.
1508. Willems SM, Mohseny AB, Balog C, et al. Cellular/intramuscular myxoma and grade I myxofibrosarcoma are characterized by distinct genetic alterations and specific composition of their extracellular matrix. J Cell Mol Med. 2009 Jul;13(7):1291-301. Cited in: PubMed; PMID 19320777.
1509. Willén H, Akerman M, Carlén B. Fine needle aspiration (FNA) in the diagnosis of soft tissue tumours; a review of 22 years experience. Cytopathology. 1995 Aug;6(4):236-47. Cited in: PubMed; PMID 8520003.
1510. Wilson TJ, Howe BM, Stewart SA, et al. Clinicoradiological features of intraneural perineuriomas obviate the need for tissue diagnosis. J Neurosurg. 2018 Oct;129(4):1034-1040. Cited in: PubMed; PMID 29192862.
1512. Wong DD, Low IC, Peverall J, et al. MDM2/CDK4 gene amplification in large/deep-seated 'lipomas': incidence, predictors and clinical significance. Pathology. 2016 Apr;48(3):203-9. Cited in: PubMed; PMID 27020493.
1513. Wong NL. Fine needle aspiration cytology of pseudosarcomatous reactive proliferative lesions of soft tissue. Acta Cytol. 200246(6):1049-55. Cited in: PubMed; PMID 12462081.
1514. Wong NL, Di F. Pseudosarcomatous fasciitis and myositis: diagnosis by fine-needle aspiration cytology. Am J Clin Pathol. 2009 Dec;132(6):857-65. Cited in: PubMed; PMID 19926576.
1515. Wong YP, Chia WK, Low SF, et al. Dendritic fibromyxolipoma: a variant of spindle cell lipoma with extensive myxoid change, with cytogenetic evidence. Pathol Int. 2014 Jul;64(7):346-51. Cited in: PubMed; PMID 25047505.
1516. Wong-Arteta J, Rey M, Aragón L, et al. The utility of flow cytometry in the diagnostic work up of malignant effusions due to nonhematopoietic neoplasms. Cytometry B Clin Cytom. 2020 Nov;98(6):504-515. Cited in: PubMed; PMID 32506689.
1517. Wood BL, Arroz M, Barnett D, et al. 2006 Bethesda International Consensus recommendations on the immunophenotypic analysis of hematolymphoid neoplasia by flow cytometry: optimal reagents and reporting for the flow cytometric diagnosis of hematopoietic neoplasia. Cytometry B Clin Cytom. 200772 Suppl 1:S14-22. Cited in: PubMed; PMID 17803189.
1518. Woodruff JM, Godwin TA, Erlandson RA, et al. Cellular schwannoma: a variety of schwannoma sometimes mistaken for a malignant tumor. Am J Surg Pathol. 1981 Dec;5(8):733-44. Cited in: PubMed; PMID 7337161.
1519. Woodruff JM, Scheithauer BW, Kurtkaya-Yapicier O, et al. Congenital and childhood plexiform (multinodular) cellular schwannoma: a troublesome mimic of malignant peripheral nerve sheath tumor. Am J Surg Pathol. 2003 Oct;27(10):1321-9. Cited in: PubMed; PMID 14508393.
1520. Wozniak A, Sciot R, Guillou L, et al. Array CGH analysis in primary gastrointestinal stromal tumors: cytogenetic profile correlates with anatomic site and tumor aggressiveness, irrespective of mutational status. Genes Chromosomes Cancer. 2007 Mar;46(3):261-76. Cited in: PubMed; PMID 17171690.
1521. Wu J, Brinker DA, Haas M, et al. Primary alveolar soft part sarcoma (ASPS) of the breast: report of a deceptive case with xanthomatous features confirmed by TFE3 immunohistochemistry and electron microscopy. Int J Surg Pathol. 2005 Jan;13(1):81-5. Cited in: PubMed; PMID 15735860.
1522. Xiao J, Browning MB, Boyd KP, et al. Multimodal Therapy Including Cytoreductive Surgery and Hyperthermic Intraperitoneal Chemotherapy Can Result in Long-term Disease-free Survival in Pediatric Desmoplastic Small Round Cell Tumor With Extraperitoneal Disease. J Pediatr Hematol Oncol. 2021 Aug;43(6):228-231. Cited in: PubMed; PMID 32555030.
1523. Xie J, Pu C, Silverman JF. Fine-Needle Aspiration Cytology of Intranodal Palisaded Myofibroblastoma of the Inguinal Lymph Node. Acta Cytol. 201660(1):89-92. Cited in: PubMed; PMID 27027816.
1524. Xie Y, Zhou D, Peng L, et al. Unveiling Diagnostic Clues of NTRK-Rearranged Spindle Cell Neoplasms in Fine-Needle Aspiration Specimens. Cytopathology. 2025 Mar;36(2):170-174. Cited in: PubMed; PMID 39670651.
1525. Xu Y, Zhou T, Yu W, et al. Fine-needle aspiration of alveolar soft part sarcoma: Histologic correlation and aberrant CD68 expression. Diagn Cytopathol. 2019 Feb;47(2):114-120. Cited in: PubMed; PMID 30457206.
1526. Yamada Y, Kinoshita I, Kohashi K, et al. HIF-1α, MDM2, CDK4, and p16 expression in ischemic fasciitis, focusing on its ischemic condition. Virchows Arch. 2017 Jul;471(1):117-122. Cited in: PubMed; PMID 28477272.
1527. Yamada Y, Kuda M, Kohashi K, et al. Histological and immunohistochemical characteristics of undifferentiated small round cell sarcomas associated with CIC-DUX4 and BCOR-CCNB3 fusion genes. Virchows Arch. 2017 Apr;470(4):373-380. Cited in: PubMed; PMID 28197724.
1528. Yamaguchi U, Hasegawa T, Hirose T, et al. Sclerosing perineurioma: a clinicopathological study of five cases and diagnostic utility of immunohistochemical staining for GLUT1. Virchows Arch. 2003 Aug;443(2):159-63. Cited in: PubMed; PMID 12836021.
1529. Yamamoto H, Yoshida A, Taguchi K, et al. ALK, ROS1 and NTRK3 gene rearrangements in inflammatory myofibroblastic tumours. Histopathology. 2016 Jul;69(1):72-83. Cited in: PubMed; PMID 26647767.
1530. Yamashita K, Kohashi K, Yamada Y, et al. Primary extraskeletal osteosarcoma: a clinicopathological study of 18 cases focusing on MDM2 amplification status. Hum Pathol. 2017 May;63:63-69. Cited in: PubMed; PMID 28235629.
1531. Yan AC, Chamlin SL, Liang MG, et al. Congenital infantile fibrosarcoma: a masquerader of ulcerated hemangioma. Pediatr Dermatol. 200623(4):330-4. Cited in: PubMed; PMID 16918626.
1532. Yang EJ, Hornick JL, Qian X. Fine-needle aspiration of soft tissue perineurioma: A comparative analysis of cytomorphology and immunohistochemistry with benign and malignant mimics. Cancer Cytopathol. 2016 Sep;124(9):651-8. Cited in: PubMed; PMID 27159449.
1533. Yang J, Frassica FJ, Fayad L, et al. Analysis of nondiagnostic results after image-guided needle biopsies of musculoskeletal lesions. Clin Orthop Relat Res. 2010 Nov;468(11):3103-11. Cited in: PubMed; PMID 20383617.

1534. Yang S, Zhao C, Zhang Y, et al. Mediastinal fetal rhabdomyoma in nevoid basal cell carcinoma syndrome: a case report and review of the literature. Virchows Arch. 2011 Aug;459(2):235-8. Cited in: PubMed; PMID 21710240.
1535. Yeow KM, Tan CF, Chen JS, et al. Diagnostic sensitivity of ultrasound-guided needle biopsy in soft tissue masses about superficial bone lesions. J Ultrasound Med. 2000 Dec;19(12):849-55. Cited in: PubMed; PMID 11127010.
1536. Yi CA, Lee KS, Choe YH, et al. Computed tomography in pulmonary artery sarcoma: distinguishing features from pulmonary embolic disease. J Comput Assist Tomogr. 200428(1):34-9. Cited in: PubMed; PMID 14716229.
1537. Yi ES, Shmookler BM, Malawer MM, et al. Well-differentiated extraskeletal osteosarcoma. A soft-tissue homologue of parosteal osteosarcoma. Arch Pathol Lab Med. 1991 Sep;115(9):906-9. Cited in: PubMed; PMID 1929787.
1538. Yong M, Raza AS, Greaves TS, et al. Fine-needle aspiration of a pleomorphic lipoma of the head and neck: a case report. Diagn Cytopathol. 2005 Feb;32(2):110-3. Cited in: PubMed; PMID 15637670.
1539. Yoshida A, Arai Y, Kobayashi E, et al. CIC break-apart fluorescence in-situ hybridization misses a subset of CIC-DUX4 sarcomas: a clinicopathological and molecular study. Histopathology. 2017 Sep;71(3):461-469. Cited in: PubMed; PMID 28493604.
1540. Yoshida A, Goto K, Kodaira M, et al. CIC-rearranged Sarcomas: A Study of 20 Cases and Comparisons With Ewing Sarcomas. Am J Surg Pathol. 2016 Mar;40(3):313-23. Cited in: PubMed; PMID 26685084.
1541. Yoshida A, Sekine S, Tsuta K, et al. NKX2.2 is a useful immunohistochemical marker for Ewing sarcoma. Am J Surg Pathol. 2012 Jul;36(7):993-9. Cited in: PubMed; PMID 22446943.
1542. Yoshida A, Wakai S, Ryo E, et al. Expanding the Phenotypic Spectrum of Mesenchymal Tumors Harboring the EWSR1-CREM Fusion. Am J Surg Pathol. 2019 Dec;43(12):1622-1630. Cited in: PubMed; PMID 31305268.
1543. Younan Y, Martinez A, Reimer N, et al. Combined classical spindle cell/pleomorphic lipoma spectrum imaging and clinical data. Skeletal Radiol. 2018 Jan;47(1):51-59. Cited in: PubMed; PMID 28823067.
1544. Yu Y, Demierre MF, Mahalingam M. Anaplastic Kaposi's sarcoma: an uncommon histologic phenotype with an aggressive clinical course. J Cutan Pathol. 2010 Oct;37(10):1088-91. Cited in: PubMed; PMID 19638066.
1545. Zafar A, Wang W, Liu G, et al. Molecular targeting therapies for neuroblastoma: Progress and challenges. Med Res Rev. 2021 Mar;41(2):961-1021. Cited in: PubMed; PMID 33155698.
1546. Zaharopoulos P, Wong JY. Fine-needle aspiration cytology in fibromatoses. Diagn Cytopathol. 19928(1):73-8. Cited in: PubMed; PMID 1551369.
1547. Zajdela A, Zillhardt P, Voillemot N. Cytological diagnosis by fine needle sampling without aspiration. Cancer. 1987 Mar;59(6):1201-5. Cited in: PubMed; PMID 3815294.
1548. Zámecník M, Michal M. EMA+ cells in dermatofibrosarcoma protuberans. A study of 11 tumors suggesting perineurial cell differentiation. Cesk Patol. 2002 Apr;38(2):55-62. Cited in: PubMed; PMID 12426982.
1549. Zee SY, Wang Q, Jones CM, et al. Fine needle aspiration cytology of dermatofibrosarcoma protuberans presenting as a breast mass. A case report. Acta Cytol. 200246(4):741-3. Cited in: PubMed; PMID 12146044.
1551. Zelger B, Weinlich G, Zelger B. Perineuroma. A frequently unrecognized entity with emphasis on a plexiform variant. Adv Clin Path. 2000 Jan;4(1):25-33. Cited in: PubMed; PMID 10936896.
1552. Zelger BW, Zelger BG, Plörer A, et al. Dermal spindle cell lipoma: plexiform and nodular variants. Histopathology. 1995 Dec;27(6):533-40. Cited in: PubMed; PMID 8838333.
1553. Zeppa P, Errico ME, Palombini L. Epithelioid sarcoma: report of two cases diagnosed by fine-needle aspiration biopsy with immunocytochemical correlation. Diagn Cytopathol. 1999 Dec;21(6):405-8. Cited in: PubMed; PMID 10572273.
1554. Zeppa P, Vigliar E, Cozzolino I, et al. Fine needle aspiration cytology and flow cytometry immunophenotyping of non-Hodgkin lymphoma: can we do better? Cytopathology. 2010 Oct;21(5):300-10. Cited in: PubMed; PMID 20132132.
1555. Zhang H, Erickson-Johnson M, Wang X, et al. Molecular testing for lipomatous tumors: critical analysis and test recommendations based on the analysis of 405 extremity-based tumors. Am J Surg Pathol. 2010 Sep;34(9):1304-11. Cited in: PubMed; PMID 20679883.
1557. Zhang S, Gong Y. From cytomorphology to molecular pathology: maximizing the value of cytology of lymphoproliferative disorders and soft tissue tumors. Am J Clin Pathol. 2013 Oct;140(4):454-67. Cited in: PubMed; PMID 24045541.
1558. Zhang Y, Renberg S, Papakonstantinou A, et al. Diagnosing gastrointestinal stromal tumors: The utility of fine-needle aspiration cytology versus biopsy. Cancer Med. 2022 Jul;11(14):2729-2734. Cited in: PubMed; PMID 35301817.
1559. Zhang Y, Wessman S, Wejde J, et al. Diagnosing synovial sarcoma by fine-needle aspiration cytology and molecular techniques. Cytopathology. 2019 Sep;30(5):504-509. Cited in: PubMed; PMID 31161693.
1560. Zhao Z, Paquette C, Shah AA, et al. Fine Needle Aspiration Cytology of Diffuse-Type Tenosynovial Giant Cell Tumors. Acta Cytol. 201761(2):160-164. Cited in: PubMed; PMID 28324880.
1561. Zhao Z, Takano A, Lim AST, et al. Metastatic alveolar rhabdomyosarcoma on the fine-needle aspiration cytology of cervical lymph node in an elderly patient, with FISH confirmation: A case report. Malays J Pathol. 2020 Apr;42(1):115-119. Cited in: PubMed; PMID 32342940.
1562. Zhao Z, Yin Y, Zhang J, et al. Spindle cell/sclerosing rhabdomyosarcoma: case series from a single institution emphasizing morphology, immunohistochemistry and follow-up. Int J Clin Exp Pathol. 20158(11):13814-20. Cited in: PubMed; PMID 26823695.
1563. Zheng K, Yu XC, Xu M, et al. Surgical Outcomes and Prognostic Factors of Myxoid Liposarcoma in Extremities: A Retrospective Study. Orthop Surg. 2019 Dec;11(6):1020-1028. Cited in: PubMed; PMID 31721459.
1564. Zhou H, Guo M, Gong Y. Challenge of FNA diagnosis of angiomyolipoma: A study of 33 cases. Cancer Cytopathol. 2017 Apr;125(4):257-266. Cited in: PubMed; PMID 28152270.
1565. Zhu P, Sun K, Lao IW, et al. Expanding the Spectrum of NUTM1 -Rearranged Sarcoma : A Clinicopathologic and Molecular Genetic Study of 8 Cases. Am J Surg Pathol. 2024 Aug;48(8):930-941. Cited in: PubMed; PMID 38946048.
1566. Zreik R, Soyalp K, Ruiz S, et al. Ultrasound-guided fine-needle aspiration of a posterior neck dedifferentiated liposarcoma with MDM2 fluorescence in situ hybridization performed on a Pap-stained smear. Diagn Cytopathol. 2015 Apr;43(4):320-4. Cited in: PubMed; PMID 25132684.
1567. Zreik RT, Carter JM, Sukov WR, et al. TGFBR3 and MGEA5 rearrangements are much more common in "hybrid" hemosiderotic fibrolipomatous tumor-myxoinflammatory fibroblastic sarcomas than in classical myxoinflammatory fibroblastic sarcomas: a morphological and fluorescence in situ hybridization study. Hum Pathol. 2016 Jul;53:14-24. Cited in: PubMed; PMID 26980036.

Subject index

Bold page numbers indicate the main discussion(s) of the topic.

D

The IAC-IARC-WHO Cytopathology Reporting Systems

Lung

International Academy of Cytology – International Agency for Research on Cancer – World Health Organization Joint Editorial Board. WHO Reporting System for Lung Cytopathology. Lyon (France): International Agency for Research on Cancer; 2022. (IAC-IARC-WHO cytopathology reporting systems series, 1st ed.; vol. 1). https://publications.iarc.who.int/620.

Pancreaticobiliary system

International Academy of Cytology – International Agency for Research on Cancer – World Health Organization Joint Editorial Board. WHO Reporting System for Pancreaticobiliary Cytopathology. Lyon (France): International Agency for Research on Cancer; 2022. (IAC-IARC-WHO cytopathology reporting systems series, 1st ed.; vol. 2). https://publications.iarc.who.int/621.

Lymph node, spleen, and thymus

International Academy of Cytology – International Agency for Research on Cancer – World Health Organization Joint Editorial Board. WHO Reporting System for Lymph Node, Spleen, and Thymus Cytopathology. Lyon (France): International Agency for Research on Cancer; 2024. (IAC-IARC-WHO cytopathology reporting systems series, 1st ed.; vol. 3). https://publications.iarc.who.int/644.

Soft tissue

International Academy of Cytology – International Agency for Research on Cancer – World Health Organization Joint Editorial Board. WHO Reporting System for Soft Tissue Cytopathology. Lyon (France): International Agency for Research on Cancer; 2026. (IAC-IARC-WHO cytopathology reporting systems series, 1st ed.; vol. 4). https://publications.iarc.who.int/651.

WHO Classification of Tumours Online

The content of this new, innovative, and comprehensive cytopathology reporting series is also available in a convenient digital format, at https://tumourclassification.iarc.who.int